LAPAROSCOPIC
SURGERY ATLAS

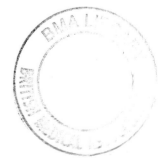

LAPAROSCOPIC SURGERY ATLAS
Volume 2

Prof. C. Palanivelu MS, DNB, MCh (GE), FRCS Ed., FACS

Chair, Division of Surgical Gastroenterology
and Minimal Access Surgery
Director, Digestive Diseases Research and
National Training Institute
GEM Hospital, Coimbatore, India

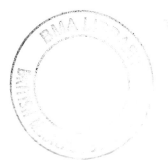

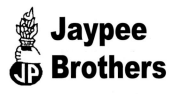

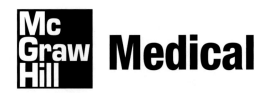

© 2008, C. Palanivelu

First published in India in 2008 by

Corporate Office
4838/24 Ansari Road, Daryaganj, **New Delhi** - 110002, India, +91-11-43574357

Registered Office
B-3 EMCA House, 23/23B Ansari Road, Daryaganj, **New Delhi** 110 002, India
Phones: +91-11-23272143, +91-11-23272703, +91-11-23282021,
+91-11-23245672, Rel: +91-11-32558559 Fax: +91-11-23276490, +91-11-23245683
e-mail: jaypee@jaypeebrothers.com, Visit our website: www.jaypeebrothers.com

First published in USA by The McGraw-Hill Companies, 2 Penn Plaza, New York, NY 10121.
Exclusively worldwide distributor except South Asia (India, Nepal, Sri Lanka, Bhutan, Pakistan, Bangladesh, Malaysia).

ISBN-13: 978-0-07-160193-1
ISBN-10: 0-07-160193-7

Dedicated to

My beloved parents

Late Shri P. Chinnusamy and Mrs. Kaliammal

also to my family

ever loving Jaya, wife

Priya, daughter

Senthilnathan, son-in-law

Praveen Raj, son

Master Mukhil, grand son

also

to my Teachers

and

my Patients

who made this possible

Contents

Volume 1

Section I : General Laparoscopy

Section II : Esophagus And Diaphragm

Volume 2

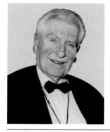

Foreword

"To become educated, read good books and visit good masters."

Is that famous maxim available for modern surgical education?

A surgical operation can be compared to a journey inside the human body. In this journey, the navigator must fulfil three essential requirements to obtain his licence: a perfect knowledge of anatomy; a perfect choice of strategies and a perfect mastery of the surgical techniques. Since the beginning of the 18ᵗʰ century (birth of modern surgery), the apprentice-surgeons were looking for good books and good teachers to learn surgical anatomy. The constant improvements in the field of imaging technology all along the 20ᵗʰ century have lead to the production of books at levels close to perfection. Though books are satisfactory for describing surgical techniques, they cannot entirely replace the role of a mentor. The fine gesture and hand movements of the surgeon cannot be shown in textbooks. In open surgery, only the first assistants can witness the surgery in the depth of the operating field. The introduction of movie cameras into the operating theatre has improved the situation. But the camera man has to be well trained to record these procedures without disturbing the operating team. But most often the surgeon is disturbed in the process of recording. Books still were the principle companion of the surgeon to learn the techniques of conventional surgery with some help from videos.

Many things have changed since the introduction of laparoscopic surgery. The constraints of recording the surgery have been entirely removed and we are able to record high quality videos with the help of advanced imaging technology. The fundamental requirements for surgical techniques remain the same in laparoscopic surgery.

Improved magnification with the laparoscope has resulted in better understanding of the anatomy. It permits better determination of the plane of dissection during surgery. Conduction of regular training programmes with the international experts has become much easier at present. The surgeon can demonstrate the entire technique along with continuous explanation of the procedure and provide technical tips. Live interaction during the procedure is also possible. The surgeries can be broadcasted all around the world. The recorded videos can also be stored in libraries for further training. The audiovisual documents are now the principal companions of the surgeon in learning laparoscopic surgery.

Does that mean books have lost their major interest in that domain? A "yes" answer could be possible 15 years ago, when laparoscopic surgery was introduced. I was ready to admit that modern technologies can replace the traditional printed material that was too static and difficult to update frequently. But with experience, I have abandoned that opinion. During these 15 years, the major leaders in laparoscopic surgery have created specialized training centres and have documented thousands hours of laparoscopic procedures. They have published their results following the actual methodology. Their experiences are mature and stable enough to be printed in the form of book along with the photographs to become further a definitive milestone in the history of laparoscopic surgery.

Professor C. Palanivelu was among the very first in India and the world to embark on the voyage of laparoscopic surgery. He is among the top ten world leaders who created a laparoscopic training centre. His GEM Foundation is a leading and recognized centre of excellence in laparoscopic surgery. He is riding in the front row of the developers laparoscopic surgery not only as a terrific operator but also as a very good teacher. His books present the best of his teaching. The two volumes compile the entire current concepts in the field of laparoscopic surgery and the personal opinions and concepts of the author. The chapters are well balanced and cover the complete spectrum of the present indications of what it is possible to be done by laparoscopic approach. Each chapter treats the topics in an exhaustive manner. The writing is clear and pleasant to read because it has often the style of conversations in the operating theatre. Plenty of excellent and informative pictures are included along with the text at the right positions. The present work fulfils perfectly the above mentioned tasks: a close up picture on what is to day the State of the Art in Laparoscopic Surgery and also a milestone in the history of the development of laparoscopic surgery. It is the best key to open the door of the Gem Foundation training centre. These books are the best guides not only for the beginners but also for the experts looking for learning more advanced procedures. These have to be among the major reference books for the residents in training as they are absolutely **"text book and atlas".** They give an immense credit to the author and his team.

Professor C. Palanivelu, prominent Master-Teacher in laparoscopic surgery, provides an additional reason to the world community of laparoscopic surgeons to pay a great tribute to the Indian surgeons for their huge contribution in the development of minimally invasive surgery.

"To become educated, read good books and visit good masters."

The surgeons looking for good education in laparoscopic surgery will now know the books that they have to read and the master they have to visit.

Jacques PÉRISSAT, MD, FACS,

Professor Emeritus of Surgery

Université Victor Segalen Bordeaux FRANCE

Membre de l'Académie Française de Chirurgie

Honorary Fellow of the American Surgical Association

Past-President of the International Federation Societies Endoscopic Surgeons

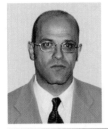

Foreword

Over recent years minimal access surgery has evolved very rapidly owing to the efforts of a group of laparoscopic surgeons across the world that have taken up the task of standardizing basic procedures and encompassing a variety of complex surgical procedures. This textbook is a testimony of such evolution, attesting to the remarkable progress of minimal access surgery. It consists of an up-to-date collection of minimal access procedures that covers a wide array of operations. Procedures included range from the access into the abdomen to obtain a pneumoperitoneum, to the performance of a laparoscopic liver resection or a Whipple's procedure.

In each chapter, the author brings us a description of the disease process, treatment options and a clear account of the technical steps of the surgical procedures. Illustrations are clearly depicted and an impressive collection of surgical photographs demonstrates the extensive experience of the author. The historical notes described in several of the chapters give a perspective of the evolution of this field. It is through this approach that Dr. Palanivelu puts together a thorough explanation that encompasses all aspects of the pathologic process.

This is a merger of a textbook and an atlas of surgery, and thus emerges as an excellent educational tool for surgeons in training and experienced surgeons alike. This work is truly representative of the best laparoscopic surgery practices today.

Horacio J. ASBUN, MD, FACS,
Director, Minimal Access Surgery
John Muir/Mt Diablo Health System
California, USA

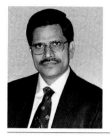

Preface

It is a matter of great pleasure for me that my previous books **"Art of Laparoscopic Surgery - Basic and Advanced Techniques"**, **"CIGES Atlas of Laparoscopic surgery"**, **"Palanivelu's Textbook of Surgical Laparoscopy"** and **"Operative manual on Laparoscopic Hernia surgery"** have all been well accepted by the surgical fraternity. The constant support from the surgeons has encouraged me to comeout with an entirely new book in the field of laparoscopic surgery. The aim of this book is to provide the readers with the entire information on the current concepts of the field of minimal invasive surgery.

The basic principles of laparoscopic surgery have been well established along with the technical details of the basic procedures like cholecystectomy, appendicectomy and fundoplication. The key focus of current laparoscopic surgery is advanced procedures for cancers of the digestive system. Cancers of the digestive system such as esophagus, colon and stomach have been successfully treated by laparoscopy. The current publications on laparoscopic colorectal surgery proved beyond doubt about the oncological safety of these minimally invasive procedures. Apart from minimally invasive surgical oncology the current focus is also on procedures like laparoscopic repair of inguinal and ventral hernias. The main objective of bringing out this book is to provide an in depth, practical, up to date guide on surgical laparoscopy for the benefit of surgical fraternity.

I have explained all the procedures based on my more than decade long experience in the field of laparoscopic surgery along with the practical aspects that I have learnt from various national and international conferences. I have also added certain innovative techniques based on my experience. I am glad to say that few of the procedures explained in following chapters have been done for the first time in the history of laparoscopic surgery. I am confident that this book will help the surgeons to grasp the concept of current laparoscopic surgery and the technical details of the various procedures.

The book has been divided in two volumes to make the size of the book manageable. Each chapter describes in detail the thought process, decision-making and the requisite advanced techniques with adequate number of illustrative diagrams and color photographs.

Volume I deals with various aspects of the basics of laparoscopic surgery and alos contains chapters on esophagus, stomach duodenum and gall bladder.

Volume II contains chapters on Common bile duct, liver, pancreas, spleen, colon, hernia, urology and gynecology.

I always remind myself of the famous quote;

" Look behind you at what you have already accomplished
Look up and believe that the sky is the limit
Look down to make sure you're on the right path
Look ahead and claim success in everything you do."

C. PALANIVELU, MS, DNB, MCh (GE), FRCS Ed., FACS

Acknowledgements

I would like to thank my family members Jaya, Praveen, Priya and Senthilnathan who have tolerated me for my prolonged absence from home and showered me with their love and affection. It is from Master Mukhil, my grandson from whom I rejuvenate my energy, after tedious and prolonged work in the hospital.

My immense thanks goes to Dr. R. Parthasarathi, for his meticulous editorial work along with compiling scores of color photographs and illustrations in specific order to add glitter to this rich material, spread over this manual. I would like to thank Dr. S. Venkatachalam, my anesthetsist for his valuable contributions in the chapter on anesthetic management. I also thank Dr. S. Rajapandian for preparing the color illustrations that is spread over the entire textbook.

I would like to acknowledge all my dedicated team members Dr. P.S. Rajan, Dr. K. Sendhilkumar, Dr. R. Senthilkumar, Dr. G.S. Maheshkumar, Dr. A. Roshan Shetty, Dr. S. Senthilkumaran, Dr. P. Senthilnathan, Dr. M. Vijay Kumar, Dr. Anand Prakash, Dr. Alfie Kavalakat, Dr. Kalpesh Jani, Dr. Rangarajan, Dr. Sai Krishna Vittal and Dr. Madhan Kumar for their support and help in bringing this exhaustive book. My sincere appreciation goes to Sister Malathy Hariharan for her expert assistance in the operating theatre since the day one of my laparoscopic surgery carrier.

My special thanks goes to Dr. S.V. Kandasami, Dr. S. Sadasivam, Dr. Sunil Mathew, Dr. Kaleel-ur-Rehman, Dr. Neelayathatchi and Dr. V.G. Mohan Prasad for their continued support in all my endevours. I am also thankful to Mr. R.Venkatachalam for his valuable technical guidance and Mr. S. Thangapandi for his wonderful job of aligning the jumbled manuscript in a neat and presentable form. I am also thankful to Mrs S. Jaya for helping in typing the manuscript.

C. PALANIVELU, MS, DNB, MCh (GE), FRCS Ed., FACS

GEM Hospital, Coimbatore, India

SECTION ⑤

Common Bile Duct

43

Laparoscopic Bile Duct Injury and Management

INTRODUCTION

Since its introduction in the late 1980s, laparoscopic cholecystectomy rapidly became the standard treatment for patients with symptomatic gallstones. Biliary injuries during laparoscopic cholecystectomy are an important cause for morbidity and it was thought that the incidence of these injuries would reduce with the increasing experience of the surgeons. But these injuries have not yet reached the levels that were prevailing in the era of open cholecystectomy. An important and disturbing aspect of these injuries is their occurrence in the hands of highly experienced and competent surgeons even after the knowledge about the inherent risks of bile duct injury and its associated complications.[1] Numerous reports have been published describing the mechanism of injuries, treatment approaches, and factors influencing the long-term results of patients with bile duct injuries during laparoscopic cholecystectomy.[2-5] As these injuries are more complex when compared to

injuries following open surgeries they have a significant long term health implications for the patients and the society in general.[6]

CLASSIFICATION OF INJURIES

Strasberg classification[7]

Type A : Bile leak from a main duct still in continuity with the common bile duct

These injuries are either due to cystic duct stump leaks or leaks from small bile ducts in the liver bed. The cystic duct stump leak can occur due to increased pressure in the biliary system due to a retained stone.[6] The leak from the liver bed can be due to extensive dissection especially in cases of dense inflammation. These are the least serious types of injuries of the bile duct. Decompression of the biliary tract by ERCP and stenting usually stops the leak.

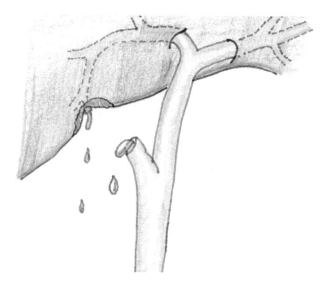

Figure 1 : Type A Injury : Bile leak from a main duct still in continuity with the common bile duct

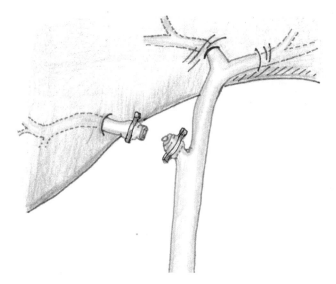

Figure 2 : Type B Injury : Occlusion of part of biliary tree

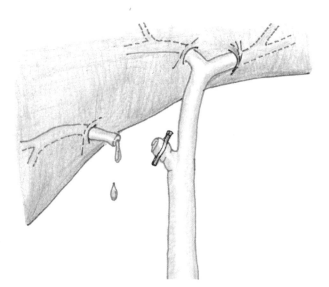

Figure 3 : Type C Injury : Bile leak from duct not in communication with main ductal system

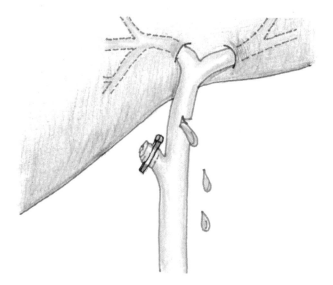

Figure 4 : Type D Injury : Lateral injury to extrahepatic ducts

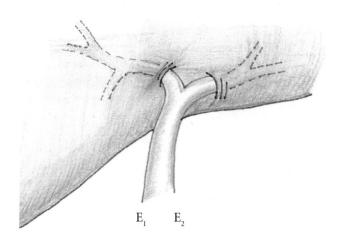

Figure 5 : Type E Injury (confluence intact)

E_1 - >2cm of common hepatic duct stump

E_2 - <2cm of common hepatic duct stump

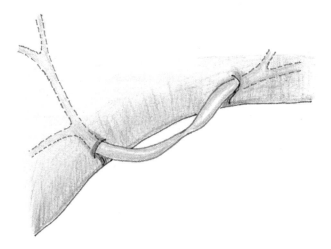

Figure 6 : Type E_3 Injury: Destroyed confluence, R & L hepatic duct intact

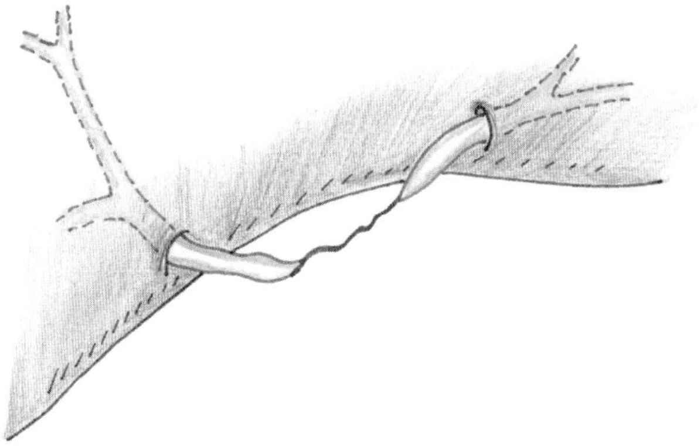

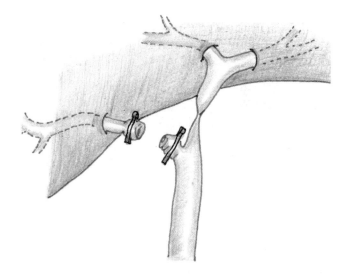

Figure 7 : Type E_4 Injury : Destroyed confluence, R & L hepatic ducts separated

Figure 8 : Type E_5 Injury : Combined hepatic duct and aberrant duct injury

In our experience, we had five cases of Type A Biliary injury. These patients developed biliary peritonitis between 6th and 8th post operative day. Out of these, two patients had biliary leak through all the ports. In all the cases relaparoscopy was done after thorough peritoneal toilet, large drainage tube kept in the subhepatic space in addition to sub diaphragmatic and pelvic cavity. After complete recovery endoscopic stenting was required in three cases. Six cases of biliary leak following subtotal cholecystectomy from our series and two cases done by other surgeons were managed by ERCP with sphincterotomy and stenting.

Two of our patients had developed collection in the sixth postoperative day following subtotal cholecystectomy. The drains had been removed on the second day as the drainage tube did not show any bile leak. Ultrasound showed collection in the subdiaphragmatic area which was drained by relaparoscopy. No definite source of the leak could be identified. The patients recovered completely in one week.

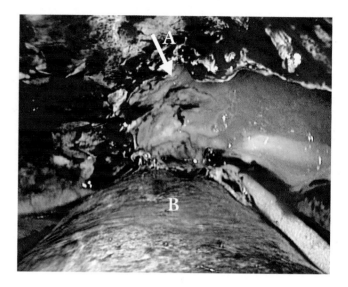

Figure 10 : Large subdiaphragmatic cavity after sucked out the content

A - Cavity
B - Right lobe of liver

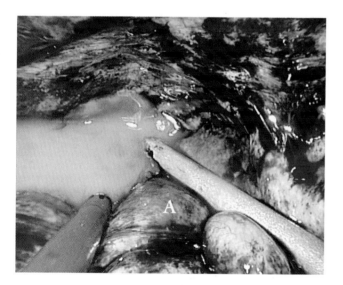

Figure 9 : Aspiration of biliary collection

A - Right lobe of liver

In our series we had one accessory bile duct leaks presented with peritubal bile leak. Both cases presented on the first postoperative day. Relaparoscopy, peritoneal toileting and suturing of the accessory duct near the liver bed were done and the patient recovered uneventfully. If accessory duct leak is not associated with peritonitis in the presence of drainage tube, it can be usually managed by ERCP and stenting. Three cases of accessory duct injury was recognized intraoperatively and managed by suturing.

Type B : Occlusion of part of biliary tree

In about 1 - 2% of patients cystic duct enters the right duct, which in turn joins the main ductal system. Such an aberrant duct might mimic the cystic duct and may be divided. Injury to aberrant right sectoral ducts appears to be a more frequent complication associated with laparoscopic cholecystectomy than was seen during the era of open cholecystectomy.[8, 9] At times the right anterior or posterior sectoral duct may also be divided. In these types of injuries, both ends of the duct are ligated and do not result in bile leak. Most of these patients are asymptomatic and the concerned segment of the liver atrophies. When the affected portion of the liver is large, they present with pain or cholangitis in the occluded segment. We have no experience with this type of injury.

Type C : Bile leak from duct not in communication with main ductal system

These types of injuries are almost always due to transection of aberrant right hepatic duct. This is similar to type B injuries, but the proximal part of the duct is not ligated and persistent bile leak is usually associated with this type of injury. These patients are usually diagnosed early when compared to type B injuries due to collection of bile in the abdominal cavity. The ERCP findings in these type of injuries might be interpreted as normal as the leak may not be seen arising from the common bile duct. HIDA scan and PTC may be needed at times to demonstrate exact location of these leaks and also to plan the corrective surgery.

We had four cases of Type C injury. Four cases were managed by through peritoneal lavage and drainage, while 2 needed open Roux-en-Y hepatico jejunostomy after 6 weeks.

Type D : Lateral injury to extrahepatic ducts

These are major injuries due to laceration or injury to the main extrahepatic ducts like common bile duct, common hepatic duct right and left hepatic duct. If these are diagnosed at the time of the surgery, primary closure over a T tube usually heals the laceration. These injuries can present later due to the occurrence of biliary strictures after healing of the laceration. These are most often due to associated vascular injuries and can progress to Type E injuries.

Injury can also happen when the diathermy gets conducted to the common hepatic duct or common bile duct if the dissection instrument accidentally touches the clips. This will lead to delayed leak and bilioma formation. Two of our cases presented like this between 7 and 12th POD. Both the cases were managed by laparoscopic drainage. A small rent was

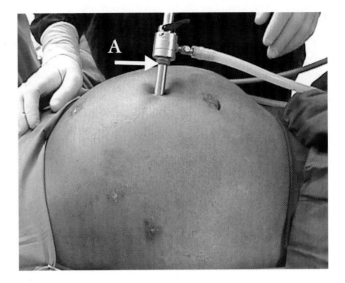

Figure 11 : Relaparoscopy. Previous lap chole ports are seen

A - Supraumbilical port

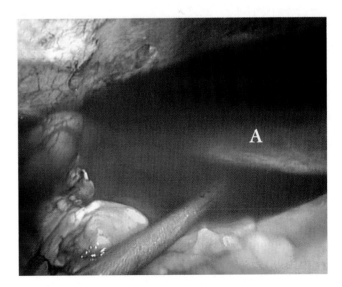

Figure 12 : Biliary peritonitis. Aspiration of bile

A - Right lobe of liver

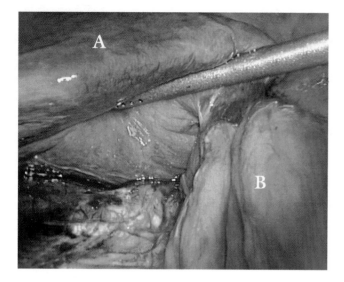

Figure 13 : Adhesion of duodenum to the gall bladder fossa

A - Right lobe of liver
B - Duodenum

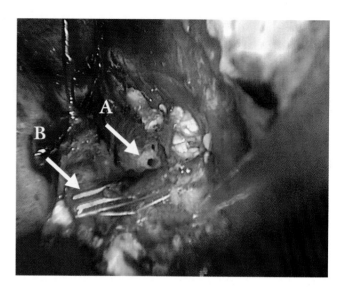

Figure 14 : Rent in the common hepatic duct

A - Rent in CHD
B - Clipped cystic duct

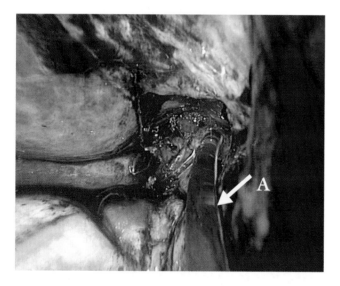

Figure 15 : Feeding tube being introduced in the common hepatic duct through the rent

A - Feeding tube

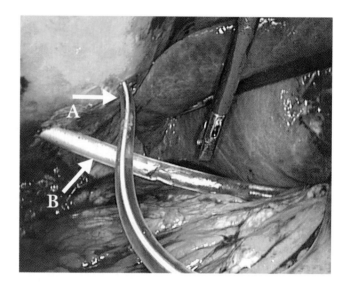

Figure 16 : Drain to the gallbladder fossa

A - Feeding tube taken out through the separate stab
B - Drainage tube in the gall bladder fossa

visible in common hepatic duct. A feeding tube (6 F) was inserted through the rent along with drains in subhepatic and sub diaphragmatic space. The feeding tube was removed after 10 days. There is no stricture of the bile duct on follow up over 3 years.

A 45 year aged female patient developed biliary peritonitis due to injury of the common hepatic duct. Relaparoscopy revealed a rent in the common hepatic duct, a T tube was placed through the rent at the site of laceration and sutured. The T tube was removed after 8 weeks. One year later the patient was operated for stricture of CBD and hepaticojejunostomy was done by open method.

Post op collection, Intoraop showing rent in the left hepatic duct, palacememt of tube thorugh the rent.

Type E: These are the most ominous injuries of all and they result in complete separation of the hepatic parenchyma from the lower ducts and duodenum. It may be due to stenosis or complete loss of ductal tissue. The documented incidence of injuries to the proximal bile duct appear to occur at a higher rate than those that occur before the introduction of laparoscopy.[10, 11] The sub classification of Bismuth can be applied to type E injuries classification. Another disturbing aspect of these proximal injuries is the association of vascular injuries along with it. The right hepatic artery which is close to the cystic duct might be interpreted as the cystic artery and divided. The vascular insult may occur even without division of the vessels. Extensive dissection to expose the extrahepatic duct system might also result in devascularization of the common bile duct. These might present as late biliary strictures. The importance of arterial ischemia as a potential etiologic factor of failed initial repairs after bile duct injury has been studied extensively.[12-14]

Bismuth's Classification	
I	>2cm of common hepatic duct stump
II	<2cm of common hepatic duct stump, confluence intact
III	Destroyed confluence, R & L hepatic duct intact
IV	Destroyed confluence, R & L hepatic ducts separated
V	Combined hepatic duct and aberrant duct injury.

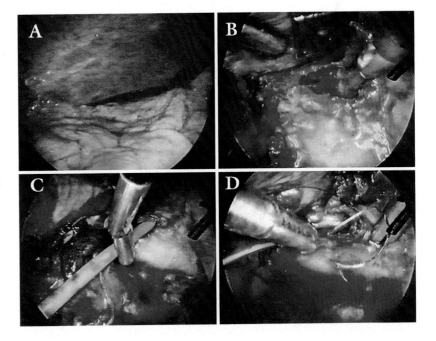

Figure 17 : Left hepatic injury - Laparoscopic Management

A - Biliary collection in the peritoneal cavity
B - Rent in the left hepatic duct was identified
C - Insertion of feeding tube
D - T tube was inserted and sutured in place

Four cases were referred to us following laparoscopic cholecystectomy. Three cases were Type III and one case was Type II injury. All the cases were treated by hepaticojejunostomy with interval of 6-8 weeks. All patients recovered well. One patient continues to have recurrent cholangitis which subsides after a course of antibiotics. As the ducts are not dilated yet and the patient is free from jaundice we are continuing the conservative management.

ETIOLOGY FOR BILIARY TRACT INJURY

Misidentification of common bile duct,[15] cautery injuries to the bile duct and improper or failed application of clips to the cystic duct are the major causes of ductal injury. Once the common bile duct is isolated and dissected, it is clipped and divided accidentally causing a major biliary injury.

1. Experience

Lack of experience has been termed as the major cause for bile duct injury (Learning curve effect). These injuries can occur when the surgeon progress beyond the learning curve and starts to perform these

surgeries at a regular interval when they tend to be over confident about their technique.

2. Misidentification of common bile duct as cystic duct

Misidentification of the common bile duct for the cystic duct can occur due to faulty dissection techniques, aberrant anatomy and in complicated situations like acute cholecystitis. The technique of laparoscopic cholecystectomy has also been postulated as a cause of biliary injuries. The method of traction of infundibulum superiorly can place the common bile duct and the cystic duct in alignment creating a favorable setting for the division of common bile duct. Rather this can be avoided if the traction widens the Calots triangle delineating the cystic duct and bile duct junction more clearly.

3. Faulty dissection in Techniques

The infundibular technique of Calots triangle dissection often described was associated with about 80% of injuries in a study involving patients who had undergone laparoscopic cholecystectomy by this

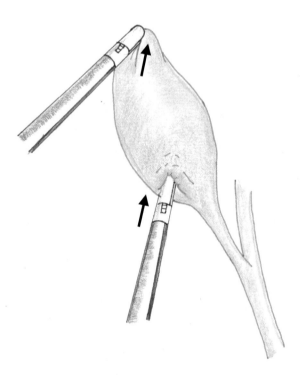

Figure 18 : Improper traction on infundibulum causing malalignment of cystic duct with common bile duct. Cystic duct appears parallel and continuous with common bile duct

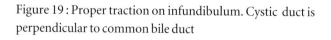

Figure 19 : Proper traction on infundibulum. Cystic duct is perpendicular to common bile duct

technique. In this technique the cystic duct is isolated by dissection on the front and back of Calot's triangle and after isolation it is traced on to the gall bladder. Identification of the cystic duct is by the appearance of the flaring of the duct to become the infundibulum. This flare was a conclusive evidence of the infundibular cystic duct junction and was supposed to help in safe dissection. But in cases of acute inflammation, the mistaken flare was identified when the common bile duct was followed to the inflammatory mass in which the cystic duct was hidden (hidden cystic duct syndrome). This technique is unreliable and should not be used alone for anatomic identification of the ducts. Factors such as short cystic duct, large stone in Hartmann's pouch, tethering of gall bladder to common bile duct and smaller caliber common bile duct can also lead to injuries if this technique is used.

Injury to the biliary structures in the liver bed can also occur if the plane of separation of the gall bladder from the liver bed is done in a deeper plane, especially in cases of acute cholecystitis where the dissection is difficult. Excessive traction may align the cystic duct with the common bile duct leading to the conclusion that the common bile duct is the cystic duct. Failure of adequate traction (hard cirrhotic liver) gives poor visualisation of the hepatic hilum also may be high risk for bile duct injury.

4. Due to clips

Apart from misidentification, failure of clips applied to the cystic duct (either due to loosening of the clips, division of the duct distal to the clip, inclusion of other tissues within the clip and thermal necrosis) might also lead to ductal injuries. When applying clip to the cystic duct, it is essential to see the both arms of the clip carefully. After the application, it has to be verified that that the clip occludes the duct completely. For occlusion of wide and thick cystic ducts, ligation with sutures, endoloop or endosuturing is preferred over clips. One should not handle the area where the clip is applied, after the application. At the end of the procedure it is ideal to check the clips gently in doubtful cases.

5. Due to cautery

Cautery should not be applied close to the clips and unnecessary handling of the tissues in the area of clip should be avoided as far as possible. Excessive use of cautery to control bleeding in the area of Calots triangle may also lead to thermal injuries. The loss if insulation in dissection instruments might lead to accidental burns either in the extra hepatic biliary system or in any of the hollow viscus. Some of these injuries may occur late in the post operative period. For example extensive dissection of a misidentified common bile duct with cautery might lead to devascularisation of the duct, resulting in delayed biliary structures.

6. Aberrant anatomy

The congenital anomalies of the extra hepatic biliary system are very common and these can cause disasters if they are not recognized properly during dissection. For example an aberrant duct that joins the hepatic duct might be identified as the cystic duct joining the hepatic duct and may be divided.

7. Difficult cases

It has been documented that the incidence of biliary injuries is 3 times more common during laparoscopic cholecystectomy for conditions like acute cholecystitis and gangrene of the gall bladder when compared to elective surgery. Dense inflammation, adhesions, loss of tissue plane, excessive bleeding during dissection that prevent proper identification of the structures are some of the factors that result in increased incidence of biliary injuries. Following the technique of modified subtotal cholecystectomy Type II in cases with difficult Calot's triangle dissection has been the safest approach in our experience. For detailed description of the technique refer chapter 42.

HOW TO PERFORM SAFE DISSECTION OF CALOT'S TRIANGLE ?

Two different views exist on the technique of safe dissection of Calot's triangle which includes the "Infundibular technique" and the recent "Critical view technique." The disadvantage of the infundibular technique has already been described.

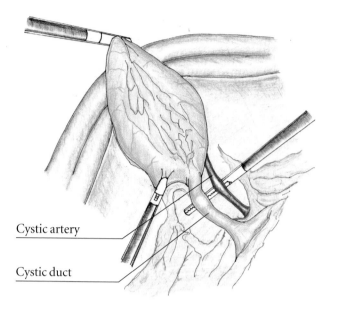

Cystic artery

Cystic duct

Figure 20 : Critical view of safety. Complete dissection of calot's triangle

The **"Critical View of Safety"** described by Strasberg requires complete dissection of Calot's triangle free of fat, fibrous and areolar tissue and separation of the base of the gall bladder from liver bed.[1,16] It is usually necessary to dissect from both ventral and dorsal aspects using a variety of dissection techniques such as gentle dissection with finer instruments using electrocautery, blunt dissection and irrigation. At completed dissection there should be only 2 structures seen to be entering into the gall bladder that is the cystic duct and cystic artery. If this critical view is not obtained then it is better to resort to intra operative cholangiogram to identify the structures. Staying close to the gall bladder during the clearance of Calot's triangle is the key for safe dissection.

The other safety precautions that have to be taken are the setting of adequate cautery level, maintenance of the equipments and insulation. When using cautery the instruments should always be directed away from the important structures such as bile duct.

Role of Intra operative Cholangiogram?

Traditionally intraoperative cholangiography has been advocated as a routine procedure for all cholecystectomies, in order to accurately define the biliary anatomy and to detect intraductal stones.[17,18] Though routine cystic duct cholangiograms have been shown by some to reduce the incidence of biliary injury, there are inherent problems associated with it. The cholangiogram must be interpreted correctly for proper identification. The images can be misinterpreted and still injuries occur even after cholangiogram.

Cholangiogram of "Doom"

The usual misinterpretation is visualization of only the lower part of the biliary tree without filling the proximal ducts. In reality this means that the common bile duct has been cannulated and a clip has been placed across it and hence contrast cannot flow proximally into hepatic ducts. Failure to fill the proximal ducts must be interpreted as abnormal finding until proven otherwise.

Similarly accessory right hepatic duct can be cannulated which might lead to confusion. If these abnormalities are not detected during cholangiogram, then the surgeon might proceed to division of these ducts.

It has been now shown that the routine intra operative cholangiography yields very little useful clinical information over and above that which is obtained with selective policies. No difference was found in the rates of major or minor bile duct injuries between the two policies, although injuries were more likely to be noted immediately if intra operative cholangiography was performed. We do cholangiogram in selective cases. Most of the cholangiograms in our centre are done to rule out CBD stones in doubtful cases rather than to identify the anatomy.

Prevention of bile duct injuries

It should be remembered that more importance must be given in prevention of these injuries than to repair of these injuries. The following are some of the basic safety precautions that help in avoiding biliary injury.

1. To operate after adequate training and supervision

2. Proper selection of simple cases during early phase

of the career. It is advisable to seek the advise of the surgeon available in the theatre if one come across a situation like this.

3. Follow proper dissection techniques

4. Identification of structures properly before clipping or division

5. Performing modified subtotal chgolecystectomy II in cases of difficult dissection in the Calot's triangle

6. Identification of risk factors that might lead to injuries
   a. Chronically inflamed and scared tissue
   b. Bleeding around the Calot's triangle obscuring the view
   c. Excessive fat in the portal area
   d. Presence of acute cholecystitis
   e. Obesity (relatively lower risk factor)
   f. Altered anatomy - presence of congenital variations in the anatomical positions

7. Proper use of energy sources in the area of dissection and adherence to safety precautions

8. Placement of a drainage tube is case of difficult dissection

MANAGEMENT OF BILIARY INJURIES

Proper management of iatrogenic bile duct injuries is mandatory to avoid immediate or late life threatening sequelae, such as recurrent cholangitis and biliary cirrhosis with portal hypertension. Most often these patients mainly suffer from the additional morbidity associated with hasty and incomplete repairs done in the primary centers and the late referrals to tertiary centres after the injury has occurred. Immediate recognition, assessment of the injury and deciding on the type of intervention will place in the patients in a safe path to recovery.

What to do when we suspect bile duct injuries ?

The most important factor is the recognition of these injuries. Early recognition and treatment of the injury reduces the severity of the injury and improves the outcome. Only less than 50 % of the injuries are recognized during the surgery.[19] It is better to perform an intra operative cholangiogram to assess the nature of injury. Although intra operative cholangiogram does not prevent the incidence of bile duct injury, it increases the chances of recognition. Immediate repair of the injury is the best possible treatment option provided the expertise of the surgeon is adequate. Assistance should be sought from a surgeon with experience in bile duct repair as this definitely increases the chances of cure.

Management of injuries recognized post operatively

Patients with obvious injury will have persistent bile leakage through drainage tube. General malaise, abdominal pain, nausea and vomiting, abdominal distension, ileus, jaundice with or without cholangitis and fever and altered liver function tests are better considered as indicators of bile leak until proved other wise. If this policy is followed then most of the injuries can be detected as early as possible. But these symptoms are often under evaluated by the primary surgeon and at the time of diagnosis the patient usually develops bilioma and biliary peritonitis. It is unfortunate that the majority of bile duct injuries go unrecognized and may present weeks to months or even years later.[20] (1) Recurrent cholangitis, (2) Secondary biliary cirrhosis ascites and (3) Ascites (4) esophageal varices are the late clinical manifestation of an unrecognized biliary injury.

Diagnosis

Ultrasound may be helpful in detecting subhepatic fluid collection (bilioma) but it may some times miss the injury and smaller collections. CT scan will offer a better view of the nature and extent of the injury and the presence of collection and other relevant detail, eg., presence of vascular injury, extent of damage to the liver after long duration and subhepatic fluid collection (bilioma). Failure of dye excretion into the small bowel due to block or presence of radionucleotide in the fluid collection may indicate injury in scintiscan.

But the exact nature and extent of injury can be documented only by endoscopic retrograde cholangio pancreaticogram (ERCP). ERCP will also allow for placement of stent to decompress the ductal system

Immediate Management on recognition

If facilities and expertise are available then the following options can be considered after complete assessment of the degree of injury.

Type	Management - Immediate
A	Suture of the cystic duct or application of loop + Adequate Drainage Reduction of intrabiliary pressure by post operative ERCP/stenting (if needed)
B	Not often found during surgery
C	Accessory right hepatic duct or segmental hepatic duct Less than 3mm : Ligation of the both levels Greater than 5mm : Primary or Roux en Y Hepaticojejunostomy
D	Less than 50 % of circumference : Primary repair with T Tube + Adequate drainage Avulsion of cystic duct : Primary repair with T Tube + Adequate drainage More than 50 % of circumference, thermal injury : Roux en Y Hepaticojejunostomy
E	Hepaticojejunostomy

These procedures are better attempted in a setup where biliary reconstructive procedures are routinely carried out. If this is not the condition, then the patients are better managed by adequate drainage by a large sized drain and referral to a tertiary centre.

especially in A and D type of injuries. The cholangiogram may be normal in certain injuries like B and C as the area of damage is not in continuity with the biliary system. Percutaneous Transhepatic Cholangiogram (PTC) will be helpful in detection of these lesions and placement of catheter during this evaluation my help in identification of the accessory hepatic duct and right and left hepatic duct during the surgery.

The role of hepatic angiography in these situations has been evaluated completely as the presence of vascular injury will have a definitive impact on the postoperative mortality and morbidity.[21] Angiography should be performed in suspected cases to rule out concomitant vascular injury. Vascular injury can be suspected if there is significant hemorrhage during the surgery, seeing multiple clips on radiographs, significant elevation of transaminases in the postoperative period.

In a study of 18 cases of failed initial repair of bile duct injury, 61 % of patients had coexisting arterial injury in 11 patients (61%). The patients with arterial injuries developed strictures after a longer duration when compared to development of strictures in patients without arterial injury. The possible cause for strictures in patients without arterial injury was probably due to faulty repair techniques, whereas in patients with arterial injury the reason for the development of late strictures was due to vascular compromise. In these patients ischemia due to previous injury has caused failure of the successful anastomosis. This study stresses the need for assessment of the vascular compromise in assessing the success of the repairs.[12]

Treatment

Successful management requires multidisciplinary approach with experts in biliary surgery, therapeutic endoscopy, and interventional radiology. The first attempt to repair the injury carries the highest success rate. The aim of treatment is the reestablishment of bile flow. Surgery is the gold standard and ERCP of PTC is preferred in selected patients as a 'bridging' procedure to decompress the biliary system and to relieve cholangitis before definitive

Type	Management - Postoperative
A	Drainage of collection + reduction of intrabiliary pressure by ERCP/stenting
B	Symptomatic patients: 　　Hepaticojejunostomy, 　　Segmental hepatic resection, if anastomosis not possible 　　(only for recurrent cholangitis not manageable conservatively) Asymptomatic: 　　Diagnosed after long duration : No treatment is required 　　Recently diagnosed, drains a large portion of liver : Bypass procedures
C	Drainage of collection $\pm$ biliary enteric anastomosis Resection of the liver, if the drainage segment is small
D	ERCP + Stent as initial treatment (usually resolves) No recovery: Same as immediate management
E	Due to strictures, clip occlusion : Balloon dilation, Stents Hepaticojejunostomy for patients not responding to nonoperative treatment or ductal separation

therapy. Management depends on the type of injury, the type of initial management and its result, and the time elapsed since the initial operation or repair.

Lessons learnt from few cases

There is no cause for concern if a patient shows evidence of minor biliary injury in the postoperative period (by increased drain output), if the drain is functioning well, ultrasound shows no evidence of collection of bile either subhepatic or sub diaphragmatic space and no cholangitis. We have managed about six patients in this manner.

In one of our patients of laparoscopic cholecystectomy for acute cholecystitis, biliary leak was noted by the side of the drainage tube due to blockage of the tube by omentum. We decided to perform relaparoscopy as we thought that the collection might lead to infection, pericholedochal fibrosis and futher complications. ERCP and stenting was perfomed on the next day followed by relaparoscopy. It revealed bile collection in the subhepatic and

subdiaphragmatic area and the tube was found to be kinked. There was a biliary leak midway at the lateral border of the gall bladder fossa and 4-0 vicryl sutures were placed above and below the accessory duct. The patient was discharged on third postoperative day. If this patient had managed by conservative methods the collection would have increased and lead to other complications

Ultrasound guided aspiration of the biliary collection has been advocated by some. We would like to stress the importance of a thorough peritoneal lavage with adequate breaking of loculations in this setting. Unless this is performed the patient might continue to have persistent episodes of fever and collection. A highly skilled hepatopancreaticobiliary surgeon had performed a difficult laparoscopic cholecystectomy for more than 5 hours and drainage tube was not kept as the surgeon was very confident of his technique.

Patient developed biliary peritonitis and ultrasound showed evidence collection of bile in the sub diaphragmatic, subhepatic and pelvic area. Ultrasound

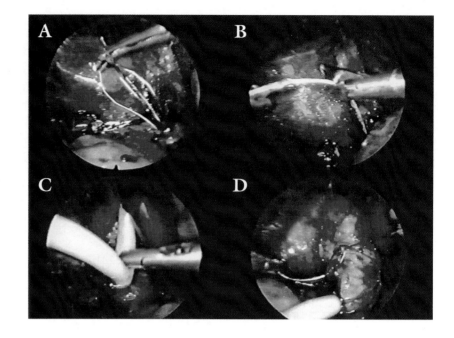

Figure 21 : Laparoscopic removal of broken ERCP basket from the CBD

A - CBD was opened stone extracted and basket is being pulled out

B - Basket wire was cut using heavy non insulated scissor

C - Placement of T tube

D - Suturing of CBD

guided aspiration was done on 5th and 8th post operative day. ERCP and stenting was done on 12th postoperative day. Subsequently USG guided aspiration was again done and a tube was placed in the right hypochondrium (under ultrasound guidance). Due to continued sepsis, patient was referred to our institution. CT scan showed multiple collections throughout the peritoneal cavity.

Relaparoscopy was done in our hospital on 32nd postoperative day. Pneumoperitoneum was created by open Hasson technique. Three additional trocars were placed at the epigastric, left iliac, right lumbar region. 7x 5cm collection of pus was removed from the lateral side of the pelvis along with infected tissue and slough from the subhepatic areas and thorough peritoneal lavage was done. The patient was discharged in the 4th day.

Even though there was no bile leak in this patient, the persistence of infected fluid was due to incomplete aspiration under US guidance. In presence generalized peritonitis and biliary collection, it is better to do laparotomy or relaparoscopy for adequate

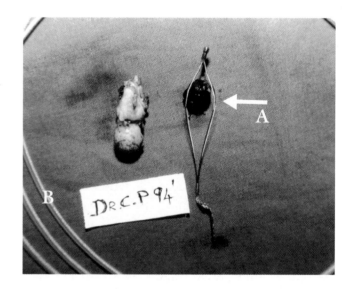

Figure 22 : Extracted broken ERCP Basket from the common bile duct

A - Basket with stone

B - Basket wire

peritoneal toileting and placement of a large drainage tube. Subsequently ERCP may be done to evaluate the site and nature of injury, to plan further course of treatment cholangitis. If the collection and sepsis worsen due to lack of adequate drainage it may produce secondary irreparable damage to the common duct. This patient was operated for common duct stricture after 6 months and hepatico jejunostomy was performed.

We had operated on a patient with impacted Dormia basket in the common bile duct following attempted stone extraction through ERCP in 1994. We successfully extracted the impacted basket through laparoscopy. After choledochotomy and removal of the basket, the common bile duct was closed over a T tube. The patient had an uneventful recovery.

CONCLUSION

Biliary injuries following laparoscopic cholecystectomy is a significant problem that can lead to disastrous consequences, if proper dissection techniques and safety precautions are not followed. High degree of suspicion is important for recognition of these injuries. Once recognized these must be promptly referred to tertiary centers for appropriate management, as the first repair is the best repair for these injuries. Improper management often leads to high morbidity in the form of biliary strictures and its complications.

References

1. Strasberg SM, Eagon CJ, Drebin JA T. The "hidden cystic duct" syndrome and the infundibular technique of laparoscopic cholecystectomy-the danger of the false infundibulum. J Am Coll Surg 2000; 191:661-667.

2. Schlumpf R, Klotz HP, Wehrli H, Herzog U. A nation's experience in laparoscopic cholecystectomy. Prospective multicenter analysis of 3722 cases. Surg Endosc 1994; 8(1):35-41.

3. Sutherland F, Launois B, Stanescu M, et al. A refined approach to the repair of postcholecystectomy bile duct strictures. Arch Surg 1999; 134(3):299-302.

4. Lillemoe KD, Melton GB, Cameron JL, et al. Postoperative bile duct strictures: management and outcome in the 1990s. Ann Surg 2000; 232(3):430-41.

5. Topal B, Aerts R, Penninckx F. The outcome of major biliary tract injury with leakage in laparoscopic cholecystectomy. Surg Endosc 1999; 13(1):53-6.

6. Strasberg SM, Hertl M, Soper NJ. An analysis of the problem of biliary injury during laparoscopic cholecystectomy. J Am Coll Surg 1995; 180(1):101-25.

7. Soper NJ, SM S. Avoiding and classifying common bile duct injuries during laparoscopic cholecystectomy. In Phillips EH, Rosenthal RJ, eds. Operative strategies in laparoscopic surgery. New York: Springer - Verlag, 1995. pp. 65 - 72.

8. Lillimoe KD, Petrofski JA, Choti MA. Isolated right segmental hepatic duct injury: A diagnostic and therapeutic challenge. J Gastrointest Surg 2000; 2:168-177.

9. Meyers WC, Peterseim DS, Pappas TN. Low insertion of hepatic segmental duct VII-VIII is an important cause of major biliary injury or misdiagnosis. Am J Surg 1996; 171:187-191.

10. Jarnigan WR, LH. B. Operative repair of bile duct injuries involving the hepatic duct confluence. Arch Surg 1999; 134:769-775.

11. Buanes T, Mjaland O, Waage A. A population-based survey of biliary surgery in Norway. Relationship between patient volume and quality of surgical treatment. Surg Endosc 1998; 12:852-855.

12. Koffron A, Ferrario M, Parsons W. Failed primary management of iatrogenic biliary injury: Incidence and significance of concomitant hepatic arterial disruption. Surgery 1999; 130:722-28.

13. Majno PE, Pretu R, Mentha G, P. M. Operative injury to the hepatic artery. Consequences of a biliary-enteric anastomosis and principles for rational management. Arch Surgery 1996; 131:211-215.

14. Gupta N, Solomon H, Fairchild R, DL K. Management and outcome of patients with combined bile duct and hepatic artery injuries. Arch Surg 1998; 133:176 -181.

15. Davidoff AM, Pappas TN, Murray EA. Mechanisms of major biliary injury during laparoscopic cholecystectomy. Ann Surg 1992; 215:196-208.

16. Strasberg SM, Herd M, Soper NJJ. An analysis of the problem of biliary injury during laparoscopic cholecystectomy. Am Coll Surg 1995; 180:101 -125.

17. Mirizzi P. Operative cholangiography. Surg Gynecol Obstet 1937; 65:702-710.

18. Mills JL, Beck DE, FJ H. Routine operative cholangiography. Surg Gynecol Obstet 1985; 161:343-5.

19. Richardson MC, Bell G, Fullarton GM. Incidence and nature of bile duct injuries following laparoscopic cholecystectomy: an audit of 5913 cases. West of Scotland Laparoscopic Cholecystectomy Audit Group. Br J Surg 1996; 83(10):1356-60.

20. LH. B. Hilar and intrahepatic biliary enteric anastomosis. Surg Clin North Am 1994; 74:845-863.

21. Chapman WC, Halevy A, Blumgart LH, IS. B. Postcholecystectomy bile duct strictures. Arch Surg 1995; 130:597-604.

44

Laparoscopic Treatment of Common Bile Duct Stones

INTRODUCTION

When laparoscopic surgery was introduced in 1988, it was soon accepted as a gold standard procedure and was embraced by all surgeons worldwide. But the concept of laparoscopic common bile duct exploration is still surrounded by mystery due to perceived difficulties and dangers associated with the procedure. Now with the technological advancements in imaging and instrumentation technology, laparoscopic common bile duct exploration is emerging as the primary treatment option in centers were facilities and adequate expertise are available. Currently the role of routine preoperative ERCP is being questioned and minimal access surgery is moving towards a single stage laparoscopic CBD exploration either through transcystic or choledochotomy approach.[1,2]

Courvoisier described the first conventional common bile duct exploration in 1889 for ductal stones.[3]

Hamskehr introduced routine "T" tube drainage after surgical exploration of the common bile duct. It was Mirizzi, an Argentinean surgeon who developed the art of intraoperative cholangiography. The advent of intraoperative choledochoscope and the routine use of intraoperative cholangiogram have dropped the incidence of residual stones to almost nil. Endoscopic sphincterotomy first described by Classen provided a worthy alternative to choledochotomy by conventional approach.[4] The first laparoscopic cholecystectomy was reported by Philip Mouret in 1988 in France.[5] The common bile duct exploration was attempted as a logical extension of the procedure and Jacobs et al reported the first laparoscopic common bile duct exploration in 1991[6] (interestingly, hundred years after Courvoisier described the first conventional common bile duct exploration in 1889).[2]

COMMON BILE DUCT STONES

The natural history of ductal stones have not been defined clearly, but most of the stones pass through the ampulla of Vater. The incidence of CBD stones in patients undergoing laparoscopic cholecystectomy is around 10% and these can cause complications such as jaundice, acute cholangitis and pancreatitis.[7] The diagnosis of common bile duct stones usually pose a problem as most of the investigative modalities like ultrasound and biochemical parameters are not accurate. Magnetic resonance imaging is the latest non invasive imaging technique which could play a major role in the diagnosis of common bile duct stones.[8] Though intraoperative ultrasound has been shown to have a high level of sensitivity and specificity, intraoperative cholangiogram still remains the gold standard.[9]

TREATMENT OPTIONS

When choosing the modality and timing of intervention in patients with common bile duct, it is important to identify all factors including the patients age, associated comorbid illness, his ability to withstand general anesthesia, number of stones, their location and size of the stones as well as the diameter of the common bile duct. There are several treatment options available for CBD stones such as preoperative ERCP, sphincterotomy, ERCP and biliary drainage with endoprosthesis, Open and laparoscopic exploration and postoperative ERCP.

The other treatment options that complement the above mentioned options are shock wave lithotripsy (intracorporeal/extracorporeal), laser lithotripsy, per oral cholangioscopy, percutaneous stone extraction and dissolution therapy. The surgeon has to choose among these treatment options and tailor the approach to the individual.

PATIENT MANAGEMENT

The clinical situations of patients who present with common bile duct stones can be divided into three main categories.

1. Diagnosed preoperatively
2. Diagnosed intraoperatively
3. Diagnosed postoperatively

1. Stones Diagnosed Preoperatively

The general trend of management of these patients is by preoperative ERCP, stone extraction followed by laparoscopic cholecystectomy if all the facilities are available.[10-13] But now single stage laparoscopic common bile duct exploration and cholecystectomy is emerging as a primary and cost effective treatment modality with least morbidity, as the additional morbidity and cost of the ERCP is avoided in this approach. Laparoscopic common bile duct exploration can be performed either by the transcystic approach or by choledochotomy.

Severe, complicated calculus disease and poor condition of patients are contraindications for laparoscopic bile duct exploration. Patients who are deeply jaundiced with impaired renal function, those with cholangitis or severe pancreatitis due to ampullary impaction and poor-risk patients (cardio-respiratory disease) are best treated by endoscopic sphincterotomy and stone extraction in the first instance. Laparoscopic cholecystectomy (LC) is undertaken once the condition of the patient has improved. Biliary drainage procedures are advocated for patents with large dilated CBD, multiple impacted tones, non removable impacted CBD stones, retained stones not amenable to ERCP and obstruction secondary to tumor.

2. Ductal Calculi Discovered During Surgery

Decision making is relatively easy when stones are discovered intraoperatively. The three options that are available are (a) to continue with laparoscopic CBD exploration, (b) to convert to open procedure and complete CBD exploration or (c) to leave the stones in place for subsequent ERCP

If the surgeon is experienced, the most appropriate treatment is the combined laparoscopic stone extraction and cholecystectomy. The single-stage laparoscopic treatment is a more cost-effective option than postoperative endoscopic stone extraction and avoids the necessity for a sphincterotomy, which is an important consideration in young and middle-aged patients.

In patients in whom a ductal calculus is not dealt with at the time of cholecystectomy, a small cannula is inserted into the common duct through the cystic duct is recommended. In addition to providing an excellent access for postoperative cholangiography, a guide wire can be easily inserted through the cannula down the bile duct into the duodenum, thereby facilitating endoscopic sphincterotomy in the postoperative period.

3. Ductal Calculi Discovered After Surgery

These patients are best managed by post operative ERCP and stone extraction which is considered as the least morbid procedure. Even in the best possible hands of endoscopists as failure rate of 10% in stone retrieval has been reported.[14] In these situations we have to opt either for laparoscopic or open exploration.

REVIEW OF LAPAROSCOPIC TREATMENT OPTIONS

The laparoscopic treatment options for CBD stones basically consists of initial intraoperative cholangiogram, entering the CBD, removal of stones by a combination of techniques like basketing and using balloons. This is followed by verification of ductal clearance either by choledochoscope or intraoperative cholangioscopy or both. Finally the access route (transcystic or choledochotomy) is closed with a T tube. The technique applied in a individual patient may be a combination of these steps. The following paragraphs will briefly describe the concepts of each approach. The indications, contraindications advantages and disadvantages of each will be discussed. The exact technique of surgery will be discussed later.

Transcystic Approach to CBD

After performance of intraoperative cholangiogram the same incision can be enlarged to gain access into CBD. The incision should be made closer to the CBD, so that it involves lesser cystic duct dilatation. Before attempting this technique the cholangiogram should be studied properly for the anatomy of the cystic duct junction.

The opening and the cystic duct is dilated with either bougies or balloon catheters that are passed over a guide wire. The cystic duct is dilated just enough to allow for the extraction of the largest

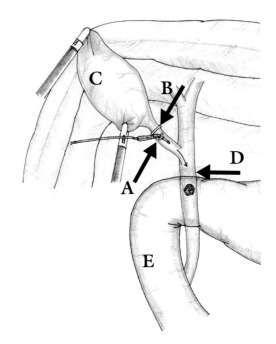

Figure 1 : Transcystic extraction of CBD stone

A - Baloon catheter is introduced in the cystic duct
B - Sentinel clip
C - Gall bladder
D - Common Bile duct
E - Duodenum

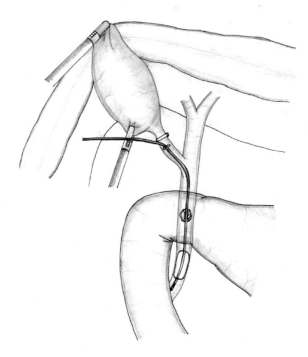

Figure 2 : Tip of the balloon catheter introduced beyond the the and the baloon is inflated

calculus in the common bile duct. Another technique has been described that uses a "plastic peel away introducer sheath" one size larger than the choledocho-scope. This allows multiple entries of the choledocho-scope without damaging valves.[15] This is most helpful for removing multiple stones from the cystic duct. Dilatation of the duct beyond 8mm can lead to splitting of CBD. The cystic duct dilatation may not necessary in more than 50% of the patients as it is generally dilated to the size of the duct that passed into the CBD. The stones that are present in the proximal duct cannot be approached through transcystic route.

The ideal patients for transcystic exploration are small sized stone (<8mm or diameter less than or equal to diameter of cystic duct), limited number of stones, stones located below the cystic duct junction and

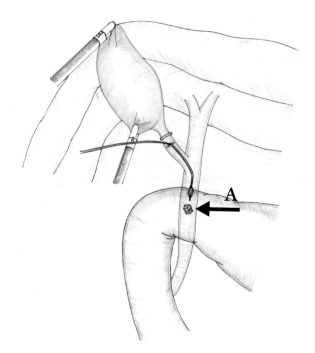

Figure 3 : Basket is introduced in the CBD through the cystic duct

A - Stone in the common bile duct

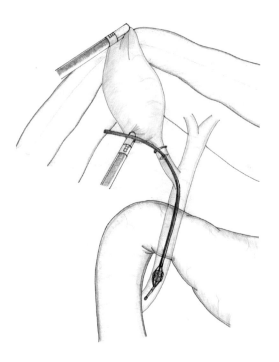

Figure 4 : Basketing of the CBD stone

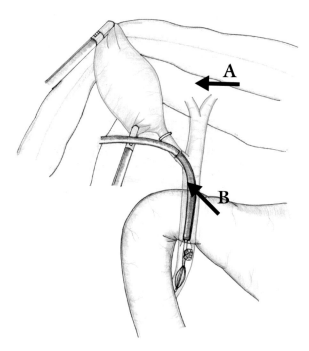

Figure 5 : Choledochoscope introduced through the cystic duct after dilatation into the CBD

A - Choledochoscope
B - Basket

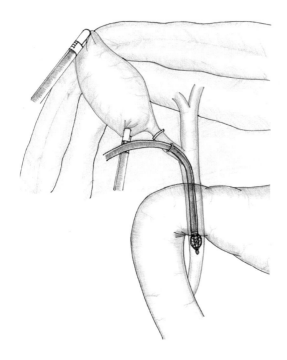

Figure 6 : Basketing and extraction of the stone under choledochoscopic view

Antegrade Approach

Laparoscopic antegrade sphincterotomy was first reported by DePaula and Curet et al.[17,18] In this technique, an endoscopic sphincterotome is introduced antegrade of either via cystic duct or CBD and guided through ampulla. A side viewing duodenoscopy confirms the position of sphincterotome before sphincterotomy. Indications for these techniques have been described as multiple large CBD stone, patients with common hepatic and intrahepatic stones, as a drainage procedure in elderly patients with incompletely cleared duct and patients with papillary stenosis. The main advantage is the possible biliary drainage procedure if needed without the risk of producing pancreatitis. We do not have any experience in this type of technique.

a patent cystic duct. The limiting factors include anatomic features related to the cystic duct such as small size, tortuous duct, obstructive cystic valve, rupture of cystic duct during instrumentation and low level of insertion of cystic duct.[16]

Choledochotomy Approach

A longitudinal incision just the size of the largest stone is made over the anterior aspect of the common bile duct just below the insertion of the cystic duct. The main advantage of the choledochotomy is the ability to visualise the proximal tree. This technique is preferable for patients with dilated common bile duct >10mm, calculi >1cm, multiple calculi, calculi that require lithotripsy secondary to impaction, failed transcystic exploration and intrahepatic calculi that are inaccessible by transcystic approach. The supposed disadvantage of this approach is the possible stricture of the common bile duct.

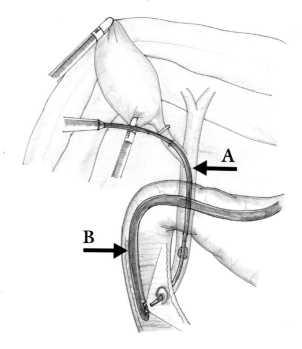

Figure 7 : Antegrade sphincterotomy

A - Endoscopic sphincterotome
B - Side view duodenoscope

Factors influencing duct exploration approach

Factor	Trancystic Approach	Choeldochotomy Approach
Single stone	+	+
Multiple stones	+	+
Stones < 6mm diameter each	+	+
Stones > 6mm diameter each	-	+
Intrahepatic stones	-	+
Diameter of cystic duct < 4mm	-	+
Diameter of cystic duct > 4mm	+	+
Diameter of common bile duct < 6mm	+	-
Diameter of common bile duct >6mm	+	+
Cystic duct entrance - lateral	+	+
Cystic duct entrance - posterior	-	+
Cystic duct entrance - distal	-	+
Inflammation - mild	+	+
Inflammation - marked	+	-
Suturing ability - poor	+	-
Suturing ability - good	+	+

Adopted from Joseph Petelin [7, 20]

Removal Methods

Once the CBD is opened, the removal of the stones can be performed by using any of the following methods. Smaller stones can be just flushed into the duodenum by injection of saline through cholangiogram catheter. If this fails, various other options are available. The stones can be extracted through the dormia basket by radiological guided approach. Alternatively balloon sweep of the CBD from above and below can also be done. Some surgeons use choledochoscope for extraction of stones from the CBD with a dormia basket through the working channel.

Closure of the Access Opening

The access opening in the cystic duct or the common bile duct can be closed in multiple ways. The cystic duct opening may be closed with a drainage tube that passes through it which will act as decompression tube and as a route for postoperative cholangiogram.[15, 19] The choledochotomy is usually closed over a T tube made of latex.[7, 20] Some surgeons prefer silicon T tubes, as they have been reported to have decreased incidence of bacterial colonization.[21-24] But this material does not provide enough tissue reaction and has to be removed after a long interval, after surgery.

Alternatively the choledochotomy can be closed primarily in situations where the post operative cholangiogram and choledochoscopy does not reveal any residual stones and there is no evidence of any distal obstruction or edema of the ampulla. Numerous studies have shown that this technique is a safe method of closure of the choledochotomy.[25-27] The use of biliary endoprosthesis has been reported for the treatment of biliary and cystic duct leaks following cholecystectomy, in the post operative period. The same concept has been used by some in closure of the choledochotomy and cystic duct opening.[28, 29] These methods ensure complete decompression and also serve as a guide for intubation of ampulla if need arises for ERCP.

ROLE OF ERCP AT PRESENT SITUATION

ERCP was not in routine preoperative use during the open surgery era, as none of the randomized studies proved that its routine use was superior to conventional common duct exploration. After laparoscopic cholecystectomy surgeons resorted to the routine use of preoperative ERCP and sphincterotomy even in case of slightest suspicion of stones so that these patients could be managed by endoscopic stone removal or by conventional method. This routine preoperate use of ERCP is being questioned now as it is not an absolutely safe and effective method.[30-32] It has been shown that the clearance rate of endoscopic sphincterotomy is 90%.[14] ERCP is associated with life threatening complications such as bleeding (3%) pancreatitis (5%) duodenal perforation (1%) and late papillary stenosis (10-33%) and a small but significant mortality of 1-2%.[14] Pancreatitis is a well recognized complication of ERCP and sphincterotomy, where as this can be completely avoided by the supraduodenal exploration of the common bile duct as the papilla in totally undisturbed.

Considering these, it would be advisable to do ERCP selectively in patients who are deeply jaundiced with impaired renal function, cholangitis due to ampullary impaction and poor risk patients. The routine use of preoperative ERCP in patients of CBD stones is gradually wading of with increasing experience of the laparoscopic surgeons.

TECHNIQUE OF LAPAROSCOPIC CBD EXPLORATION

Preoperative preparations

The standard preoperative work-up includes ultrasound examination and LFT (bilirubin, transaminase, alkaline phosphates). Antibiotics are administered routinely at the induction of anaesthesia. As the majority of these patients are elderly, chemoprophylaxis with heparin against deep venous thrombosis and use of antithrombotic graduated elastic stockings is advisable.

Theatre setup

The theatre setup for laparoscopic CBD exploration is very crucial as the imaging equipments, instruments and disposables needed for this procedure is numerous and should be available in perfect condition before attempting this procedure. Without the availability of the guide wires, balloons (which are not used routinely in the operative room) a chaotic environment will prevail in the operation theatre.

It is always better to have two camera systems, that can capture the image from the laparoscope and choledoscope separately. The monitors should show the combined image of the laparoscopic and choledochoscopic camera in PIP (Picture in Picture). This is invaluable when the surgeon manipulates the choledochoscope with laparoscopic instruments to obtain a clear view of the stone. Presence of a video mixer that integrates these images into one image is essential. The theatre personnel should be well trained to use all the monitors, cameras and the imaging system, as this surgery involves proper set up of the theatre with monitors displaying outputs from 2 cameras, integration of the picture through video mixer and the necessary documentation and recording that has to be performed during the procedure.

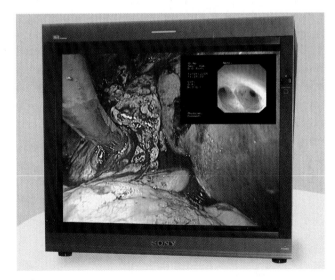

Figure 8 : Picture in picture view of laparoscopy and choledochoscopy

We routinely use a pediatric endoscope for intraoperative stone localization instead of using the routine choledochoscope (Ultra slim 5.2 mm Olypmus Exera). The manipulation of these scopes which have 4 degrees of freedom of movements is much better when compared to conventional choledochoscope with only 2 degrees of freedom. Wire baskets are available that can be inserted through the pediatric endoscopes for removal of stone. This can be used for in common bile ducts that are more than 7-8mm diameter.

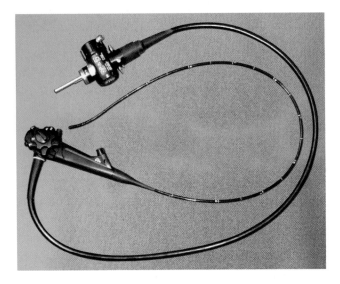

Figure 9 : Ultra slim 5.2 mm Olypmus Exera scope

The following check list acts as a very useful reminder. These instruments are mainly needed for bile duct exploration and it would be a better idea to store all these instruments in a separate mobile trolley and bring this trolley inside the theatre during the surgery.

1. Two cameras with two monitors
2. Fluoroscope (C-arm type)
3. Balloon-tipped catheters (4 French preferred)
4. Sigura type baskets
5. 0.035 inch diameter long (>90 cm) guidewire
6. Mechanical over-the-wire dilators (7-12 French)
7. Atraumatic grasping forceps (for choledochoscope manipulation)
8. Flexible choledochoscope with light source
9. Electrohydraulic or pulsed dye lithotripter
10. T-tube (transductal) or C-tube (Transcystic)
11. Stent (straight, 7 French or 10 French)

Team set up and port position

Patient positioning is essentially the same as laparoscopic cholecystectomy. An operating table which allows fluoroscopy is extremely advantageous for intraoperative cholangiogram and exploration. The monitors are placed on either sides of the patients head end. The pneumoperitoneum is created by Veress needle and the ports are placed identical to that of lap cholecystectomy. 5th trocar for the Olsen forceps and the flexible endoscope is placed directly over the position of the common duct.

Intraoperative cholangiogram

After the initial dissection in Calot's triangle, retraction is maintained on the fundus of the gall bladder. The cystic duct is dissected down bluntly close to its junction with the common duct. A clip (sentinel clip) is placed at the junction with the gallbladder neck. An incision is made on the larger portion of the cystic duct closer to the common duct, leaving adequate length of cystic stump for closure. A clamp is used to milk the cystic duct from its junction with the common duct to clear out any stones. This maneuver facilitates successful passage of catheter and also prevents the inadvertent pushing of the stones into the common duct. Cholangiogram is performed using Olsen clamp and the anatomy of the biliary tract, nature of CBD stones, their number, shape and location is assessed. A short cystic duct lying perpendicular to the CBD is an ideal position for intra operative cholangiogram. Long cystic duct lying parallel to the CBD that opens at an acute angle is a difficult situation.

After performing IOC, the method of approach of the CBD stone can be decided. I usually prefer choledochotomy for common bile duct exploration as the size of the stones encountered in this part of the world are usually larger. The treatment decisions can be based on the stone size and location as per the recommendations advocated by Petelin.[7]

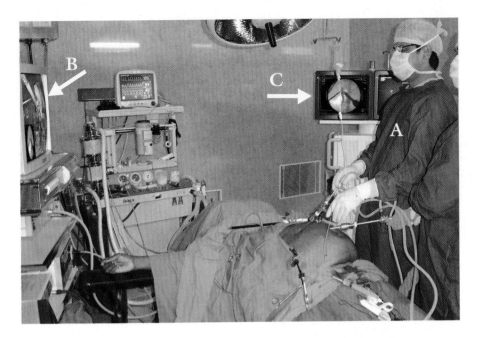

Figure 10 : Team setup for CBD exploration

A - Surgeon
B - Laparoscopic monitor with PIP of C arm image
C - C arm fluroscope

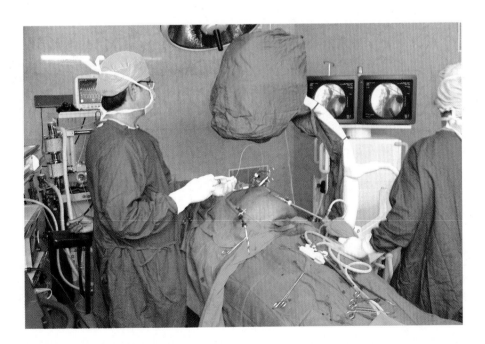

Figure 11 : Performing per operative cholangiogram

Transcystic Approach

The gall bladder is retracted towards the diaphragm through the right lateral port and the cystic duct is dilated to allow for removal of the stone. Either over the wire mechanical dilators or balloon dilators is used for the dilatation of the cystic duct. Care should be taken to prevent splitting or laceration of common bile duct, cystic duct during this maneuver. It is advisable to limit the dilatation upto 8mm to prevent this complication.

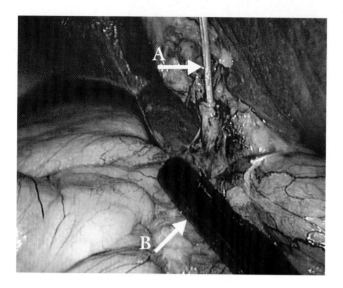

Figure 12 : Transcystic extraction of CBD stone

A - Basket introduced in the cystic duct

B - Laparoscopic ultrasound probe is used to locate the stone

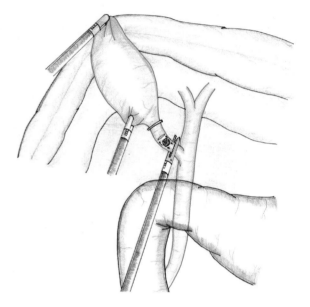

Figure 14 : Milking of remaining stone in the cystic duct after basket extraction

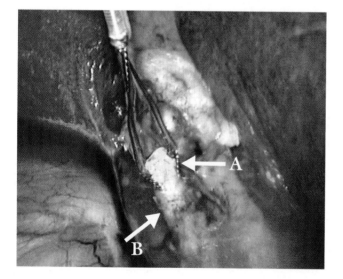

Figure 13 : Extraction of CBD stone through transcystic approach

A - Stone with in the basket

B - Cystic duct

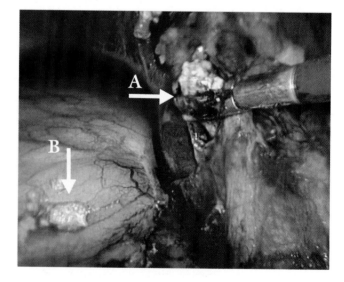

Figure 15 : Milking of remaining stone in the cystic duct after basket extraction

A - Stone is milked out from the cystic duct

B - CBD stone extracted by basket

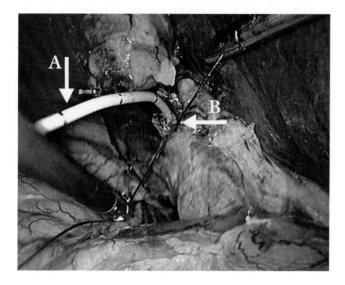

Figure 16 : Decopression tube introduced in the CBD through cystic duct

A - Decompression tube
B - Ligation of cystic duct

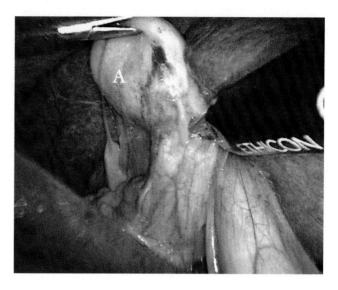

Figure 17 : Separation omental adhesion from the CBD

A - Gall bladder

Choledochotomy

If choledochotomy is decided as the method of approach to the duct, the catheter used for the cholangiogram is left in situ and minimal dissection of the common duct is performed to expose the anterior wall of the common bile duct. Stay sutures are not necessary. The incision of the anterior wall of the common bile duct is made low down in a vertical oblique fashion and should not exceed 1 cm in length. It may require extension if the stone is large, but in practice we have observed that choledochotomy wounds (by virtue of the high elastin content of the bile duct) can be stretched to allow delivery of stones whose diameters are even 30%-50% greater than the size of the wound. Bleeding from the cut edges is controlled by precise soft electrocoagualtion. At this stage, saline is injected forcibly through the cystic duct cannula. This may result in escape of the stone, which is then picked by the spoon forceps and retrieved.

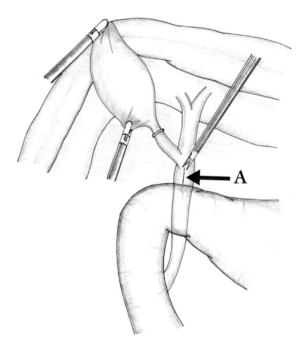

Figure 18 : Choledochotomy using scissor

A - Vertical opening in the CBD

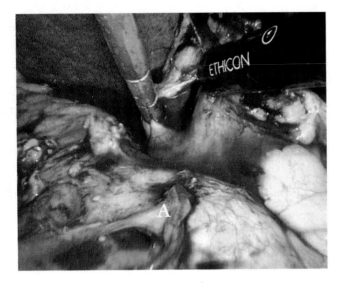

Figure 19 : Choledochotomy. Opening of CBD using harmonic scalpel

A - Duodenum

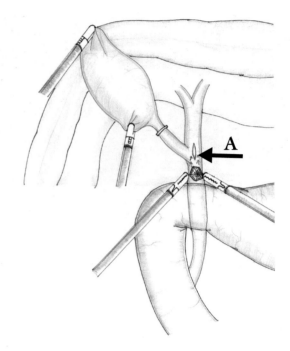

Figure 20 : Milking out the CBD stone

A - Choledochotomy

Stone extraction

The method of extraction of the stone is either of the two approaches. The following few maneuvers like suction, milking out the duct, irrigation, and use of balloon and Dormia basket can result in successful extraction of stones.

Suction

In choledochotomy we usually resort to suction extraction. This step consists of insertion of a suction device just inside the choledochotomy with the tip pointing towards the ampulla. Low suction is applied and this causes the stones to adhere the suction tip. Following delivery through the choledochotomy, the stone is transferred to a spoon forceps and removed. The duct can be often completely cleared by this simple technique.

Milking out

Two round-ended atraumatic graspers are used to straddle the common duct which is massaged between the two instruments in a proximal direction, starting at the lower end. Once the stone has reached the choledochotomy one of the graspers is used to occlude the bile duct above choledochotomy while the other eases the stone out. We have found this technique to be useful for large calculi.

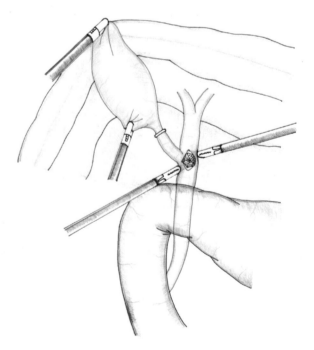

Figure 21 : Extraction of CBD stone

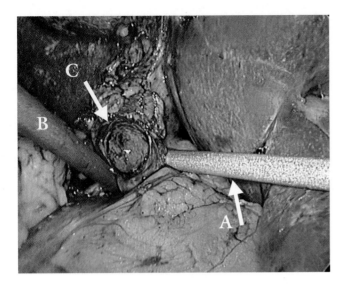

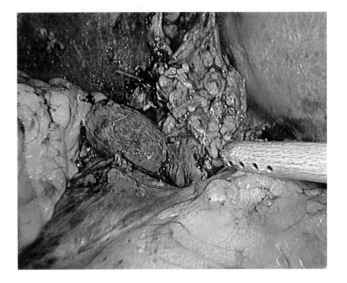

Figure 22 : Milking out the CBD stone

A - Suction nozzle from the epigastric port
B - Grasping forceps from right subcostal port
C - Partially extruding stone

Figure 23 : Extracted CBD stone

Irrigation

Saline is irrigated through a suction catheter in the transcystic approach. This is more effective in patient with smaller stones as it flushes the stones into duodenum. In case of choledochotomy this vigorous irrigation flushes the stone out of the CBD through the incision. An intravenous injection of 1mg glucagon relaxes the ampulla which further facilitate down flushing of stones into the duodenum.

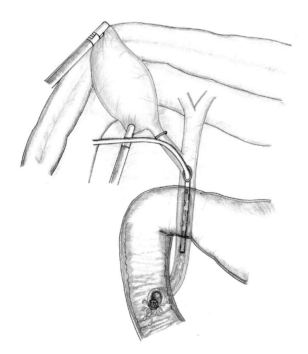

Figure 24 : Flushing out the CBD stone into the duodenum by forceful saline irrigation using suction catheter

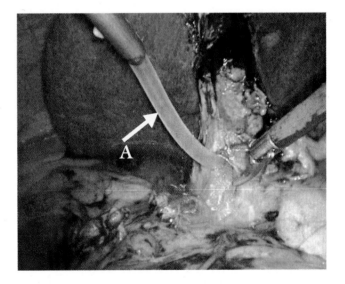

Figure 25 : Irrigation and washing of proximal CBD using suction catheter for debris and remaining stones and fragments

A - Suction catheter from right subcostal port

Balloon manipulation

The standard Fogarty Balloon is passed through the separate port for Oslen forceps and guided through the choledochotomy or the cystic duct. The balloon is guided into the CBD to pass across the ampulla and lie in the duodenum. The balloon is inflated and withdrawn till it produces resistance which indicates the level of the sphincter. The balloon is deflated, withdrawn for about 1cm for it to pass through the ampulla and again reinflated. The tip of the balloon now lies in the distal CBD and is slowly withdrawn maintaining the inflated position to extract the stones. This process is repeated 2-3 times to ensure complete clearance of the distal common bile duct.

Basket maneuvers

In some patients the Dormia basket is introduced into the abdomen through the 5th port and guided into the cystic duct opening or the choledochotomy opening. The basket is guided to the distal end of the common bile duct and slowly withdrawn while the wires of the basket are opened and closed to catch any stone fragments. The presence of stones in the basket is denoted by the inability of the basket to close completely.

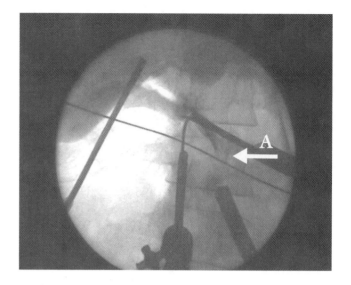

Figure 27 : Under C arm fluroscope guidance basketing the stone

A - Basket with the CBD stone

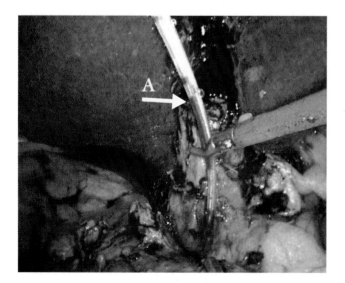

Figure 26 : CBD exploration using basket

A - Basket inserted through the choledochotomy

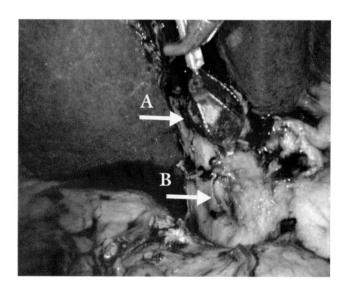

Figure 28 : Extraction of CBD stone using basket

A - Stone in the basket

B - Choledochotomy

We routinely use the fluoroscope for extraction of the stone with the basket and balloon. The CBD is filled with contrast medium and the stone manipulated with the Dormia basket under vision to capture the stones. Once the stone is caught between the wires of the basket, the basket is removed along with the scope in sweeping motion. This maneuver is repeated until the entire CBD is free of stones.

Choledochoscope

We use the pediatric endoscope (160 Exera 5.2mm outer diameter, 2.8 mm working channel) for the choledochoscopic examination and extraction of stone. The advantage of using the pediatric endoscope has been already described in the previous paragraphs. The endoscope is connected to the second camera and the output from this endoscopic camera is relayed to the monitors through a video mixer. The PIP view of the choledochoscope and the laparoscope is very useful for manipulation of the stone.

The endoscope is inserted through the 5th port through a 7mm trocar. The trocar is withdrawn after the scope enters the abdomen to facilitate in easy manipulation of the scope. The scope is usually held by the assistant at the cannula insertion site and it has to be manipulated continually to keep the stone in view. The torque of the scope by the surgeon and the assistant has to be in unison, which is the most difficult part when routine choledochospoes are used. Once the scope enters the cystic duct or the common bile duct it is kept in position by a blunt grasper and a continuous flow of saline at low pressure is connected to the working channel. This distends the CBD and maintains the field of vision clear.

Once the stone is seen, the irrigation is temporarily disconnected and the wire basket is inserted through the choledochoscope, till it exists through the working channel. The basket is manipulated along with the tip of the endoscope till the stone fragments are caught between the wires of the basket. The endoscope along with the basket containing the stone is gradually brought out of the cystic duct. This is then removed by stone holding forceps. Once distal clearance is over, the choledochoscope is gently guided into the proximal position of the duct and the same procedure repeated till complete clearance is achieved.

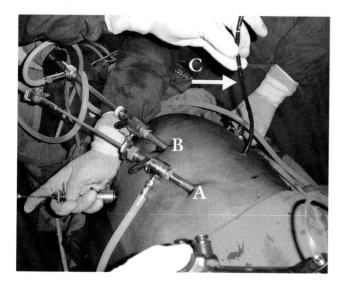

Figure 29 : Choledochoscope is introduced by enlarging the right subcostal port

A - Epigastric working port
B - Umbilical camera port
C - 5.2 mm olympus scope is introduced directly into the peritoneal cavity

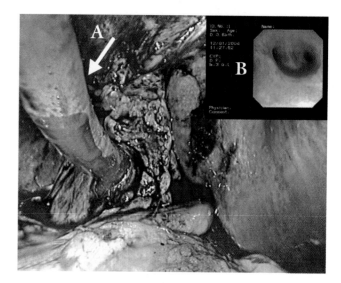

Figure 30 : Choledochoscope visualization of the proximal bile duct

A - Choledochoscope
B - Choledochoscopic view of right and left hepatic duct and the confluence

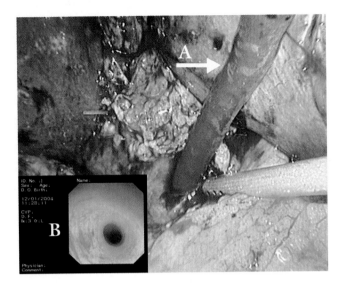

Figure 31 : Visualization of distal CBD using Choledochoscope

A - Choledochoscope in the CBD

B - Distal CBD

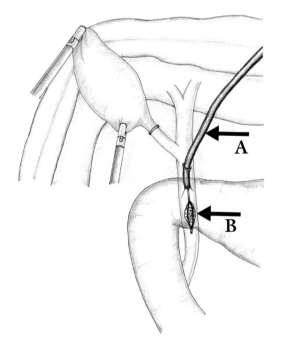

Figure 32 : Basketing of CBD stone using Choledochoscope

A - Choledochoscope

B - Basket with the stone

Occasionally we use intraoperative lithotripsy to dislodge a fragment an impacted stone from the distal end of the common bile duct.

Problems expected during common duct exploration

1. Patient temperature may drop due to irrigating fluids. Use of warm fluid for irrigation may avoid this complication.

2. 6th port for caudal traction of the Hepatoduodenal ligament may be needed.

3. Difficulty in identification of the CBD can be managed by

    a. Meticulous dissection of the cystic duct down to common duct.

    b. Needle aspiration.

    c. Intraoperative ultrasound.

Completion Cholangiogram and Choledochoscope

The endoscopic evaluation of the compete biliary tree is performed to rule out any biliary stone along with the cholangiogram. The cholangiogram can be performed through the trancystic route or through the tube after closure of the choledochotomy.

Closure of the Access Opening

In cases of access through the cystic duct approach, the same opening in the cystic duct can be used for tube drainage to decompress the CBD. This provides adequate drainage (300 ml/day) and is excellent for postoperative cholangiograms over T tube.

The T tube closure of choledochotomy is usually applied in our series. The latex tube is taken into the abdominal cavity through the 10mm epigastric port. We routinely use latex on tube as it aids in tract formation around the tube. The horizontal limb of the T tube is trimmed to a total length of 1.5cm and filleted.

The incision in the common bile duct is then closed by two to three interrupted 4/0 absorbable sutures (Polysorb, coated Vicryl) after insertion of a T tube. The T-Tube is placed and pushed cephalad to lessen the chances of inadvertent dislodgment during suturing process. The sequence for suture placement

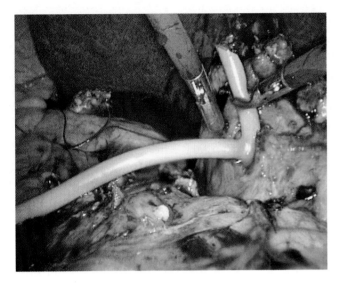

Figure 33 : Insertion of 'T' tube in the CBD

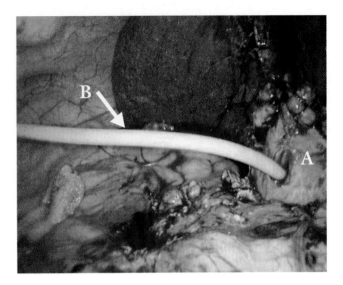

Figure 34 : Position of 'T' tube

A - CBD

B - 'T' tube

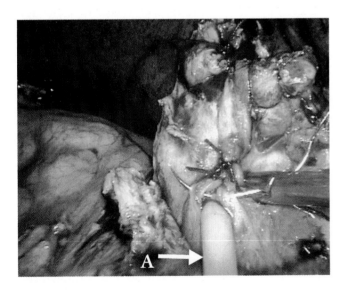

Figure 35 : Suturing of CBD after placing the 'T' tube using 4 0 vicryl

A - 'T' tube

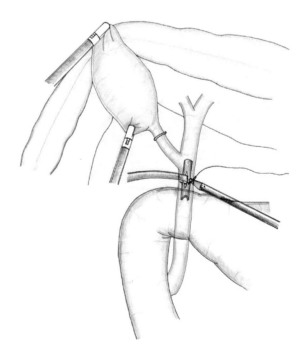

Figure 36 : Suturing of CBD after placing the 'T' tube

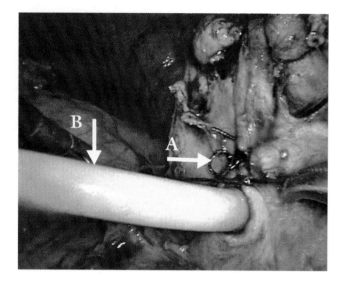

Figure 37 : Completion of suturing

A - Interrupted vicryl suture

B - 'T' tube

is outlined in figures. The distal end of the tube (which is inside the peritoneal cavity at this stage of the surgery) is usually closed with a ligature, a clip or clamp as continuous seepage of bile stains the abdomen. Approximating the wound from the distal end of the choledochotomy is preferred as it is visualized well in laparoscopic approach, in contrast to conventional surgery. After cholecystectomy long limb is brought out through the lateral port. When suturing has been competed, saline is injected though the cystic duct cannula or T-tube to ensure a water tight seal closure.

During certain situations, we resort to primary closure of the choledochotomy with absorbable sutures. This permits early recovery of the patient as the T tubes significantly reduces the mobility of the patient. T tubes are usually left for 6 weeks and are often uncomfortable. Complete clearance of the entire biliary system demonstrated by intra operative cholangiogram and choledochoscopy is an indication for primary closure. There should not be any evidence of pancreatitis or ductal edema in such

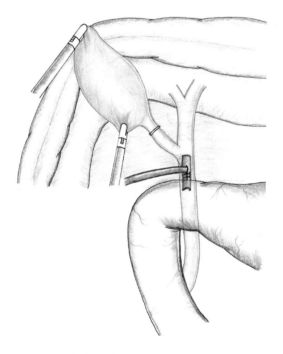

Figure 38 : Completion of suturing after placing 'T' tube

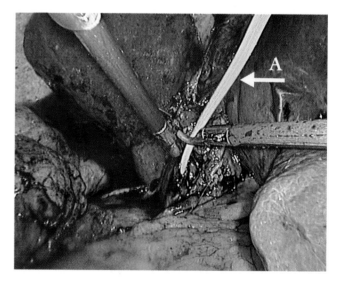

Figure 39 : Placement of stent into the CBD

A - Stent in introduced in the CBD through extra 3mm port

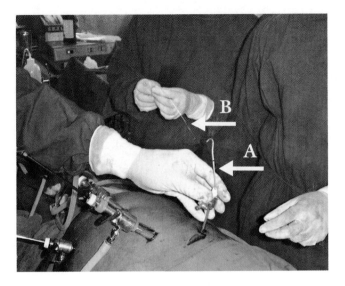

Figure 40 : External view of placement of CBD stent

A - Stent in the 3mm trocar

B - Guide wire is being pulled out to retain the stent

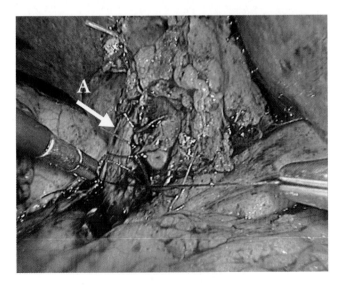

Figure 41 : Primary closure of CBD

A - Interrupted vicryl stitches

patients. We have not encountered any problems in this selective approach of primary suturing of choledochotomy.

The cholecystectomy is completed as routine. At the end of the procedure, the T tube is brought out through a separate stab incision on the side and a subhepatic drain placed. The wounds are closed with 3-0 vicryl and pneumoperitoneum deflated.

Post operative management

The patient was treated with antibiotics and continuous drainage of T tube in the post operative period. The T tubes are usually left undistributed for a period at 2-3 weeks. The patient is usually discharged at 5th day after assessment of the bio-chemical parameters, post op cholangiogram and the clinical status. The T tube is usually removed in the outpatient department after discharge.

Prevention of biliary injury

Repeated insertion of the basket and balloon might lead to biliary tract injury; several recommendations have been advocated to prevent these injuries.

1. Avoid repeated instrumentation when obstructive valves are detected

2. Introduce all instruments through the cystic duct into the CBD under fluoroscopic guidance

3. Insert all instruments as parallel as possible with the CBD, avoiding a perpendicular approach

4. Use a soft, atraumatic Dormia basket or balloon catheter

5. Avoid dilatation of nondilated cystic duct and use laparoscopic choledochotomy in such cases when feasible

6. Perform routinely control cholangiographic examination at the end of the procedure to detect any contrast material extravasation which might signal the presence of a biliary tract injury.

WHEN TO CONVERT TO OPEN SURGERY

The laparoscopic common bile duct exploration must not be continued indefinitely as this might lead to further complications. Conversion to open approach should be considered in situations like failure to progress beyond due to difficult anatomy or unsuspected pathology such as Mirrizzi and uncontrollable bleeding that obscures the field of vision.

LAPAROSCOPIC BILIARY DRAINAGE PROCEDURES

Laparoscopic choledochoduodenostomy

Indications

1. Grossly dilated common duct.
2. Short distal stricture with proximal dilatation.

Procedure

Principles of choledochoduodenostomy are the same as conventional Surgery. Side to side choledochoduodenostomy, described by Gliedman and Gold is indicated for any type of common bile duct obstruction except in cases of injury and malignancy. Avoiding circumferential mobilisation and transection does not compromise the blood supply and larger anastomosis, minimises the chances of leakage.

The common bile duct is incised longitudinally with a scalpel, knife hook or harmonic scalpel beginning at the point at which it transverses the duodenum posteriorly and extending proximally of 2.5cm. After extraction, both proximal and distal ducts are thoroughly rinsed with warm saline for clearing debris and infected fluid.

The duodenum is incised longitudinally along its superior border for a distance of approximately 1.5cm. A single layered anastomosis is performed using 4 0 vicryl, positioning the knots on the inner side. Knots should be placed with 2mm gap and adequate tightness. There is no need for T-tube drainage in these patients. If the duct is less than 2cm, the duct is transected and end to side anastomosis is performed. This is indicated for distal bile duct injury, malignant obstruction and duodenum is not suitable for choledochoduodenostomy. Gallbladder should be left intact during the entire anastomosis as this is the primary method of upward traction on the gall bladder with ligation in continuity of the cystic duct. After completion of anastomosis, cholecystectomy is performed.

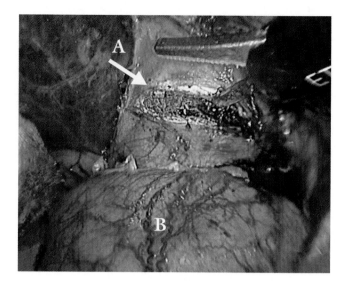

Figure 42 : Transverse opening of the Dilated CBD using harmonic scalpel

A - Opening in the CBD, stone is seen
B - Duodenum

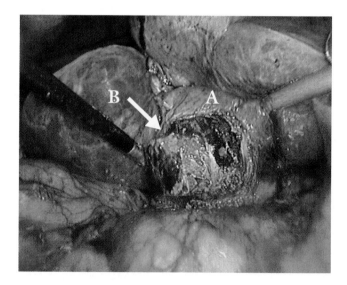

Figure 43 : Milking out of large CBD stone

A - CBD
B - Stone

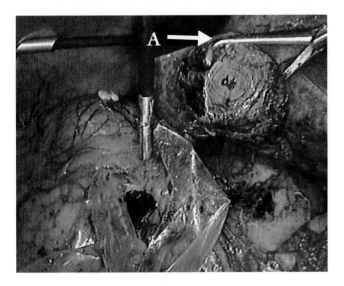

Figure 44 : Extraction is placed in the endobag

A - 10 mm right angle is used to grasp the stone

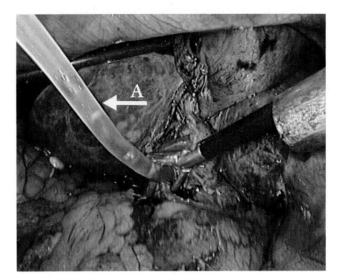

Figure 45 : Irrigation of proximal CBD

A - Suction catheter

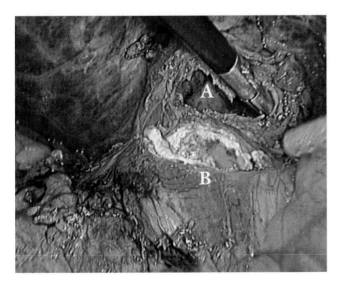

Figure 46 : Transverse opening in the duodenum for anastomosis

A - CBD

B - Duodenum

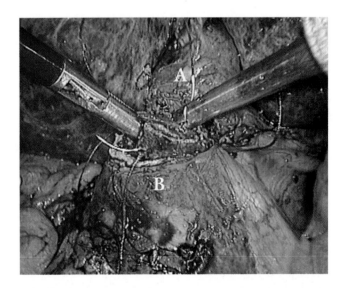

Figure 47 : Cholechoduodenal anastomosis using continuous vicryl Sutures

A - CBD

B - Duodenum

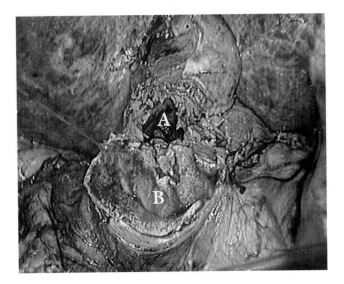

Figure 48 : Completion of posterior layer anastomosis

A - CBD
B - Duodenum

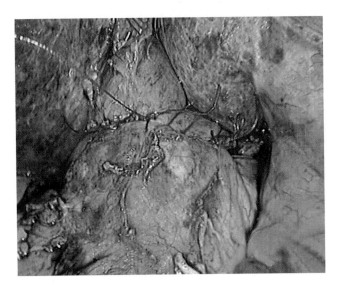

Figure 49 : Completion of Choledochoduodenostomy

Laparoscopic Choledochojejunostomy

Grossly dilated proximal common duct with long distal stricture in association with chronic pancreatitis choledochojejunal Roux en Y anastomosis may be performed.

DISCUSSION

From the initial series of laparoscopic common bile duct exploration, numerous reports have been published. In the hands of experienced surgeons the results of the technique have shown a success rate of more than 90% and mortality less than 1% with minimum complications and recurrence. Though most of the surgeons have preferred transcystic routes, we routinely use choledochotomy approach as we find the approach is better suited for our patients as the size of the CBD stones generally tend to bigger when compared to western population.

The mean operative time for these surgeries is around 1½ hours. The length stay of these patients also varies from 1 to 7 days depending on the associated co-morbid factors. The usual complications that have found were, nausea, diarrhea, urinary infection and complications associated with T tube such as dislodgment, infection around the T tube site. These complications are generally less when compared to open approach for common bile duct stones.

We have performed 225 laparoscopic common bile duct exploration till now in our institute. We routinely follow a policy of selective intra operative cholangiogram in our patients and the incidence of incidental common bile duct stones is not known.

Laparoscopic CBD exploration was attempted in 225 patients and successfully completed in 218 patients. The mean operative time for our patients undergoing laparoscopic CBD exploration was 90 minutes (45 mts to 180 mts) and the mean length of stay was 2.3 days (3 days (2-5 days). The ductal exploration was done by the choledochotomy route in 196 (87%) patients and the transcystic route in 19 (13%) patients. T tubes were placed in 180 (91%) patients for closure of this common bile duct and the remaining 16 patients underwent primary closure of the common bile duct.

Sing-Stage versus Two-Stage Procedure

Intervention	Advantages	Disadvantages
Single-stage approach Lap cholecystectomy Combined with laparoscopic CBD exploration	Single admission Shorter hospital stay Economical	Requires expertise and the necessary equipments. Contraindicated in high risk patients Not suitable for poor anesthetic risk patients
Two-stage approach Lap cholecystectomy Combined with either or Postoperative ERCP	Easier procedure Takes shorter time, better in high risk patients No need for specialized equipment	Lengthier stay Two separate procedures Skilled endoscopist and Preoperative ERCP ERCP suite necessary 10 % of ERCPs may fail to retrieve the stone, which might require second surgery.

Seven patients had to undergo open exploration of the common bile duct to retrieve the stones. Out of 180 patients who underwent T tube closure, 3 patients had retained stones which were removed by ERCP later. There were no major complications such as bile leaks, or mortality in our series.

The laparoscopic common bile duct exploration is now preferred as a single stage treatment for patients with common bile duct stones and the use of peroperative ERCP is increasingly challenged due to the small but significant incidence of complications.

A randomized, prospective trial of ERCP followed by laparoscopic cholecystectomy versus laparoscopic cholecystectomy with laparoscopic common bile duct exploration revealed equivalent success rates and patient morbidity between the 2 groups. The single stage treatment offered lower cost and shorter hospital stay.[11] In a smiliar study of 80 patients randomized to laparoscopic common bile duct exploration and laproscopic cholecystectomy followed by post op ERCP (40 each), duct clearance was 100% in the laparoscopic group compared with 93% in the ERCP group. The laparoscopic group showed a decrease in operative time and shorter hospital stay.[12] In a multicenter prospective randomized trial comparing two-stage (preoperative endoscopic retrograde cholangiography and stone extraction followed by

laparoscopic cholecystectomy during the same hospital admission 150 patients) vs single-stage management (laparoscopic cholecystectomy with lap CBD exploration 150 pateints) of patients with gall-stone disease and ductal calculi by E.A.E.S, the single stage group had significantly shorter hospital stay (6.4 vs 9.5 days). They concluded that in fit patients (ASA I and II), single-stage laparoscopic treatment is the better option, and preoperative Endoscopic sphincterotomy and extraction should be confined to poor-risk patients-i.e., those with cholangitis or severe pancreatitis.[13]

CONCLUSION

Laparoscopic common bile duct exploration can be performed safely and effectively through laparoscopy. But it requires a highly specialized skill in advanced laparoscopic surgeries and also special imaging equipments, two cameras and a series of extraction devices like basket and balloon. ERCP may not be required in all patients with bile duct calculi as most of these can be removed by single stage procedure with added benefits like shorter hospital stay and costs. In a ideal setup where all the facilities are available, a single-stage approach with very low morbidity would be optimal, but it is currently not possible in all hospitals. But as the technology improves and more surgeons get trained in advanced laparoscopic surgeries this will be possible in the next few years. Till then every hospital and surgeon should have a management protocol based on their expertise, presence of experienced endoscopist and the facilities available in the hospital to treat the patients of common bile duct stones.

References

1. Cuschieri A, Croce E, Faggioni A, et al. EAES ductal stone study. Preliminary findings of multi-center prospective randomized trial comparing two-stage vs single-stage management. Surg Endosc 1996; 10(12):1130-5.

2. Shuchleib S, Chousleb A, Mondragon A, et al. Laparoscopic common bile duct exploration. World J Surg 1999; 23(7):698-701; discussion 702.

3. Courvoiser L. CASUISTISCH. Statististische Beitrage zur Pathologie und Chirurgie der Gallenwege Leipzig: Vogel; 1890; 387:57-58.

4. Classen M, Demling L. Endoscopic sphincterotomy of the papilla of vater and extraction of stones from the choledochal duct. Deutsche Medizinische Wochenschrift 1974; 99:469-467.

5. Mouret P. How I developed laparoscopic cholecystectomy. Ann Acad Med Singapore 1996; 25(5):744-7.

6. Jacobs M, Verdeja JC, Goldstein HS. Laparoscopic choledocholithotomy. J Laparoendosc Surg 1991; 1(2):79-82.

7. Petelin JB. Laparoscopic common bile duct exploration. Surg Endosc 2003; 17(11):1705-15.

8. Guibaud L, Bret PM, Reinhold C, et al. Diagnosis of choledocholithiasis: value of MR cholangiography. AJR Am J Roentgenol 1994; 163(4):847-50.

9. Leijonmarck CE. Laparoscopic management of common bile duct stones. Eur J Surg 2000; Suppl 585:22-6.

10. Memon MA, Hassaballa H, Memon MI. Laparoscopic common bile duct exploration: the past, the present, and the future. Am J Surg 2000; 179(4):309-15.

11. Liberman MA, Phillips EH, Carroll BJ, et al. Cost-effective management of complicated choledocholithiasis: laparoscopic transcystic duct exploration or endoscopic sphincterotomy. J Am Coll Surg 1996; 182(6):488-94.

12. Rhodes M, Sussman L, Cohen L, Lewis MP. Randomised trial of laparoscopic exploration of common bile duct versus postoperative endoscopic retrograde cholangiography for common bile duct stones. Lancet 1998; 351(9097): 159-61.

13. Cuschieri A, Lezoche E, Morino M, et al. E.A.E.S. multicenter prospective randomized trial comparing two-stage vs single-stage management of patients with gallstone disease and ductal calculi. Surg Endosc 1999; 13(10):952-7.

14. Cotton PB, Lehman G, Vennes J, et al. Endoscopic sphincterotomy complications and their management: an attempt at consensus. Gastrointest Endosc 1991; 37(3):383-93.

15. Hunter JG, Soper NJ. Laparoscopic management of bile duct stones. Surg Clin North Am 1992; 72(5):1077-97.

16. Gigot JF, Navez B, Etienne J, et al. A stratified intraoperative surgical strategy is mandatory during laparoscopic common bile duct exploration for common bile duct stones. Lessons and limits from an initial experience of 92 patients. Surg Endosc 1997; 11(7):722-8.

17. DePaula AL, Hashiba K, Bafutto M, et al. Laparoscopic antegrade sphincterotomy. Surg Laparosc Endosc 1993; 3(3):157-60.

18. Curet MJ, Pitcher DE, Martin DT, Zucker KA. Laparoscopic antegrade sphincterotomy. A new technique for the management of complex choledocholithiasis. Ann Surg 1995; 221(2):149-55.

19. Phillips EH. Controversies in the management of common duct calculi. Surg Clin North Am 1994; 74(4):931-48; discussion 949-51.

20. Petelin JB. Laparoscopic choledochotomy for treatment of common bile duct stones. Surg Endosc 1998; 12(4):367-8.

21. Lygidakis NJ. Operative risk factors of cholecystectomy-choledochotomy in the elderly. Surg Gynecol Obstet 1983; 157(1):15-9.

22. Lygidakis NJ. Incidence of bile infection in biliary lithiasis. Effects on postoperative bacteremia of choledochoduodenostomy, T-tube drainage, and primary closure of the common bile duct after choledochotomy-a prospective clinical trial. Am Surg 1984; 50(5):236-40.

23. Lygidakis NJ. Choledochotomy for biliary lithiasis: T-tube drainage or primary closure. Effects on postoperative bacteremia and T-tube bile infection. Am J Surg 1983; 146(2):254-6.

24. Koivusalo A, Makisalo H, Talja M, et al. Bacterial adherence and biofilm formation on latex and silicone T-tubes in relation to bacterial contamination of bile. Scand J Gastroenterol 1996; 31(4):398-403.

25. Decker G, Borie F, Millat B, et al. One hundred laparoscopic choledochotomies with primary closure of the common bile duct. Surg Endosc 2003; 17(1):12-8.

26. Ha JP, Tang CN, Siu WT, et al. Primary closure versus T-tube drainage after laparoscopic choledochotomy for common bile duct stones. Hepatogastroenterology 2004; 51(60):1605-8.

27. Zhang LD, Bie P, Chen P, et al. [Primary duct closure versus T-tube drainage following laparoscopic choledochotomy]. Zhonghua Wai Ke Za Zhi 2004; 42(9):520-3.

28. Fanelli RD, Gersin KS. Laparoscopic endobiliary stenting: a simplified approach to the management of occult common bile duct stones. J Gastrointest Surg 2001; 5(1):74-80.

29. Martin CJ, Cox MR, Vaccaro L. Laparoscopic transcystic bile duct stenting in the management of common bile duct stones. ANZ J Surg 2002; 72(4):258-64.

30. Rijna H, Borgstein PJ, Meuwissen SG, et al. Selective preoperative endoscopic retrograde cholangiopancreatography in laparoscopic biliary surgery. Br J Surg 1995; 82(8):1130-3.

31. Schmitt CM, Baillie J, Cotton PB. ERCP following laparoscopic cholecystectomy: a safe and effective way to manage CBD stones and complications. HPB Surg 1995; 8(3):187-92.

32. Vitale GC, Larson GM, Wieman TJ, et al. The use of ERCP in the management of common bile duct stones in patients undergoing laparoscopic cholecystectomy. Surg Endosc 1993; 7(1):9-11.

45

Laparoscopic Choledochal Cyst Excision

INTRODUCTION

Choledochal cysts are congenital bile duct anomalies. These cystic dilatations of the biliary tree can involve the extrahepatic biliary radicles, the intrahepatic biliary radicles, or both. In 1723, Vater and Ezler published the anatomic description of a choledochal cyst.

In 1959, Alonzo-Lej produced a systematic analysis of choledochal cysts, reporting on 96 cases.[1] He devised a classification system, dividing choledochal cysts into 3 categories, and outlined therapeutic strategies. Todani has since refined this classification system to include 5 categories.

PATHOPHYSIOLOGY

No strong unifying etiologic theory exists for choledochal cysts. The pathogenesis probably is multifactorial. In many patients with choledochal cysts, an anomalous junction between the common bile duct and pancreatic duct can be demonstrated.[2] This occurs when the pancreatic duct empties into the common bile duct more than 1 cm proximal to the ampulla. Some series, such as the one published by Miyano and Yamataka in 1997, have documented such anomalous junctions in 90-100% of patients with choledochal cysts. This abnormal union allows pancreatic secretions to reflux into the common bile duct, where the pancreatic proenzymes become activated, damaging and weakening the bile duct wall. Defects in epithelialization and recanalization of the developing bile ducts and congenital weakness of the ductal wall also have been implicated. The result is formation of a choledochal cyst.

These anomalies are classified by Todani and coworkers. Five major classes of choledochal cysts exist (i.e, types I-V), with subclassifications for types I and IV (ie, types IA, IB, IC; types IVA, IVB).[3]

1. **Type I** cysts are the most common and represent 80-90% of choledochal cysts. They consist of saccular or fusiform dilatations of the common bile duct, which involve either a segment of the duct or the entire duct.

    i. **Type IA** is saccular in configuration and involves either the entire extrahepatic bile duct or the majority of it.

    ii. **Type IB** is saccular and involves a limited segment of the bile duct.

    iii. **Type IC** is more fusiform in configuration and involves most or all of the extrahepatic bile duct.

2. **Type II** choledochal cysts appear as an isolated diverticulum protruding from the wall of the common bile duct. The cyst may be joined to the common bile duct by a narrow stalk.

3. **Type III** choledochal cysts arise from the intraduodenal portion of the common bile duct and are described alternately by the term choledochocele.

4. **Type IVA** cysts consist of multiple dilatations of the intrahepatic and extrahepatic bile ducts.

    Type IVB choledochal cysts are multiple dilatations involving only the extrahepatic bile ducts.

5. **Type V** (Caroli disease) consists of multiple dilatations limited to the intrahepatic bile ducts.

INCIDENCE

Choledochal cysts are much more prevalent in Asia than in Western countries. Approximately 33-50% of reported cases come from Japan, where the frequency in some series approaches 1 case per 1000 population.

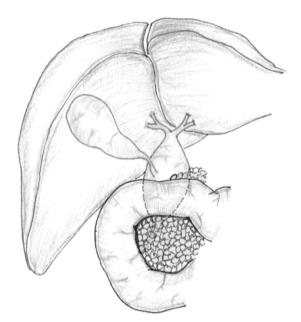

Figure 1 : Type Ia cyst

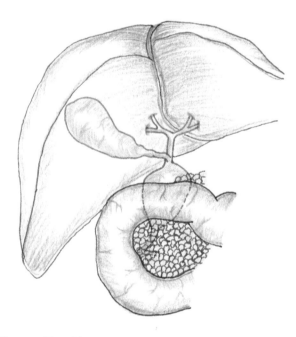

Figure 2 : Type I b cyst

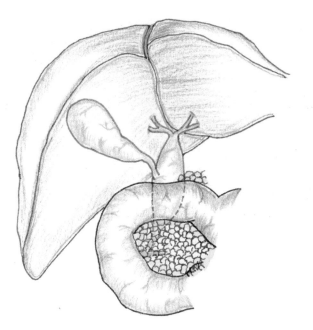

Figure 3 : Type Ic cyst

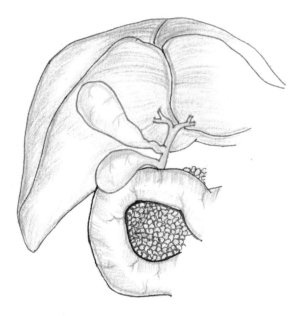

Figure 4 : Type II cyst

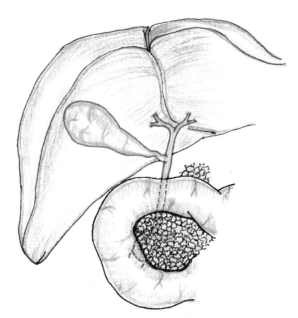

Figure 5 : Type III cyst

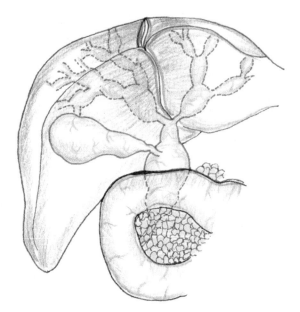

Figure 6 : Type IVa cyst

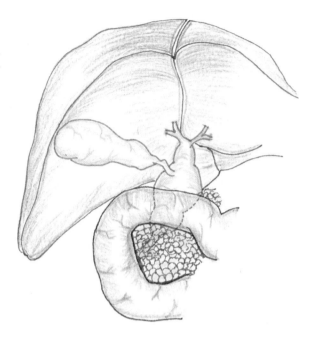

Figure 7 : Type IVb cyst

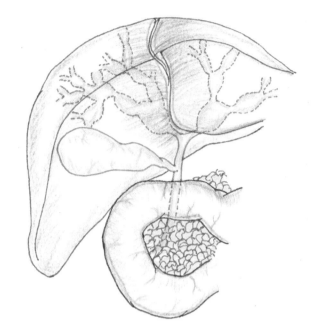

Figure 8 : Type V cyst

The development of complications depends on the age of the patient at the time of presentation. Infants and children may develop pancreatitis, cholangitis, and histologic evidence of hepatocellular damage. Adults in whom subclinical ductal inflammation and biliary stasis may have been present for years may present with one or more severe complications such as hepatic abscesses, cirrhosis, portal hypertension, recurrent pancreatitis, and cholelithiasis. Cholangiocarcinoma is the most feared complication of choledochal cysts, with a reported incidence of 9-28%.

CHOLEDOCHAL CYST AND MALIGNANCY[6]

Malignancy in choledochal cyst can arise from the distal CBD, the wall of the cyst (even after successful drainage at cystoenterostomy), or the intrahepatic bile ducts. The risk of cancer appears to be related to the age of the patient; it is high (>20 times) compared with that of the healthy population. Risk of detecting a biliary tree malignancy in a resected cyst is 0.7% in patients who undergo surgery before the age of 10 years, 6.8% in patients who undergo

surgery at the age of 11-20 years, and 14.3% in patients who undergo surgery after the age of 20 years.

More than half of the cancers arise from the cyst wall, even after successful internal drainage. Total cyst excision has not prevented the risk of malignancy in the remaining bile ducts.[6,7,21] Malignancy can develop many years after excision of the cyst, and it can develop in areas of the biliary tree remote from the cyst such as the gallbladder and terminal common duct, which is left behind after excisional surgery.

Any type of cyst is susceptible to malignancy, but the greatest prevalence is observed with types I, IV, and V. Factors thought to contribute to the development of malignancy include prolonged bile stasis and chronic inflammation of the cyst wall.[8] Inflammatory and metaplastic changes increase with patient age, and they are frequently observed in association with carcinoma of the bile duct. The increased risk of biliary tract malignancy, even after surgery, warrants close surveillance in any case of choledochal cyst.

Sex

Choledochal cysts are more prevalent in females than males, with a female-to-male ratio in the range of 3:1 to 4:1.

Age

Most patients with choledochal cysts are diagnosed during infancy or childhood, although the condition may be discovered at any age. Approximately 67% of patients present with signs or symptoms referable to the cyst before the age of 10 years.

CLINICAL PRESENTATION

The history varies according to the age at presentation. Choledochal cysts can present dramatically in infancy. The clinical manifestations in older children and adults are more protean.[4]

1. Infants

   i. Infants frequently present with jaundice and acholic stools. In early infancy, this may prompt a workup for biliary atresia.

   ii. In addition, infants with choledochal cysts often have a palpable mass in the right upper quadrant of the abdomen, accompanied with hepatomegaly.

2. Children

   i. Children diagnosed after infancy typically have a clinical picture of intermittent biliary obstruction or recurrent bouts of pancreatitis[5].

   ii. Those with a biliary obstructive pattern can still present with a palpable right upper quadrant mass and jaundice.

   iii. Children whose primary manifestation is pancreatitis may pose some difficulty in arriving at the correct diagnosis. These patients frequently have only intermittent attacks of colicky abdominal pain. Biochemical testing reveals elevated amylase and lipase concentrations, which lead to the proper diagnostic workup.

3. Adults

   i. Adults with choledochal cysts can present with one or more severe complications.

   ii. Frequently, adults with choledochal cysts complain of vague epigastric or right upper quadrant pain and can develop jaundice or cholangitis.

   iii. The most common symptom in adults is abdominal pain.

   iv. A classic triad of abdominal pain, jaundice, and a palpable right upper quadrant abdominal mass has been described in adults with choledochal cysts but is found in only 10-20% of patients.

Physical: A right upper quadrant mass may be palpable. This is observed more frequently in infancy and early childhood. Patients who develop pancreatitis present with nonspecific midepigastric or diffuse abdominal pain.

INVESTIGATIONS

Biochemical investigations

1. No laboratory studies are specific for the diagnosis of a choledochal cyst. An elevated white blood cell count, with increased numbers of neutrophils and immature neutrophil forms may be observed in the presence of cholangitis.

2. Liver function tests may be useful in narrowing the differential diagnosis. Hepatocellular enzyme and alkaline phosphatase levels may be elevated. None of these tests are specific for the diagnosis of a choledochal cyst.

3. Serum amylase and lipase concentrations may be increased in the presence of pancreatitis. Serum amylase concentrations also may be elevated in biliary obstruction and cholangitis.

Imaging Studies

1. **Abdominal ultrasonography** is the test of choice for the diagnosis of a choledochal cyst. Ultrasound is useful in the antenatal period as well, according to Chen and coworkers (2004), and can demonstrate a choledochal cyst in a fetus as early as the beginning of the second trimester.[9,10] Caroli disease has also been detected antenatally with ultrasound by Sgro and colleagues (2004).

2. **Abdominal CT scan and MRI** help to delineate the anatomy of the lesion and of the surrounding structures.[13] These tests also can assist in defining the presence and extent of intrahepatic ductal involvement. In 2004, Yu and associates published a series of 64 patients in whom magnetic resonance cholangiopancreatography was particularly valuable for defining anomalous pancreaticobiliary junctions.

3. **Invasive diagnostic studies:** When noninvasive measures (eg, ultrasound, CT scan, MRI) fail to sufficiently delineate the anatomy, endoscopic retrograde cholangiopancreatography (ERCP). should be performed.[14] These studies are particularly helpful in demonstrating the presence of an anomalous pancreatobiliary junction and in delineating associated extrahepatic or intrahepatic strictures and stones.[15] In case ERCP fails to delineate the full extent of the cyst and anomalous insertion of the pancreatic duct, we always perform peroperative cholangiogram. This is particularly useful when the cyst is very large.

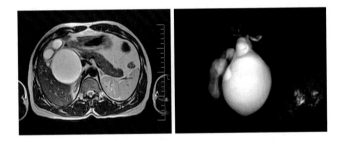

Figure 9 : MRI shows Type Ia choledochal cyst

SURGICAL MANAGEMENT[16]

Treatment of choledochal cysts is surgical, except in type V with multiple intrahepatic cysts, which can benefit from medical management for variable periods of time. In the past, aspiration and external drainage were used extensively because most patients were quite sick, and a simple quick procedure was convenient. These external drainage procedures of the biliary tree were unsuccessful because of numerous complications, including repeated cholangitis and biliary fistula.

Internal drainage, either with cystoduodenostomy or cystojejunostomy with Roux-en-Y biliary reconstruction, were used in the past. These procedures left the cyst behind, and the free reflux of pancreatic enzymes into the cyst via the anomalous pancreatico-biliary junction resulted in a high incidence of calculi, recurrent cholangitis, anastomotic strictures, and carcinoma arising from the cyst.[17] Of patients treated with either cystoduodenostomy or cystojejunostomy, 65% remained symptomatic, and 40% required repeat surgery at a later date. Recurrent cholangitis and chronic inflammation in the remaining cyst eventually produces metaplasia that leads to malignant transformation.

Total excision of the cyst in types I, II, and IV, followed by reconstruction of the biliary tree with hepaticojejunostomy in a Roux-en-Y fashion has been widely accepted as the procedure of choice in treating choledochal cysts. This procedure implies an excision of the distal terminal choledochal duct. Consequently, it blocks the reflux of pancreatic enzymes into the biliary tract, therefore decreasing the incidence of carcinoma of the bile duct.

Total excision of the cyst is possible in virtually all infants and young children.[18] In older patients with repeated cholangitis and marked pericystic inflammation, this disease may be best managed with resection of the anterolateral part of the cyst followed by an endocystic resection of the lining, leaving the back wall adjacent to the portal vein in place, as reported by Lilly in 1977. This technique also appears to be most useful in patients who have previously undergone cystoenterostomy and who require repeat surgery because of recurrent cholangitis. This technique makes the dissection less hazardous.

Perioperative cholangiography via a puncture of the cyst or via the gallbladder is always obtained. It outlines the exact anatomy of the choledochal cyst and its relationship with the pancreas. Cholecystectomy is routinely performed at the same time.

Biliary reconstruction can be performed with a Roux-en-Y hepaticojejunostomy as high as possible, near the hilum of the liver.[17] Some authors, including Raffensperger and Shamberger, have interposed a reversed segment of jejunum to prevent reflux. This idea has not been universally accepted. No stents are routinely necessary.

The surgical management for each choledochal cyst type is as follows:

1. **Type I:** The treatment of choice is complete excision of the involved portion of the extrahepatic bile duct. A Roux-en-Y hepaticojejunostomy is performed to restore biliary-enteric continuity.

2. **Type II:** The dilated diverticulum comprising a type II choledochal cyst is excised entirely. The resultant defect in the common bile duct is closed over a T-tube.

3. **Type III (Choledochocele):** The choice of therapy depends upon the size the cyst. Choledochoceles measuring 3 cm or less can be treated effectively with endoscopic sphincterotomy. Lesions larger than 3 cm typically produce some degree of duodenal obstruction. These lesions are excised surgically through a transduodenal approach. If the pancreatic duct enters the choledochocele, it may have to be reimplanted into the duodenum following excision of the cyst.

4. **Type IV:** The dilated extrahepatic duct is completely excised and a Roux-en-Y hepaticojejunostomy is performed to restore continuity. Intrahepatic ductal disease does not require dedicated therapy unless hepatolithiasis, intrahepatic ductal strictures, or hepatic abscesses are present. In such instances, the affected segment or lobe of the liver is resected.

5. **Type V (Caroli disease):** Disease limited to one hepatic lobe is amenable to treatment by hepatic lobectomy. When this occurs, the left lobe usually is affected.[12] Hepatic functional reserve should be examined carefully in all patients before committing to such therapy. Patients with bilobar disease who begin to manifest signs of liver failure, biliary cirrhosis, or portal hypertension may be candidates for liver transplantation.

OPERATIVE TECHNIQUE

Preoperative preparation

Patients with jaundice or cholangitis should be assessed carefully for normal blood coagulation parameters. Other preparations are same as for routine surgery. Prophylactic antibiotics should be administered immediately prior to induction of anaesthesia and continued postoperatively for 24 hours.

Intraoperative cholangiography should be available. Harmonic Scalpel is an ideal tool for Hemostatic dissection.

Positioning and operating team

Under general anaesthesia, the patient is positioned supine with a small sand bag under the right hypochondrium to elevate the hilum. CO_2 pneumoperitoneum is established by Veress needle or open Hasson technique.[19] Camera port (10mm) is placed at the umbilicus as a blind primary trocar. There after all other trocars are placed under visual guidance. Totally 6 ports are made. At the level of the upper border of the first part of duodenum, right hand working port (10mm) is placed in the epigastrium slightly to left of the midline. Left hand working port 5mm in placed at the right midclavicular line, slightly lower than the right hand working port. Fundal retraction port (5mm) is placed at the right anterior axillary line, just below the lower border of the liver. Epigastric port (3 or 5mm) is used to hold the cyst anteriorly in the beginning and, later to lift the quadrate lobe during the reconstruction phase. Left lumbar port is used as retraction port for duodenum and head of pancreas.

Adequate working space is easily obtained by lifting fundus of the gall bladder cranially and transverse colon and duodenum caudally. A general inspection of the abdomen is performed, specifically assessing for portal hypertension, character of the liver, size of the spleen, and status of the pancreas.

Mobilisation of Duodenum and Head of pancreas

The peritoneum over the cyst just proximal to the first part of duodenum is incised transversely and the first part of the duodenum is mobilized well down to expose the retropancreatic cyst extension. The peritoneal incision is extended laterally to mobilize the hepatic flexure and the second part of duodenum upto the third part. Kocherisation of the duodenum and the head of pancreas is performed well medially.

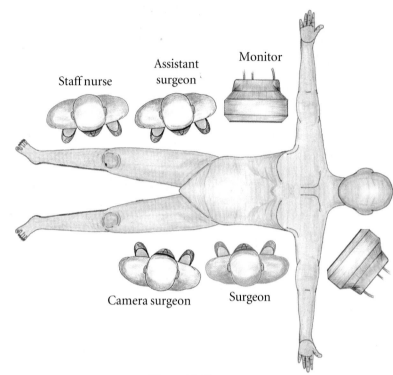

Figure 10 : Team setup

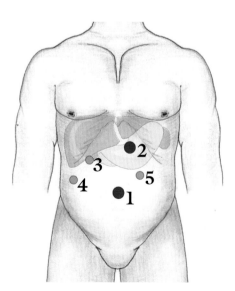

Figure 11 : Port position

No.	Instruments	Place
1	Camera	Umbilicus 10mm
2	Right hand working port	Epigastric 10mm
3	Left hand working port	Right subcostal 5mm
4	Gall bladder retracting port	Right lateral 5mm
5	Duodenum retracting port	Left pararectus 5mm

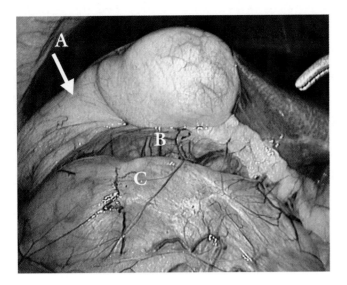

Figure 12 : Large choledochal cyst

A - Gall bladder shifted laterally by tthe cyst

B - Choledochal cyst

C - Duodenum

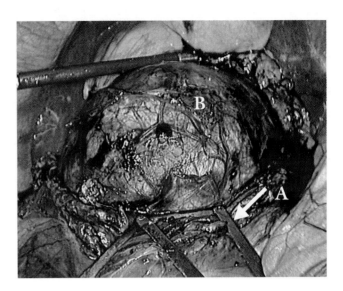

Figure 14 : Completely mobilized duodenum

A - 5mm liver retractor used to retract the duodenum caudally

B - Choledochal cyst after peritoneal reflection

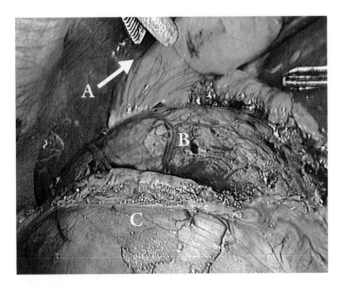

Figure 13 : Mobilization of duodenum

A - Gall bladder retracted cranially

B - Choledochal cyst

C - Duodenum

The hepatic artery is identified and protected during dissection, as it may be adherent to the medial side of the cyst. Displacement of the artery may occur depending upon the dilatation of the choledochal cyst. Small cysts may be mobilized circumferentially without decompression. Hepatic artery dissection away from the cyst is much easier before decompression.

Peroperative Cholangiogram

Operative cholangiogram is performed by inserting needle percutaneously into the cyst. 10-15ml of bile is aspirated before injecting the contrast dye. Increase of pressure within the cyst may cause spread of bacteria into the systemic circulation in presence of cholangitis.

Anomalous insertion of the pancreatic duct into the dilated bile duct and the lower limit of the cyst should be assessed before mobilizing the cyst caudally. Injury to the pancreatic duct opening, known to cause pancreatitis, should always be avoided.

Decompression of the cyst

The anterior wall is incised transversely across the cyst on the medial aspect and the hepatic vessels are carefully dissected away from the cyst. The dissection is kept close to the cyst wall in order to avoid injury to the vessels. In some cases we found numerous vessels running over the cysts, particularly in patients who had evidence of repeated inflammation. Apart from increased vascularity, they are vulnerable to bleed during dissection. In two patients, the hepatic arteries and its branches such as gastro duodenal artery and right gastric artery were identified on the wall of the cyst where the cyst was enlarged more than 10cms in diameter. 5mm curved Harmonic Scalpel is highly useful in this maneuver.

Transection of the distal common duct

Medial and the lateral cyst walls are incised first and finally the posterior cyst wall is incised. The dissection posteriorly to separate the cyst wall from the portal vein is a very crucial step in this operation. One assisting grasper in the epigastric port is used to lift up the cyst anteriorly.

Two hand technique is highly useful. Blunt and sharp dissection is alternatively used to separate the cyst wall from the portal vein. In ¾th of the cases, it is easily separable. Sometimes, we may need to inject saline between the cyst wall and the vein to create a plane before attempting dissection.

Lilly technique: Occasionally, the cyst adheres densely to the portal vein secondary to long-standing inflammatory reaction. In this situation, a complete, full-thickness excision of the cyst may not be possible. Lilly devised a technique, in which the serosal surface of the adherent cyst wall is leaving behind the portal vein while the mucosa of the cyst wall is removed by curettage or cautery fulguration. Theoretically, this removes the risk of malignant transformation in that segment of the cyst.

If cholangiogram reveals absence of anomalous pancreatic duct, the dilated cyst is excised entirely upto the narrowed common duct. If cholangiogram reveals insertion of the pancreatic duct into the cyst, the choledochal cyst is excised just proximal to its opening and is oversewn carefully avoiding injury to the anomalous pancreatic duct.

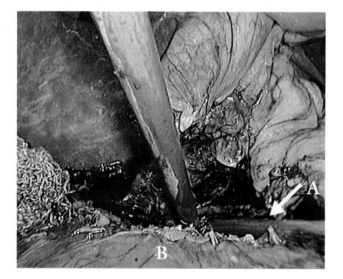

Figure 15 : Decompression of the cyst

A - 5 mm suction canula
B - Duodenum

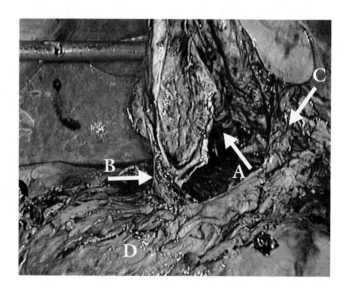

Figure 16 : Posterior mobilization of the cyst after division of the lower end of the common duct

A - Posterior wall of the cyst
B - Normal distal end of CBD
C - Right hepatic artery
D - Posterior wall of part I duodenum

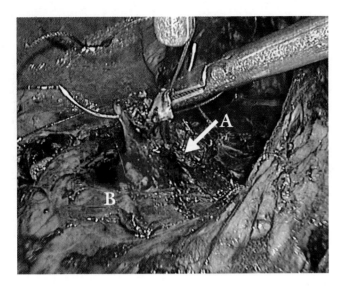

Figure 17 : Suturing of the distal end of CBD

A - Distal end of CBD

B - Posterior wall of duodenum

divided. The cystic-common duct junction is always excised. If the confluence is uninvolved with cystic dilatation, anastomosis between common hepatic duct and Roux-en-y jejunal anastomosis is formed.

If the cystic dilatation continues intrahepatically, the common hepatic duct is divided close to its confluence and hepatico-jejunostomy is performed. If the right and left hepatic ducts are grossly dilated with a good length of extra-hepatic portion, then both the ducts can be individually anastomosed to the Roux - en y loop. If the cystic dilatation involves the bifurcation then bifurcation resection can be performed and both right and left hepatic ducts can be anastomosed individually to the Roux-en-y loop.

Laparoscopic Hepaticojejunostomy reconstruction

Roux-en-y loop is created either extracorporeally by extending the umbilical port or intracorporeally[19] using endo GIA Stapler. An appropriate loop is

If the cyst extends more distally upto the ampulla, it is always advisable to do Kocherisation before attempting dissection distally. The retractor in the left lumbar port is used to grasp the duodenum and retract caudally and to the left. The entire cyst is visualized by this maneuver. Once the distal portion of the cyst dissection is completed, division of cyst and closure of the distal stump should be performed sequentially. The cyst is lifted up anteriorly by grasper using through the epigastric or lateral trocar. The medial wall is incised and a suture is applied using 2-0 vicryl. The division and suturing is sequentially placed. If not, after complete division, subsequent suture placement is difficult as the divided end tends to retract. A continuous suturing is always preferred.

Mobilisation of the cyst proximally

The transected cyst is dissected free from the portal vein posteriorly and hepatic artery medially until a normal caliber common hepatic duct is found. At this stage, the cystic duct is clipped or ligated and

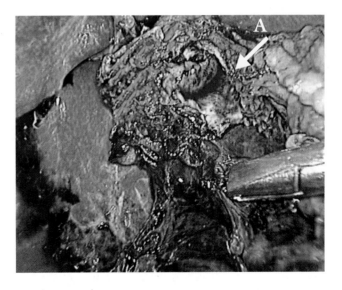

Figure 18 : Cyst was excised completely

A - Proximal divided end at the level of confluence

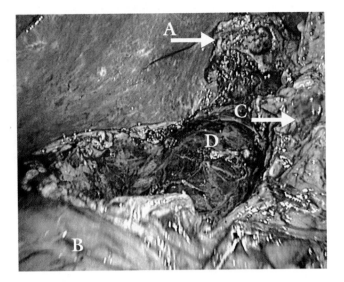

Figure 19 : After excision of the choledochal cyst

A - Proximal divided end (common hepatic duct)

B - Duodenum

C - Right hepatic artery

D - Portal vein

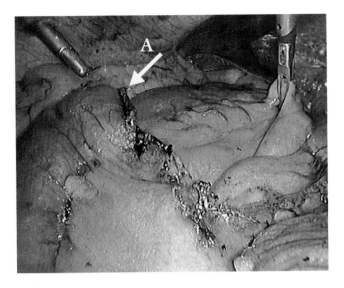

Figure 20 : Division of jejunum using Endo GIA stapler for Roux en Y loop

A - Divided distal end of jejunum

chosen with a good arterial arcade and adequate length of mesentery to reach the hilum without tension. The long limb of the Roux-en-y loop is transplaced into the subhepatic space, through a window in the mesocolon.

Lateral enterotomy is made equal to the width of the proximal divided hepatic duct, stitches are started at the lateral corner, the first being a U stitch. If the hepatic ducts are thick walled, 2- 0 vicryl is preferred. Majority of them are thin walled and so 4-0 vicryl is preferred. End to side hepaticojejunostomy is performed by continuous suture. In case of narrow proximal duct, interrupted stitches are preferred. Once the posterior stitches are placed, a Ryle's tube is passed across the stoma and anterior wall anastomosis is completed. By this maneuver narrowing of the stoma is avoided, the same tube is used as decompression tube to prevent anastomatic leak.

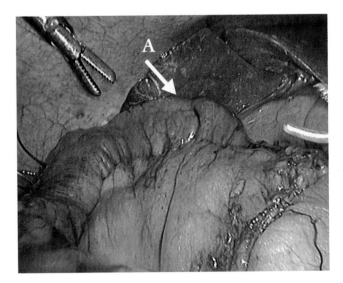

Figure 21 : Distal end of divided jejunum is taken to the supracolic compartment through the window in the mesocolon

A - Long limb of Roux-en-Y loop

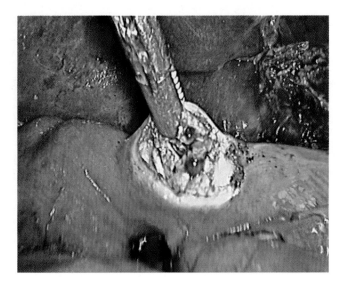

Figure 22 : Jejunotomy in the long limb for anastomosis

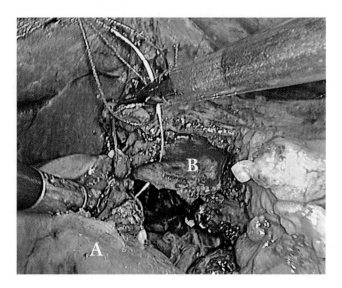

Figure 23 : Performing posterior layer of hepatico jejunos-tomy using 4 0 vicryl

A - Jejunum
B - Proximal end of common hepatic duct

Cholecystectomy

Once the reconstructive part is over, then comes removal of gall bladder. Till the final stage, the gall bladder should be intact for traction.

I have not excised the confluence in any of the patients and there was no need for double duct anastomosis. Jejunal continuity is re-established with an end to side anastomosis, 35-40cms distal to the hepatico-jejunal anastomosis. Advantages with this method of reconstruction include free flow of gastric and duodenal contents, without reflux into the long limb. Percutaneous transjejunal decompression tube protects the anastomosis. Even if leakage occurs it is easily manageable due to distal diversion of gastric and duodenal contents.

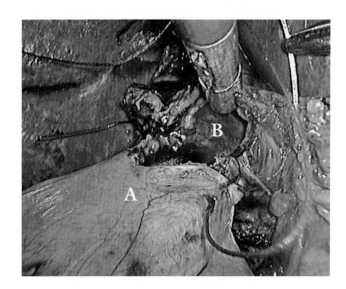

Figure 24 : Completion of posterior layer of hepaticojejunostomy

A - Jejunum
B - Proximal end of common hepatic duct

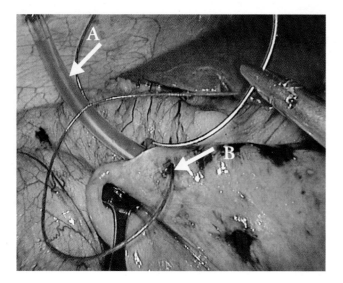

Figure 25 : Decompression tube (Ryle's tube) is taken into the peritoneal cavity and placed into the jejunum by a small stab and fixed by purse string suture

A   -   Decompression tube
B   -   Purse string stitch using catgut

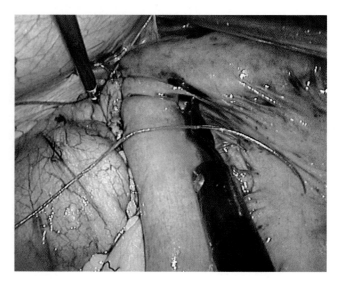

Figure 26 : Fixing the jejunal loop to the lateral abdominal wall using the same catgut

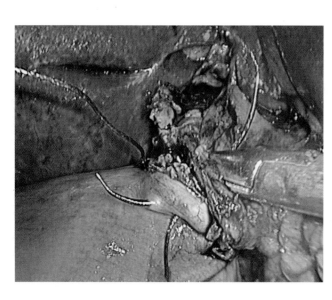

Figure 27 : Hepaticojejunostomy -anterior layer, continuous Vicryl stitches

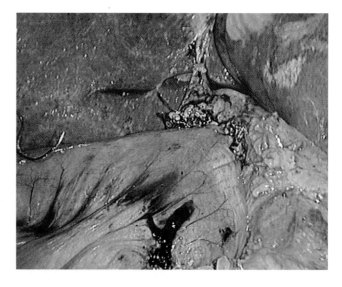

Figure 28 : Completion of hepaticojejunostomy

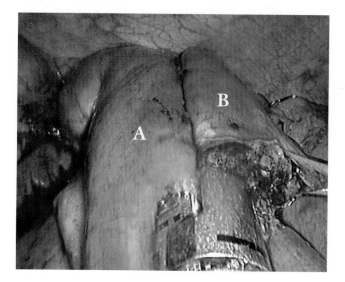

Figure 29 : Side to side jejunojejunostomy using Endo GIA stapler

A   -   Proximal divided end of jejunum
B   -   Distal end of jejunum

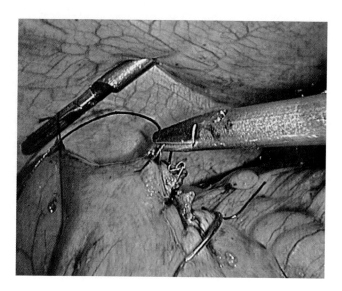

Figure 30 : Closure of the stapler entry wound

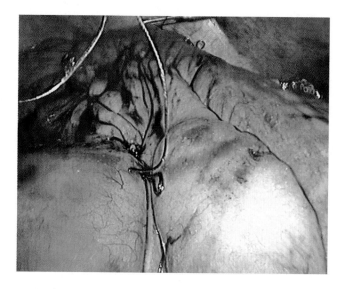

Figure 31 : Closure of the mesenteric defect to prevent internal herniation

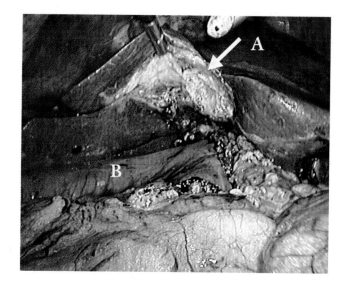

Figure 32 : Position of the long limb of the Roux-en-Y loop after completion of the surgery

A   -   Gall bladder bed after cholecystectomy
B   -   Long limb of Y loop

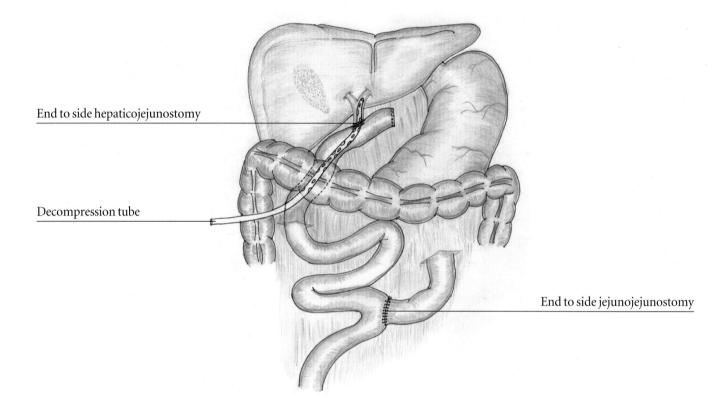

End to side hepaticojejunostomy

Decompression tube

End to side jejunojejunostomy

Figure 33 : Diagram shows the anastomosis of hepatico jejunostomy

RESULTS

Our Experience 1996 - 2005

Total number of patients - 26

Type I	A	3
	B	1
	C	19
Type II		3
Male		7
Female		19
Malignant transformation		1

Our first case of laparoscopic choledochal cyst excision was performed in the 1996. In the first operation, we could excise the entire cyst, reconstruction was performed through laparotomy as we were not comfortable due to placement of trocars at different locations. In the same year the third procedure was completed entirely by laparoscopic approach successfully.

Malignant Transformation

In one of our patient aged 32 years, during the initial dissection, we found that the medial wall of the cyst appeared densely adherent to the hepatic artery. Laparotomy was done and with difficulty, the choledochal cyst was excised and hepaticojejunostomy was performed. There was papillary projection on the mucosal layer which on biopsy proved to be adenocarcinoma. This was not included in the above series.

Anastomotic Leak

No anastomotic leak in our series. All patients were given liquid diet on the 2nd postoperative day and soft solid diet 3-4 days from the day of surgery. Mean hospital stay was 5-6 days.

Cholangitis

No evidence of cholangitis in this series. Only one patient complained pain in the epigastric region at an interval of 6 months - suggestive of acid peptic disease and unlike cholangitis.

Bleeding

During dissection, we had no bleeding from the vessels. During anastomosis, while taking stitches on the posterior wall of the hepatic duct, we had needle puncture of the portal vein which was controlled by compression for a short while after removal of the needle. Otherwise, these procedure is totally bloodless.

We had a complication related to placement of transjejunal stent. We had to perform laparotomy for bleeding noticed in the decompression jejunostomy tube. There was drop of Hb & BP on the 2nd postoperative day. Immediately laparotomy done which revealed a small spurt of arterial bleeding at the entry of tube into the jejunum. The purse string suture was not tightly holding tube and hence there was bleeding on the mucosal side.

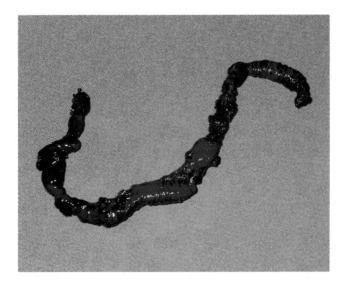

Figure 34 : Blood clot in the jejunum

Post Surgical Complications

As there are very few reports of laparoscopic excision of choledochal cyst, we don't have long term results. There are reports available following conventional approach.

1. Cholangitis

i.   In 1996, Miyano et al reported a 2.3% incidence of cholangitis after cyst excision.

ii. In 1995, Todani and Watanabe et al found cholangitis in 10 patients in their 25-year review of 97 patients who underwent cyst excision.

iii. In contrast, Chijiiwa et al (in 1993 and 1994) found that 88% of patients who previously underwent cystoenterostomy had cholangitis.

2. Biliary stone formation

i.   In 1993 and 1994, Chijiiwa et al reported a 25% rate of choledocholithiasis and a 33% rate of hepatolithiasis after cystoenterostomy.

ii. In a 1997 publication, Yamataka et al reported stone formation in 3 of the 18 patients who underwent previous cyst excision. Two patients had stones at the porta hepatis, and one patient had stones at both the porta hepatis and within the left lobe of the liver.

iii. Stones can be observed in the intrapancreatic bile duct. Usually, cholangitis and stone formation are observed in the same patient. These complications are thought to result from many factors, including the following:

 a. Stricture of anastomosis

 b. Residual debris in the intrahepatic bile duct

 c. Dilated intrahepatic duct, especially in type IV and type V choledochal cysts

3. Anastomotic stricture

i.   Apart from technical errors, anastomotic strictures may be a progressive phenomenon after surgery.

ii. In a 1993 report, Hata et al found a 4.1% rate of anastomotic strictures. A few weeks after an adequate anastomosis, the diameter of the anastomoses usually reduces in size to 70-80% of that at the time of the operation.

iii. Such a reduction in the anastomotic diameter may result from excessive devascularization of the duct during dissection. A wide anastomosis as far up as the hepatic hilum may prevent such an anastomotic stricture.

4. Residual debris in the intrahepatic bile ducts

Residual debris is commonly observed in older patients. Debris left within the intrahepatic duct or pancreatic duct during cyst excision may be responsible for post excisional stone formation and pancreatitis.

5. Intrahepatic bile duct dilatation

Dilatation usually regresses after cyst excision and hepaticojejunostomy in young patients. In older patients and adults, this dilatation tends to persist. Dilatation and residual debris may cause cholangitis and stone formation. Some authors recommend endoscopic examination of the duct during surgery to clean out all the debris.

6. Malignancy

i. The risk of carcinoma in the retained cyst approaches 50% in patients treated with cysto-enterostomy. Overall, the risk is approximately 20 times greater than the incidence in the general population.

ii. Total cyst excision had been promising in eliminating the risk of cancer development. However, sporadic cases of carcinoma in the intrahepatic ducts and distal common duct after complete cyst excision have been reported (Ohi, 1990; Todani, 1995).

iii. In a 1997 report, Yamataka et al have recommended excision of the intrapancreatic terminal choledochus.

iv. With regard to intrahepatic ducts, adequate bile drainage may prevent malignant transformation.

CONCLUSION

In summary, total excision of the cyst with adequate bile drainage is the standard treatment for choledochal cysts. Long-term follow-up is necessary to detect any late complications, especially the development of malignancy.

Our Contribution

1. Society of American Gastrointestinal Endo Surgery, Atlanta, USA, March 29-31, 2001 (Video library)

References

1. Alonso Ley F, Rever WB, Pessagno DJ 1959. Congenital cysts with a report of 2 and analysis of 94 cases. International Surgery (Abstract) 108:1-30

2. Yu ZL, Zhang LJ, FU JZ.Anomalous Pancreato biliary junction.Analysis &treatment principles. Hepatobiliary pancreat Dis Int 2.Feb;3(1)136-9

3. Todani T,Watanbe Y,Narisive M, Tabuchi K,Okajima K.1977 Congenital bile duct cysts.Classification and operative procedures and review of thirty seven cases arising from choledochal cyst.American Journal of Surgery134,263-269

4. Gigot JF, Nagorney DM,Farnell MB, Moir C,Ilstrup D 1996. Bileduct cyst in adults.A changing spectrum of presentation.Journal of Hepato biliary pancreatic Surgery 3 : 405-411.

5. Attman MS, Halls JM, Douglas AP, Renner IG 1978. Choledochal cyst presenting as acute pancreatitis. American Journal of Gastroenterology 70:514-519

6. Ishibashi T, Kasahara K, Yasuda Y, Nagai H, Kamazewa K 1997. Malignant change in the biliary tract after excision of choledochal cyst. British journal of Surgery 84: 1687-1691

7. Fieber SS, Nance FC : Choledochal cyst and neoplasm: Comprehensive review of 106 cases and presentation of two original cases.Am Surg Nov : 63(11):982-87

8. Reveille RM, Van Steigmann G, Everson GT 1990. Increased secondary bile acids in choledochal cyst. Possible role in biliary metaplasia and carcinoma. Gastroenterology 99:525-527

9. Chen CP, Cheng SJ, Chang TY. Prenatal diagnosis of choledochal cyst using ultrasound and Magnetic Resonance Imaging. Ultrasound Obs Gynaecol 2004 Jan;23(1):93-4

10. Gallivan EK, Crombleholme TM, D'Alton ME: Early Prenatal diagnosis of Choledochal cyst. Prenet Diag 1996 Oct; 16(10)934-7

11. Laparoscopic Assisted minimally invasive treatment of choledochal cyst.J Laparoendosc Adv.Surg Tech A 1999. Oct 9(5):415-18

12. Musante F, Derchi LE, Bonoti p 1982. CT Cholangiography insuspected Caroli's disease.Journal of Computed Assisted Tomography 6:482-485

13. Hogland M, Muren C, Baijisen M W 1990. Computed Tomography with intravenous cholangiography contast. A method of visualisingcholedochal cyst . European journal of Radiology 10 : 159-161

14. Lindberg CG, Hammerstrom LE, Holmin T, Lindsted C: Cholangiographic appearance of choledochal cyst. Abdom Imaging 1998 Nov-Dec ; 23 (5)

15. Nagi B, Kochhar R, Bhasin D: Endoscopic retrograde cholangiopancreatography in the evaluation of anomalous junction of pancreatobiliary duct and related disorders. Abdom Imaging 2003 Dec:28(6) 847-52

16. Powell CS, Sawyer JL, Raynolds VH 1981. Management of adult choiledochal cyst. Annals of Surgery 193: 666-676

17. Chijiiwa K, Koga A : Surgical managemnt & long term follow up of patients with choledochal cyst. Am J Surg 1993 Feb; 165(2):238-40

18. Jordan PH, Goss JA, Rosenberg WR: Some consideration for management of choledochal cyst AM J Surg 2004 Jun; 187(6)73-7

19. Laparoscopic treatment of congenital choledochal cyst.Surg Endosc 1998 Oct: 12(10) 1268-71 Shimura H, Tanaka M, Shimura S, Mizumeb K

20. Chijuiva K, Tanaka M 1994. Late complications after excisional operation in patients with choledochal cyst.Journal of American College of Surgeons 179:139-144

21. Yamamoto J, Shimamura Y, Ohtani J, Ohtani H, Yano M et al 1996. Bile duct carcinoma arising from the anastomatic site of hepatico-jejunostomy after the excision of congenital biliary dilatation .A case report. Surgery 119: 476-479

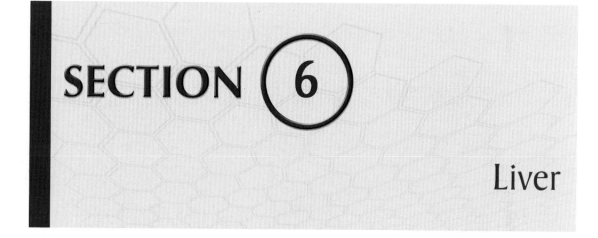

SECTION 6

Liver

46

Laparoscopic Hepatic Surgery

INTRODUCTION

Liver surgery has always been considered a difficult proposition. Consequently, it is a matter of no surprise that laparoscopic liver surgery was initiated a fair while after this technology was first introduced. The fields that laparoscopy has played a major therapeutic role in the treatment of liver diseases are in the management of liver cysts and tumors.

Laparoscopic management of simple (benign) hepatic cyst was first reported in 1991 by two separate groups (Fabiani P et al and Paterson-Brown S et al). However, laparoscopy was used before this for diagnosis of this condition. The first use of diagnostic laparoscopy for hepatic cyst was documented in 1955. In fact, laparoscopic ultrasonography was used for diagnosis of liver disorders as early as in 1989. Regarding the liver tumors M.Gagner et al reported the application of this minimally invasive approach and successfully performed the first liver resection

for a focal nodular hyperplasia. Since then many studies have established the safety and feasibility of laparoscopic liver surgery.

SURGICAL ANATOMY OF LIVER

Understanding the surgical anatomy of the liver, its segments, attachments, vascular pattern and biliary drainage is essential for performing laparoscopic surgeries on the liver. Liver is the latest as well as the most difficult intrabdominal organ to come under the purview of laparoscopic surgery. This section deals with the basic architecture of the liver, modern concepts of its anatomy and relations to the surrounding structures.

Liver is the largest parenchymal organ[1] in the body weighing between 1200 and 1800 g in the adult. The greater part of the liver occupies the right hypochondrium enclosed within the rib cage on the right side and this explains the fact that liver is difficult to approach both in open surgery as well in laparoscopic surgery. Topographically, liver extends from the 5th rib in the midclavicular line to the right costal margin.

SURFACES OF THE LIVER AND THEIR RELATIONS

Liver has got three distinct surfaces[6] which are posterior, antero superior and inferior. Posterior surface is related to the ventral part of the diaphragm and the surgically important bare area of the liver forms part of the posterior surface of liver. Three anatomic entities that relate to the posterior surface are the retrohepatic part of the IVC, the right adrenal gland and the upper pole of the right kidney.

The anterosuperior surface of the liver lies opposite to the dome of the diaphragm, pericardium, pleura and the anterior part of the rib cage. The superior surface is covered by peritoneum except for the attachment of the falciform ligament.

Inferior surface, otherwise called the visceral hepatic surface is the most important of all the surfaces from the surgical point of view. The space under the right lobe is the subhepatic space of Morrison, the most important of the sub-diaphragmatic spaces and the space under the left lobe is the lesser sac. The structures that are related to the inferior surface are the gall bladder, right adrenal gland, right kidney, right renal vessels, head of pancreas, proximal part of the pancreatic neck, first and second part of the duodenum, common bile duct, portal vein, hepatic artery, IVC and hepatic flexure of the colon. The portal structures namely portal vein, bile duct and hepatic arteries enter and leave the liver from inferior surface of the liver. Together with the surrounding fossa and tissues, it forms capital "H" configuration,[2] which can be well made out during laparoscopic exposure.

PERITONEAL ATTACHMENTS OF THE LIVER

The liver is covered by the visceral peritoneum on all its surfaces except over a part of posterior surface which is called the bare area of the liver.[3] Here, the liver is in direct contact with the diaphragm. The liver is supported by a handful of ligaments[4,5] which are nothing but the reflections of the peritoneal coverings to the diaphragm and to the abdominal wall.

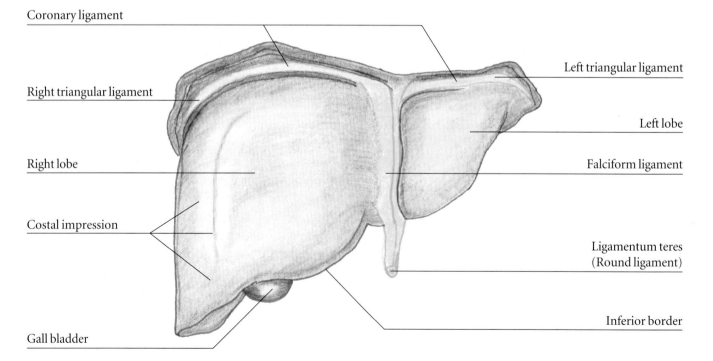

Figure 1 : Anterior view of liver

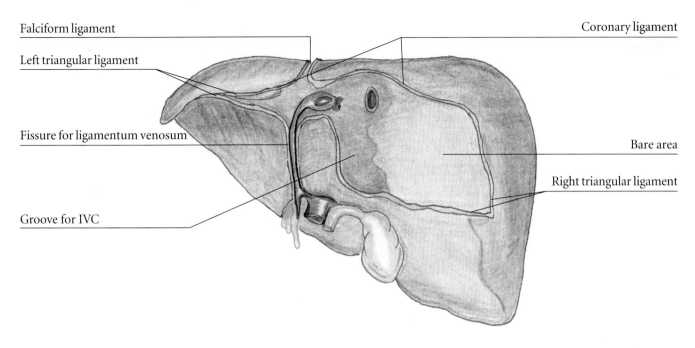

Falciform ligament

Left triangular ligament

Fissure for ligamentum venosum

Groove for IVC

Coronary ligament

Bare area

Right triangular ligament

Figure 2 : Posterior view of liver

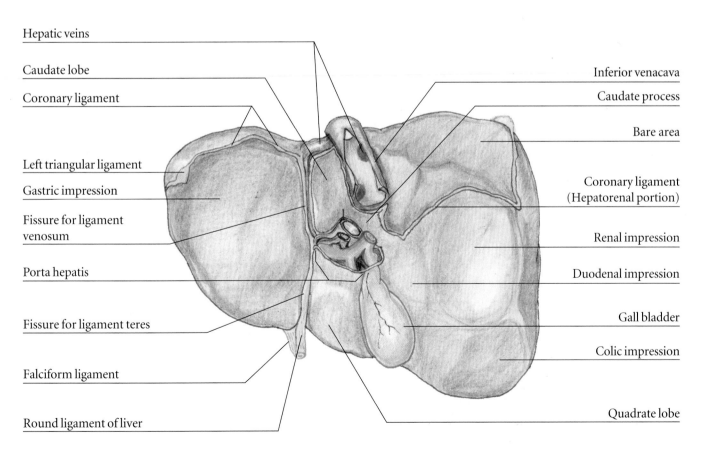

Hepatic veins

Caudate lobe

Coronary ligament

Left triangular ligament

Gastric impression

Fissure for ligament venosum

Porta hepatis

Fissure for ligament teres

Falciform ligament

Round ligament of liver

Inferior venacava

Caudate process

Bare area

Coronary ligament (Hepatorenal portion)

Renal impression

Duodenal impression

Gall bladder

Colic impression

Quadrate lobe

Figure 3 : Visceral surface of liver

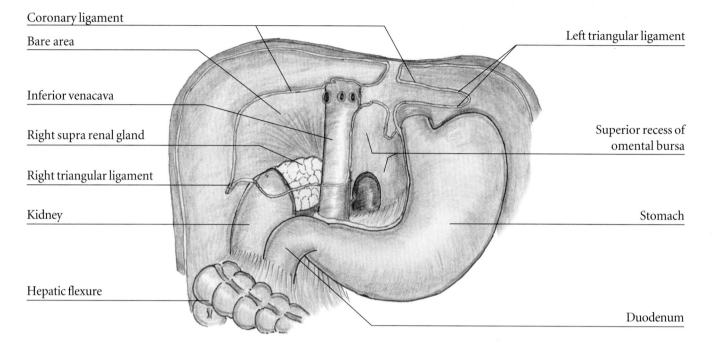

Coronary ligament

Bare area

Inferior venacava

Right supra renal gland

Right triangular ligament

Kidney

Hepatic flexure

Left triangular ligament

Superior recess of
omental bursa

Stomach

Duodenum

Figure 4 : Bed of liver

The falciform ligament is a sickle-shaped double layered fold of peritoneum that runs from the umbilicus and anterior abdominal wall to the superior surface of the liver. The free margin of the falciform ligament houses the ligamentum teres (round ligament) which is the obliterated left umbilical vein. The ligamentum teres runs through the portoumbilical fissure on the inferior surface of the liver and gets attached to the terminal part of the left branch of portal vein. This anatomical fact assumes significance from the fact that this pathway from the portal vein to the obliterated left umbilical vein is opened up due to the raised portal pressure (like in cirrhosis) producing engorgement of veins around the umbilicus, a condition referred to as 'caput medusae'.

On the posterosuperior surface of the liver, the falciform ligament divides to form the right and left anterior coronary ligaments.[7] These ligaments define the anterior border of the bare area of the liver. The posterior borders of the bare area are formed by the right and left posterior coronary ligaments, which are the reflections of the diaphragmatic peritoneum. On the left, the anterior and posterior coronary ligaments are small and merge almost immediately into the left triangular ligament which attaches the slender tapering left portion of the liver to the diaphragm. On the right, the coronary ligaments merge to form a small right triangular ligament. In addition, the posterior coronary ligament during its course is reflected on the upper part of the right kidney to form the hepato renal ligament. To mobilize the right lobe, the right coronary and right triangle ligaments need to be divided whereas left triangular and coronary ligaments are divided to mobilize the left lobe.

PORTA HEPATIS AND THE HILAR PLATE

Porta hepatis, otherwise called hepatic hilum contains portal vein, hepatic artery and bile duct. These structures are placed in the free border of the lesser omentum (hepatoduodenal ligament) wherein the portal vein is situated posteriorly, the hepatic duct at its anterolateral border and the hepatic artery at its anteromedial border. Porta hepatis lies in the transverse fissure on the inferior surface of the liver, sandwitched between the quadrate lobe anteriorly and caudate lobe posteriorly.

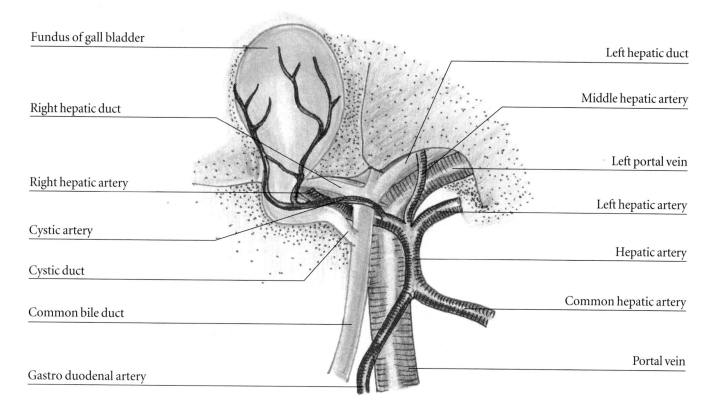

Figure 5 : Porta hepatis - relationship

The Glissonian capsule[17] near the porta hepatis fuses with the connective tissue surrounding the vascular and biliary elements to constitute the plate system. Three plate systems are defined which include hilar plate[22] above the biliary confluence, the cystic plate related to the gall bladder and the umbilical plate situated above the umbilical portion of the left portal vein.

By the technique of lowering of hilar plate, wherein the Glisson's capsule on the posterior border of the quadrate lobe is incised, the hilar plate is dissected to expose the left hepatic duct. This maneuver is of particular importance during surgery for high bile duct strictures and hilar cholangiocarcinoma. Similarly, umbilical plate dissection will lead to the segment III duct and vein.

Portal Vein

Portal vein is formed by the confluence of superior mesenteric vein and splenic vein behind the neck of the pancreas. It ascends in the hepatoduodenal ligament to the porta where it divides into right and left branches. Portal vein supplies 75% of blood supply to the liver. Right branch which is short and wide immediately enters the parenchyma and divides into anterior and posterior sectorial branches. Anterior branch divides further to supply segments V & VIII whereas posterior branch supplies segments VI & VII. Left branch which is long and narrow has a different set of branches. Basically it consists of two parts namely transverse part and umbilical part.[18] Branch to the caudate lobe arises from the transverse part which at the level of umbilical fissure turns sharply to become umbilical part. Segmental branches to segments II, III & IV arise from the umbilical part. Ligamentum teres is attached to the umbilical part of the left branch,[3] which can be opened up in case of portal hypertension and is responsible for the development of dilated veins around the umbilicus.

Intrahepatic biliary tract

At the hilum, the right and the left duct unites to form the common hepatic duct. On the right side,

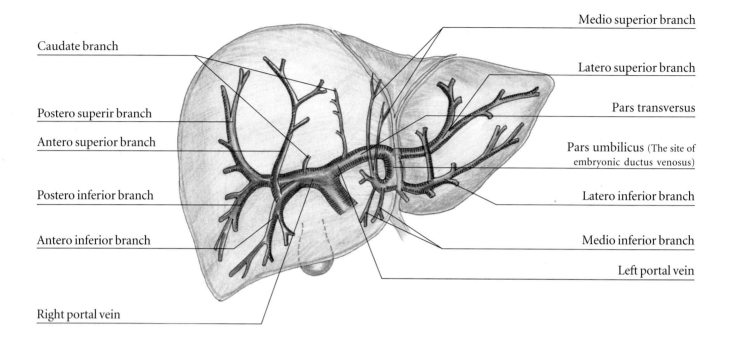

Caudate branch

Postero superir branch

Antero superior branch

Postero inferior branch

Antero inferior branch

Right portal vein

Medio superior branch

Latero superior branch

Pars transversus

Pars umbilicus (The site of embryonic ductus venosus)

Latero inferior branch

Medio inferior branch

Left portal vein

Figure 6 : Intrahepatic distribution of hepatic portal vein

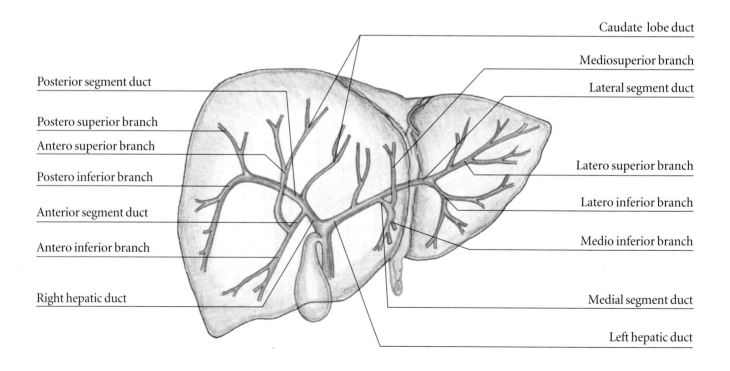

Posterior segment duct

Postero superior branch

Antero superior branch

Postero inferior branch

Anterior segment duct

Antero inferior branch

Right hepatic duct

Caudate lobe duct

Mediosuperior branch

Lateral segment duct

Latero superior branch

Latero inferior branch

Medio inferior branch

Medial segment duct

Left hepatic duct

Figure 7 : Intrahepatic distribution of the bile ducts

the branching pattern resembles the portal vein[19] with the biliary radicals lying superior to the portal vein branches. On the left side, the duct divides into lateral segment duct which supplies segments II & III and medial segment duct which supplies segment IV. Left duct has more extrahepatic course and hence left side hepaticojejunostomy is easier.

Hepatic artery

Hepatic artery supplies 25% of blood supply to the liver. Branching pattern of the hepatic artery correlates with that of the bile duct except the fact that it is inferior to bile duct.[20]

Hepatic veins

Anatomy of the hepatic veins is altogether different from the above structures which forms the portal triad. Right hepatic vein, the largest one drains segment V, VI, VII & part of VIII. Middle hepatic vein which divides the liver into 2 functional lobes drains segments IV, V & part of VIII. Left hepatic vein drains the left lateral segments II & III.

All the hepatic veins drain into the retrohepatic portion of the inferior vena cava.[21] These veins and the

IVC can be approached laparoscopically through the superior surface of the liver by incising the superior layer of the coronary ligament. Caudate lobe drains through small independent branches to IVC directly.

ANOMALIES OF THE BILIARY TREE[23]

The biliary and hepatic anatomy detailed above can at times be altered. It is essential for the surgeon to be familiar with the anomalies of the biliary tree which will prevent unnecessary complications during hepatic surgeries. By far, the intra as well as extrahepatic biliary ductal anatomy is the one which has varied anomalies. This section is devoted to the anomalies of the intrahepatic biliary anatomy whose knowledge is essential for the hepatic resectional procedures.

The constitution of a normal biliary confluence by union of the right and left hepatic ducts as described above is seen in about 72% of the cases (Healey and Schroy 1953). A triple confluence of right anterior and posterior sectoral ducts and left hepatic duct is seen in 12% of cases. In addition any of the sectoral duct on the right side may join the left duct or the

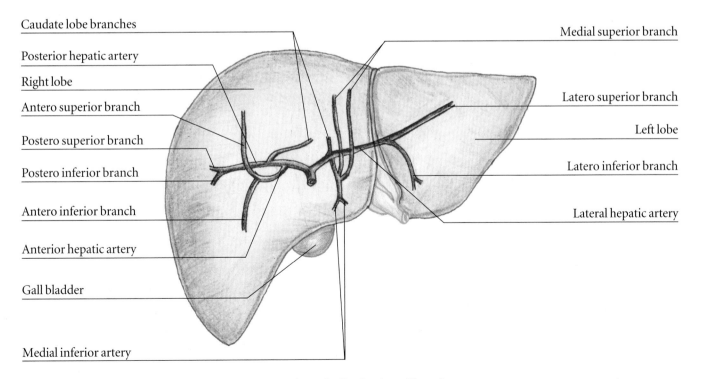

Figure 8 : Intrahepatic distribution of hepatic artery

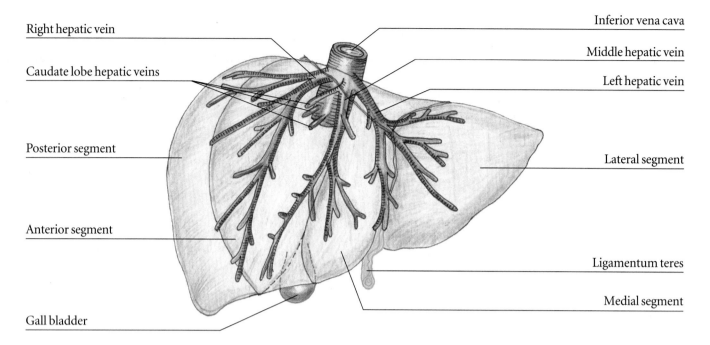

Right hepatic vein

Caudate lobe hepatic veins

Posterior segment

Anterior segment

Gall bladder

Inferior vena cava

Middle hepatic vein

Left hepatic vein

Lateral segment

Ligamentum teres

Medial segment

Figure 9 : Intrahepatic distribution of hepatic portal vein

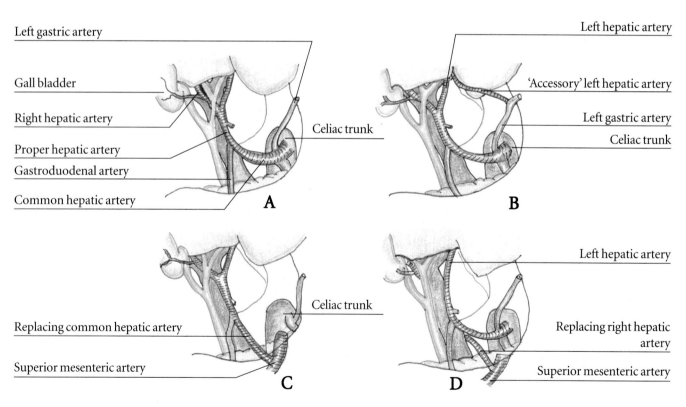

Left gastric artery

Gall bladder

Right hepatic artery

Proper hepatic artery

Gastroduodenal artery

Common hepatic artery

Celiac trunk

A

Left hepatic artery

'Accessory' left hepatic artery

Left gastric artery

Celiac trunk

B

Replacing common hepatic artery

Superior mesenteric artery

Celiac trunk

C

Left hepatic artery

Replacing right hepatic artery

Superior mesenteric artery

D

Figure 10 : Hepatic artery variations

A - Normal pattern   B - Access left hepatic artery arising from the left gastric artery   C - Replacing common hepatic artery arising from the superior mesenteric artery   D - Replacing right hepatic artery arising from the superior mesenteric artery

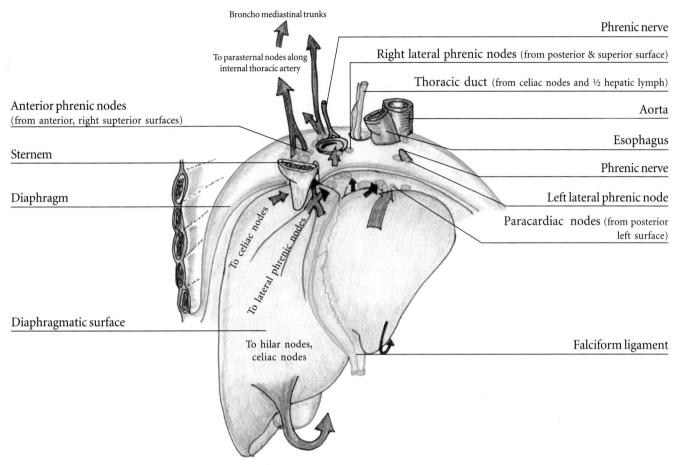

Broncho mediastinal trunks

To parasternal nodes along
internal thoracic artery

Phrenic nerve

Right lateral phrenic nodes (from posterior & superior surface)

Thoracic duct (from celiac nodes and ½ hepatic lymph)

Aorta

Esophagus

Phrenic nerve

Left lateral phrenic node

Paracardiac nodes (from posterior
left surface)

Anterior phrenic nodes
(from anterior, right supterior surfaces)

Sternem

Diaphragm

Diaphragmatic surface

To celiac nodes

To lateral phrenic nodes

To hilar nodes,
celiac nodes

Falciform ligament

Figure 11 : Superficial lymphatic drainage o f the liver. About one half of the drainage is to the thoracic duct

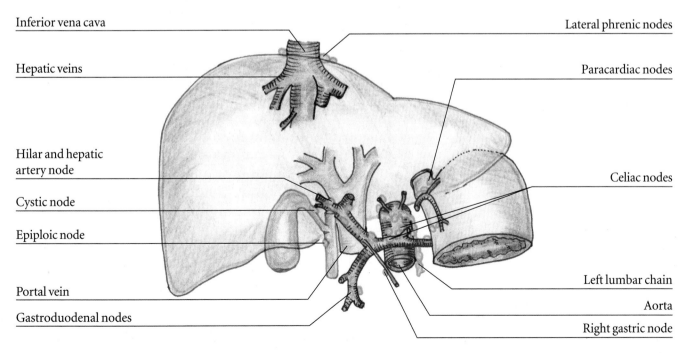

Inferior vena cava

Hepatic veins

Hilar and hepatic
artery node

Cystic node

Epiploic node

Portal vein

Gastroduodenal nodes

Lateral phrenic nodes

Paracardiac nodes

Celiac nodes

Left lumbar chain

Aorta

Right gastric node

Figure 12 : Deep lymphatic drainage of liver. The superficial and deep lymphatics anastomose freely

common hepatic duct. Other rare anomalies include the absence of confluence and the right posterior sectoral duct joining the neck of the gall bladder.

Intrahepatic bile duct variations are also common. These are mainly due to the ectopic drainage of various segments. The segments with ectopic drainage include IV, V, VI & VIII. Care should be taken to precisely identify these variations to avoid biliary injury and leak.

FUNCTIONAL SURGICAL ANATOMY

The understanding of the internal architecture of the liver has witnessed sea of changes during the last century. Traditionally, liver is divided into right and left anatomical lobes by the attachment of the falciform ligament. Based on the external appearance, the liver has four lobes namely right, left, quadrate and caudate. The concept of functional anatomy of the liver,[8,9,10] dividing it into lobes and segments based on the hepatic arterial blood supply, portal venous blood supply, biliary drainage and hepatic venous drainage changed the outlook of the hepatic surgery.

Although many authors[11,12,13] have described the segmental anatomy, we follow the most widely practiced system formulated by Couinaud in 1954.[11]

Couinaud segmentation system is based on the distribution in the liver of both the portal vein and the hepatic veins. According to this system, the liver is divided into four sectors by the three hepatic veins. The plane through which these hepatic veins passes is called portal scissurae. The main scissura which contains the middle hepatic vein divides the liver into right and left lobes. The plane of this scissura extends from gall bladder bed to the junction of middle hepatic vein and inferior vena cava. This line is called as Cantlie's line. Right scissura further divides the right lobe into an anteromedial and postero lateral sectors, while the left scissura divides the left lobe into medial and lateral sectors.

The planes containing the portal pedicles are called hepatic scissurae. Eight segments are described, one for the caudate lobe (Segment I), three on the left (Segments II, III & IV) and four on the right (segments V, VI, VII, VIII). Each segment has

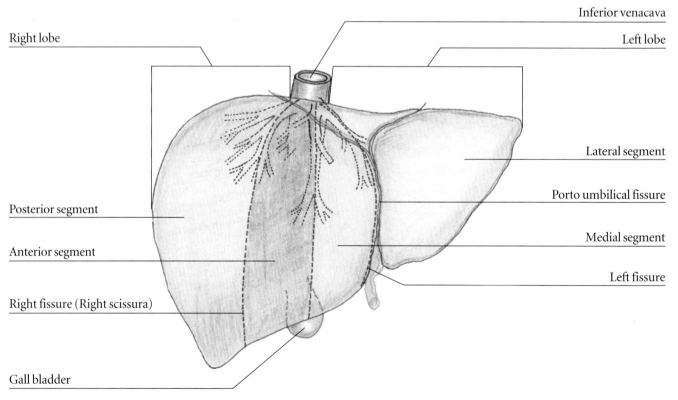

Figure 13 : Segments of liver

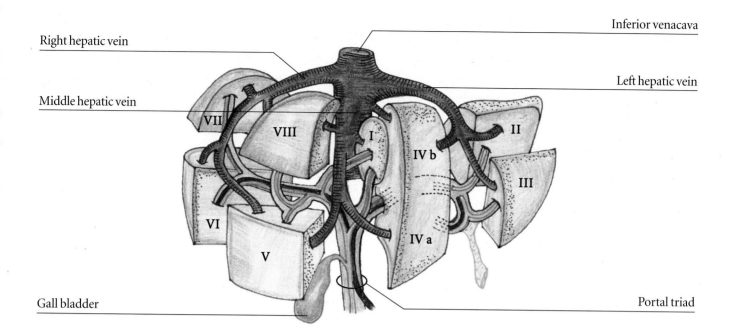

Figure 14 : Couinaud segmentation system of liver

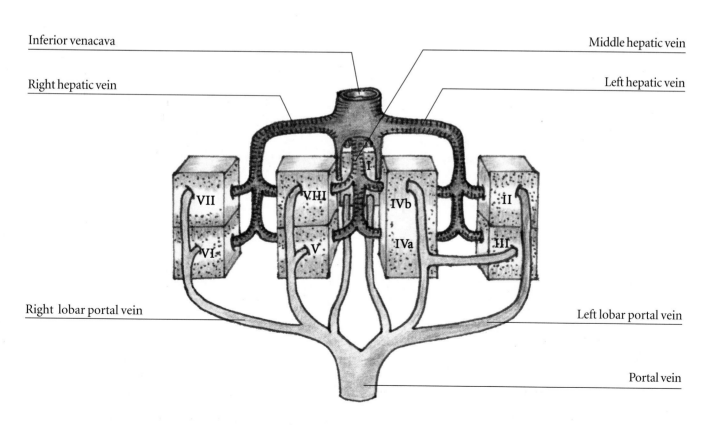

Figure 15 : Functional representation of hepatic segments

independent and separate branches from portal veins and hepatic artery and has a separate biliary and hepatic venous drainage. Caudate lobe[14,15,16] is supplied by both the branches of portal vein, hepatic artery and bile duct while the venous drainage is by short hepatic veins which drain directly in to the IVC. A well defined avascular plane exists between these segments so that liver resections can be performed along this plane with minimal blood loss and bile leakage.

DIAGNOSIS AND PREOPERATIVE WORKUP

The approach to the diagnosis of liver tumors will be influenced by the age and sex of the patient and whether or not the lesion is symptomatic. It is seldom possible to make a specific diagnosis of mass lesion in the liver solely on clinical grounds since these features are often non specific. However, a detailed history and clinical examination will aid in making a correct diagnosis using modern imaging systems. With rapid advances in medical technology, new imaging modalities and refinements in the existing imaging systems are being employed to detect very small lesions of even less than 0.5cm in the liver. Here in this section, a brief overview of the imaging modalities used to detect the liver tumors is discussed.

HEPATIC IMAGING

Ultrasound - Conventional, Doppler, Intraoperative, Contrast enhanced
CT scan - Conventional, spiral
CTAP - CT Arterial Portography
CTHA - CT Hepatic Arteriography
MRI - Magnetic Resonance Imaging
PET - Positron Emission Tomography

Abdominal Sonography

Ultrasound abdomen is the preliminary investigation for any hepatic tumors. It is radiation free and economical[24] with good patient acceptability rate. Doppler ultrasound with colour coding[25] provides us the information regarding the vascular pattern of the tumor and its relation to major vessels. Intraoperative ultrasound[26-29] is now routinely performed in all patients undergoing liver resection since it detects impalpable and inaccessible tumors. Moreover, it can detect tumors of even 3mm in size which is difficult to make out in CT or MRI scan.[30,31] In addition, intraoperative monitoring of liver tumors using ultrasound is now the routine practice during local ablative therapies like radiofrequency ablation and cryoablation.

CT Scan

With the advent of spiral CT,[32] the diagnosis of liver tumors is simplified as it offers many advantages. The image acquisition is faster[33-37] (less than 10 sec) and three dimensional images and thinner slices can be obtained in single breath hold of the patient. Spiral CT also allows the acquisition of three different perfusion phases[38] (arterial, venous and equilibrium phases) which is critical in the assessment of vascularity of the lesion. Computed tomography arterial portography (CTAP) yields high sensitivity in thedetection of hepatic metastasis. Ionising radiations[39,40] and the contrast induced allergic reactions[41,42] are the two major limiting factors against which the CT scan should be judiously and carefully used.

Magnetic Resonance Imaging

The sensitivity and specificity of picking up liver tumors by the MRI exceeds that of the CT scan or ultrasound.[43-56] At the same time it doesn't carry any ionising radiation and the gadolenium contrast that is used in MRI imaging is generally considered safe. Small hepatocellular carcinoma and hepatic metastasis are clearly made out in MRI scan. Our present indications for MRI scan include those lesions that are unclear in CT or Ultrasound imaging especially in case of suspected metastasis.

Other modalities

Hepatic angiography though less commonly employed now is useful in evaluating the tumor invasion into major hepatic artery. It is more accurate in this aspect when compared to CT scan. Additionally, it is also useful for chemoembolisation of large, unresectable tumors.

Positron Emission Tomography is being more frequently used nowadays, which has yielded high sensitivity in the detection of hepatic metastasis from colorectal cancer.[57-59] However the pick up rate for hepatocellular carcinoma is poor with the sensitivity ranging from 50% to 70%.[60-62]

To summarise, a handful of imaging modalities are available to diagnose liver tumors. Abdominal sonography continues to be the first line of investigative tool while CT scan and MRI offer fine details about the tumor pathology in addition to detecting small tumors not diagnosed by ultrasound. Newer techniques like PET scan is coming into vogue and their use in hepatic imaging will be defined in the years to come.

PRE OPERATIVE ASSESSMENT

Assessment of the status of the liver before surgery is an indispensible part of the workup for liver tumors. The plan of action for any hepatic tumors depend on the functional status of the liver, associated cirrhosis and viral markers besides patient and tumor variables. Hence, it is imperative that the liver should be fully evaluated for its functional reserve. But unfortunately, there is no single test till date that accurately assess the hepatic reserve and the functional status. However, there are a few clinical scoring systems and liver function tests that will guide us to assess its functions which will be discussed here.

Liver function tests to assess hepatic reserve[63]

Clearance/Tolerance tests

Aminopyrine breath test

Indocyanine Green (ICG) retention

Bromsulpthalein (BSP) retention

Galactose tolerance

Bile acid tolerance

Beta Hydroxy butyrate

Functional Imaging/Blood flow: uptake/clearance

Reticuloendothelium

Gold

Sulphur colloid

Rose Bengal

HIDA scan

Neogalactosyl albumin (NGA)

Galactosyl serum albumin (GSA)

Scoring Systems - Child's Score

The fact that liver failure accounts for more that 50% of deaths[64-68] following hepatic resection underlines the importance of assessing the hepatic reserve. This figure holds good for both hepatocellular carcinoma and colorectal metastasis in most of the reported series.[64-68]

Over the years many scoring systems have been developed to know the functional status of the liver, but Child's clinical scoring system has stood the test of the time and it emerges as the single most reliable scoring system. Though many modification to the original Child's scoring system have come into vogue, the most widely used one is the Child-Pugh modification (Table 1).

Table 1. Child - Pugh Scoring System

Variable	Degree		
	1	2	3
Ascites	None	Controlled	Tense
Encephlopathy	Absent	State I-II	State III-IV
Albumin (g/c)	> 3.5	3-3.5	< 3
Bilirubin (mg/dc)	< 2	2-3	> 3
Prothrombin time	< 4	4-6	> 6

Child Pugh class	Total points
A	5-6
B	7-9
C	10-15

The outcome of hepatic resection closely follows the Child Pugh classification. Franco et al[69] demonstrated that the mortality for a Child class A patient undergoing liver resection was 3.7% versus 16.7% for both Child class B & C patients. Based on these studies, it is generally recommended that liver resection is advocated for patients with Child A class whereas other modalities of treatment are employed for child B & C patients. Unfortunately the positive predective value of the Child score for liver resections has been shown to be quite variable especially for Child's A patients. Hence to overcome the limitations of Child Pugh scoring systems, various biochemical and imaging studies are designed to assess some specific aspects of liver function. These tests will only augment Child-Pugh assessment but will not replace it. Of the innumerable tests available, the one that is now routinely adopted is Indocyanine green (ICG) retention test.

Indocyanine Green (ICG) retention test

ICG is a tricarbocyanine dye that binds to albumin and alpha-1 lipoproteins. It is actively transferred into the liver parenchymal cells which is then secreted into the bile. The fact that it is solely removed from the circulation by the liver[70] is used to assess the function of the liver. By convention, the amount of dye retained in the plasma at 15 minutes after its injection into peripheral vein (ICG-15) is used to calculate the status of the liver. Clearance is considered to be impaired when 15% or more of the dye remains within the plasma, 15 minutes following the injection of 0.5mg/kg of ICG.

Volumetric Studies

Volumetric studies are generally employed for larger lesions undergoing major hapatectomies. For segmentectomies, bisegmentectomies and subsegmentectomies, analysis of the post resection remnant liver volume is not mandatory until and otherwise the situation warrants. However in case of major hepatic resections like lobectomies and hepatectomies, volumetric assessment of the liver that is to be resected and remnant liver is mandatory.

As major hepatic resections involve removal of substantial portion of the liver, there should be enough liver parenchyma left after resection to take care of the function of the entire liver. To assess this critical liver volume to be resected or to be left out, volumetric studies are being routinely performed. Here computerized tomography is most often used which calculates accurately the volume of the resected and remnant liver. Okanoto et al (1984) observed a close relation between CT volumetric measurements of the liver and tumor and the ICG 15 retention test. These measurements could predict the safe limits of hepatectomy in patients with impaired liver function. It may mandate a decision to either avoid a liver resection that carries an unacceptable risk or to perform preoperative portal vein embolisation on the side to be resected in order to induce hypertrophy of the contralateral liver. Though there are wide variations in the amount and rate of regeneration of liver following liver resections, there is a consensus among most hepatic surgeons that there should be at least 20% of the liver volume to be left out in healthy patients and 40% in cirrhotic patients if one is contemplating hepatic resection.

SPECIAL INSTRUMENTS FOR LIVER RESECTION

Liver is the last and latest organ in the abdomen to be conquered by laparoscopy. It took a while to widely adopt minimally invasive approach to liver tumors basically because of its size, location and vascularity. Before venturing into the laparoscopic management of liver tumors, the surgeon should be familiar with the open hepatic resections. Not only the surgeon should be highly skilled with adequate experience, but also he or she should be equipped with modern gadgets available for liver surgery. Of late, a wide variety of instruments have become available which have made liver surgeries bloodless, and hitherto impossible resections possible. The knowledge of the functional anatomy of the liver, the acquintence of operative skills and the availability of specialized instruments are critical to the performance of safe and successful hepatic surgery. This section will highlight some of the armamentarium which will be of immense help towards bloodless liver surgery.

Special instruments for liver resection
1. Ultrasonic Shears
2. Argon Plasma Coagulation (APC)
3. Cavitational Ultrasonic Surgical Aspirator (CUSA)
4. Laparoscopic Ultrasound
5. Electrothermal Bipolar Vessel Sealer (Ligasure)
6. Vascular Staplers
7. Tissue Link
8. Water Jet

Ultrasonic Shears (Harmonic Scalpel)

Harmonic scalpel® (Ethicon Endo-Surgery, USA) works on the principle of ultrasonic vibrations. The device composes of a generator, handpiece and blade.[71] The microprocessor in the generator pulses the acoustic system in the hand piece with an AC current. The electric pulsing of the piezoelectric crystals results in the vibration of the transducer at the rate of 55.5 KHz which is transmitted to the tip of the instrument. There are four configurations available at the tip namely scissors, hook, spatula and ball. The common configuration which is found to be useful is the scissors type wherein the lower blade is the active one, which vibrates in longitudinal axis at the rate of 55.5 KHz. The upper blade, called tissue pad is an inactive one which helps in grasping the tissues and also prevents the vibrational energy from spreading further. The mechanism of coagulation and cutting[72] is simple. Ultrasurgical devices denature protein by the transfer of mechanical energy to the tissues which is sufficient to break tertiary hydrogen bonds and by the generation of heat from internal tissue friction that results from the high frequency vibration of the tissue. The coagulum that is formed[73] seals the blood vessels by coapting and tamponading the vessel wall.

Harmonic scalpel offers many advantages when compared to the electrocautery.[74] The lateral thermal damage is minimal (2mm)[75] and can coagulate

vessels upto 5mm in diameter.[76] Moreover, the maximal temperature reached during its working is 80° C, which is well below the 250° to 400° C temperatures achieved with electrocautery and laser surgery. It can be used in dividing the liver parenchyma and small vessels and biliary cannaliculi, although it is not advisable for dividing larger vessels. One more likable feature is that it never produces fumes or smoke except for a transient mist[77-78] which settles down quickly.

Cavitational Ultrasonic Surgical Aspirator (CUSA)

A second mechanism for cutting tissues is by cavitation, which uses the same principle of ultrasonic vibration used by harmonic scalpel.[79] But the difference is in two aspects. One is the frequency which is 23KHz for CUSA[80] while harmonic scalpel vibrate at the rate of 55.5KHz.[71] The other is the geometry of the vibrating blade which consist of a hollow circular titanium tube with a conical hollow tip. To and fro vibration of the tip produces vacuoles inside the cell which expands and fragments the cell.[81] Continuous suction removes the cellular debris and paves way for newer tissue contacts. CUSA is very useful in parenchymal division and at the same time low water content tissues like blood vessels and bile ducts are left undivided. This tissue specific action helps in dividing the liver parenchyma and securing the blood vessels and ducts which can be clipped or stapled and divided.[82-85] Using laparoscopic CUSA probe, bloodless parenchymal division is thus possible and even major resection are now being performed with bloodless field.

Argon Plasma Coagulation (APC)

Argon Plasma Coagulation[86] is mainly used for surface coagulation at the denuded areas. In case of hepatic resection, the divided surface is coagulated with APC so that surface ooze is prevented. APC works in a similar fashion as that of the electrocautery. Argon is an inert, noncombustible gas which conducts electricity better than the air. Thus, a beam of argon gas can be used to conduct electricity between the eletrode and the tissue that can be used for coagulation without the probe touching the tissue. Since argon gas cannot go beyond the solid tissue, the electric current meets the tissue interface and fulgurates only the surface. Care should be taken during its use in laparoscopic surgeries as gas embolism is a possibility. There are cases on record where air embolism has occurred from APC usage especially during laparoscopic procedures as there is no vent for argon gas to escape out. Hence during the use of APC, one of the trocars should be opened so that the argon gas can escape freely to the outside. Moreover APC should not be used for larger, visible feeding vessels for the above mentioned risk of embolism.

Electrothermal Bipolar Vessel Sealer (EBVS) - Ligasure

Ligasure[87] is a modified version of bipolar electrocautery which is more precise and safe compared to electrocautery. It consists of 2 jaws between which the electric current flows. It is devised in such a way that it coagulates the tissue at four places and cuts in between.[88] Lateral spread is very minimal, even less than the harmonic scalpel. There are no active surfaces exposed outside the jaws and hence there is less chance of accidental injury to the surrounding tissue. Its principle use is in parenchymal division[90] and also in division of smaller blood vessels and bile ducts upto 7mm diameter. Clinical results with EBVS in laparoscopic and open procedures demonstrate it to be safe and effective in reducing operative time.[89]

Laparoscopic Ultrasound

Laparoscopic ultrasound has now become an indispensable tool during major hepatic resections. The advantages of intraoperative ultrasound are many fold which are highlightened in the table. Laparoscopic ultrasound probes uses higher frequencies (7.5 MHz) compared to conventional ones and hence the resolution is better. It avoids unnecessary laparoto-

mies[97-100] and at the same time necessary resections are done with ease.[110]

Advantages of laparoscopic ultrasound
1. Greater sensitivity and specificity in detecting smaller lesions
2. Better definition of the location of the lesions
3. Detection of tumor thrombus and tumor invasion
4. Defines the relation of hepatic vasculature and bile duct to the tumor
5. Detection of peritoneal tumor deposits
6. Assessment of the operability of the tumor.
7. Guidance of laparoscopic radiofrequency ablation and other ablative techniques

Laparoscopy has obvious shortcomings in evaluating the tumor as it eliminates the surgeon's ability to palpate structures and lesions. Laparoscopic ultrasound attempts to restore some of the tactile feed back while providing important information as in open procedures.

It has been suggested that laparoscopic intraoperative ultrasound should be routinely used in colorectal cancer surgery and hepatic resections.[101,102] Apart from its use during resectional procedures, laparoscopic intraoperative ultrasound (IOUS) is now increasingly employed in various ablative techniques as well.[107-109] Its role in liver surgery is exemplified from the fact that no other preoperative investigation[91-94] has been able to duplicate the sensitivity and specificity of laparoscopic IOUS in the identification of occult lesions.[103-106] The table given compares the sensitivity, specificity and accuracy of

Comparison of imaging modalities available in evaluating liver tumors[95-96]

	Arteriography	CT	Preop US	IOUS	Exploration
Sensitivity	38	49-66	41-68	78-94	66-77
Specificity	57	94-95	96-97	95-100	94-95
Accuracy	39	58-76	73-75	84-95	81-94

different imaging modalities that are available to detect liver tumors.

CURRENT PERSPECTIVE IN LAPAROSCOPIC LIVER SURGERY

With available technology, laparoscopic hepatic surgery is becoming more and more popular. Laparoscopic approach is an ideal way to treat simple cysts and hydatid cysts. The peripherally situated benign tumors have been successfully managed by laparoscopic wedge or segmental excision at many centres world wide. Of late major anatomical hepatic resections like right and left hepatic resections have been performed successfully at few centres. Laparoscopic donor hepatectomy also have been successfully done recently.

The reasons for slow progress of laparoscopic liver surgery are the associated technical difficulties and concern about the intraoperative hazards of bleeding and gas embolism. Laparoscopic liver surgery presents unique technical challenges and hemorrhage control from large intrahepatic vessels may be difficult. Cases of gas embolism have been reported and this potentially lethal complication adds to the concerns associated with laparoscopic liver surgery.

The advent of technological refinements, experience in laparoscopic and hepatic surgery and application of the principles of oncologic surgery has expanded the role of laparoscopic liver resections. Increasing data suggest that immune function is better preserved after laparoscopic than after open surgery. This may confer a survival advantage to a person undergoing laparoscopic procedure over the open approach.

Indications

Laparoscopic surgery has been used for treating congenital liver cysts (CLC), adult polycystic liver disease (APLD), hydatid liver cysts, neoplastic liver cysts such as liver cystadenoma, benign hepatic tumors and selectively hepatic malignant tumors.

1. Cystic Liver Disease

Laparoscopic management of CLCs has been increasingly reported, but not all CLCs are amenable to laparoscopic treatment.[111,112] Again, a strict selection of patients is mandatory, the best candidates

for a laparoscopic approach being large, superficial, accessible cysts at the liver surface, located in the anterior segments of the right liver or in the left lateral liver segments.[113] Deeply seated and posterior liver cysts are difficult to reach during laparoscopic exploration.

Wide fenestration technique (Lin procedure) by deroofing the cyst wall using electrocatuery or preferably harmonic shears is a key factor to avoid cyst recurrence, but great care should be taken to stay 1cm away from the parenchymal liver edge in order to avoid bleeding from liver parenchyma.

With proper selection of patients and type of cystic liver disease and meticulous and aggressive surgical techniques, the laparoscopic approach appears to be the gold standard treatment for patients suffering from CLC.

2. Adult polycystic liver disease (APLD)

Adult polycystic liver disease is a rare condition which is difficult to treat, because highly symptomatic cystic hepatomegaly is often associated with severely impaired quality of life and with complicated clinical presentation. The purpose of any treatment option is to reduce significantly the mass effect of this huge polycystic hepatomegaly with a minimal morbidity in order to achieve long-term relief of symptoms and to improve the quality of the patient's life. Wide fenestration is applicable to only APLD type I. Currently, the most appropriate therapeutic approach for APLD remains controversial between open fenestration technique, open partial liver resection or liver transplantation.[114,115] The role of laparoscopy in the management of APLD is very limited.

3. Liver cystadenoma

Liver cystadenoma is a rare cystic neoplasm, characterized by a certain tendency to malignant transformation to cystadenocarcinoma. Complete excision of the lesion is thus the only successful mode of therapy in order to cure the patient, by reducing the possibility of progressive symptomatic enlargement, or secondary infection and of possible malignant transformation. Though open hepatic resection remain the mainstay of surgical therapy for neoplastic liver cysts, in selected cases of lesions located within the liver, laparoscopic approach can be offered.

4. Benign hepatocellular tumors

The indications for surgical resection of benign liver tumors have been progressively restricted and tailored according to each type of liver tumor. Liver haemagioma and focal nodular hyperplasia (FNH) are considered as benign and indolent disease with no risk of malignant transformation or complicated clinical presentation during natural history[116]. Despite a large representation of these tumors in the reported laparoscopic series of liver resection for hepatocellular tumors, these lesions should not be resected even by laparoscopy unless they are responsible for specific disease related symptoms such as pain or compression due to large lesions or in case of enlarging tumor.

Cherqui et al[117] have emphasized the role of laparoscopically guided biopsy to improve diagnostic accuracy before going to laparoscopic resection. But liver cell adenoma (LCA) should be resected irrespective of the presence of symptoms or the tumor size and location because of the risk of its malignant transformation. Selection of patients and liver tumors is a key factor for success of laparoscopic liver resection. The best indications are small, superficial, peripheral lesions, located in the left lateral segments or in the anterior segments of the right part of the liver. Large tumors, tumors close to the hepatic veins or the inferior vena cava, centrally or posteriorly located tumors in the right part of the liver are not ideal candidates for laparoscopic resection. However, the use of a hand-assisted technique was recently reported to facilitate safe access to the posterior and superior part of the right liver.

5. Malignant Tumors

Minimally invasive approach was applied in the managements of malignant hepatic tumors only recently. The reason for reluctancy on the part of surgical fraternity is the concern of complete tumor removal. Of late, studies have shown the feasibility of laparoscopic approach in the managements of malignant liver tumor. Hepatocellular carcinoma and colorectal malignancies which are operable can be offered laparoscopic approach as an alternate to open surgery. But adequate tumor clearance should be obtained in all such cases.

Hepatic Resections

The vast majority of laparoscopic liver resections reported in the literature are minor resections, limited to wedge resections or to removal of one or two liver segments. Left lateral segmentectomy is the anatomical liver resection that is most easily reproducible laparoscopically. Only very few major hepatectomies were done laparoscopically, most of them being performed through the hand-assisted approach.[118-122] Laparoscopic hepatectomy is a technically demanding operation, requiring complex and expensive equipment and instrumentation. Improved instrumentation has contributed to safer laparoscopic hepatectomy although none of these instruments are yet perfect. Intraoperative laparoscopic ultrasonography permits clear visualization of the extent of tumors and their relationship to the hepatic vascular anatomy and permits identification of the plane of resection. The development of flexible ultrasound probes allows the tumor to be visualized. The introduction of the ultrasound scalpel has greatly improved the ability to maintain haemostasis during laparoscopic surgery.

Harmonic Ace (Ethicon), a new version of harmonic scalpel is highly effective in hepatic transection including control of small vessels. This along with CUSA helps in hepatic transection without blood loss. Argon beam coagulator has also shown to reduce blood loss. It allows for rapid and diffuse superficial coagulation at the plane of transection with little carbonization of liver tissue. The use of linear staplers to transect the main hepatic veins makes the parenchymal resection safer and faster.

Intraoperative control of major intrahepatic vessels and application of total vascular isolation techniques though described in open approach are difficult to achieve laparoscopically. Hand-assisted laparoscopic surgery has been developed to facilitate major hepatic resections by improving liver exposure and vascular control and this increases the safety of the procedure.

Gas embolism is a specific potential risk of laparoscopic liver resection, but has never been reported outside the use of the argon beam coagulator.[123] Great care must be applied when using the argon beam coagulator laparoscopically.[124] Major bleeding is also a well-known concern during liver resection and is more difficult to control laparoscopically, being responsible for half of the conversions in the reported series.[119] For this reason, the Pringle maneuver has been used quite often during laparoscopic liver resection as reported by Cherqui et al.[121] Several clinical series have demonstrated the safety and the tolerance of the Pringle manoeuvre when performed laparoscopically.[121,122,125-127] However, this manoeuvre does not seem to be necessary any longer for minor hepatectomies. Biliary leaks and other complications of liver resections should be prevented by precise intrahepatic dissection and clipping. Conversion to an open procedure should not be considered a failure but rather as a good surgical judgment to maintain the safety of the procedure.

A few series comparing laparoscopic with open minor hepatic resections for benign and malignant liver diseases have been reported to date. The laparoscopic group was demonstrated to be associated with a similar complications rate, a decreased blood loss and the usual postoperative functional benefits of minimally invasive surgery.

Advantages

In addition to the usual benefits associated with any minimally invasive approach like less post operative pain, shorter hospital stay, better cosmesis and wound relates problems, laparoscopy offers some other additional advantages when applied to liver malignancies. First the postoperative course after hepatectomy is improved in the cirrhotic patient mainly due to decreased postoperative ascites because of the preservation of abdominal wall allowing a better collaterals venous drainage and improved post operative kinetics of the diaphragm.[128-130] Second, minimal scarring and less adherences, leading to enhanced feasibility of repeat liver resection or transplantation whenever necessary.[131] Third, improved post operative immunity, especially cellular immunity, largely involved in the anti-tumor response.[132,133]

CONCLUSION

A significant benefit of laparoscopic approach for liver resection is the avoidance of a large, disabling subcostal incision, responsible for early and late complications and inconvenience (pain, infection, dehiscence, muscular relaxation, sensitive defect, etc). The laparoscopic approach is an attractive alternative to open surgery for treating liver tumors. Minimally invasive liver surgery is feasible, safe and reproducible. It has to be performed only in highly specialized centres where the necessary equipments are available. In addition the surgeon should be an expert in both hepatic and advanced laparoscopic surgeries.

References

1. Zeret KS. Embyonic development of the liver. In : Arias IM, editor. The liver-biology and pathobiology. 4th edition. Philadelphia : Lippincott Williams & Wilkins; 2001

2. Skandalakis JE, Gray SW, Skandalakis LJ et al. Surgical anatomy of the liver and associated extrahepatic structures. Part 2 - surgical anatomy of the liver

3. Ger R. Surgical anatomy of the liver. Surg Clin N Am 1989;69:179-93

4. Williams PL, Bannister LH, Berry MM, et al, editors. Gray's anatomy of the human body. 38th edition. Edinburgh (UK): Churchill Livingstone; 1995. p.90

5. Basmajian JV, Slonecker CE. Grant's method of anatomy. 11th edition. Baltimore (MD): Williams & Wilkins; 1989. p.76

6. Surgical anatomy of the liver, Surgical Clinics of North America, liver surgery current concepts, April 2004, p 415

7. Mirilas P. Skandalakis JE. Benign anatomical mistakes : right and left coronary ligaments. Am Surg 2002;68:832-5

8. Rex H. Beitrage sur Morphologie der Saugerleber. Morphol Jahrb 1888;14:517

9. Cantlie J. On a new arrangement of the right and left lobes of the liver, J Anat 1897;32:4

10. Bradley O. A contribution to the morphology an development of the mammalian liver. J Anat Physiol 1909;43:1

11. Couinaud C. Lobes et segments hepatiques : note sur l'architecture anatomique et chirurgicale du foie, Presse Med 1954;62:709

12. Goldsmith NA, Woodburne RT. Surgical anatomy pertaining to liver resection. Surg Gynecol Obstet 1957;105:310

13. Bismuth H. Surgical anatomy and anatomical surgery of the liver. World J Surg 1982;6:3-9

14. Healey JE Jr, Schroy PC, Sorensen RJ. The Intrahepatic distribution of the hepatic artery in man. J Int Coll Surg 1953;20:133

15. Michels NA. Newer anatomy of the liver. Philadelphia: WB Saunders; 1965

16. Madding GF, Kennedy PA. Trauma to the liver. Philadelphia: WB Saunders; 1965

17. Couinaud C. Le foie. Paris: Masson et Cie; 1957

18. Hjortsjo CH. The topography of the Intrahepatic duct system. Acta Anat 1951;11:599-615

19. Champetier J. Les voies biliares. In : Chevrel JP, editor. Anatomie Clinique, vol.2: Letronc. Paris: Springer-Verlag France; 1994. p. 407-20

20. Healey JE Jr, Schwartz SI. Surgical anatomy. In : Schwartz SI, editor. Diseases of the liver. New York : McGraw-hill; 1964

21. Nakamura S, TsuzukiT. Surgical anatomy of the hepatic veins and the inferior vena cava. Surg Gynecol Obstet 1981;152:43-50

22. Blumgard, Diseases of the liver and biliary tract, Surgical anatomy of the liver, p 14

23. Blumgard, Diseases of the liver and biliary tract, Surgical anatomy of the liver, p 19

24. Hoff L. Introduction. In: Hoff L, editor. Acoustic characterization of contrast agents for medical ultrasound imaging. Dordrect (Netherlands): Kluwer Academic Publishers; 2001. p 1-6

25. Ralls PW, Jeffrey RB Jr, Kane RA, Robbin M. Ultrasonography. Gastroenterol Clin North Am 2002;31(3):801-25

26. Benson MD, Gandhi MR. Ultrasound of the Hepatobiliary-pancreatic system. World J Surg 2000;24(2):166-70

27. Zacerl J, Scheuba C, Imhof M, Zacherl M, Langle F, Pokieser P, et al : Current value of intraoperative sonography during surgery for hepatic neoplasms. World J Surg 2002; 26(5):550-4

28. Machi J, Sigel B, Zaren HA, Kurohiji T, Yamashita Y. Operative ultrasonography during Hepatobiliary and pancreatic surgery. World J Surg 1993;17(5):640-5

29. Machi J, Sigel B. Intraoperative ultrasonography. Radiol Clin N Am 1992;30(5): 1085-103

30. Conlon R, Jacobs M, Dasgupta D, Lodge JP. The value of intraoperative ultrasound during hepatic resection compared with improved preoperative magnetic resonance imaging. Eur J Ultrasound 2003;16(3):211-6

31. Jarnagin WR, Bach AM, Winston CB, Hann LE, Heffernan N, Loumeau T, et al. What is the yield of intraoperative ultrasonography during partial hepatectomy for malignant disease? J Am Coll Surg 2001;192(5):577-83

32. Padhani AR, Dixon AK. Whole body computed tomography: recent developments. In:Grainger RG, Allison DJ, Adam A, Dixon AK, editors. Diagnostic radiology-a textbook of medical imaging, 4th edition, vol.1 London: Churchill Livingstone; 2001. p81-99

33. Silverman PM. Preface. In: Silverman PM. Editor. Multislice computed tomography – a practical approach to clinical protocols. Philadelphia: Lippincott Williams and Wilkins; 2002. p. xiii

34. Teefey SA, Hildeboldt CC, Dehdashti F, Siegel BA, Peters MG, Heiken JP et al. Detection of primary hepatic malignancy in liver transplant candidates: prospective comparison of CT, MR imaging, US and pet. Radiology 2003;226(2):533-42

35. Laghi A, Iannaccone R, Rossi P, Carbone I, et al. Hepatocellular carcinoma: detection with triple-phase multi-detector row helical CT in patients with chronic hepatitis. Radiology 2003;226(2):543-9

36. Klingenbeck-Regn K, Schaller S, Flohr T, Ohnesorge B, Kopp AF, Baum U. Subsecond multi-slice computed tomography; basics and applications. Eur J Radiol 1999;31(2):110-24

37. Kang HK, Jeong YY, Choi JH, Choi S, Chung TW, Seo JJ, et al. Three-dimensional multi-detector row CT portal venography in the evaluation of portosystemic collateral vessels in liver cirrhosis. Radiographics 2002;22(5);1053-61

38. Funke M, Kopka L, Grabbe E. Biphasic contrast-enhanced multislice helical CT of the liver. In: Silverman PM, editor. Multislice computed tomography – a practical approach to clinical protocols. Philadelphia: Lippincott Williams and Wilkins; 2002. p. 35-8

39. Wong K, Paulson EK, Nelson RC. Breath-hold three-dimensional CT of the liver with multidetector row helical CT. Radiology 2001;215(1):55-62

40. Rydberg J, Buckwalter KA, Caldemeyer KS, Philips MD, et al. Multisection CT : scanning techniques and clinical applications. Radiographics 2000; 20(6):1787-806

41. Grainger RG. Intravascular radiological iodinated contrast media. In: Grainger RG, Allison DJ, Adam A, Dixon AK. Editors. Diagnostic radiology-a textbook of medical imaging. Vol.1. 4th edition. London:Churchill Livinstone; 2001 p.27-41

42. Katayama H, Yamaguchi K, Kozuka T, Takashima T, Seez P, Matsuura K. Adverse reactions to ionic and non-ionic contrast media. A report from the Japanese Committee on the Safety of Contrast Media. Radiology 1990;175(3):621-8

43. Larson RE, Semelka RC, Bagley AS, Molina PL, Brown ED, Lee JK. Hypervascular malignant liver lesions: comparison of various MR imaging pulse sequences and dynamic CT. Radiology 1994;192(2):393-9

44. Low RN. MR imaging of the liver using gadolinium chelates. Magn Reson Imaging 1997;7(1); 56-67

45. Low RN. MR imaging of the liver using gadolinium chelates. Magn Reson Imaging Clin N Am 2001;9(4):717-43

46. Miller WJ, Baron RL, Dodd GD 3ʳᵈ, Federle MP. Malignancies in patients with cirrhosis: CT sensitivity and specificity in 200 consecutive transplant patients. Radiology 1994;193:645-50

47. Oi H, Murakami T, Kim T, Matsushita M, Kishimoto H, Nakamura H. Dynamic MR imaging and early-phase helical CT for detecting small Intrahepatic metastases of hepatocellular carcinoma. AJR Am J Roentegenol 1996;166(2):369-74

48. Pedro MS, Semelka RC, Braga L. MR Imaging of hepatic metastases. Magn Reson Imaging Clin N Am 2002;10(1):15-29

49. Rode A, Bancel B, Douek P, Chevallier M, Vilgrain V, Picaud G, et al. Small nodule detection in cirrhotic livers: evaluation with US, spiral CT and MRI and correlation with pathologic examination of explanted liver. J Comput Assist Tomogr 2001; 25(3):327-36

50. Semelka RC, Shoenut JP, Kroeker MA, Greenberg HM, Simm FC, Minuk GY, et al. Focal liver disease: comparison of dynamic contrast-enhanced CT and T2-weighted fat-suppressed, FLASH and dynamic gadolinium-enhanced MR imaging at 1.5T Radiology 1992;184(3):687-94

51. Semelka RC, Shoenut JP, Ascher SM, Koreker MA, Greenberg HM, Yaffe CS, et al. Solitary hepatic metastasis: comparison of dynamic contrast-enhanced CT and MR imaging with fat-suppressed T2-weighted, breath-hold T1-weighted FLASH, and dynamic gadolinium-enhanced FLASH sequences. J Magn Reson Imaging 1994;4(3):319-23

52. Semelka RC, Worawattanakul S, Kelekis NL, John G, Woosley JT, Graham M, et al. Liver lesion detection, characterization, and effect on patient management; comparison of single phase spiral CT and current MR techniques. J Magn Reson Imaging 1997;7(6):1040-7

53. Semelka RC, Helmberger TK, Contrast agents for MR imaging of the liver. Radiology 2001;218(1):27-38

54. Semelka RC, Braga L, Armao D, Martin DR, Bader T, Beavers KL, et al. Liver. In: Semelka RC, editor. Abdominal-pelvic MRI. New York: Wiley-Liss; 2002. p.33-317

55. Yamashita Y, Mitsuzaki K, Yi T, Ogata I, Nishiharu T, Urata J, et al. Small hepatocellular carcinoma in patients with chronic liver damage: prospective comparison of detection with dynamic MR imaging and helical CT of the whole liver. Radiology 1996;200(1):79-84

56. Libberecht L, Bielen D, Verslype C, Vanbeckevoort D, Pirenne J, Nevens F, et al. Focal lesions in cirrhotic explant livers; pathological evaluation and accuracy of pretransplantation imaging examinations. Liver Transpl 2002;8(9):749-61

57. Kinkel K. Lu Y, Both M, Warren RS, Thoeni RF. Detection of hepatic metastases from cancers of the gastrointestinal tract by using noninvasive imaging methods (US, CT, MR Imaging PET): a meta-analysis. Radiology 2002:224(3):748-56

58. Desai DC, Zervos EE, Arnold MW, Burak WE. Mantil J, Martin EW Jr. Positron emission tomography affects surgical management in recurrent colorectal cancer patients. Ann Surg Oncol 2003;10(1):59-64

59. Rydzewski B, Dehdashti F, Gordon BA, Teefey SA, Strasberg SM. Siegel BA. Usefulness of intraoperative sonography for revealing hepatic metastases from colorectal cancer in patients selected for surgery after undergoing FDG PET. Am J Roentgenol 2002;178:353-8

60. Johnson DL, Martin WH, Delbeke D. Other gastrointestinal tumors. In: Delbeke D. Martin WH, Patton JA, Sandler MP, editors. Practical FDG imaging – a teaching file. New York: Springer-Verlag; 2002. p 236-79

61. MacManus MP, Hicks RJ, Matthews JP, Hogg A, McKenzie AF, Wirth A, et al. high rate of detection of unsuspected distant metastases by PET in apparent stage III non-small-cell lung cancer: implications for radical radiation therapy. Int J Radiat Oncol Biol Phys 2001;50(2):287-93

62. Hsia TC, Shen YY, Yen RF, Kao CH, Changlai SP. Comparing whole body 18F-2-deoxyglucose positron emission tomography and technetium-99m methylene diophosphate bone scan to detect bone metastases in patients with non-small cell lung cancer. Neoplasma 2002;49(4):267-71

63. Vijay P., Khatri, Philip D. Schneider. Liver Surgery: Modern Concepts and Techniques. Surgical Clinics of North America, April 2004, Vol84, Number 2, p360

64. Kanematsu T, Takenaka K. Matsumata T, Furuta T, Sugimachi K, Inokuchi K. Limited hepatic resection effective for selected cirrhotic patients with primary liver cancer. Ann Surg 1984;199(1):51-6

65. Lee CS, Sung JL, Hwang LY, Sheu JC, Chen DS, Lin TY, et al. Surgical treatment of 109 patients with symptomatic and asymptomatic heaptocelular carcinoma. Surgery 1986; 99(4):481-90

66. Tso J1, Asbun HJ, Hughes KS, Abaubara S, August DA, Azurin A, et al. Hepatoma registry of the Western world. Repeat hepatic Resection Registry. Cancer Treat Res 1994; 69:21-31

67. Arii S, Okamoto E, Imamura M. Registries in Japan: current status of hepatocellular carcinoma in Japan. Liver Cancer Study Group of Japan. Semin Surg Oncol 1996;12(3): 204-11

68. Nonami T, Nakao A, Kurokawa T, Inagaki H, Matsushita Y, Sakamoto J, et al. Blood loss and ICG clearance as best prognostic markers of psot-heaptectomy liver failure. Hepatogastroentrology 1999;46(27):1669-72

69. Franco D, Capussotti L, Smadja C, Bouzari H, Meakins J, Kemeny F, et al. Resection of hepatocellular carcinomas. Results in 72 European patients with cirrhosis. Gastroenterology 1990;98(3):733-8

70. Wheeler HO, Cranston WI, Meltzer JI. Hepatic uptake and biliary excretion of indocyanine green in the dog. Proc Soc Exp Biol Med 1958;99-236

71. Amaral JF. Laparoscopic application of an ultrasonically activated scalpel. Gastrointest Clin North Am 1993;3:381-392

72. Mueller W. The advantages of laparoscopic assisted bipolar high frequency surgery. Endosc Surg 1993;1:96-96

73. Pearce JA. Cutting and coagulating processes. In: Pearce JA, ed. Electrosurgery. New York: Wiley:62-128

74. Hambley R, Debda PA. Abell E, et al. Wound healing of skin incisions produced by ultrasonically vibrating knife, scalpel, electrosurgery and carbon dioxide laser. J Dermatol Surg Oncol 1988;14:11

75. Meltzer RC, Hoenig DM, Chrostek C, et al. Porcine seromyotomies using an ultrasonically activated scalpel. Surg Endosc 1194:8:253

76. Hoenig DM, chrostek CA, Amaral JF. Laparosonic coagulating shears: alterntive method of hemostatic control of unsupported tissue. J Endourol 1996;10:431-433

77. Marinkovic S, Chrostek CA, Amaral JF, Surgical laparoscopic energy and lateral thermal damage. Minimally Invs Ther 1994;4:333

78. Ott DE, Moss E, Matrinez K. Aerosol exposure from an ultrasonically activated (harmonic) device. J am Assoc Gynecol Laparosc 1998:5:29-32

79. Zucker et al. Text book of surgical laparoscopy. Electro cautry and special instruments. 72.

80. Hodgson WJ, Poddar PK, Mencer EJ, et al. Evaluation of ultrasonically powered instruments in the laboratory and clinical setting. Am J Gastroenterol 1979;72:133-140

81. Vaxquez Jm, Eisenberg E, O'Steen KG, et al Laparoscopic ablation of endometriosis using the cavitational ultrasonic surgical aspirator. J Am Assoc Gynecol Laparosc 1993;1:36-42

82. Hodgson WJ, Morgan J, Byrne D, et al. Hepatic resections for primary and metastatic tumors using the ultrasonic surgical dissector Am J Surg 1992;163:246-250

83. Fasano VA, Zemi S, Frego L, et al. Ultrasonic aspiration in the surgical treatment of intracranial tumors. J Neurosurg Sci 1981;25:35-40

84. Chopp RT, Shah BB, Addonizio JC. Use of ultrasonic surgical aspirator in renal surgery. Urology 1983;22:157-159

85. Transberg KG, Rigotti P, Brackett KA, et al. Liver resection: a comparison using the Nd-YAG laser, an ultrasonic surgical aspirator or blunt dissection, Am J Surg 1986; 151;368-373

86. The plasma scalpel : a new thermal knife lasers surg Med 1982; 2(1):101-6

87. Heneford BT, Mathews BD, Sing RF, Backus C, P rat B, Greene FL, Surg. Endosc 2001. 15:799-801

88. Kennedy JS, Stranmoahn PL, Taylor KD, Chandla JG, Surg Endosc 1998; 12:876-878

89. Peterson SL, Stranahan PL, Schmaltr D, Mihaichuk C, Cospify N, Surg Technol lat 2002; 10:55-60

90. Horgan PG. A novel technique for parenchymal division during hepatectomy, Am J Surg 2001, 181:236-237

91. Ravikumar TS, Buenaventura S, salem RR et al. Intraoperative ultrasonography of liver: detection of occult liver tumors and treatment by cryosurgery. Cancer Detect Prev 1994;18:131-8

92. Wernecke K, Rummeny E, Bongartz G, et al. Detection of hepatic masses in pateitns with carcinoma: comparative sensitivities of sonography, CT and MR imaging. AJR Am J Roentgenol 1991;157:731-9

93. Clarke MP, Kane RA, Steele G Jr, et al. Prospective comparison of preoperative imaging and intraoperative ultrasonography in the detection of liver tumors. Surgery 1989;106:849-55

94. Knol JA, Marn CS, Francis IR, et al. Comparisons of dynamic infusion and delayed computed tomography, intraoperative ultrasound, and palpation in the diagnosis of lvier metastases. Am J Surg 1993;165:81-8

95. Machi J, Sigel B. Operative ultrasound in general surgery. Am J Surg 1996;172:15-20

96. Boggs RR, Rouch DA, Chua GT. Intraoperative ultrasound of hepatic tumors. Indiana Med 1992;85:496-8

97. Bismuth H. Castaing D, Garden J. The use of intraoperative ultrasound in surgery of primary liver tumors. World J Surg 1987;11:610-4

98. Parker G, Lawrence W, Horsley S, et al. Intraoperative ultrasound of the liver affects operative decision making. Ann surg 1989;209:569-77

99. Haider MA, Leonhardt C, Hanna SS, et al. The role of intraoperative ultrasonography in planning the rsection of hepatic neoplasms. Can Assoc Radiol J 1995;46:98-104

100. Cervone A, Sardi A, Conaway GL. Intraoperative ultrasound (IOUS) is essential in the management of metastatic colorectal liver lesions. Am Surg 2000;66:611-5

101. Hartley JE, Kumar H, Drew PJ, et al. Laparoscopic ultrasound for the detection of hepatic metastases during laparoscopic colorectal cancer surgery. Dis Colon Rectum 2000;43:320-4

102. Barbot DJ, Marks JH, Feld RI, et al. Improved staging of liver tumors using laparoscopic intraoperative ultrasound. J Surg Oncol 1997;64:63-7

103. Cuschieri A. Laparoscopic management of cancer patients. J R Coll Surg Edinb 1995;40: 1-9

104. Hunderbein M, Rau B, Schlag PM. Laparoscopy and laparoscopic ultrasound for staging of upper gastrointestinal tumors. Eur J Surg Oncol 1995;21:50-5

105. Gouma DJ, De Wit LT, Nieveen van Dijkum E, et al. Laparoscopic ultrasonography for staging of gastrointestinal cancer: comparative accuracy with traditional procedures. Surg Laparosc Endosc 1995;5:176-82

106. Golretti O, Buccianti P, Chiarugi M, et al. Laparoscopic sonography in screening metastases from gastrointestinal cancer: comparative accuracy with traditional rpoceudres. Surg Laparosc Endosc 1995;5:176-82

107. Machi J, Oishi AJ, Mossing AJ, et al. Hand-assisted laparoscopic ultrasound-guided radiofrequency thermal ablation of liver tumors: a technical report. Surg Laparosc Endosc Percutan Tech 2002;12:160-4

108. Cuschieri A, Bracken J, Boni L. Initial experience with laparoscopic ultrasound-guided radiofrequency thermal ablation of hepatic tumors. Endoscopy 1999;31:318-21

109. Machi J, Uchida S, Sumida K et al. Ultrasound-guided radiofrequency thermal ablation of liver tumors: percutaneous, laparoscopic, and open surgical approaches. J Gastrointst Surg 2001;5:477-89

110. John TG, Grieg JD, Crosbie JL, et al. Superior staging of liver tumors with laparoscopy and laparoscopic ultrasound. Ann Surg 1994;220:711-9

111. Gigot JF, Legrand M, Hubens G, et al. Laparoscopic treatment of nonparasitic liver cysts: adequate selection of patients and surgical technique. World J Surg 1996;2O: 556-61.

112. Morino M, Garrone C, Fcsta V, Miglietta C. Traitement coelioscopique des kystes non parasitaires du foie. Ann Chir 1996;5O:419-30.

113. Couinaud C. Le Foie. Etudes Anatomiques et Chirurgicales. Paris: Masson, 1957.

114. Starzl TE, Reyes J, Tzakis A, Mieles L, Todo S, Gordon R. Liver transplantation for polycystic liver disease. Arch Surg 1990;125:575-7.

115. Lang H, Woellwarth JV, Oldhafer KJ, et al. Liver transplantation in patients with polycystic liver disease. Transplant Proc 1997:29:2832-3.

116. Trastck VF, Van Heerden JA, Sheedy PF, Adson MA. Cavernous hemangioma of the liver: resect or observe? Am J Surg 1983;145:49-53.

117. Cherqui D, Rahmouni A, Charlotte F, et al. Management of focal nodular hyperplasia and hepatocellular adenoma in young women: a series of 41 patients with clinical, radiological and pathological correlations. Hepatology 1995;22:1674-81.

118. Descottes B Lachachi F, Sodji M, et al. Early experience with laparoscopic approach for solid liver tumors: initial 16 cases. Ann Surg 2000;232:641-5.

119. Descottes B, Glineur D, Lachachi F, et al. Laparoscopic liver resection of benign liver tumors: results of a multicenter European experience. Surg Endosc 2003; 17: 23-30.

120. Huscher CGS, Lirici MM, Chiodini S. Laparoscopic liver resections. Semin Laparosc Surg 1998;5:204-10.

121. Cherqui D, Husson E, Hammoud R, et al. Laparoscopic liver resections: a feasibility study in 30 patients. Ann Surg 2000;232:753-62.

122. Huscher CGS, Lirici MM, Chiodini S, Recher A. Current position of advanced laparoscopic surgery of the liver. J R Coll Surg Edinb 1997;42:219-25.

123. Croce E, Azzola M, Russo R, Golia M, Angelini S, Olmi S. Laparoscopic liver tumor resection with the Argon Beam. Endosc Surg 1994;2:186-8.

124. Hashizume M, Takenaka K, Yanaga M, et al. Laparoscopic hepatic resection for hepatocellular carcinoma. Surg Endosc 1995:9:1289-91.

125. Farges O, Jagot P, Kirstettcr P, Marty J, Belghiti J. Prospective assessment of the safety and benefit of laparoscopic liver resection, j Hepatobiliary Pancreat Surg 2002;9:242-8.

126. Lesurtel M, Cherqui D, Laurent A, Tayar C, Fagniez PL. Laparoscopic versus open left lateral hepatic lobectomy: a case control study, j Am Coll Surg 2003;2:236-42.

127. Decaillot F, Cherqui D, Leroux B, et al. Effects of portal triad clamping on haemodynamic conditions during laparoscopic liver resection. Br J Anaesth 2001;87:493-6.

128. Abdel-Atty MY, Farges O, Jagot P, Belghiti J. Laparos opy extends the indications for liver resection in patients with cirrhosis. Br J Surg 1999;86:1397-400.

129. Frazee RC, Roberts JW, Okeson GC, et al. Open versus laparoscopic cholecystectomy. A comparison of postoperative pulmonary function. Ann Surg 1991.; 213: 651-3; discussion 653-4.

130. Laurent A, Cherqui D, Lesurtel M, Brunetti F, Tayar C, Fagniez PL. Laparoscopic liver resection for subcapsular hepatocellular carcinoma complicating chronic liver disease. Arch Surg 2003; 138:763-9; discussion 769.

131. Burpee SE, Kurian M, Murakame Y, Benevides S, Gagner M. The metabolic and immune response to laparoscopic versus open liver resection. Surg Endosc 2002;16:899-904.

132. Tsuchiya Y, Sawada S, Yoshioka I, et al. Increased surgical stress promotes tumor metastasis. Surgery 2003; 133:547-55.

133. Vittimbcrga FJ Jr. Foley DP, Meyers WC, Gallery MP.Laparoscopic surgery and the systemic immune response. Ann Surg 1998;227:326-34.

47

Laparoscopic Management of Benign Non-parasitic Hepatic Cysts

INTRODUCTION

Hepatic cysts are rare. They are usually fortuitous discoveries by the surgeon when operating for some other conditions. With the easy availability and use of non-invasive imaging tools, especially ultrasonography, their frequency is rising. However, most cases are either detected incidentally during imaging or when they become symptomatic. The most common non-parasitic hepatic cyst is the congenital or developmental cyst.[1] These can be further divided into sporadic and polycystic variants. Polycystic liver disease is distinct from simple liver cyst and has a genetic basis. The causative gene in polycystic kidney disease has recently been characterized[2] and is likely to be responsible for polycystic disease of the liver and other organs.[3] Whereas childhood polycystic disease is inherited as an autosomal recessive disorder and affects mainly the liver and the kidney, adult polycystic disease is inherited as an autosomal dominant disorder and affects the spleen, pancreas, ovaries, lungs and kidneys apart from the liver. An isolated form of adult polycystic liver disease has also been identified.[4] However, since laparoscopy plays a role in the management of primarily sporadic hepatic cysts, only this disease shall be discussed in detail here.

Classification of Cystic Lesions of the Liver

A. Congenital Hepatic Cysts:

 (i) Sporadic

 (ii) Polycystic liver disease.

B. Post-traumatic cysts: Pseudocysts.

C. Ductal Origin:

 (i) Choledochal cyst.

 (ii) Caroli's disease.

 (iii) Bile duct duplication.

D. Parasitic: Echinococcal cyst (hydatid disease)

E. Neoplastic:

   (i)   Primary

          (a) Cystadenomas

          (b) Cystadenocarcinomas

          (c) Cystic sarcomas

   (ii) Metastatic

HISTORICAL PERSPECTIVES

The first case of non-parasitic cystic disease of the liver was reported by Bristowe in 1856[5] and he stressed on its association with polycystic liver disease. Michel recoded the first sporadic non-paracytic hepatic cyst in the same year. Lin et al first described the technique of fenestration or deroofing of the cysts in 1968.[6] Laparoscopic management was first reported in 1991 by two separate groups.[7,8] However, laparoscopy was used before this for diagnosis of this condition. The first use of diagnostic laparoscopy for hepatic cyst was documented in 1955.[9] In fact, laparoscopy ultrasonography was used for diagnosis of liver disorders as early as 1989.[10]

SYNONYMS

Biliary cyst, non-parasitic cyst of the liver , benign hepatic cyst, congenital hepatic cyst, unilocular cyst of the liver, solitary cyst of the liver.

INCIDENCE

The true incidence of this disease is difficult to estimate as it is usually is asymptomatic in most of the patients. Between 1-5% of the population may have asymptomatic disease, with an increasing incidence with age.[11,12] The female to male ratio is 1.5:1 in asymptomatic simple cysts but increases to 9:1 for symptomatic or complicated cysts.[13] The cysts are larger in adults older than 50 years of age and in women.[12]

ETIOLOGY

Several theories have been proposed to explain the development of congenital hepatic cysts. The most prevalent theory is an aberration in the embryologic bile duct differentiation. Normally, there is an excess of bile duct formation in the embryo, most of which undergoes degeneration during differentiation. Failure of the normal degeneration of the bile ductules in the embryo may be responsible for the cystic lesions of the liver. Another theory proposes that some aberrant bile duct loses communication with the biliary tree during development and this results in obstruction and inflammatory hyperplasia with subsequent dilatation.

SURGICAL PATHOLOGY

The cyst is spherical or ovoid and varies in size from a few mm. to several cms. It is unilocular and does not communicate with the biliary system. As it grows, it causes atrophy of the hepatic parenchyma, sparing the vessels and bile ducts, which may then protrude and produce folds on the inner aspect of the cyst. In absence on intracystic bleeding, the cyst fluid is clear and contains water and electrolytes without bile acids and bilirubin, similar to the normal secretion of the biliary epithelium. In majority of the patients, the cyst is solitary. However, rarely, they can be multiple, making gross differentiation from polycystic liver disease difficult. The cyst wall is lined by a single layer of cuboidal or columnar epithelium, similar to bile ducts.

CLINICAL FEATURES

Most cases are asymptomatic, with clinical symptoms occurring in only 5% of patients. Symptoms present in the later stages of life with the mean age of onset of symptoms being in the fifth decade. The commonest symptoms include abdominal pain, feeling of fullness or early satiety. Patients present clinically with abdominal pain, mass or pressure effects in equal proportions. Only cysts of fairly large dimensions may cause sufficient hepatomegaly as to be palpable. Sudden severe upper abdominal pain may occur due to intracystic bleeding, perforation or torsion of a peduculated cyst. Pressure on the adjacent stomach may cause early satiety, vomiting and weight loss.

Complications of Congenital Hepatic Cysts

1. Intracystic bleeding.
2. Cyst perforation.
3. Torsion of peduculated cyst.
4. Infection.
5. Malignant degeneration.
6. Compression of inferior vena cava.
7. Fistulization into the duodenum.
8. Communication with an intrahepatic duct.
9. Cholestasis due to CBD compression.
10. Portal hypertension due to portal vein compression.

INVESTIGATIONS

1. **Blood tests:** Usually normal, except rarely in late cases where a majority of the liver has undergone pressure atrophy.

2. **Ultrasonography (USG):** The gold standard. In addition to the diagnosis, provides information about the cyst wall, fluid content and surrounding liver content.

3. **Computed Tomography (CT):** Accurate imaging, only when some confusion persists after USG.

4. **MRI:** Not done routinely.

5. **Radionuclide liver scan :** shows 'cold' areas in the liver. No extra information.

6. **White blood cell (WBC) scan:** This is to confirm infected cyst.

7. **Chest X-ray & Barium Examination of the**

GIT: - To assess the mass effect of the cyst on adjacent organs - not very useful.

8. **Angiography:** It shows avascular lesions - not much role after the advent of CT & Color Doppler USG.

9. **Hydatid serology:** This is to differentiate from hydatid cysts, especially in patients belonging to areas endemic for echinococcosis.

10. **Laparoscopic Ultrasound:** For the detection of deep-seated small cysts.

DIFFERENTIAL DIAGNOSIS

It is usually easy to distinguish congenital hepatic cysts from other cystic lesions of the liver like abcess, necrotic malignant tumour, large hemangioma and hematomas. However, three lesions may sometimes be confused with congenital hepatic cysts.

Firstly, hepatic metastases of neuroendocrine tumors can sometimes be difficult of differentiate from congenital hepatic cysts.

Secondly, hydatid cysts may be confused with congenital hepatic cysts under the following circumstances:

1. Hydatid disease may occur in a patient belonging to a non-endemic area.

2. Unilocular, non-calcified hydatid cysts.

3. Two or more contiguous liver cysts may mimic septations of hydatid cyst.

4. Intracystic clots in congenital hepatic cysts may mimic hydatid cyst with split wall or daughter cysts.

5. Negative serology in hydatid patients.

	Congenital Hep. Cyst	Hydatid Cyst
Septations	Absent	Common
Calcifications	Absent	Common
Split Walls	Absent	Possible
Cyst-biliary Communication	Absent	Possible
Serological Test	Negative	Positive (Usually)

In such cases, microscopic examination of the aspirated cystic fluid is the confirmatory test.

Thirdly, multiple congenital hepatic cysts may be confused with polycystic disease of the liver. In polycystic disease, usually, kidney is also affected. Moreover, either a parent or a sibling of a patient of polycystic disease may be a known sufferer of the same disease.

TREATMENT

Intervention for simple cysts is indicated only in symptomatic patients. Surgery is the mainstay of therapy. Since the first reported use of laparoscopy in the management of this disease, it has become the procedure of choice.[14,15,16]

Team Set-up

The operating surgeon and the camera surgeon stand on the left of the patient facing the monitor, while the assistant surgeon stands on the left.

Ports

1. 10mm camera port in the umbilicus or supra-umbilically, depending on the position of the cyst.

2. 10 mm right hand working port in the left upper quadrant of the patient, the exact site determined by the size and location of the cyst.

3. 5 mm left hand working port in the right upper quadrant of the patient.

Instruments

Apart from the routine set, we use a special trocar-cannula set designed by ourselves for spillage-free decompression of the cyst because hydatid cyst can easily mimic a congenital hepatic cyst, with only histopathological examination of the cyst wall and cytological examination of the fluid providing the final diagnosis. For excision of the cyst wall, a good bipolar cautery forceps, the Harmonic Scalpel or Ligasure is needed.

Operative Technique

After the introduction of the camera port, the cyst is identified. The right and left hand working ports are

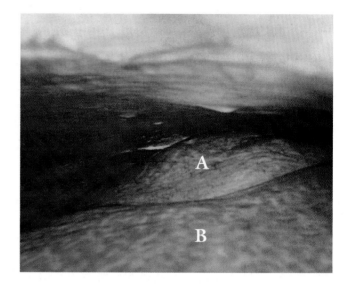

Figure 1 : Large cyst in the segment VII and VIII

A - Cyst
B - Liver

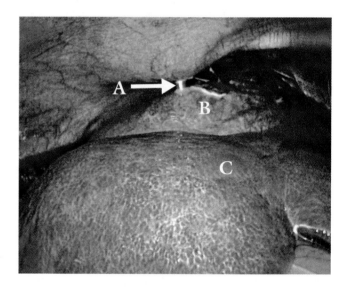

Figure 2 : 5 mm trocar is introduced into the cyst under laparoscopic guidance

A - 5 mm trocar
B - Cyst
C - Liver

inserted under vision. The Veres needle is used to puncture the cyst and aspirate fluid to confirm the absence of biliary staining. Alternately, if a hydatid cyst cannot be ruled out, the hydatid trocar-cannula specially designed by us is used for punctured and aspirating the cyst. Once the possibility of hydatid cyst is ruled out, the cyst wall is excised using Harmonic Scalpel or Ligasure 2-3mm from the hepatic parenchyma-cyst wall junction. If a large part of cyst is extending above the liver, excision of the cyst wall will result in wide opening of the cyst cavity and no further procedure is required. If the cyst wall is largely intrahepatic, excision of the external cyst wall will create a small opening in the cyst wall relative to the size of the cyst cavity. In such cases, we prefer to obliterate the cavity by omentopexy. After confirming hemostasis, a drain is placed intra-abdominally as there can be a temporary serous secretion from the cyst.

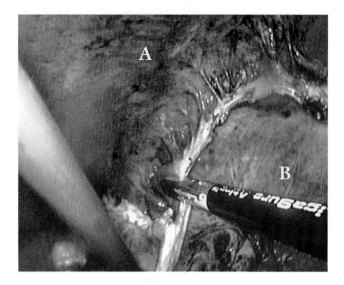

Figure 4 : Marsupialization of cyst is done using Ligasure

A - Diaphragm

B - Cyst cavity

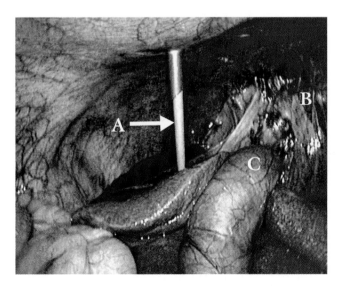

Figure 3 : Contents of the cyst is aspirated. Area of the liver occupied by the cyst is seen

A - 5 mm suction cannula

B - Collapsed cyst

C - Gall bladder

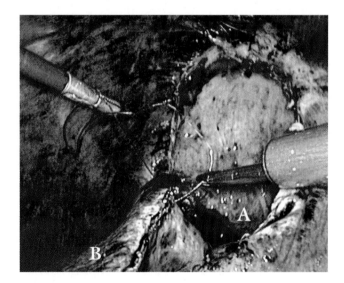

Figure 5 : Edges of the liver surface is sutured using 2 0 vicryl, continuous stitches for hemostasis and to prevent bile leak

A - Cyst cavity

B - Liver

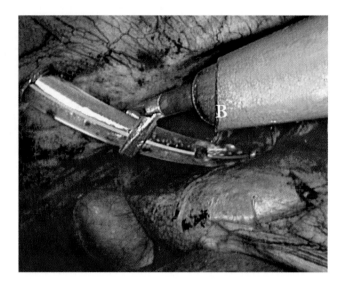

Figure 6 : Placement of drainage tube in the subdiaphragmatic space

RESULTS

We have performed laparoscopic fenestration of simple hepatic cysts in 27 patients of which there were 22 males and 5 females. Of the 27 patients, 17 patients were symptomatic complaining of distension of abdomen; vague abdominal pain, aching in nature or heaviness in the upper abdomen. In 11 patients, simultaneous cholecystectomy was performed for incidental cholelithiasis. Omentopexy was carried out in 16 patients. All our patients had a single cyst. Right sided cysts were overwhelmingly common, constituting 20 of our patients, with only 7 patients having a cyst in the left lobe of the liver.

In addition to this, we have come across five patients in whom there was a thick walled cyst in the right lobe of the liver. Thick yellow fluid was aspirated containing shiny flecks, which on microscopy were proved to be cholesterol crystals. Histopathological examination of the excised cyst wall established a diagnosis on intra-hepatic choledochal cysts, sequestered from the biliary tree.

The follow-up period has ranged from 12 years to two months with an average follow-up of 7.2 years. There have been no recurrence till date.

DISCUSSION

The detection of cysts had increased with the advent and routine use of ultrasound and CT scan. They may also present as a result of complications described above. Even in large cysts, surgical intervention is indicated only in symptomatic patients. However, before surgical therapy, hydatid disease must be ruled out, especially, in patients residing in endemic areas or having traveled from endemic areas. Other cystic lesions must also be excluded such as cystadenoma and cystadenocarcinoma where cyst septations, papillary structures or multiloculated cystic formation may be seen radiologically.[17,18]

Though the common age of presentation is late in life, giant hepatic cyst has been diagnosed in the fetus in-utero.[19] Expectant management by repeated trans-uterine aspirations till term followed by laparoscopic management in the neonatal period has been advised. Despite improvement in imaging techniques, the probability of preoperatively mistaking a hydatid liver cyst for a simple liver cyst remains about 5%.[20] Therefore, laparoscopic fenestration, planned for a liver cyst could be performed unintentionally for an undiagnosed hydatid liver cyst. The risk of misdiagnosing a hydatid liver cyst for a simple liver cyst, especially in the presence of a solitary cyst, should be considered before laparoscopic fenestration is performed. Due to this reason, we advocate using the Palanivelu Hydatid System for spillage-free aspiration of the fluid in all suspicious cases. Intraoperative aspiration of cyst fluid before fenestration can minimize this risk, thus avoiding severe intraoperative and late complications.

Percutaneous aspiration of cyst content is the simplest treatment for symptomatic, non-parasitic cysts. However, this is associated with a high rate of recurrence[17,30,31] as well as a considerable risk of infection. Non-surgical management in the form of percutaneous aspiration under USG guidance followed by injection of sclerosant like ethanol or minocycline has been advocated.[21-24] Cyst sclerosis has been found to have a success rate of 65-95% in obliteration of the cyst and in the relief of symptoms produced by the cyst with a fairly low complication rate.[22,25-28] It is essential to rule out cystadenoma, malignancy, biliary communication and infection before attempting sclerotherapy. Surgery is indicated if the above conditions cannot be ruled out, in the presence of biliary communication, in those cysts where sclerosis has been ineffective and in cases of recurrence. Complications of ethanol sclerosis include severe abdominal pain during injection due to extravasation of ethanol into peritoneal cavity, transient neuropsychiatric disorders due to absorption of ethanol into the blood and cyst inflammation. Minocycline is associated with lesser complications making it a more popular sclerosant. The drawback of this method is absence of histopathological confirmation of the diagnosis. Though long-term follow-up is not available, medium-term results over a median of 35-41 months are good.[29]

Surgical procedures described for treatment for liver cysts include intra-operative aspiration, unroofing, cystojejunostomy, total excision of cyst, partial liver resection, hepatic lobectomy and liver transplantation. Since the first report of laparoscopic management of congenital hepatic cyst, it has become the preferred mode of management of this disease.

Indications of laparoscopic management of benign non-parasitic hepatic cysts:[23,32-35]

1. Symptomatic or complicated cyst located in the anterior liver segments - III, IV, V & VI.

2. A dominant enlarged symptomatic cyst of polycystic liver disease located in the above segments.

3. Cyst-biliary communication.

4. Failure of sclerosis.

5. Recurrent cyst after sclerosis or prior laparoscopic management.

The contra-indications to laparoscopic management have also been defined:[23, 32, 34,36,37]

1. When cystadenoma or malignancy is suspected.

2. Posteriorly located cysts.

3. Multiple small cysts.

4. Previous upper abdominal surgery (relative contraindication).

Author	Patients (n)	Patients Requiring Conversion (n)	Maximum Follow-up (Months)	Recurrence (n)
Fabiani et al (1991)[7]	4	0	15	0
Albrink et al (1994)[56]	4	0	-	0
Morino et al (1994)[33]	4	0	22	1
Gigot et al (1996)[54]	17	2	48	3
Zacherl et al (1996)[57]	4	0	41	0
Cala et al (1996)[58]	3	0	6	0
Koperna et al (1997)[59]	10	1	-	1
Emmermann et al (1997)[36]	18	1	43	2
Martin et al (1998)[34]	13	0	80	1
Diez et al (1998)[60]	9	0	36	1
Marks et al (1998)[37]	10	1	67	0
Palanivelu et al (2005)	27	0	144	0

Laparoscopic management of the cyst consists of cyst fenestration wherein the protruding wall of the cyst is widely excised to allow the cyst to drain intraperitoneally and cyst excision. Though cyst excision has been performed for congenital solitary hepatic cysts,[34,38,39,51] it may be difficult if the cyst is large and is centrally placed because of the proximity of biliary radicles and blood vessels. The excised edge must be oversewn or cauterized for Hemostasis, and the cyst cavity must be inspected for the presence of bile. If a biliary communication is found, it should be oversewn as well. Leaving viable cyst-lining epithelium behind allows for the possibility that another cyst will form; however, these cysts are usually small and only rarely require subsequent treatment. Wide unroofing, or cyst fenestration has been reported to have good results.[1,50] Though laparoscopic modality of management had its detractors,[40] its benefits found it becoming a popular mode of management of this disease. Besides achieving similar results as open surgery with fewer complications, shortened hospital stay and reduced sick leave, laparoscopy offers the advantage of inspecting the inner surface of the cyst wall for signs of malignancy and biopsies of suspicious lesions to be taken.[41] Various methods have been described as adjuvant to laparoscopic fenestration to achieve lasting relief. This includes injection of ethanol into the residual cyst cavity,[42,43] fulguration of the cyst cavities by electrocoagulation or argon beam coagulation,[44] and placement of an omental transpositional flap onto the cyst cavity itself.[45] According to Emmerson et al,[45] omental flap keeps the cyst cavity open to the abdomen and also resorbs some of the fluid produced by the cystic epithelium.

However, some authorities,[46] that simple cysts do not require ablation of the residual cyst lining or omentoplasty. We believe that if partial cyst excision has removed more than 50% of the estimated surface area of the cyst, no further therapy other than intraperitoneal drainage of the residual cyst is necessary. The adjuvant maneuvers are required only is less surface area is excised or the majority of the cyst resides within the liver parenchyma.

Laparoscopic ultrasound has been found to be useful for intraoperative management, providing information not available with CT or traditional USG and significantly affecting operative strategy.[47,48]

Complications of laparoscopic management of hepatic cysts have ranged from 0-15% and include dyspnea, pleural effusion, ascites, hemorrhage, infection and subhepatic bile collection.[41] Biliary cystadenoma is a very rare hepatic neoplasm, accounting for fewer than 5% of cystic neoplasms of the liver; regardless of the various diagnostic modalities, such a lesion may be difficult to distinguish preoperatively from a cystadenocarcinoma. The incidental finding of biliary cystadenoma after laparoscopic fenestration of a cystic hepatic lesion requires an open hepatic resection.[49]

Laparoscopic deroofing (combined with omentoplasty and/or oversewing) of uncomplicated liver cysts is associated with a recurrence rate of 10-25%, with less morbidity and mortality as compared to open surgery.[52,53,] Recurrence of a simple hepatic cyst following laparoscopic deroofing have been attributed to failure in ablating the secreting lining of the cyst wall; and in providing adequate measures to prevent early closure of the cyst such as may occur when the resected window is relatively small as compared to the overall size of the cyst cavity.[50] Factors predicting failure included previous surgical treatment, deepsited cysts, incomplete deroofing technique, location in the right posterior segments of the liver, and a diffuse form of PLD with small cysts.[54]

Complicated cysts such as infected cysts or bleeding into cysts can be managed similarly.[46] The source of bleeding is usually the stretched capsule; thus, unroofing and partial cyst excision are likely to be curative.

Thus, laparoscopic management of symptomatic solitary nonparasitic liver cysts is permanently successful in a large majority of cases when diagnosis is correct.[55]

CONCLUSION

Laparoscopic management of congenital hepatic cysts is the gold standard. It is associated with minimum morbidity and good long-term outcome. The major advantages of laparoscopic surgery are also availed, namely less pain, earlier mobilisation, shorter convalescence and high acceptibility by patients.

References

1. Beecherl EE, Bigam DL, Langer B, Gallinger S. Cystic disease of the liver. In: Zuidema GD, Yeo CJ (eds). Shackelford's Surgery of the Alimentary Tract. Vol. III, 5th edition. W.B. Sauders Company 2002: 447-460.

2. The European Polycystic Kidney Disease Consortium. The polycystic kidney disease 1 gene encodes a 14kb transcript and lies within a duplicated region on chromosome 16. Cell 1994; 77:881-94.

3. Van Adelsberg JS, Frank D. The PKD1 gene produces a developmentally regulated protein in mesenchyme and vasculature. Nature Medicine 1995; 1:359-64.

4. Pirson Y, Lannoy N, Peters D etal. Isolated polycystic liver disease as a distinct genetic disease, unlinked to polycystic kidney disease 1 and polycystic kidney disease 2. Hepatology 1996, 23:249.

5. Schwartz SI. Cysts and Benign Tumours. In: Zinner MJ, Schwartz SI, Ellis H (eds.) Maingot's Abdominal Operations, Vol. II, 10th edition. Prentice Hall International Inc. 1997: 1547-1559.

6. Lin TY, Chen CC, Wang SM. Treatment of non-parasitic cystic disease of the liver: a new approach to therapy with polycystic liver. Ann Surg 1968; 168:921-7.

7. Fabiani P, Katkhouda N, Iovine L, Mouiel J. Laparoscopic fenestration of biliary cysts. Surg Laparosc Endosc. 1991 Sep;1(3):162-5.

8. Paterson-Brown S, Garden OJ. Laser-assisted laparoscopic excision of liver cyst. Br J Surg. 1991 Sep;78(9):1047.

9. Heissing A. Report on a case of diagnosis of liver cyst by laparoscopy. Dtsch Med J. 1955 Apr 15;6(8):267-9.

10. Fornari F, Civardi G, Cavanna L, etal. Laparoscopic ultrasonography in the study of liver diseases. Preliminary results. Surg Endosc. 1989;3(1):33-7.

11. Caremani M, Benci A, Maestrini R, etal. Abdominal cystic hydatid disease (CHD): Classification of sonographic appearance and response to treatment. J. Clin. Ultrasound, 24:491,1996.

12. Larsen KA. Benign lesions affecting the bile ducts in the postmortem cholangiogram. Acta Pathologica, Microbiologica et Immunologic Scandinavica 1961, 51:47-62.

13. Moreaux J, Bloch P. The solitary biliary cyst of the liver. Archives Francaises des Maladies de l'Appareil Digestif 1971, 60:203-24.

14. Krahenbuhl L, Baer HU, Renzulli P etal. Laparoscopic management of nonparasitic symptom-producing solitary hepatic cysts. J Am Coll Surg. 1996 Nov;183(5):493-8.

15. Marvik R, Myrvold HE, Johnsen G, Roysland P. Laparoscopic ultrasonography and treatment of hepatic cysts. Surg Laparosc Endosc. 1993 Jun;3(3):172-4.

16. Hansman MF, Ryan JA Jr, Holmes JH 4th, etal. Management and long-term follow-up of hepatic cysts. Am J Surg. 2001 May;181(5):404-10.

17. Edwards JD, Eckhauser FE, Knol JA, Strodel WE, Applemann HD. Optimizing surgical management of symptomatic solitary hepatic cysts. Am Surg 1987; 53:510-4.

18. Ishak KG, Willis GW, Cummins SD, Bullock AA. Biliary cystadenoma and cystadenocarcinoma. Report of 14 cases and review of the literature. Cancer 1977; 38:322-38.

19. Tsao K, Hirose S, Sydorak R, etal. Fetal therapy for giant hepatic cysts. J Pediatr Surg. 2002 Oct; 37(10):31.

20. Giuliante F, D'Acapito F, Vellone M etal. Risk for laparoscopic fenestration of liver cysts. Surg Endosc. 2003 Nov;17(11):1735-8.

21. Cellier C, Cuenod CA, Deslandes P etal. Symptomatic hepatic cysts: Treatment with single-shot injection of minocycline hydrochloride. Radiology 1998, 206:205.

22. Montorsi M, Torzilli G, Fumagalli U etal. Percutaneous alcohol sclerotherapy of simple hepatic cysts: Results from a multicentre survey in Italy. HPB Surg. 1994, 8:89.

23. Moorthy K, Mihssin N, Houghton PW. The management of simple hepatic cysts: sclerotherapy or laparoscopic fenestration. Ann R Coll Surg Engl. 2001 Nov; 83(6):409-14.

24. Eriguchi N, Aoyagi S, Tamae T, Treatments of non-parasitic giant hepatic cysts. Kurume Med J. 2001; 48(3):193-5.

25. Simonetti G, Profili S, Sergiocomi GL etal. Percutaneous treatment of hepatic cysts by aspirations and sclerotherapy. Cardiovascular Interventional Radiology 1993,16:81-4.

26. Yamada N, Shinzawa H, Ukai K etal. Treatment of symptomatic hepatic cysts by percutaneous instillation of minocycline hydrochloride. Digestive Diseases and Sciences 1994, 39:2503-9.

27. Tanaka Y, Ogino M, Tokuda H etal. Examination of percutaneous minocycline hydrochloride injection therapy for hepatic cyst by one puncture method. Nippon Shokakibyo Gakkai Sasshi 1996, 93:828-36.

28. Tikkakoski Tm Makela JT, Leinonen S etal. Treatment of symptomatic congenital hepatic cysts with single-session percutaneous drainage and ethanol sclerosis: technique and outcome. Journal of Vascular Intervention and Radiology 1996, 7:235-9.

29. Pozniczek M, Wysocki A, Bobrzynski A eta. Sclerosant therapy as first-line treatment for solitary liver cysts. Dig Surg. 2005 Jan; 21(5-6):452-454.

30. Sanchez H, Gagner M, Rossi RL et al. Surgical management of nonparasitic cystic liver disease. Am J Surg 1991; 161:113-8.

31. Saini S, Mueller PR, Ferrucci JT Jr, et al. Percutaneous aspiration of hepatic cyst does not provide definitive therapy. AJR Am J Roentgenol 1983; 141:559-60.

32. Gigot JF, Legrand M, Hubens G etal. Laparoscopic treatment of nonparasitic liver cysts: Adequate selection of patients and surgical technique. World Journal of Surgery, 1996; 20:556-61.

33. Morino M, De Giuli M, Festa V etal. Laparoscopic management of symptomatic nonparasitic cysts of the liver. Indications and results. Ann Surg. 1994 Feb;219(2):157-64.

34. Martin IJ, McKinley AJ, Currie EJ etal. Tailoring the management of nonparasitic liver cysts. Ann Surg. 1998 Aug;228(2):167-72.

35. Tan YM, Ooi LL, Soo KC etal. Does laparoscopic fenestration provide long-term alleviation for symptomatic cystic disease of the liver? ANZ J Surg. 2002 Oct;72(10):743-5.

36. Emmermann S, Zornig C, Lloyd DM etal. Laparoscopic treatment of nonparasitic cysts of the liver with omental transposition flap. Surg Endosc 1997; 11:734-6.

37. Marks J, Mouiel J, Katkhouda N etal. Laparoscopic liver surgery: A report of 28 patients. Surg Endosc 1998:12:331-4.

38. Libutti SK, Starker PM. Laparoscopic resection of a nonparasitic liver cyst. Surg Endosc. 1994 Sep;8(9):1105-7.

39. Kanya L, Botos A, Bezsilla J, etal.Laparoscopic surgery of focal lesions of the liver. Acta Chir Hung. 1999;38(2):187-9.

40. Ganti AL, Sardi A, Gordon J.Laparoscopic treatment of large true cysts of the liver and spleen is ineffective. Am Surg. 2002 Nov;68(11):1012-7.

41. Klingler PJ, Gadenstatter M, Schmid T, etal. Treatment of hepatic cysts in the era of laparoscopic surgery. Br J Surg 1997; 84:438-44.

42. Jeng KS, Yang FS, Kao CR, Huang SH. Management of symptomatic polycystic liver disease: laparoscopic adjuvant with alcohol sclerotherapy. J Gastroenterol Hepatol 1995; 10:359-62.

43. Tanaka S, Watanabe M, Akagi S, et al. Laparoscopic fenestration in combination with ethanol sclerotherapy prevents a recurrence of symptomatic giant liver cyst. Surg Lap Endosc 1998; 8:453-6.

44. Que F, Nagorney DM, Gross JB, Torres VE. Liver resection and cyst fenestration in the treatment of severe polycystic liver disease. Gastroenterology 1995; 108:489-94.

45. Emmermann A, Zornig C, Lloyd DM, et al. Laparoscopic treatment of nonparasitic cysts of the liver with omental transposition flap. Surg Endosc 1997; 11:734-6.

46. Nagorney DM. Surgical management of cystic disease of the liver. In: Zacherl J, Scheuba C, Imhof MLong-term results after laparoscopic unroofing of solitary symptomatic congenital liver cysts. LH, Fong Y (eds): Surgery of the Liver and Biliary Tract, Vol. II, 3rd ed.; 1261-74.

47. Schachter P, Sorin V, Avni Y, etal. The role of laparoscopic ultrasound in the minimally invasive management of symptomatic hepatic cysts. Surg Endosc. 2001 Apr;15(4):364-7.

48. Marvik R, Myrvold HE, Johnsen G, Roysland P. Laparoscopic ultrasonography and treatment of hepatic cysts. Surg Laparosc Endosc. 1993 Jun;3(3):172-4.

49. Fiamingo P, Veroux M, Cillo U, Incidental cystadenoma after laparoscopic treatment of hepatic cysts: which strategy? Surg Laparosc Endosc Percutan Tech. 2004 Oct;14(5):282-4.

50. C Y Chan, C H J Tan, S P Chew, C H The. Laparoscopic fenestration of a simple hepatic cyst. Singapore Med J 2001 Vol 42(6) : 268-270.

51. Kammula US, Buell JF, Labow DM, Surgical management of benign tumors of the liver. Int J Gastrointest Cancer. 2001;30(3):141-6.

52. Gloor B, Ly Q, Candinas D. Role of laparoscopy in hepatic cyst surgery. Dig Surg. 2002;19(6):494-9.

53. Tocchi A, Mazzoni G, Costa G, Symptomatic nonparasitic hepatic cysts: options for and results of surgical management. Arch Surg. 2002 Feb;137(2):154-8.

54. Gigot JF, Legrand M, Hubens G, Laparoscopic treatment of nonparasitic liver cysts: adequate selection of patients and surgical technique. World J Surg. 1996 Jun;20(5):556-61.

55. Zacherl J, Scheuba C, Imhof M. Long-term results after laparoscopic unroofing of solitary symptomatic congenital liver cysts. Surg Endosc. 2000 Jan;14(1):59-62.

56. Albrink MH, McAllister EW, Rosemurgy AS, etal. Laparoscopic management of cystic disease of the liver. The American Surgeon, 1994; 60:262-6.

57. Zacherl J, Imhof M, Fugger R, etal. Laparoscopic unroofing of symptomatic congital liver cysts. Surg Endosc 1996; 10:813-5.

58. Cala Z, Cvianovic B, Perko Z, etal. Laparoscopic treatment of nonparasitic cysts of spleen and liver. J Laparoendosc Surg, 1996:6:387-91.

59. Koperna T, Vogl S, Satzinger U, etal. Nonparasitic cysts of the liver: Results and options of surgical treatment. W J Surg, 1997; 21:850-5.

60. Diez J, Decoud J, Gutieerez L, etal. Laparoscopic treatment of symptomatic cysts of the liver. Br J Surg, 1998; 85:25-7.

61. Palanivelu C. Laparoscopic management of simple hepatic cysts.In: C.Palanivelu: CIGES Atlas of Laparoscopic Surgery.2 nd edition, Jayprr broyhers medical publishers (p) Ltd, 2003: 213-216

62. Palanivelu C. Laparoscopic management of simple hepatic cysts. C.Palanivelu. Palanivelu's Textbook of Surgical Laparoscopy. Gem digestive diseases foundation,1 st edition,2002:397-398

48

Laparoscopic Management of Hydatid Cysts of the Liver

HISTORY

Hydatid disease has been known to mankind since the earliest times. Hippocrates described 'livers full of water'. Hydatid is Greek for 'drop of water' while echinococcosis means 'hedgehog berry' in the same language. It was postulated to be of animal origin in the later part of the eighteenth century. The term 'echinococcus' was coined by Rudolphi in the first decade of the nineteenth century. The life cycle of the parasite was elucidated by Haubner in 1855 and it was confirmed as a zoonosis in 1862 by Krabbe and Finsen.[1]

Surgery remains the mainstay of treatment for hepatic echinococcosis. Several non-surgical options have been explored. Medical therapy consists of albendazole alone or in combination with praziquantel by which stabilization of the disease has been reported.[2-6] In endemic countries with scarce surgical resources, a percutaneous approach of aspiration, injection and re-aspiration (PAIR) has been advocated by WHO in selected cases.[7] Modifications of this technique have been developed to address a few of its shortcomings. Saremi described a percutaneous approach in which a special cutting instrument is used to fragment and evacuate daughter cysts and laminated membrane while the cavity is continuously irrigated with scolecidals.[8] Percutaneous evacuation of cyst content (PEVAC) using a large bore catheter has been advocated by Schipper etal.[9] Drug therapy in the form of oral albendazole is given for specific conditions in liver hydatid, viz. (1) widely disseminated hydatid disease, (2) localized disease in poor surgical risk patients, (3) ruptured cysts, and (4) patients in whom significant intraoperative spillage has occurred.[8,10] A variety of surgical procedures are done for hydatid cysts of the liver, which are tailored to suit each individual case. These include marsupialization, closed total cystectomy, partial pericystectomy, partial pericystectomy with capitonnage, modified capitonnage, partial pericystectomy with omentoplasty, anatomical and nonanatomical liver resections.[1,8,11-13]

The first report of laparoscopic treatment of hydatid cyst of the liver was published in 1994[14] by Bickel et al followed soon there after by the first report of anaphylactic shock complicating laparoscopic treatment of hydatid cysts of liver.[15] In fact, an exaggerated fear of anaphylaxis seemed to discourage surgeons from more widely adopting minimal access techniques for the treatment of hydatid cysts.[16] However, gradually reports started appearing in the world literature detailing laparoscopic management of liver hydatid disease.[17-27] Various laparoscopic techniques described are total pericystectomy, puncture and aspiration of contents followed by marsupialization, unroofing and drainage, unroofing and omentoplasty, and omentoplasty using helical fasteners.[20,22,24,25,27,28-30] We use a special trocar-cannula system designed by ourselves to prevent spillage of hydatid fluid for laparoscopic management of hydatid cysts.

INTRODUCTION

Hydatidosis caused by Echinococcus granulosus is an endemic parasitic disease in Mediterranean countries, North Africa, Spain, Greece, Turkey, Portugal, Middle East, Australia, New Zealand, South America, Baltic areas, the Philippines, Northern China and the Indian sub-continent. However, physicians and surgeons worldwide may encounter the disease sporadically because of increased travel and immigration.[11,31] In India, hydatid disease is common in most of the states of which Andhra Pradesh and Tamil Nadu predominate.[56]

There are four species of Taenia echinococcus that are known to cause disease:

1. Echinococcus granulosus
2. Echinococcus multilocularis.
3. Echinococcus oligartus.
4. Echinococcus vogeli.

Parasitosis caused by Echinococcus multilocularis which is also called as malignant hydatidosis is found in central and eastern Europe, Japan, Canada and USA. The definitive hosts are the red fox, arctic fox, dog and cat while the intermediate hosts are various members of the rodent family. Human disease is rare but life-threatening. Echinococci oligarthus and vogeli are mainly confined to South America and are rarely known to cause human disease.

DEVELOPMENT IN THE INTERMEDIATE HOST

Human hydatid disease is commonly caused by the parasite Echinococcus granulosus that has the dog as the definitive host and sheep as the intermediate host. Humans are accidental intermediate hosts. Once within man or other intermediate host, the ingested eggs hatch in the duodenum to release oncospheres (true larvae) that burrow into the jejunal submucosa and enter veins or lymphatics. They reach the liver, which acts as an effective filter for most of the larvae; if, however, that barrier is overcome, the larvae pass through the inferior vena cava into the right side of the heart and then to the lungs. If the worm is not trapped in either the liver or lungs, or if it travels in lymphatics and bypasses the liver and lungs, it may lodge virtually anywhere in the body, most notably in the peritoneum, spleen, kidneys, heart, brain, spine, bony skeleton, and muscles. Not every larva develops; over 90% are overcome by the host reaction.

The hydatid cyst has three layers: (a) the outer pericyst, composed of modified host cells that form a dense and fibrous protective zone; (b) the middle laminated membrane, which is acellular and allows the passage of nutrients; and (c) the inner germinal layer, where the scolices (the larval stage of the parasite) and the laminated membrane are produced.

The inner germinal layer or the endocyst is the active part of the cyst, producing brood capsules which release protoscolices. Most of the brood capsules and scolices pinch off from the germinal layer and precipitate to the bottom of the fluid to become hydatid sand, which is just visible to the naked eye. The hydatid sand floating within the cyst may contain as many as 400,000 protoscolices per ml. and an average cyst contains up to 500 ml of such sand.

Daughter vesicles (brood capsules) are small spheres that contain the protoscolices and are formed from rest of the germinal layer. Before becoming daughter cysts, these daughter vesicles are attached by a pedicle to the germinal layer of the mother cyst. At gross examination, the vesicles resemble a bunch of grapes.

Scolices, which are infectious miniature adult tapeworms, possess a dual potential. If they are ingested by a primary host the apical region of the scolex evaginates and the organism attaches within a crypt of Lieberkuhn in the host's proximal small bowel, where it develops into the adult worm. However, if the scolex is deposited in a favorable milieu such as the peritoneal cavity or tracheobronchial tree after cyst rupture it may form a new hydatid cyst.

Those parts of the endocyst that become isolated from the nourishing hydatid fluid degenerate, forming a gelatinous amber-colored structure called matrix which may have a pseudotumoral appearance on ultrasound or CT. Because matrix is amorphous and yellow, it can be confused with pus by the surgeon. Matrix is most common in older patients who on average have harbored the parasite longer than the young. Lesions in the lung usually do not develop matrix, probably because enlargement of the cysts is relatively unrestricted until they become large enough that further growth is inhibited by the chest wall, mediastinum, or diaphragm.

The host tissue adjacent to the cyst mounts a chronic inflammatory reaction. As this subsides, scar tissue forms arounds the cyst. This is the pericyst (ectocyst) and it protects the fragile hydatid much like a tire protects an inner tube. The pericyst, which is not demonstrable by ultrasound or CT unless it is thickened or calcified, becomes thicker as the cyst enlarges. Blood vessels are obliterated within the developing pericyst, but bile ducts are not. Eventually the increasingly substantial pericyst becomes a hindrance to further enlargement of the endocyst, forcing it to become redundant within the confines of the pericyst.

Cysts and pericysts in the liver may calcify. Calcification of the pericyst, which can develop at all stages of the life cycle of hydatids, is found in nearly one-third of liver cysts. Pericyst calcification does not always indicate that the cyst is dead, but calcification of the endocyst does. When ruptured, the older mother cyst nearly always dies, but daughter cysts often survive. Perhaps 10-30% of cysts die and disintegrate without treatment. Exophytic growth of the cyst with extrahepatic extensions may rupture or may separate and grow as individual hydatid cyst. Left untreated, the cyst grows and follows one of several courses: form fistulas into adjacent organs or the biliary system, ruptures into the peritoneal cavity causing seeding of multiple daughter cysts throughout the peritoneal cavity, developing daughter cysts within or rarely, dying *de novo*. Older cysts have an increased risk of exogenous daughter cyst formation, which is an important factor for recurrence of disease after surgery.[9,33]

In many patients with *E. granulosus* infection, there are numerous cysts, depending on the number of ova ingested and the number that survive: two or more cysts may be present in the same or different organs. Estimates of multiple cysts vary widely: 5-25% in some series, 30-60% in others. On average, lesions are over twice as likely to be solitary as multiple and multiorgan involvement occurs in 10-15% of patients. Multiple cysts are more common in the liver than in the lungs and elsewhere (except in metastatic hydatidosis), but, even when multiple, are distinct from the alveolar "malignant" cysts of *E. multilocularis*. Despite the frequency of multiple cysts, it should be remembered that a solitary cyst in any location within the body might well be a hydatid cyst (it may truly be the only cyst present or it may not be possible to recognize others clinically or by diagnostic imaging).

Location of Hydatid Disease in Humans	
Location	**Frequency (%)**
Liver	55-75
Lung	18-35
Peritoneal Cavity	10-16
Kidney	1-4
Spleen	2-3
Uterus, Adnexa	0.5-1.5
Retroperitoneum	0.5-1.5
Pancreas	0.3-0.8
Others	0.1-3

INCIDENCE

The incidence of E. granulosus infestation in endemic areas ranges from 1-220 cases per 100,000 inhabitants, while the incidence of E. alveolaris ranges from 0.03-1.2 cases per 100,000 inhabitants, making it a much more rare form of echinococcosis. Infestation with E. Vogeli is the most rare form of echinococcosis and is reported mainly in the southern parts of South America. In India, hydatid is reported from practically all the parts of the country. However, Tamil Nadu and Andhra Pradesh, especially the Madurai district of the former, have a higher incidence of the disease.

CLINICAL PRESENTATION

Many hydatid cysts remain asymptomatic, even into advanced age. Parasite load, the site, and the size of the cysts determine the degree of symptoms. A history of living in or visiting an endemic area must be established. Also, exposure to the parasite through the ingestion of foods or water contaminated by the feces of a definitive host must be determined.

Though the common mode of infection is the unhygienic practice of consuming unwashed or improperly washed infected raw fruits and vegetables, direct contact with infected dogs is also another means of contracting the disease, especially in children.[1]

The age group most commonly affected is the third and fourth decade.[36-39] However in non-endemic areas, all the age groups are usually equally affected with the average age of presentation being older.[1,10] Literature reports equal infestation in both sexes[1,36,37] or predominant female infestation.[10,38]

Abdominal pain was the commonest mode of presentation (51.5% of cases) in this study which has also been reported by other authors.[10,38] Echinococcal infestation should be suspected in patients who present with an abdominal mass, pain, fever, jaundice, or anaphylaxis.[12] However, in non-endemic countries, most of the cases are asymptomatic and are detected fortuitously.[1,11,12]

The most common pathology was a single cyst in the right lobe of liver.[10,11,36] Most symptomatic cysts are larger than 5 cm in diameter.

Symptoms due to pressure usually take a long time to manifest, except when they occur in the brain or the eyes.

HYDATID DISEASE OF THE LIVER

Pressure effects are initially vague. They may include nonspecific pain, cough, low-grade fever, and the sensation of abdominal fullness. As the mass grows, the symptoms become more specific because the mass impinges on or obstructs specific organs.

In the liver, the pressure effect of the cyst can produce symptoms of obstructive jaundice and abdominal pain. With biliary rupture, the classic triad of biliary colic, jaundice, and urticaria is observed. Passage of hydatid membranes in the emesis (hydatid emesia) and passage of membranes in the stools (hydatid enterica) may occur rarely.

Secondary complications may occur as a result of infection of the cyst or leakage of the cyst. Infection of the cyst can occur either as a primary infection or as a secondary infection following an episode of a leak into the biliary tree leading to a cystobiliary fistula. Minor leaks lead to increased pain and a mild allergic reaction characterized by flushing and urticaria. Major rupture leads to a full-blown anaphylactic reaction, which is fatal if not treated promptly. A rupture into the biliary tree can lead to obstruction by the daughter cysts, producing cholangitis. Rupture into the bronchi can lead to expectoration of cyst fluid.

Skin: Apart from the above mentioned manifestations like jaundice, urticaria and erythema, spider

Clinical Features of Hepatic Hydatid Disease
Asymptomatic
Hepatomegaly
Jaundice
Urticaria
Malaise
Abdominal Pain
Abdominal Mass
Fever
Anorexia
Cough

Complications of Hepatic Hydatid Cysts

1. Rupture	A.	Intraperitoneal
	B.	Intrabiliary
	C.	Intrapleural
	D.	Intrabronchial
	E.	Into adjacent Organs
2. Pressure Effects	Obstructive Jaundice, Budd-Chiari Syndrome	
3. Organ Dysfunction	Cholangitis, Biliary Cirrhosis	
4. Secondary Infection		
5. Spread, Recurrence	A.	Spontaneous Rupture of Cyst
	B.	Iatrogenic Puncture, Surgical Inoculation
6. Allergic Reactions	A.	Urticaria
	B.	Brochospasm
	C.	Anaphylaxis
	D.	Eosinophilia

angiomas may be seen as a result of portal hypertension secondary to either biliary cirrhosis or obstruction of the inferior vena cava.

Vital signs: Fever could be a sign of secondary infection or allergic reaction. Hypotension is observed with anaphylaxis secondary to a cyst leak.

Abdomen: The most common sign is abdominal tenderness. Hepatomegaly may be present or a mass may be felt. Tender hepatomegaly is a sign of secondary infection of the cyst, especially when coupled with fever and chills. Ascites is rare. Splenomegaly can be the result of either splenic echinococcosis or portal hypertension.

INVESTIGATIONS

1. Routine hematology - Elevated total leucocyte count, eosinophilia.

2. Casoni's intradermal test - Due to the low sensitivity and specificity as well as risk of anaphylactic reaction, Casoni's intradermal test is considered obsolete now.

3. Immunological serology
   i. Indirect haemagglutination test (IHA)
   ii. Complement fixation test (CFT)
   iii. Latex agglutination test (LT)
   iv. Bentonite flocculation test (BFT)
   v. Indirect fluorescent antibody test (IFAT)
   vi. Immunoelectrophoresis (IEP)
   vii. Counterimmune electrophoresis (CIE)
   viii. Double diffusion test (DD)
   ix. Enzyme linked immunosorbent assay (ELISA)
   x. Radioallergosorbent test (RAST)
   xi. Basophil degranulation test (BDT)

For individual patients, the strategy for serological diagnosis should be initial screening with a highly sensitive test like IHA or LT, followed by confirmation by a highly specific test like IEP, DD test, ELISA or RAST. A positive IEP test highly specific for active infection (cross-reaction with Taenia solium cysticercosis only). ELISA and RAST are simple to perform and useful for population surveys. The only serological test that has a role in monitoring progress after surgical treatment of hydatids is CFT because it reverts to negative within 12 months of cure. Recently, reports have suggested that BDT has a high sensitivity and that it becomes negative within a week of cure.

4.   Imaging studies

i.   Plain X-ray abdomen: The only sign on a plain Xray would be an elevated right hemdiaphragm.

ii. Ultrasonography (USG): USG, due to its easy availability, affordability and diagnostic sensitivity is the initial imaging test of choice. Its role includes: (1) Screening in endemic areas and in family members. (2) First line diagnostics. (3) Interventional non-operative procedures. (4) IOUS. (5) Monitoring treatment and during follow-up.

iii.Intra-operative ultrasound (IOUS): IOUS is useful for localization and management of small, nonpalpable or deep-seated cysts.

iv. Computerised tomography (CT): CT gives the maximum information of the position and extent of intra-abdominal hydatid disease.

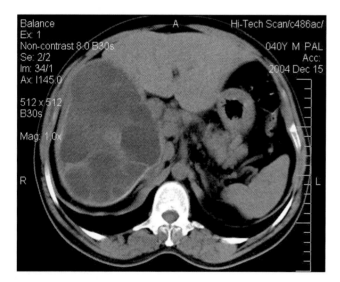

Figure 1 : CT picture shows hydatid cyst with daughter cysts in segment 6 of the liver.

v.   Magnetic resonance imaging (MRI): MRI does not yield any extra-information as compared to CT and is much costlier.

vi. Endoscopic retrograde cholangiography (ERC): ERC has a diagnostic and therapeutic role to play when combined with sphincterotomy in cases of biliary rupture of hydatid cyst.

vii Magnetic resonance cholagiopancreato-graphy (MRCP): MRCP is a new investigative modality for non-invasive visualization of the pancreato-biliary complex. It may have a limited role in the diagnosis of biliary rupture of hydatid cyst.

CLASSIFICATION OF HYDATID CYSTS

There are two classification systems used by clinicians worldwide while discussing hydatid disease – the WHO classification and the Gharbi classification, both based on ultrasonographic findings. Though the WHO classification is more elaborate, the Gharbi classification is more popular due to its simplicity and ease of application.

Gharbi Classification of Hydatid Cysts	
Type I	pure fluid collection - univesicular cyst
Type II	fluid collection with a split wall - detached laminated membrane - 'water lily' sign
Type III	fluid collection with septa - daughter cysts
Type IV	heterogenous appearance - presence of matrix - mimics a solid mass
Type V	reflecting thick walls - calcifications

WHO Classification	
CE1 :	Unilocular, simple cyst with uniform anechoic content. Cyst may exhibit fine echoes due to shifting of brood capsules which is often called hydatid sand ("snow flake sign").
CE2 :	Multivesicular, multiseptated cysts; cyst septations produce "wheel-like" structures, and presence of daughter cysts is indicated by "rosette-like" or "honeycomb-like" structures. Daughter cysts may partly or completely fill the unilocular mother cyst.
CE3 :	Unilocular cyst which may contain daughter cysts. Anechoic content with detachment of laminated membrane from the cyst wall visible as floating membrane or as "water-lily sign" which is indicative of wavy membranes floating on top of remaining cyst fluid.

CE4 : Heterogenous hypoechoic or hyperechoic degenerative contents. No daughter cysts. May show a "ball of wool" sign which is indicative of degenerating membranes.

CE5 : Cysts characterized by thick calcified wall that is arch shaped, producing a cone shaped shadow. Degree of calcification varies from partial to complete.

MEDICAL MANAGEMENT

Albendazole and Praziquantel are the two drugs used commonly for medical management of hepatic hydatid disease.

The indications of medical management are: Patients with

1. Widely disseminated hydatid disease.
2. Localized disease who are poor surgical risks.
3. Ruptured cysts.
4. Significant intraoperative spillage.

Recommended drugs and dosage

1. Albendazole in a curative dose of 10mg/kg body weight in two equal divided doses for 28 day. The cycle is repeated three times separated by 2-weeks intervals.
2. Praziquantel in a dosage of 40mg/kg body weight once a week as an adjunct to albendazole. It is more effective for E. alveolaris infestation.

Overall, chemotherapy may be effective in some 30-40% of patients. It is most effective for pulmonary hydatid, less so for liver infections and essentially ineffective for diseases of the bone, brain, eye and other sites.

NON-OPERATIVE INTERVENTION

PAIR (Puncture, Aspiration, Injection, Re-aspiration)[41]

PAIR was proposed in 1986 by the Tunisian team that first used it in a prospective study. Guidelines for the treatment of hydatid disease including PAIR, have been proposed by the WHO in 1996.

Technique

- Serological tests - baseline value is obtained.
- Prophylaxis with albendazole is given.
- Puncture and parasitological examination (if possible) or fast test for antigen detection in cyst fluid is carried out.
- 10-15 cc of cystic fluid is aspirated.
- Cyst fluid is tested for bilirubin.
- If bilirubin present: stop the procedure. If no bilirubin present: aspirate all cystic fluid.
- 95% ethanol solution or hypertonic saline (1/3 of the amount of aspirated fluid) is injected.
- Reaspiration of protoscolicide solution after 5 minutes.

Indications:

1. Non-echoic lesion < 5 cm in diameter.
2. Cysts with daughter cysts and/or with detachment of membranes.
3. Multiple cysts if accessible to puncture.
4. Infected cysts.
5. Pregnant women.
6. Children >3 years old.
7. Patients who fail to respond to chemotherapy alone.
8. Patients in whom surgery is contraindicated.
9. Patient who refuse surgery.
10. Patients who relapse after surgery.

Contraindications

1. Non-cooperative patients and inaccessible or risky location of the cyst in the liver.
2. Cyst in spine, brain and/or heart.
3. Inactive or calcified lesion.
4. Cysts communicating with the biliary tree.
5. Cysts open into the abdominal cavity, bronchi and urinary tract.

Benefits

1. Minimal invasiveness.
2. Reduced risk compared with surgery.
3. Confirmation of diagnosis.

4. Removal of large numbers of protoscolices with the aspirated cyst fluid.

5. Improved efficacy of chemotherapy given before and after puncture (probably because of an increased penetration of antihelminthic drugs into cysts re-filling with hydatid fluid).

6. Reduced hospitalization time.

7. Cost of the puncture and chemotherapy usually less than that of surgery or chemotherapy alone.

Risks

1. Same risks as any puncture (haemorrhage, mechanical lesions of other tissues, infections) - blind procedure.

2. Anaphylactic shock or other allergic reactions

3. Secondary echinococcosis caused by spillage

4. Chemical (sclerosing) cholangitis if cysts communicate with the biliary tree

5. Sudden intracystic decompression, thus leading to biliary fistulas

6. Persistence of satellite daughter cysts

7. Systemic toxicity of alcohol or hypertonic saline in case of large cysts (total volume injected must be carefully calculated)

SURGICAL MANAGEMENT

All patients are treated with albendazole 10mg/kg/day for at least two weeks pre-operatively before subjecting them to surgery and this is continued post-operatively for four weeks.

Laparoscopic Management

We have developed a new technique of laparoscopic management of hydatid cysts using a special instrument designed by ourselves.

The Palanivelu Hydatid System (PHS)

The PHS consists of a trocar and cannula along with 5mm and 3 mm reducers.

Trocar

The trocar is 29 cms long. It is hollow throughout its length. Tip is pyramidal shaped with each facet of the pyramid bearing a fenestration to enable any fluid leaking on its insertion to be sucked into its hollow body by the suction connected in the other end. Its long shaft also bears two fenestrations opposite to each other at a distance of 17 cms from the tip.

Cannula

The cannula is 26 cms long with an inner diameter of 12mm. It has two side channels - one for gas

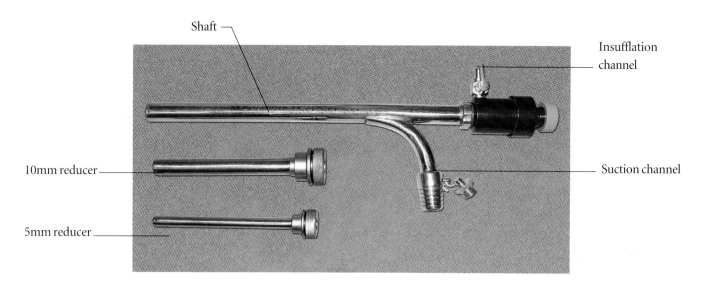

Figure 2 : Palanivelu hydatid trocar system - Cannula and reducer

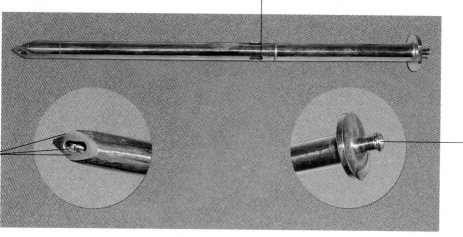

3 holes in the shaft (at the same level where the suction channel present in the cannula)

3 holes in the pyrimidal tip

Suction channel

Figure 3 : Palanivelu hydatid trocar system - Trocar

insufflation and another for suction. The suction channel has an inner diameter of 10 mm. Its outer nozzle is designed so that the suction tube can be fitted onto it in an airtight manner.

Principle of PHS

The cannula has two side-channels - one for CO_2 insufflation and another for suction. The suction side-channel has an outer diameter of 12 mm and an inner diameter of 10 mm. By connecting a powerful suction machine to this wide channel, a strong vacuum seal is created between the rim of the cannula and the surface of the hydatid cyst. This is essential in preventing spillage of hydatid fluid when the trocar is subsequently advanced into the hydatid cyst. The trocar is hollow to accommodate a 5 mm suction cannula which is connected to another suction machine. Once the trocar has punctured the cyst, there are two suction forces working - through the suction cannula which can be inserted into the main channel of the cannula and through the side channel of the cannula. This ensures rapid and complete evacuation of the hydatid fluid, hydatid sand and hydatid vesicle, if present.

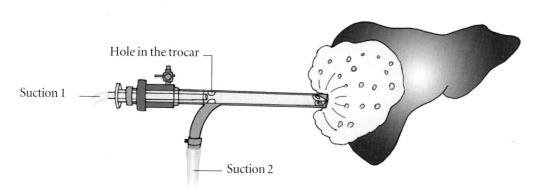

Hole in the trocar

Suction 1

Suction 2

Figure 4 : Step 1 - Pressing the cyst wall with a PHS cannula, by keeping the two separate suctions one in cannula and another in trocar

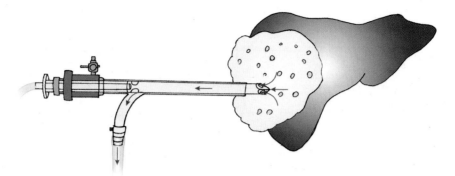

Figure 5 : Step 2 - Penetration of cyst wall with the trocar and aspiration of the cyst content

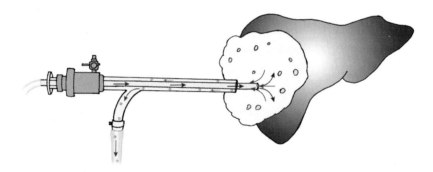

Figure 6 : Step 3 - Washing the cyst cavity with the normal saline. It will clear the remnant daugher cyst and germinal layer

Team Set-Up

For hydatid cyst in the right lobe of the liver, the patient is positioned in left lateral position with a 45 degree tilt. The surgeon stands on the left side of the patient.

In case of a hydatid cyst in the left lobe of the liver, the patient is placed in a modified lithotomy reverse Trendelenburg position with the surgeon standing between the legs of the patient.

Port Placement

For right hepatic cysts: The camera port is placed supra-umbilically and slightly to the right of midline. One 10mm port for the right hand in the epigastrium and one 5mm port for the left hand in the right hypochondrium are inserted just below the liver edge, the exact location being determined by the site of the cyst. The fourth port is a 12mm port exactly over the hydatid cyst for the hydatid trocar cannula (PHS).

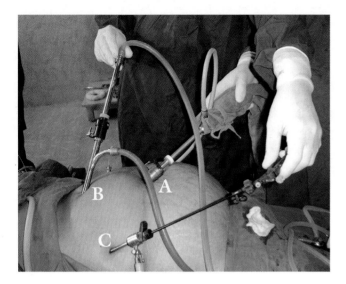

Figure 7 : Port position for right lobe hydatid cyst liver

A - Umbilical Camera port 10mm

B - Epigastric PHS port 12mm

C - Right mid clavicular working port 5mm

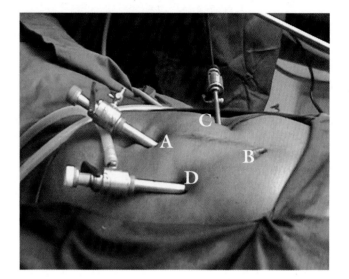

Figure 8 : Port position for left lobe hydatid cyst liver

A - Supraumbilical Camera port 10mm

B - Epigastric PHS port 12mm

C - Right mid clavicular working port 5mm

D - Left mid clavicular working port 10 mm

For left hepatic cysts: The camera port in placed supra-umbilically in the midline or just to the left of the midline. The right hand working port (10mm) is in the left hypochondrium while the left hand working port (5 mm) is in the epigastric region. The 12 mm port for PHS is inserted over the location of the cyst.

Instruments

Apart from the standard set of instruments, we use a special trocar-cannula specially designed by ourselves for spillage-free evacuation of the hydatid cyst contents. Moreover two sets of powerful suction machines are required, one for the side-channel of the PHS cannula and one for the 5mm suction cannula that is introduced through the PHS trocar or the left hand working port.

Technique

1. Uncomplicated solitary hydatid cyst

i. Mobilization of the cyst

After introducing the camera port through the umbilicus following creation of pneumoperitoneum, the hydatid cyst is identified on the surface of the liver. Any adhesions are gently separated and the cyst surface is exposed.

ii. Puncture and Aspiration of the Cyst

Step 1: The PHS trocar with cannula was introduced into the peritoneal cavity directly over the hydatid cyst. Once inside the peritoneal cavity, the trocar is withdrawn so that its tip is within the cannula. The cannula is advanced till its tip is in total contact with the hydatid cyst surface. Strong suction is applied through the side channel to create a strong negative pressure and maintain airtight contact between the cyst and the rim of the cannula.

Step 2: Thereafter, the trocar with a 5 mm. suction nozzle inside it (connected to another suction machine) is introduced into the cannula and, by steady pressure, is pushed into the cyst along with the cannula. Any fluid spillage on puncture of the cyst wall is immediately suctioned either into the body of the hollow trocar through its fenestrated tip and then into the suction cannula or into the outer cannula and thence, into the suction side-channel. A gauze piece soaked in cetrimide is wrapped around the cannula at its entry into the cyst wall.

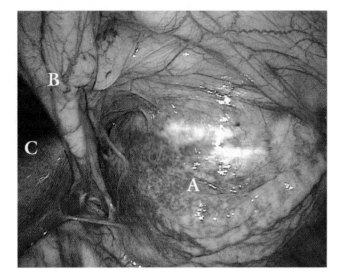

Figure 9 : Hydatid cyst left lobe liver adherent to the abdominal wall

A - Hydatid cyst
B - Falciform ligament
C - Right lobe of liver

Step 3: Once the PHS enters into the hydatid cyst, the trocar is removed and the cavity is irrigated through the main channel while maintaining continuous suction all the time simultaneously. The suction cannula connected to the separate suction machine is introduced through the right hand working port for suctioning the minimal leak if it occurs. In this way, fragments of laminated membrane, daughter cysts and debris are easily removed. Once the returning fluid is clear, CO_2 is insufflated at low pressure (3-4 mm. Hg) and another telescope is introduced into the cavity through the cannula to visualize the interior for any overt cyst-biliary communication. If the same telescope is used for intracystic visualization, it should be thoroughly cleaned before introduction into the peritoneal cavity to avoid any anaphylactic reaction. In absence of overt cyst-biliary communication (verified by absence of bile staining in the suctioned fluid and non-visualization of opening within the cyst cavity), 0.5% cetrimide is instilled into the cyst cavity as a

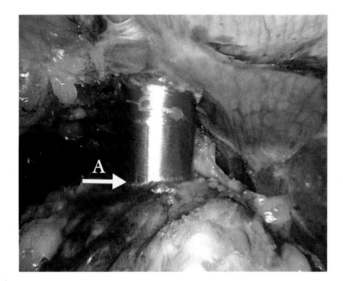

Figure 10 : Puncturing the cyst wall with PHS

A - Hydatid trocar is entered into the cyst without any spillage

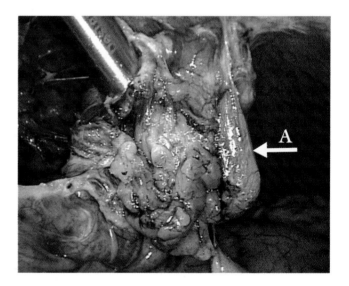

Figure 11 : Contents of the hydatid cyst was sucked out

A   - Collapsed hydatid cyst

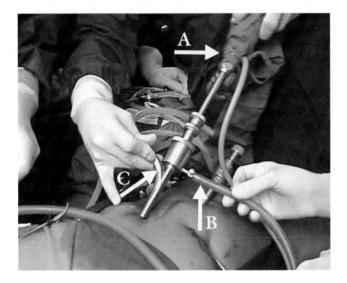

Figure 12 : Camera is introduced into the PHS to view the cyst cavity

A - Laparoscopic camera
B - Insufflation tube
C - Suction channel

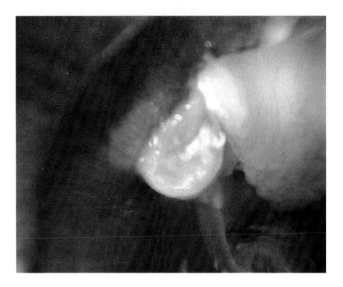

Figure 13 : View of hydatid cyst layers sucking through the side suction channel

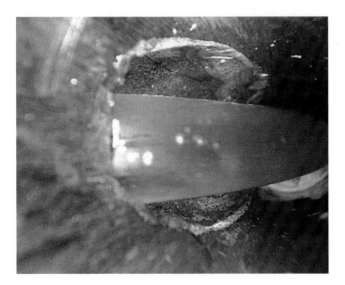

Figure 14 : To clear the remaining cyst content, 10mm suction tube can be introduced into the cyst through the suction channel of PHS under laparoscopic vision

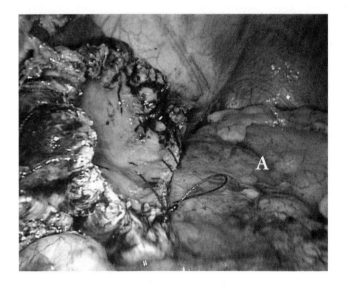

Figure 15 : After the marsupialisation of the cyst, edges were sutured with continuous stitches using 3 0 vicryl for haemostasis

A - Stomach

scolicidal agent. After 10 minutes, the scolicidal agent is sucked and the cyst is marsupialized. In case of overt signs of cyst-biliary communication, use of scolicidal agent is avoided and after marsupialization, the opening edges are sutured using 3-0 vicryl. Omentoplasty is done for all cases. Drainage tube is kept near the cyst.

Post-operatively, the cyst size is monitored by US at two weeks and 1, 3, 6, 12, 18, and 24 months. If clinically indicated, US is repeated at shorter intervals. CT scan is performed if any complication/recurrence is suspected. The primary end points were defined as complete cyst collapse by US at the end of the procedure, disappearance of cyst cavity or at least 50% reduction in cyst size at follow up imaging, and disappearance of complications such as pain, cystobiliary fistulas, vascular or biliary compression, and infection. The secondary end points of the study were recurrence of cyst cavity to >50% of its initial size, vascular or biliary compression, fistulas, pain and infection within two years after surgery, death, withdrawal from the study, or loss to follow up.

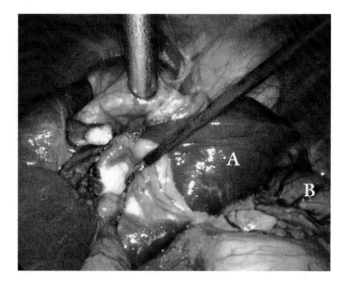

Figure 17 : Cyst was collapsed after aspiration

A - Inferior surface of left lobe

B - Stomach

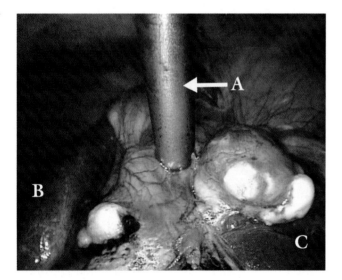

Figure 16 : Hydatid cyst involving right and left lobe of liver.

A - Cyst was punctured with PHS

B - Right lobe

C - Left lobe

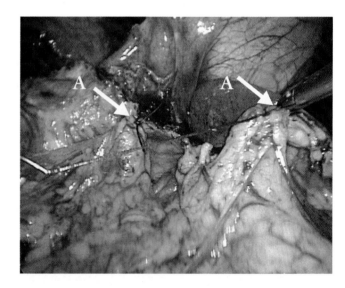

Figure 18 : After deroofing the cyst, omentum was placed and fixed to the side wall

A - Suture to the omentum and cyst wall

HYDATID CYST IN SEGMENT V

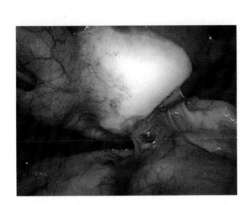

Figure 19 : Cyst in the segment V

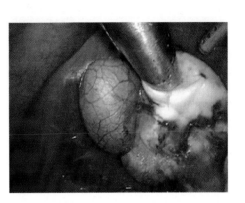

Figure 20 : Puncturing of the cyst with PHS

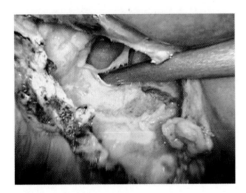

Figure 21 : Deroofing the cyst

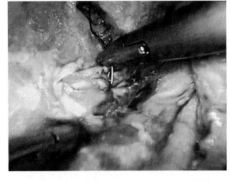

Figure 22 : Suturing of the biliary communication

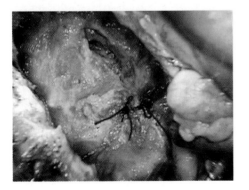

Figure 23 : Completion of suturing

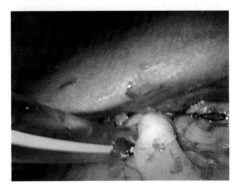

Figure 24 : Omentoplasty and DT

HYDATID CYST IN SEGMENT VI

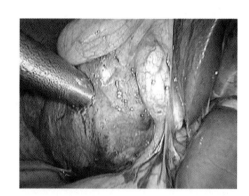

Figure 25 : Cyst in the segment VI

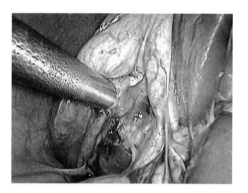

Figure 26 : Puncturing of the cyst with PHS

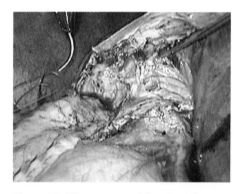

Figure 27 : Placement and fixation of omentum

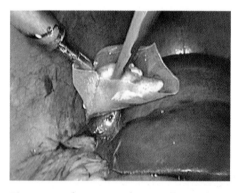

Figure 28 : Placement of cyst wall into the endobag

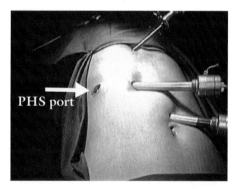

Figure 29 : Ports position

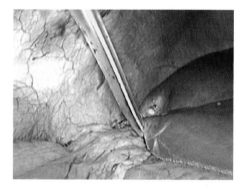

Figure 30 : Drainage is placed in the cyst after omentoplasty

HYDATID CYST IN SEGMENT VII

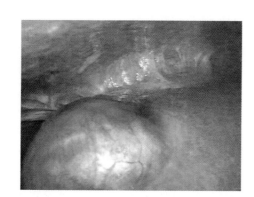

Figure 31 : Cyst in segment VII

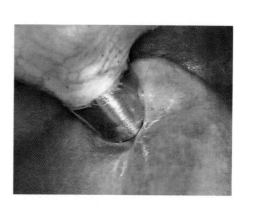

Figure 32 : Puncturing of the cyst with PHS

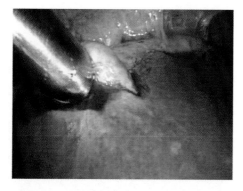

Figure 33 : Aspiration of the contents with PHS without any spillage

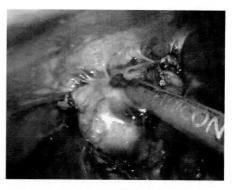

Figure 34 : Deroofing of the cyst using harmonic hook

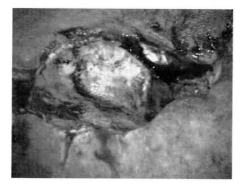

Figure 35 : Completion of Marsupialization

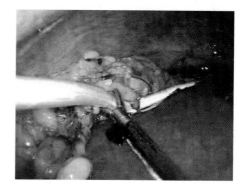

Figure 36 : Omentoplasty and keeping the drainage tube

HYDATID CYST IN SEGMENT VIII

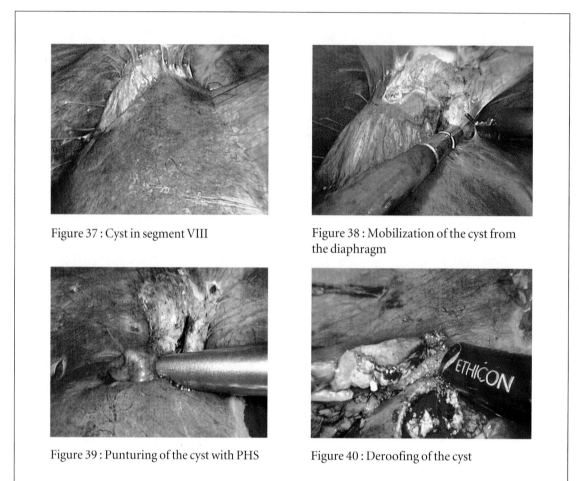

Figure 37 : Cyst in segment VIII

Figure 38 : Mobilization of the cyst from the diaphragm

Figure 39 : Punturing of the cyst with PHS

Figure 40 : Deroofing of the cyst

2. Inter-communicating cysts

Sometimes, two or more cysts are encountered such that they are communicating with each other. In such cases, frequently only one cyst will be superficial while the other(s) will be deep in the liver substance and hence, inaccessible to laparoscopic drainage. Such cases can be managed by the technique of "transcystic fenestration". This consists of draining the superficial cyst as above and the deeper cyst can be drained through the superficial cyst. In case of two cyst adjacent to each other but not communicating, the deeper cyst can be punctured through the superficial cyst in the same manner using the PHS.

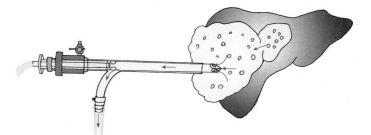

Figure 41 : In case of two communicating cyst, by puncture and aspirating the first cyst with PHS will produce the negative pressure within the cyst which will clear the second cyst

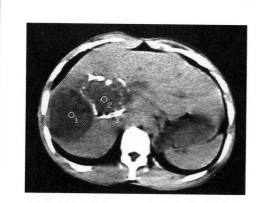

Figure 42 : CT shows two communicating cyst with calcification

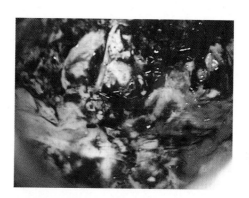

Figure 43 : After clearing the content with PHS, cyst cavity 1 is inspected

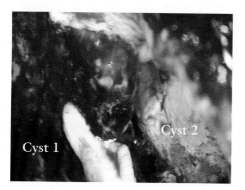

Figure 44 : Communication is visualised

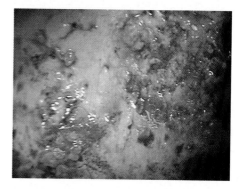

Figure 45 : Cyst cavity 2 is inspected to clear the content, calcified wall is seen

3. Cyst-Biliary Communication

Untreated hydatid cyst may rupture into the biliary system leading to obstruction, cholangitis or jaundice. Hydatid segments from the biliary system can be cleared off by two different techniques depending upon the rigidity of the hydatid cyst.

Technique One

(for patient with adequate rigid hydatid cyst)

- Preparation, ERCP and stenting if necessary
- Under Laparoscopic guidance, the Palanivelu hydatid trocar system is introduced perpendicularly into the cyst. With forced suction and simultaneous irrigation, the entire segments of germinal layer are removed. Operating laparoscope is introduced into the cyst and the confirmation of entire removal of debris is done.
- By creating negative pressure with forced suction, CBD will be cleared of the debris.
- Repeated suction and irrigation are done till the effluent is clear.
- Cholangiogram done at the end should reveal that the dye is flowing freely into the duodenum.

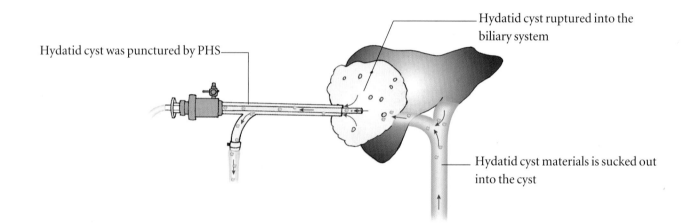

Hydatid cyst ruptured into the biliary system

Hydatid cyst was punctured by PHS

Hydatid cyst materials is sucked out into the cyst

Figure 46 : In case of hydatid cyst with biliary rupture, cyst was punctured with PHS and contents were aspirated. Aspiration creates the negative pressure within the cyst, which will suck the contents of the biliary system into the cyst. These contents were sucked out through PHS

Technique Two

This is used in small hydatid or collapsed hydatid cyst where trocar cannot be introduced into the cyst and negative pressure cannot be created.

- The cyst is opened with hook intraperitoneally and thick walled germinal layer extracted. On pressure at porta we can visualize germinal segments coming into cavity from the medial wall underflap.

- Common bile duct is dissected and choledochotomy is done. Retrograde irrigation is carried out to clear the hydatid fragments into the cavity till the fluid is clear. The lower CBD is also irrigated and 'T" tube placed, if necessary. (Figure 47 - 51)

Omentoplasty is performed. Post-operative management remains the same as for uncomplicated hydatid cysts.

HYDATID CYST WITH BILARY RUPTURE

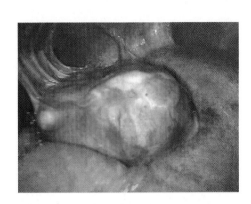

Figure 47 : Collapsed cyst in segment VI and VII

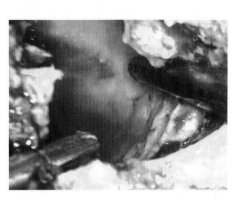

Figure 48 : Cyst contents were aspirated. Deroofing was done

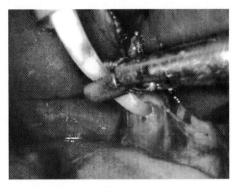

Figure 49 : Common bile duct was opened, suction catheter introduced and saline was irrigated

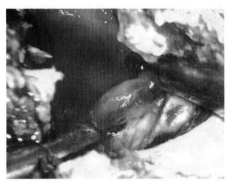

Figure 50 : Saline is coming to the cyst cavity while irrigating through the CBD

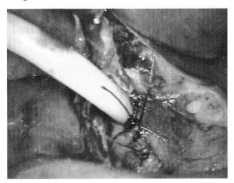

Figure 51 : ' T' tube was kept

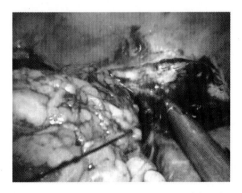

Figure 52 : Omentum was placed and fixed to the cyst wall

RESULTS

Since 1997, 66 cases have been operated using the PHS. The youngest patient was 14 years old and the oldest was 64 years old. The average age of presentation was 38.6 years. There were 55 males (83.3%) and 11 females (16.7%).

Epidemiology (Figures in brackets indicate percentage)

Total No. of Cases	66 (100)
Youngest Patient (Years)	14
Oldest Patient (Years)	64
Mean Age (Years)	38.6
Males	55 (83.3)
Females	11 (16.7)

Regarding the mode of presentation, majority of the patients (n = 34, 51.5%) presented with pain. Nearly 22.7% (n = 15) of the patients presented with non-specific complaints of nausea and dyspepsia-like symptoms. Thirteen (19.7%) patients came with presenting feature of abdominal mass or swelling. Three cases (4.6%) were discovered accidentally while screening the patients for unrelated complaints. Only one patient (1.5%) presented with fever.

Symptoms Leading to Discovery of Hydatid Disease (Figures in brackets indicate percentage)

Abdominal Pain	34 (51.5)
Nausea, Dyspepsia	15 (22.7)
Abdominal Swelling/Mass	13 (19.7)
Accidental Discovery	3 (4.6)
Fever	1 (1.5)

Most of the patients (n = 60, 90.9%) had only a single cyst while six patients (9.1%) had two cysts. The right lobe of liver was more commonly involved (n = 36, 54.5%) than the left lobe (n = 26, 39.4%). Cysts were bilateral in four cases (6.1%). Majority of the patients (n = 54, 81.9%) were uncomplicated. Of the remaining, 9 cases (13.6%) presented with cyst-biliary communication, one (1.5%) was a case of

secondarily infected cyst and two cases (3%) were recurrent cysts. Out of the recurrent cysts, one had recurred after laparoscopic attempt at removal elsewhere, while the other case was following open hydatid surgery.

Clinico-pathology (Figures in brackets indicate percentage)

Single Cyst	60 (90.9)
Multiple Cysts	6 (9.1)
Site - Right Lobe of Liver	36 (54.5)
- Left Lobe of Liver	26 (39.4)
- Bilateral	4 (6.1)
Uncomplicated Cysts	54 (81.9)
Complicated Cysts	12 (18.1)
- Cyst-biliary Communication	9 (13.6)
- Secondary Infection	1 (1.5)
- Recurrent Cysts	2 (3)
Other Organs (Spleen)	1 (1.5)

In 55 cases (83.3%), simply evacuation of the hydatid cyst by the PHS was done. In 9 cases (13.7%), this was followed by left lobectomy as the cysts were large occupying almost the entire left lobe of liver. Transcystic fenestration of underlying cyst was carried out in two (3%) of the six cases with multiple cysts while the other four were dealt with by separate insertions of PHS into individual cysts. The remnant cavity was dealt with by omentoplasty.

Type of Surgery (Figures in brackets indicate percentage)

Evacuation and Marsupialisation	55 (83.3)
Evacuation and Lobectomy	9 (13.7)
Transcystic Fenestration	2 (3)
Repeated Separate Insertion of PHS	4 (6)

The average duration of the surgery was 52 minutes. None of the patients had intra-operative anaphylactic shock.

Post-operatively, two patients (3%) had infection while nine patients (13.7%) had a minor biliary leak that stopped draining by 5-7 days.

Types of Complications (Figures in brackets indicate percentage)

Types of Complications	No.
I	2 (3)
II A	9 (13.7)
II B	0
III	0
IV	0

Out of the 66 patients, regular follow-up has been maintained in 52 patients with an average follow-up period of 5.8 years. There is no recurrence till date.

Classification by Clavien et al.[42] Grade I: alterations from the ideal postoperative course, non-life-threatening and with no lasting disability. Complications of this grade necessitate only bedside procedures and do not significantly extend hospital stay. Grade II: complications which are potentially life-threatening but without residual disability. A subdivision is made according to the requirement for invasive procedures (IIb). Grade III: complications resulting in residual long-term disability, including organ resection or persistence of life-threatening conditions. Grade IV: complications leading to patient death

DISCUSSION

Liver hydatidosis is one of the most common causes of acute abdomen in endemic regions. Echinococcal infestation should be suspected in patients who present with an abdominal mass, pain, fever, jaundice, or anaphylaxis.[34] However, in non-endemic countries, most of the cases are asymptomatic and are detected fortuitously.[1,28,34]

Ultrasonography and CT are both effective imaging modalities for the detection of liver hydatid disease.[28,34] USG is particularly useful for the detection of cystic membranes, septa, and hydatid sand while CT best demonstrates cyst wall calcification and cyst infection.[35] Certain features in US, CT or MRI may warn of biliary communication or impeding cyst rupture.[30,35] Biliary involvement may be confirmed by MRI or ERC.[1,34] Serologic tests have a sensitivity of 65-90%[28,34] but are not performed in our institution as a routine.

Surgery remains the mainstay of treatment for hepatic echinococcosis. In endemic countries with scarce surgical resources, a percutaneous approach of aspiration, injection and re-aspiration (PAIR) has been advocated by WHO in selected cases[18]. Modifications of this technique have been developed to address a few of its shortcomings. Saremi described a percutaneous approach in which a special cutting instrument is used to fragment and evacuate daughter cysts and laminated membrane while the cavity is continuously irrigated with scolecidals.[38] Percutaneous evacuation of cyst content (PEVAC) using a large bore catheter has been advocated by Schipper etal.[6] Drug therapy has a limited curative role and is used more often as an adjunct to surgery. A variety of open surgical procedures are done for hydatid cysts of the liver, which are tailored to suit each individual case. These include marsupialization, closed total cystectomy, partial pericystectomy, partial pericystectomy with capitonnage, modified capitonnage, partial pericystectomy with omentoplasty, typical and atypical liver resections.[1,28,34,37,39]

Following the first report of laparoscopic treatment of hydatid cyst of the liver was published in 1994, reports started appearing in the world literature detailing laparoscopic management of liver hydatid disease.[19-25,42-45] The indications, contra-indications, advantages and disadvantages of this technique have been elucidated[46,47] In our study, we have performed various procedures laparoscopically, viz., evacuation and marsupialization, transcystic fenestration and left lobectomy. The remnant cyst was dealt with by omentoplasty. We have used the Palanivelu Hydatid System (PHS), a specially designed trocar to obtain a totally contamination-free management of liver hydatid disease.

Laparoscopic treatment of the hepatic cysts should not be regarded as a new surgical technique. Rather, it is a new and minimally invasive access to perform established surgical techniques. As is the case for other laparoscopic operations, laparoscopic hydatid surgery follows the basic surgical principles of treating hydatid cysts of the liver: evacuation of the live cyst content, prevention of spillage, sterilization of the cavity with scolicidal agents, and management of the residual cavity. It eliminates the disadvantages of a surgical incision and shortens the hospital stay markedly.

Various Laparoscopic Apparatus

Various laparoscopic techniques described are total pericystectomy, puncture and aspiration of contents followed by marsupialization, unroofing and drainage, unroofing and omentoplasty, and omentoplasty using helical fasteners.[22,24,42,43,45,47-49] One of the problems faced in laparoscopic treatment of liver hydatid cysts is the difficulty in evacuating the particulate contents of the cyst, the daughter cysts and laminated membrane. Various instruments have been described to evacuate the contents of hydatid cysts.[21,50-55] Bickel etal initially advocated the use of a large transparent beveled cannula.[21] Later on, they modified the technique somewhat by creating a continuous vacuum inside the cannula while its tip was firmly adhered to the cyst wall.[50] An aspirator-grinder apparatus was developed by Acarli etal.[58] Saglam described a perforator-grinder-aspirator apparatus designed specifically for the evacuation of hydatid cysts.[51] A similar aspirator-grinder apparatus was described by Alper etal.[52] Kayaalp directly inserted a laparoscopic trocar into the hydatid cyst but reported greater success for anterior and unilocular cysts than for posterior and multi-locular cysts.[53] A liposuction cannula was used by Al-Shareef etal to evacuate hydatid cysts.[54] Another perforator and aspirator called the "perfore-aspirator" has been used by Zengin etal.[55] Of all these, the isolated hypobaric technique described by Bickel etal[50] is the only one which has attempted to deal with the problem of spillage. The PHS not only prevents any spillage of hydatid fluid but also assists complete evacuation of the cyst content and allows intracystic magnified visualization for cyst-biliary communication.

Advantages of PHS over other Laparoscopic Apparatus for Managing Hepatic Hydatid Disease

- PHS ensures a negative pressure vacuum seal between the outer cannula and the cyst wall which prevents spillage.
- It is possible to inspect the interior of the cyst by introducing a telescope through the PHS into the cyst.

- The cyst can be insufflated with low pressure carbon dioxide to check for any cyst-biliary communication.
- Cyst-biliary communication, if present, can be sutured within the cyst.
- Simple and complicated cyst-biliary communications can be managed with the PHS.
- Particulate cyst content, including daughter cysts, can be easily suctioned through the 10mm cannula.
- Since there is no need for any grinding apparatus, the risk of trauma to hepatic parenchyma is not there.

Cyst-Biliary Communications[58]

The frequency of this complication has been reported to be between 3.5-19%.[58-60] There are two type of cyst-biliary communications:

1. Complicated
2. Simple

Complicated cyst-biliary communications: This is also known as 'frank intra-biliary rupture'. There is rupture on both sides, viz., on the bile duct and the membrane of the cyst with a flow from the high-pressure cyst to the low-pressure biliary system. If some particulate matter (piece of membrane of small daughter cysts) enters the biliary tree, it causes cholestasis, biliary dilatation, jaundice and cholangitis.

Simple cyst-biliary communications: Rupture is present on the bile duct side but not on the cyst side. While managing the cyst, the cyst contents may become bile-stained. But, in half of the patients with this complication, there may not be any evidence of biliary communication before and during surgery. It may become manifest in the post-operative period as a biliary fistula. Centrally located cysts are more prone to this complication than the peripherally located smaller cysts.

In our series, we found cyst-biliary communication in 13.5% of our cases and all of them were managed laparoscopically.

Conservative vs. Radical Surgery

Conservative surgery consists of simple drainage, unroofing, introflexion and omentopexy while radical surgery includes partial cystectomy, pericystectomy and hepatic resections. A tailored approach is required in each patient due to variations in size, multiplicity, location and associated complications. Many authors recommend pericystectomy for hepatic hydatid disease.[61,62] The main advantage of pericystectomy in open surgery is that it can be performed without opening the cyst cavity, thus avoiding the problems of spillage and cavity management. The disadvantage is that it is associated with more blood loss and can be done only in peripherally located small cysts. In laparoscopic surgery, performing pericystectomy without prior evacuation of the cyst contents as in open surgery carries the risk of perforation and dissemination of disease during dissection. Manterola etal have reported laparoscopic pericystectomies after evacuating the cyst.[45] However, we feel that this approach neutralizes the main advantage of pericystectomy and, hence, do not recommend it.

In 9 (13.7%) of our cases, the cyst was large, occupying the entire left lobe of liver which had atrophied due to the pressure of the cyst. In this case, after evacuating the cyst using the PHS, we carried out left lobectomy laparoscopically. Prior evacuation of the cyst with the PHS ensured that there was no risk of accidental perforation with intra-abdominal dissemination of the cyst contents while performing the lobectomy.

Post-operatively, two of our patients had infection (Clavien type I complication) while nine of the patients had minor biliary leak (Clavien type II complication). All the cases responded to conservative management. Complications seen in open surgery include pleural effusions, infections, biliary fistulae, sub-diaphragmatic collection, liver abcesses.[5,37] Thus, with laparoscopic management, both the number and severity of complications decrease as compared to open surgery.

With an average follow-up of 5.8 years, we have not had any recurrences. Various reports in literature reveal a recurrence rate varying from 0.9% to 22% for open surgery.[56,57] There is an absence of adequate data in literature regarding recurrence following minimal invasive approach.

CONCLUSION

We recommend the PHS for management hepatic hydatid disease. We have found its efficacy to be optimum for preventing spillage, evacuating contents of hydatid cysts, performing transcystic fenestration and for dealing with cyst-biliary communications. The only limitation of this system is related to the anatomical relation of the cyst. At present, we do not recommend this technique for posteriorly located cysts, small cysts and cysts deep within the hepatic parenchyma.

References

1. Huizinga WKJ, Grant CS, Daar AS. Hydatid disease. In: Morris PJ, Wood WC, eds. Oxford Textbook of Surgery 2nd edition Oxford University Press, 2000: 3298-3305.

2. Schantz PM, Schwabe C. Worldwide status of hydatid disease control. J Am Vet Assoc 1969;155:2104 –21.

3. King CH. Cestodes (tapeworms) In: Mandell GL, Bennett JE, Dolin R. Principles and practice of infectious diseases. 4th ed. New York, NY: Churchill Livingstone, 1995; 2544-2553.

4. Gomez R, Marcello M, Moreno E, et al. Incidence and surgical treatment of extra-hepatic abdominal hydatidosis. Rev Esp Enferm Dig 1992;82:100 - 3.

5. Amr SS, Amr ZS, Jitawi S, Annab H. Hydatidosis in Jordan: an epidemiological study of 306 cases. Ann Trop Med Parasitol 1994;88:623 - 7.

6. Kammerer WS, Schantz PM. Echinococcal Disease. Infect Dis Clin North Am 1993;7:605 -18.

7. Magistrelli P, Masetti R, Coppola R, et al. Surgical treatment of hydatid disease of the liver: a 20-year experience. Arch Surg 1991;126:518 - 22.

8. Nahmias J, Goldsmith R, Soibelman M, et al. Three to seven year follow-up after albendazole treatment of 68 patients with cystic echinococcosis (hydatid disease).Ann Trop Med Parasitol 1994;88:295 - 304.

9. Luchi S,Vincenti A, Messina F, et al. Albendazole treatment of human hydatid tissue. Scand J Infect Dis 1997;29:165 - 7.

10. Mohamed AE, Yasawy MI, Al Karawi MA. Combined albendazole and praziquantel versus albendazole alone in the treatment of hydatid disease. Hepatogastroenterology 1998;45:1690 - 4.

11. Franchi C, Di vico B, Teggi A. Long-term evaluation of patients with hydatidosis treated with benzimidazole carbamates. Clin Infect Dis 1999;29:304 - 9.

12. Horton RJ. Albendazole in treatment of human cystic echinococcosis: 12 years experience. Acta Trop 1997;64:79 - 93.

13. Aeberhard P, Fuhrimann R, Strahm P, Thommen A. Surgical treatment of hydatid disease of the liver: an experience from outside the endemic area. Hepatogastro-enterology 1996;43:627 - 36.

14. Alfieri S, Doglietto GB, Pacelli F, et al. Radical surgery for liver hydatid disease: study of 89 consecutive patients. Hepatogastroenterology 1997;44:496 - 500.

15. Uravic M, Stimac D, Lenac T, et al. Diagnosis and treatment of liver hydatid disease. Hepatogastroenterology 1998;45:2265 - 9.

16. Men S, Hekimoglu B, Yucesoy C, et al. Percutaneous treatment of hepatic hydatid cysts: an alternative to surgery. Am J Roentgenol 1999;172:83 - 9.

17. Ustunsoz B, Akhan O, Kamiloglu MA, et al. Percutaneous treatment of hydatid cysts of the liver: long-term results. Am J Roentgenol 1999;172:91 –6.

18. Enrico Brunetti, Carlo Filice, Calum Macpherson etal. PAIR: Puncture, Aspiration, Injection, Re-Aspiration. An option for the treatment of Cystic Echinococcosis. WHO/EMC Web site. Available at www.who.int/emc-documents/zoonoses/whocdscsraph20016.html. Accessed on 15.10.2004.

19. Guibert L, Gayral F. Laparoscopic pericystectomy of a liver hydatid cyst. Surg Endosc 1995; 9:442 - 3.

20. Sever M, Skapin S. Laparoscopic pericystectomy of liver hydatid cyst. Surg Endosc 1995; 9:1125 - 6.

21. Bickel A, Eitan A. The use of a large transparent cannula, with a beveled tip, for safe laparoscopic management of hydatid cysts of liver. Surg Endosc 1995;9:1304 - 5.

22. Khoury G, Jabbour-Khoury S, Bikhazi K. Results of laparoscopic treatment of hydatid cysts of the liver. Surg Endosc 1996; 10:57 - 9.

23. Bickel A, Daud G, Urbach D, et al. Laparoscopic approach to hydatid liver cysts. Is it logical? Physical, experimental, and practical aspects. Surg Endosc 1998; 12: 1073 - 7.

24. Ertem M, Uras C, Karahasanoglu T, etal. Laparoscopic approach to hepatic hydatid disease. Dig Surg 1998; 15: 333 - 6.

25. Verma GR, Bose SM. Laparoscopic treatment of hepatic hydatid cyst. Surg Laparosc Endosc 1998; 8:280 - 2.

26. Yaghan R, Heis H, Bani-Hani K etal. Is fear of anaphylactic shock discouraging surgeons from more widely adopting percutaneous and laparoscopic techniques in the treatment of liver hydatid cyst? Am J Surg. 2004 Apr; 187(4):533-7.

27. Clavien PA, Sanabria JR, Strasberg SM. Proposed classification of complications of surgery with examples of utility in cholecystectomy. Surgery 1992;111:518 - 26.

28. Barnes SA, Lillemoe KD. Liver Abscess and Hydatid Cyst Disease. In: Zinner MJ, Schwartz SI, Ellis H, eds. Maingot's Abdominal Operations 10th edition Prentice Hill International Inc., 1997:1534-1545.

29. Cohen H, Paolillo E, Bonifacino R etal. Human cystic echinococcosis in a Uruguayan community: A sonographic, serologic, and epidemiologic study. Am J Trop Med Hyg. 1998; 59(4): 620-627.

30. Lewall DB, Nyak P. Hydatid cysts of the liver: two cautionary signs. The British Journal of Radiology 1998; 71: 37-41.

31. Chautems R, Buhler L, Gold B etal. Long term results after complete or incomplete surgical resection of liver hydatid disease. Swis Med Wkly 2003; 133:258-262.

32. Schipper HG, Lameris JS, van Delden OM etal. Percutaneous evacuation (PEVAC) of multivesicular echinococcal cysts with or without cystobiliary fistulas which contain non-drainable material: first results of a modified PAIR method. Gut 2002; 50:718-723.

33. Niscigorska J, Sluzar T, Marczewska M etal. Parasitic cysts of the liver - practical approach to diagnosis and differentiation. Med Sci Monit, 2001; 7(4): 737-741.

34. Beecherl EE, Bigam DL, Langer B etal. Cystic diseases of the liver. In: Zuidema GD, Yeo CJ eds. Shackelford's Surgery of the Alimentary Tract. 5th ed Vol III WB Saunders Company, 2000:452-460.

35. Pedrosa I, Saiz A, Arrazola J etal. Hydatid disease: radiologic and pathologic features and complications. Radiographics, 2000 May-Jun; 20(3): 795-817.

36. Gharbi HA, Hassine W, Brauner MW etal. Ultrasound examination of the hydatid liver. Radiology, 139:459-463.

37. Milicevic MN. Hydatid disease. In: Blumgart LH, Fong Y, eds. Surgery of the liver and biliary tract. 3rd edition W. B. Saunders Company Ltd, 2002:1167-1204.

38. Saremi F. Percutaneous drainage of hydatid cysts: use of a new cutting device to avoid leakage. AJR 1992; 158:83-5.

39. Filippou DK, Kolimpiris C, Anemodouras N, Rizos S. Modified capitonage in partial cystectomy performed for liver hydatid disease: Report of 2 cases. BMC Surgery 2004; 4:8.

40. Bickel A, Loberant N, Shtamler B. Laparoscopic treatment of hydatid cyst of the liver: initial experience with a small series of patients. J Laparoendosc Surg. 1994 Apr;4(2): 127-33.

41. Khoury G, Jabbour-Khoury S, Soueidi A etal. Anaphylactic shock complicating laparoscopic treatment of hydatid cysts of the liver. Surg Endosc. 1998 May;12(5):452-4.

42. Massoud WZ. Laparoscopic excision of a single hepatic hydatid cyst. Int Surg. 1996 Jan-Mar;81(1):9-13

43. Khoury G, Geagea T, Hajj A etal. Laparoscopic treatment of hydatid cysts of the liver. Surg Endosc. 1994 Sep; 8(9): 1103-4.

44. Emelianov SI, Khamidov MA. Laparoscopic treatment of hydatid liver cysts. Khirurgiia (Mosk). 2000(11):32-4.

45. Manterola C, Fernandez O, Munoz S. Laparoscopic pericystectomy for liver hydatid cysts. Surg Endosc. 2002 Mar; 16(3):521-4.

46. Sayek I, Cakmakei M. Laparoscopic management of echinococcal cysts of the liver. Zentralbl Chir. 1999;124(12):1143-6.

47. Katkhouda N, Trussler A. Laparoscopic surgery of the liver. In: Zucker KA ed. Surgical Laparoscopy 2nd edition Lippincott Williams & Wilkins, 2001:211-220.1

48. Seven R, Berber E, Mercan S etal. Laparoscopic treatment of hepatic hydatid cysts. Surgery. 2000 Jul; 128(1):36-40.

49. Altinli E, Saribeyoglu K, Pekmezci S etal. An effective omentoplasty technique in laparoscopic surgery for hydatid disease of the liver. JSLS. 2002 Oct-Dec; 6(4): 323-6.

50. Bickel A, Loberant N, Singer-Jordan J, etal. The laparoscopic approach to abdominal hydatid cysts: a prospective nonselective study using the isolated hypobaric technique. Arch Surg. 2001 Jul; 136(7):789-95.

51. Saglam A. Laparoscopic treatment of liver hydatid cysts. Surg Laparosc Endosc. 1996 Feb; 6(1):16-21.

52. Alper A, Emre A, Hazar H, etal. Laparoscopic surgery of hepatic hydatid disease: initial results and early follow-up of 16 patients. World J Surg. 1995 Sep-Oct; 19(5):725-8.

53. Kayaalp C. Evacuation of hydatid liver cysts using laparoscopic trocar. World J Surg. 2002 Nov; 26(11):1324-7.

54. Al-Shareef Z, Hamour OA, Al-Shlash S, etal. Laparoscopic treatment of hepatic hydatid cysts with a liposuction device. JSLS. 2002 Oct-Dec; 6(4):327-30.

55. Zengin K, Unal E, Karabicak I, etal. A new instrument, the "Perfore-Aspirator" for laparoscopic treatment of hydatid cysts of the liver. Surg Laparosc Endosc Percutan Tech. 2003 Apr; 13(2):80-2.

56. Amir Jahed AK, Fardin R, Farzad A, etal. Clinical echinococcosis. Annals of Surgery. 1975; 182:541-6.

57. Little JM, Hollands MJ, Ekberg H. Recurrence of hydatid disease. World J Surg. 1988; 12:700-4.

58. Acarli K. Controversies in the laparoscopic treatment of hepatic hydatid disease. HPB, 2004; 6(4):213-221.

59. Bilge A, Sozuer EM. Diagnosis and surgical treatment of hepatic hydatid disease. HPB Surg 1992; 6:57-64.

60. Berrada S, Essadki B, Zeroulai NO. Kyste hydatique du foie. Traitement par resection du dome saillant. Notre experience a propos d'une serie de 495 cas. Ann Chir 1993; 47:510-12.

61. Yorganci K, Sayek I. Surgical treatment of hydatid cysts of the liver in the era of percutaneous treatment. Am J Surg 2002; 184:63-9.

62. Belli L, Aseni P, Rondinara GF, Bertini M. Improved results with pericystectomy in normothermic ischemia for hepatic hydatidosis. Surg Gynecol Obstet 1986; 163:127-32.

49

Laparoscopic Hepatic Resection

INTRODUCTION

Laparoscopy has been in vogue in the surgical practice for nearly two decades now. As for as the liver is concerned, surgical fraternity were reluctant to apply the principles of minimal access surgery to hepatic resections for the fear of hemorrhage and bile leak. Hence laparoscopy was restricted to minor procedures like liver biopsy and fenestration of liver cysts. With the advent of modern laparoscopic hemostatic instruments and parenchymal dividing devices augmented with better understanding of the surgical anatomy as well as the pathophysiology of the hepatic tumors, laparoscopy has been incorporated albeit slowly in the management of liver tumors. Initially applied mainly to the resection of the benign tumors,[1-2] this minimal access approach has been extended to the management of malignant tumors.

Laparoscopic approach to the liver resection was first reported by Gagner[22] et al in 1992. It was a non anatomical resection for focal nodular hyperplasia. In 1995, Ferzli et al[23] reported a similar type of resection using laparoscopic approach. The first successful laparoscopic anatomical hepatic resection was reported in 1996 by Azagra et al,[24] who performed a left lateral segmentectomy in a patient with benign adenoma of liver.

To begin with, benign conditions like hemangioma and focal nodular hyperplasia were successfully resected using laparoscopic approach. But of late, lot of studies have shown that laparoscopic liver resections for malignant tumor is not only feasible but also safe. It also offers the advantages of minimally invasive approach like less postoperative pain, lesser hospital stay and early return to work. Recently studies comparing open and laparoscopic approaches to the management of the liver tumors revealed favorable outcome for laparoscopic liver resection.

The spectrum of resections that are being performed laparoscopically include segmentectomy, subsegmentectomy and wedge resection on one side and major hepatectomies and bisegmentectomies on the other side. But unlike the segmentectomies where the procedure is standardized, the steps in major hepatic resections are still evolving. Not to stop here, laparoscopic techniques are also employed in various other hepatic procedures like radiofrequency ablation of liver tumors and placement of hepatic artery infusion pumps. This section deals with the indication for liver resections, type of resections and the techniques to achieve such resections.

INDICATIONS

The indications for laparoscopic liver resections are essentially the same as that of open hepatic resections. It includes both benign conditions as well as the malignant ones.[3] But the general principles guiding the resections are different for benign and malignant tumors. In case of benign tumors, the removal of liver tissue should be kept to a minimum and indeed enucleation of many tumors is often appropriate. Such enucleative methods are employed in the management of hemangioma, adenoma and fibronodular hyperplasia. With the advent of minimal access surgery, there is a tendency to offer surgical management for many benign tumors and conditions which actually don't require such intervention. Technical feasibility of laparoscopic resections thus should not influence the management of benign tumors. Only those tumors which are symptomatic, in doubtful diagnosis or known to have malignant potential should be offered surgical management.

The operative strategy varies in case of malignant tumors. It should be guided by the principle of complete tumor removal with the current evidence suggesting that the margin of clearance should be no less than 1cm. But having said this, more often other factors have come into play to determine the extent of resection. These include the status of the liver and its functional capacity, the nature of the tumor, its size, number and position and finally the fitness of the patient to withstand major surgery.

Indications for resection in benign tumors

1. Symptomatic
2. Doubtful diagnosis
3. Tumors with known malignant potential

Common indications for liver resection[3]

1. Benign liver tumors
   i.   Haemangioma
   ii. Adenoma
   iii. Fibronodular hyperplasia
   iv. Cystadenoma

2. Malignant tumors
   i. Primary
       a. Hepatocellular carcinoma
       b. Cholangiocarcinoma
       c. Gall bladder cancer
   ii. Secondary
       a. Colorectal
       b. Neuroendocrine
       c. Secondaries from other sites

Moreover, presence of jaundice, cirrhosis and portal hypertensions will have an adverse effect during and after surgery. Jaundice will derange the functions of liver besides causing wound related complications. In cirrhotic liver, the mobilization of the liver is difficult and is associated with increased intraoperative bleeding and post operative liver failure. Hence in such patients resection should be restricted to patients with good liver function.

TYPES OF RESECTION

The amount of liver tissue that is either removed or retained determines the type of resection. The extent of the liver parenchyma that is removed is determined by various factors like the size and number of the lesions, location of the tumor and the functional status of the liver. The principles governing open liver resection holds good for laparoscopic liver resection also. Basically, liver resection can be classified as anatomical and nonanatomical. Anatomical

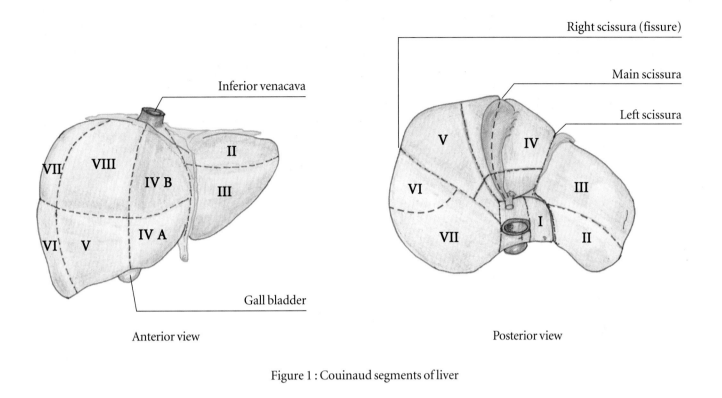

Figure 1 : Couinaud segments of liver

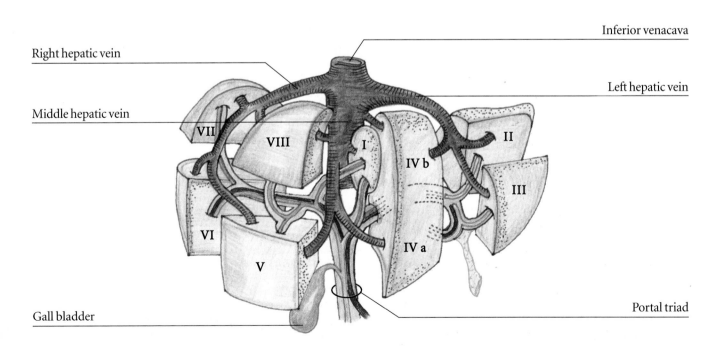

Figure 2 : Couinaud segmentation system of liver

Table 1. Major Hepatic Resections

Couinaud[4-6]	Gold Smith & Wood burne[7]	Segments Removed
Right Hepatectomy	Right Hepatic lobectomy	V, VI, VII, VIII
Left Hepatectomy	Left Hepatic lobectomy	II, III, IV
Right Lobectomy	Extended right hepatic lobectomy	IV, V, VI, VII, VIII
Left Lobectomy	Left lateral segmentlectomy	II, III
Extended Left Hepatectomy	Extended left lobectomy	II, III, IV, V, VIII

liver resections are based on the principle of segmental anatomy of the liver. Here the parenchymal division occurs at the intersegmental planes which are relatively avascular. Anatomical liver resections result in better patient outcome, improve the surgically negative margins, reduces recurrence rate and reduces intra operative blood loss. It is more physiological as it does not alter the intrahepatic blood flow, bile flow and pressure gradients.

On the contrary, non anatomic liver resections do not follow the well established intersegmental planes. Hence the plane of dissection is around the tumor which does not take into consideration the segmental anatomy of the liver. As a consequence, there is disruption of the blood flow or biliary drainage of the remaining segments. This will lead to increased post operative complications like biliary leak and haemorrhage from the resected edges. Because of all these problems, non anatomic resections are now rarely been performed except in peripherally situated benign tumors. Wedge resection is one such classical example of non anatomic resection wherein a wedge of liver parenchyma containing the tumor is removed.

The nomenclature for various types of liver resection is many fold and rather confusing. This is because of the fact that many author have described the segmental anatomy of the liver and the types of resections are based on these descriptions. Here we present a simplified classifion of liver resection, incorporating Couinaud (1957)[7] and Goldsmith and Woodburne (1957)[4-6] terminologies.

Non Anatomic Liver Resections
Wedge Resection
Enucleation
Atypical liver resection

Anatomical Liver Resection
Subsegmentectomy
Segmentectomy
Bisegmentectomy
Trisegmentectomy
Right and left Hepatectomies

The common type of laparoscopic liver resections that are routinely performed include wedge resections, segmentectomies and subsegmentectomies. A lot of studies have now been published regarding the feasibility, advantages and limitations regarding laparoscopic liver resections. Though case reports and short series have been found in the literature for major laparoscopic resections, further studies are needed to establish this minimally invasive approach to major liver resections.

LAPAROSCOPIC LIVER RESECTION - TECHNIQUE[8]

Instrumentation

Laparoscopic liver surgery requires efficient skills and high quality imaging and instruments. For better visualization of the operative field, 3 chip digital camera is very useful. Angled scope (30° or 45°)

enables the observation of the blind areas, superior, posterior and lateral surfaces of the liver and the anterior abdominal wall. Better illumination is provided by the Xenon light source. In addition, special instruments that form indispensable part of the procedure include fan shaped multi pronged liver retractor, atraumatic clip applier, harmonic shears, argon plasma coagulation, CUSA probe, ligasure, fibrin glue and vascular staplers.

An open table containing all the instruments used for conventional open liver surgery should always be kept ready. In the event of the procedure being converted into an open one, the changeover from laparoscopic table to an open one should be quick as the situation warrants.

Position and Ports

Laparoscopic liver resections are performed with the patient in supine position and legs semiflexed in modified lithotomy position. Special care is taken to prevent nerve injuries due to inadvertent compression by the operating table setup. The table is usually in reverse Trendelenberg's position and rotated sidewards as and when needed. If necessary, a sand bag is placed under the right shoulder to make the right lobe more prominent. The surgeon stands between the legs while the camera surgeon stands on the right and the first assistant on the left side of the patient. Monitor is at the head end of the patient. This patient set up is similar to the one used for fundoplication and other lower esophageal and stomach surgeries.

The access to the abdomen is usually through the umbilicus or supraumbilical area using closed Veress needle technique. Pneumoperitoneum is created using carbon dioxide insufflation and the supraumbilical trocar (10mm) is inserted. A general survey of the abdominal cavity is made after which the remaining trocars are placed under direct vision. Under normal circumstances, two working ports and two retractions with suction ports are required for hepatic resections. Though the exact placement of the trocars very with the type of resections performed, the general scheme of port placements is illustrated

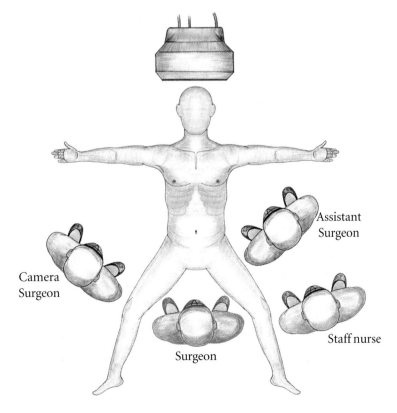

Figure 3 : Team setup

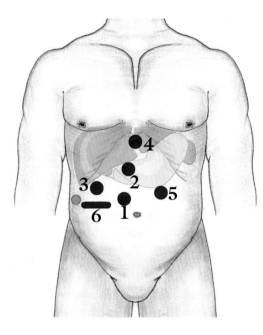

Figure 4 : Port position

No.	Instruments	Place
1	Camera	Right of supraumbilicus 10mm
2	Right hand working port	Right of midline 10mm
3	Left hand working port	Right midclavicular 5mm
4	Left lobe liver retracting port	Subxiphoid 5mm
5	Stomach retracting port	Left of supraumbilicus 5mm
6	Right lobe retraction port, Port hepatis clamp and Hand port	Right anterior axillary 5mm Extended transversely for hand port

in the figure. The camera port is usually in the supraumbilical area though it can vary. In cirrhotic patients, umbilicus is generally avoided as there might be recanalisation of the umbilical veins due to elevated portal pressure.[9] This may cause torrential bleeding during trocar placement. Two working ports, right and left are placed accordingly on either side of the camera port forming a triangulation for optimal working space. The above port position is for totally laparoscopic liver resection.

To minimise the risk of air embolism, insufflation pressure should be kept as low as possible, preferably at around 12mm Hg. In selected cases, use of an abdominal wall lift device for gaseless laparoscopy should be considered. The patients should be closely monitored for vital parameters and end tidal CO_2 levels throughout the procedure. During the use of argon plasma coagulation (APC), the intra abdominal pressure should be lowered down to the minimum, as the argon gas may raise the intraabdominal pressure facilitating the risk of gas embolism.

In addition, two more ports are placed, one at the subxiphoid level and the other at the sub costal area laterally. These ports are meant for retraction of the liver. Apart from these standard ports, additional ports for bowel retraction are placed as and when necessary. Hand port used in the later part of the surgery is placed in the right lumbar area.

KEY STEPS IN HEPATIC SURGERY

Irrespective of the type and extent of the liver resection, there are certain steps which are common to all laparoscopic liver resections. These steps closely mimic many maneuvers used in the open procedure although few differences are present.

1. Diagnostic Laparoscopy

The first step in any laparoscopic resectional procedure is the thorough evaluation of the extent of the disease and staging the disease. Nearly 40% of the tumors which were identified as resectable by preoperative investigations are found to be unresectable during diagnostic laparoscopy. Hence thorough evaluation of the tumor and its extent becomes all the more important. Initial survey looks for the presence of extrahepatic extension of the tumor, presence of ascites, status of the liver and the nodal involvement. Sometimes, mobilization of the liver and opening of the lesser sac may be necessary to assess the above mentioned features. Tumor characters like the location, extent, its relation to the vessels and ducts are made out by laparoscopic ultrasound. It uses high frequency probe (7.5MHz) and has a flexi tip to negotiate difficult and inaccessible areas. Moreover, it detects occult for the tumors which are less than 1cm in size. It also identifies the plane of division of the liver parenchyma.

2. Mobilization of the liver

The first step in the mobilization of the liver is the division of the falciform and round ligament. It can be done using harmonic scalpel, ligasure or electrocautery. Due care must be taken to coagulate the vessels in these ligaments, especially in cirrhotics. The separation of the falciform ligament[9] from the anterior abdominal wall is extended cranially so as to expose the suprahepatic, infra diaphragmatic inferior venacava. The connective tissue around the inferior venacava is cleared off by careful dissection. The divided end of the ligamentum teres (round ligament) is then used to give cranial traction of the liver so that the porta hepatis and inferior surface of the liver becomes clearly visible.

Unlike in open surgery, triangular and the coronary ligaments of the concerned side that is to be removed is divided later during the surgery once the inflow control and parenchymal division are achieved. This maneuver of dividing the ligaments lastly is very important as it provides the necessary counter

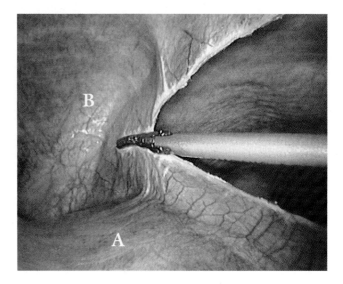

Figure 6 : Division of falciform ligament

A - Right lobe of liver

B - Diaphragm

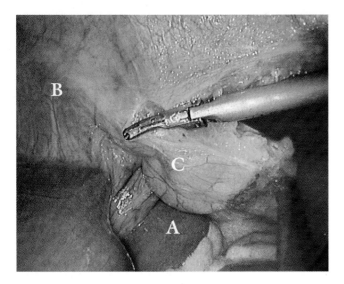

Figure 5 : Division of falciform ligament using harmonic ace

A - Left lobe of liver

B - Falciform ligament

C - Ligamentum teres

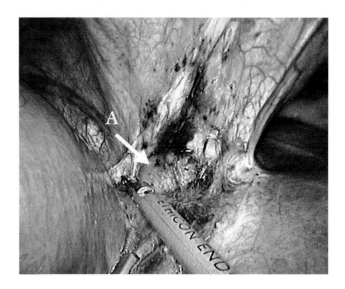

Figure 7 : Completion of falciform ligament division, infra diaphragmatic portion of inferior vena cava is seen

A - Inferior vena cava

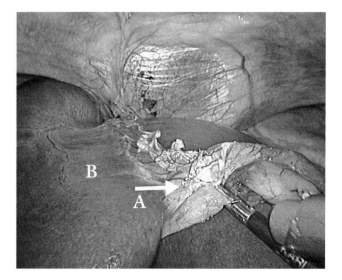

Figure 8 : Divided end of the ligamentum teres is used to hold and give traction of the right lobe of liver

A - Ligamentum teres
B - Right lobe of liver

traction and support to the liver during parenchymal division. Once the parenchyma is divided, the triangular and coronary ligaments are then divided.

3. Porta hepatis dissection - Inflow control

The next step is the inflow control which is achieved by porta hepatis dissection. The liver is cranially retracted and the porta is clearly made out. Sometimes retraction of the duodenum below is necessary to have proper exposure of the porta. The peritoneal reflection along the lateral free border of the lesser omentum is incised and dissected so as to expose the common bile duct, portal vein and the hepatic artery. The cystic duct and the artery are dissected in the Calot's triangle, clipped and divided. The divided gall bladder is then used to retract the liver cranially and removed at the end of the procedure. As the dissection proceeds towards the hilum, the right and left branches of the hepatic duct, portal vein and hepatic artery are identified. Sometimes the confluence may be intrahepatic for which lowering of the hilar plate may be needed. The concerned branches

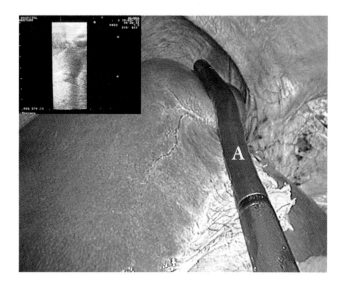

Figure 9 : Laparoscopic ultrasonographic study of the liver

A - Laparoscopic ultrasound probe

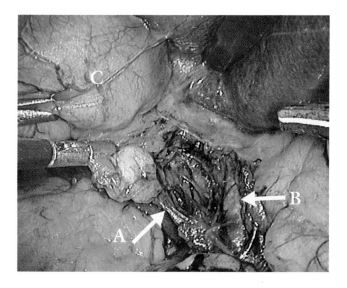

Figure 10 : Porta hepatic dissection. Cystic duct is dissected

A - Cystic duct
B - Common bile duct
C - Gall bladder

are then divided, securing the pedicle supplying the retained side of the liver. We generally follow extra-hepatic dissection to achieve inflow control. But due care should be taken to identify the anomalous anatomy present if any. At this juncture, we need to emphasis the fact that the portal triad branches to the caudate lobe should be preserved if the caudate lobe is retained. Moreover, in certain types of resections, the division of the branches is performed at the umbilical fissure and in case of segmental resections, there is no need for portal dissection at all. All these variations and modifications will be dealt in the respective sections.

4. Parenchymal division

We do not routinely use pringle maneuver. But if needed a long occlusive clamp through the lateral most port can be used to occlude the portal triad, thereby controlling the bleed. Alternatively a rubber sling with plastic tube can be used as and when necessary. We follow the anterior approach of dividing

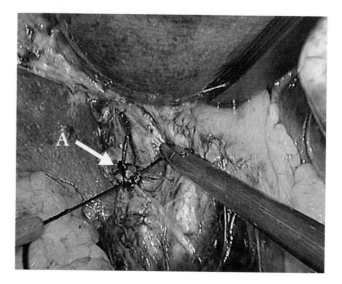

Figure 12 : Ligation of right hepatic artery

A - Right hepatic artery

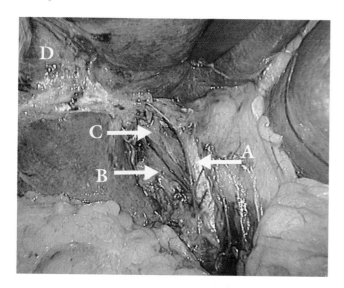

Figure 11 : Porta hepatic dissection for right hepatectomy

A - Common bile duct
B - Right hepatic artery
C - Right portal vein
D - Gall bladder bed

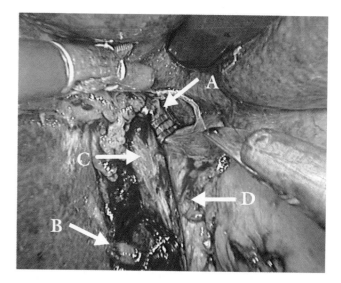

Figure 13 : Right hepatic duct is dissected, clipped and divided

A - Right hepatic duct
B - Divided end of right hepatic artery
C - Right branch of portal vein
D - Common bile duct

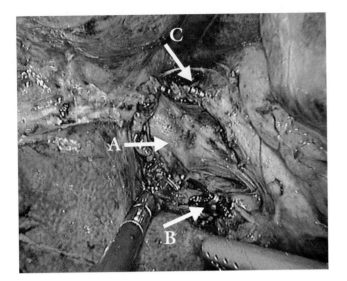

Figure 14 : Right portal vein is dissected

A - Right portal vein
B - Divided end of right hepatic artery
C - Divided end of Right hepatic duct

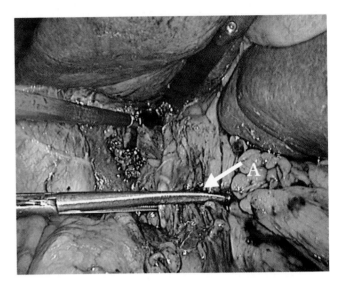

Figure 15 : Laparoscopic vascular clamp is applied to occlude the portal triad

A - Laparoscopic vascular clamp

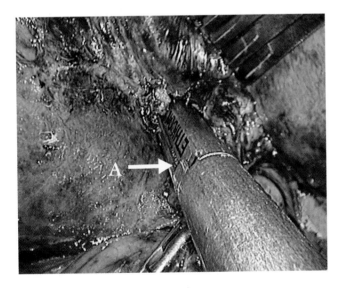

Figure 16 : Endo GIA vascular stapler is used to divide the right portal vein

A - Endo vascular stapler

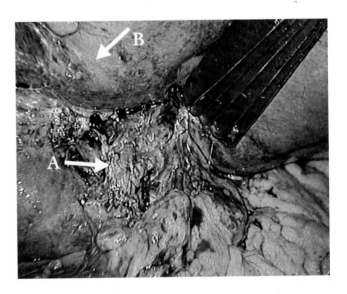

Figure 17 : Completion of portal triad dissection. Line of demarcation is seen well

A - Divided end of right portal vein
B - Line of demarcation

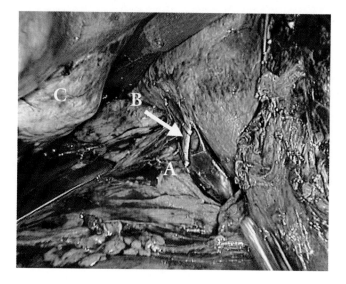

Figure 18 : Triangular ligaments are divided, short hepatic vein draining into the inferior vena cava is clipped

A - Inferior vena cava
B - Clipped vein
C - Tumor

the parenchyma before outflow control. The line of division is usually marked on the Glisson's capsule using either monopolar cautery or harmonic scalpel and the division is commenced on the anterior surface of the liver. To about 5mm in depth, the parenchyma is divided using harmonic scalpel. After this depth, the use of Cavitational Ultrasonic Surgical Aspiration (CUSA) probe will divide and suck the collagen sparse hepatocytes while leaving the ductules and vessels intact. These vessels can be divided now and then using clips or ligasure. Continuous suction during the division will keep the operative field clear. In this way, the parenchyma is divided along the entire plane to reach the posterior surface. During the division, the intraabdominal pressure is reduced to 8mm Hg to prevent gas embolism.

5. Hepatic vein division - Outflow control

As the parenchymal splitting reaches the posterior surface of the liver, the major hepatic veins are encountered. Once the hepatic vein that is to be divided is visualised, it is dissected out clearly and its

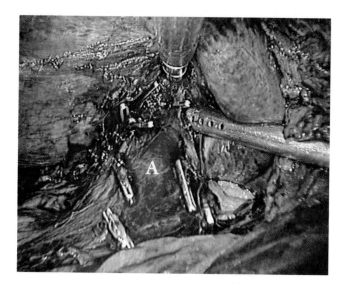

Figure 19 : Dissection of posterior surface of right lobe of liver. Retro hepatic veins are clipped and divided

A - Inferior vena cava

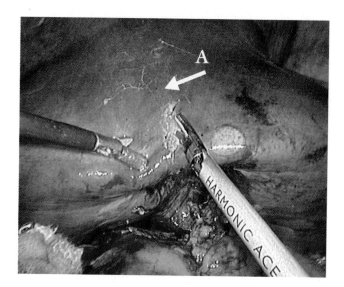

Figure 20 : Division of liver parenchyma using harmonic ace

A - Line of demarcation

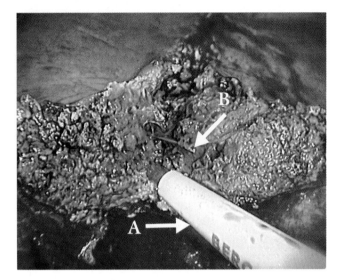

Figure 21 : Cavitional ultrasonic suction and aspiration (CUSA) is used to suck the hepatocyte

A - Laparoscopic CUSA probe
B - Exposed hepatic veins

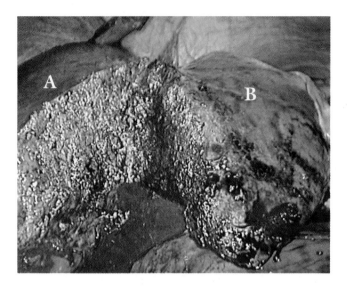

Figure 22 : Division of liver parenchyma. CUSA and harmonic ace is used for the division

A - Portion of liver with tumor
B - Normal liver

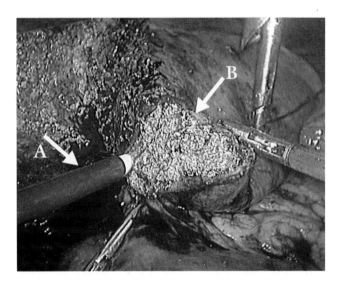

Figure 23 : Argon beam coagulation is used for surface hemostasis

A - Laparoscopic 5mm argon beam coagulation probe
B - Coagulated surface

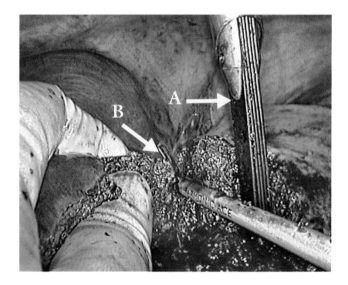

Figure 24 : Hand port is made and left hand of the operating surgeon is introduced inside the peritoneal cavity to retract the liver

A - Liver retraction is used to retractor the liver
B - Division of liver parenchyma using harmonic ace

junction with the inferior vena cava is identified. It is our practice to apply vascular stapler to divide the hepatic vein concerned. Once this is done, the remaining attachments are released and now the specimen is ready to be retrieved.

6. Specimen Retrieval

The free lying specimen should be removed in an endobag. But before that, it is imperative to check for any bleeding or bile leak from the cut surface of the liver. Any diffuse ooze from the surface can be controlled by using Argon Plasma Coagulation (APC) to the severed end. Finally, the specimen is retrieved by enlarging one of the ports taking care not to have contact with the port site. The liver specimen should be removed enbloc and not in piece meal. This facilitates proper histopathological evaluation of the tumor and its margins.

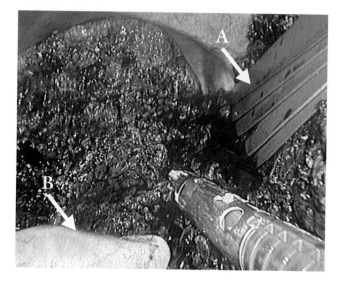

Figure 26 : Endo GIA vascular stapler is used to divide the right hepatic vein

A - Normal liver is retracted by liver retractor
B - Liver with tumor is retracted by the surgeon

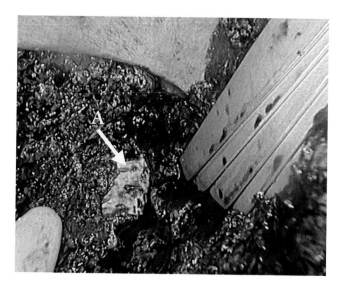

Figure 25 : Right hepatic is exposed

A - Right hepatic vein

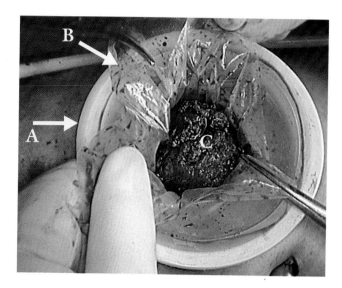

Figure 27 : Excised liver is placed in the endobag and extracted through the hand port

A - Lap disc (Ethicon)
B - Endobag
C - Excised liver

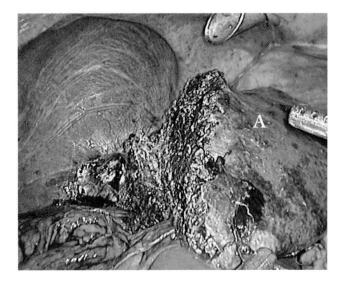

Figure 28 : Completion of right hepatectomy.

A - Remaining portion of liver

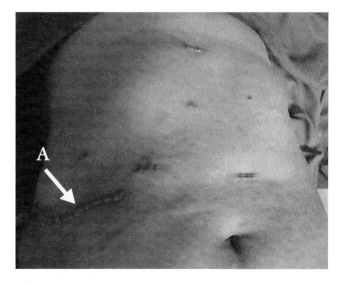

Figure 30 : Position of ports after completion of the surgery

A - Hand port

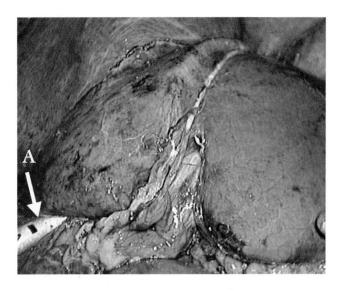

Figure 29 : Drainage tube is placed. Position of the remaining liver after right hepatectomy

A - Drainage tube

DETAILS OF INDIVIDUAL RESECTIONS

1. Right Hepatectomy

Right hepatectomy by laparoscopic approach is a major undertaking that should be taken only in centres with adequate skills and necessary armam entarium. Here segments V, VI, VII & VIII are removed. Patient is placed in reverse Trendelenberg's position with split leg table. The general scheme of port placements hold good for right hepatectomy except the fact that these ports are placed somewhat to the right. Moreover, left side table tilt is some-times necessary for proper exposure of the right lobe of the liver.

As discussed previously, the initial step is the division of the falciform ligament and ligament teres. Cra-nial traction is given to the liver and the inferior surface is exposed. Porta hepatis dissection is com-menced by incising the peritoneum over the hepatic duct. Calot's triangle is dissected out, cystic duct and artery clipped and divided separately. Depending on the situation and ease of retraction, the cranial traction of the liver is achieved by either gall bladder or ligament teres or by the use of fan shaped retractor. At the hilum, the first structure to be dissected is the common hepatic duct. The confluence of the right and left duct is made out and then the right hepatic duct is ligated using vicryl and divided.

At this point, the surgeon should be fully aware of the anatomic variations at the porta so that inadvertent biliary injury is prevented. Next in line is the hepatic artery which lies on the anteromedial aspect of the portal vein. Right hepatic artery is carefully dissected and doubly ligated using silk and divided. Left branch of the hepatic artery is duely protected and its pulsation can be felt at the umbilical fissure. Now the portal vein comes into view which is dissected all around carefully. Right branch of the portal vein is identified and divided using a vascular stapler. Branches to the caudate lobe is carefully identified and preserved. Sometimes the right anterior and posterior sectorial branch of the portal vein arise separately and these origins may be separated by as much as 2cm. It is important not to misidentify these branches during dissection. Once the portal blood supply is cut off, the colour change is visible on the surface of the liver and now it is ready for parenchymal division.

The line of division is the principle plane or the Cantlie's line passing from the gall bladder fossa to the IVC posteriorly. After marking it over the Glisson's capsule, the parenchymal division is started. Parenchyma is divided by using the methods discussed previously. The pressure at this stage is reduced to 8mm Hg and the patient is placed in Trendelenberg's position. This helps to minimize the risk of air embolism. During its splitting, the middle hepatic vein is secured and right hepatic vein is divided closed to the IVC using vascular stapler. At this stage, a hand port may be used for left hand which is used to give traction to the specimen so that the right triangular ligament, coronary ligament and the diaphragmatic attachments are divided. The retrohepatic veins draining directly into the IVC are ligated and divided before separating from the IVC. Caval ligament from the caudate lobe is also divided. After achieving hemostasis, look for any biliary leak and if not found, the specimen is retrieved as discussed in the previous section.

Left Hepatectomy

Left hepatectomy involves removal of segments II, III & IV. The essential steps involved in left hepatectomy are almost the mirror image of right hepatectomy, albeit with few variations. After dividing the round and falciform ligaments and retracting the liver cranially, porta hepatic dissection is commenced. Structures at the hilum are dissected out clearly as before. If necessary the hilar plate may be lowered to have proper visualization of the right and left branches. Moreover, the same dissection can be carried out at the umbilical fissure in which case the bridge of liver tissue between the umbilical tissue and the quadrate lobe is divided.

Generally, the left hepatic duct and portal vein has a long extrahepatic course when compared with the right side and hence the dissection on the left is easier. While dissecting the left hepatic duct, look for any anomalous drainage of right posterior or anterior sectorial duct into the left hepatic duct in which case it should be preserved and the left hepatic duct divided proximally. The left hepatic artery is ligated and divided and left branch of portal vein is divided using endovascular stapler. The branches to the caudate lobe are looked for, identified and preserved.

Once the colour change is made out on the surface, the parenchymal division is started as detailed previously. Here also the plane of division is the principle scissura (Cantlie's line). The right hepatic vein is preserved while the middle and left hepatic vein are divided. In majority of cases, the middle and left hepatic veins unite to form a common channel and drains into IVC. Once the parenchymal division reaches the anterior surface of the IVC, the gastrohepatic ligament (lesser omentum) is divided to expose the caudate lobe. The left triangular ligament is divided taking care not to injure the inferior phrenic vein which runs close to it. Also the remaining diaphragmatic attachments and the left coronary ligaments are divided. Subdiaphragmatic IVC is dissected out, the middle and left hepatic veins dissected out clearly. For this, the left lobe may need to be retracted to the right side. This exposes the ligamentum venosum which will lead to the left hepatic vein. A vascular stapler is used to divide the middle and left hepatic veins either together or separately. Finally, the left lobe is separated from the caudate lobe which frees the left lobe all around and now the specimen is ready for retrieval. In the mean time, any ooze or bile leak is checked and the cut surface is coagulated using Argon Beam Coagulation.

Left Lateral Segmentectomy (Left Lobectomy)

Removal of the anatomical left lobe (segments II & III) is far more easier when compared with major resections like right or left heptectomies. The port positions are the same except the fact that these are placed more on the left side. The round and the falciform ligaments are divided. Pedicles to the segments II & III can be ligated either at the umbilical fissure or during parenchymal division.

The plane of division is along the line of attachment of the falciform ligament to the liver surface. During parencymal splitting, the pedicles to the segments II & III are clipped or ligated and divided if not done so at the umbilical fissure. As the parenchymal division is proceeding, the left hepatic vein comes

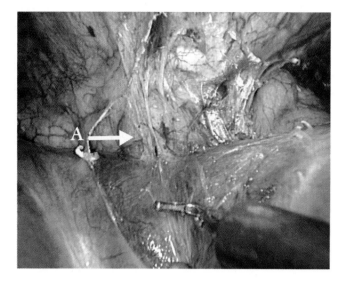

Figure 32 : Division of falciform ligament upto the diaphragm and infra diaphragmatic surface of inferior vena cava is dissected

A - Inferior vena cava

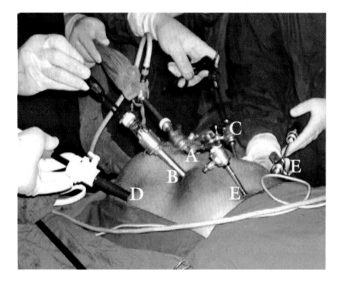

Figure 31 : Ports p[osition for left lobe resection

A - Camera port
B - Right hand working port
C - Left hand working port
D - Retracting port
E - Retracting port

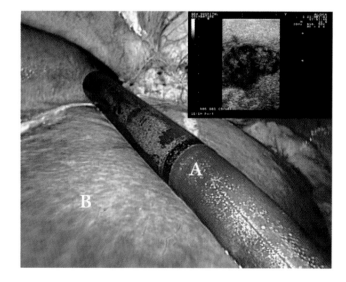

Figure 33 : Laparoscopic ultrasound examination of the liver

A - Laparoscopic ultrasound probe
B - Left lobe of liver

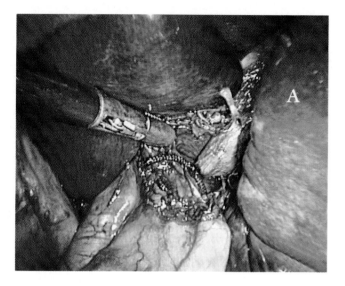

Figure 34 : Ligation and division of vein in the round ligament

A - Left lobe of liver

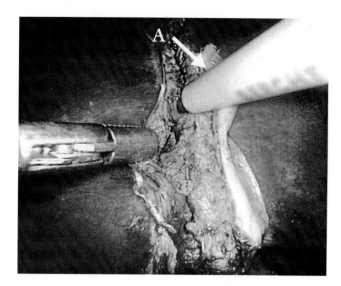

Figure 35 : Division of liver parenchyma using CUSA

A - CUSA probe

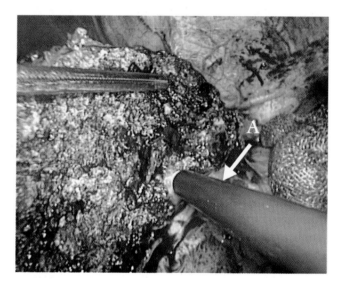

Figure 36 : After the resection of left lobe of liver, surface of the normal liver is coagulated by argon beam coagulation

A - Argon beam coagulation probe

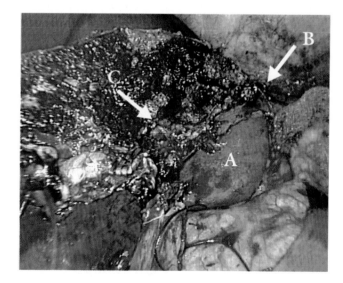

Figure 37 : Completion of left lobectomy

A - Caudate lobe f liver
B - Sutured branch of left hepatic vein
C - Clipped hepatic duct

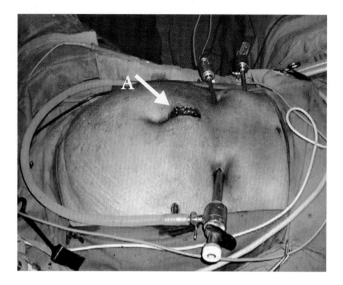

Figure 38 : Port position and size of the minilaparotomy

A - Minilaparotomy wound

into the picture which is then divided using vascular stapler. The division of the parenchyma should end anterior to the caudate lobe. Finally the left triangular ligament is divided and the specimen retrieved.

Segmentectomies

The tumors which are small and limited to a particular segment can be dealt with segmentectomy alone provided the margin of clearance in adequate. The segments that can be accessed by laparoscopic approach include segments II, III, IV, V & VI whereas segments I, VII and VIII are difficult to access.

The principles governing these segmentectomies are the same as that of major hepatic resections. Laparoscopic ultrasound probe is used to identify the pedicles as well as the plane and extent of the division. For left lobe segmentectomies (II, III, IV) the falciform and the round ligament divided and the undersurface of the liver is exposed. The pedlices can be ligated at the umbilical fissure and if not possible there, during the parenchymal division. As the parenchymal division is proceeding the corresponding hepatic vein branches of that particular segment is divided while preserving the main hepatic vein and other branches.

For segment V resection, the parenchymal division is started at the anterior surface of the liver, exactly at the Cantlie's line the right extent of the resection is at the right portal scissura. During resection, both middle and right hepatic veins should be preserved. Segment VI resection is performed with a left lateral tilt.

Bisegmentectomies

It involves removal of two adjacent segments. The common bisegmentectomies that are feasible by minimal access approach include segments II & III and V-VIII. II-III bisegmentectomy (left lateral segmentectomy) has been discussed previously. V-VIII bisegmentalectomy otherwise called right anterior sectoriectomy is just an extension of the segmental excision of the fifth segment cranially to include eighth segment. This is technically demanding since segment VIII is situated very close to the diaphragm.

Alternate Approach to liver resection - Four Hand Technique

There are many technical variations in laparoscopic liver resection. One such technique is the one developed by Kathouda and J. Mouriel.[10] Here the surgery is performed by two surgeons. One surgeon uses hand port for manipulation and with the other hand clips and divides the vessel. The second surgeon retracts the liver and sucks out the fluid and blood to make the operative field clear and accessible.

Hand port offers many advantages during laparoscopic liver resection. It reduces the parenchymal tearing due to improper traction with laparoscopic instruments. Moreover, the presence of extrahepatic disease is well made out with the hand port. During inadvertent haemorhage, the presence of hand in the abdomen will aid in rapid control of haemorrhage and also faster conversion to open surgery. The same hand port can be used for specimen retrieval also.

LAPAROSCOPIC DONOR HEPATECTOMY

Laparoscopic approach has now been recently introduced in the filed of transplantation. As the cadverci organ donors are in short supply, living donors are increasingly being used in transplantations. Cherqui et al (2002)[11] have developed a safe and reproducible method of laparoscopic living donor hepatectomy. Left lobe of the living donor is harvested as it is technically easier. This laparoscopic approach is mainly used for liver transplantation in children.[5] The delivery of the liver should be done enbloc without any damage. The harvested liver should have inflow and outflow pedicle and bile duct for proper anastomosis. This technique reduces the postoperative morbidity for the donors. A lot of animal studies[12,13,14] and few human studies[15,16,17] have shown that it is a feasible alternative to open donor hepatectomy. But further studies are needed in this aspect to recommend it as a routine procedure.

HEPATIC ARTERY INFUSION PUMPS

Laparoscopic approach is now extended to the placement of hepatic artery infusion pumps. Since about two thirds of the blood supply to hepatic metastases comes from hepatic artery, the chemotherapeutic agents can be infused directly into the hepatic artery to prevent systemic complications.

The port placements are similar to the resectional procedures. The falciform and the gastrohepatic ligaments divided and the common hepatic artery is skeletonised along its entire course. The gastroduodenal artery is divided and through the divided stump, the catheter is inserted and fixed. The catheter is connected to the pump which is placed in the subcutaneous tissue. Laparoscopic approach will be ideal in such situations which will prevent a long laparotomy scar and other wound related problems.

COMPLICATIONS

The intra and post operative complications of laparoscopic liver resection are the same as that of the open procedure with few added advantages and disadvantages. The advantages include the absence or decreased incidence of wound related complications, post operative adhesions and incisional hernia. Moreover the recovery is faster with quicker return to normal activity.

But there are a few complications that can occur during laparoscopic resectional procedures. The most troublesome is the haemorrhage from major venous structures. Minor bleeding can be controlled

laparoscopically, whereas major ones need at most times conversion to open surgery. Also since there is pneumoperitoneum, gas embolism can occur due to the opening of these major venous channels which will be detrimental.[18] In such situations put the patient in the Trendelenberg and right lateral decubitus positions and hydrate aggressively. Reducing the intraabdominal pressure and raising the CVP[19-21] will reduce such incidences. Parenchymal tearing is one another complication which can result from excessive retraction using instruments. Judicious use of laparoscopic retraction and the pressure of hand ports can reduce such complications.

Table: Complications

Intraoperative	Post operative
Major Haemorrhage	Ascites
Gas Embolism	Pleural effusion
Parenchymal tearing	Hepatic failure
Biliary injury	Haemorrhage
Diaphragmatic injury	Bile leak

DISCUSSION

Many studies have been published regarding the feasibility of laparoscopic approach to hepatic resection. Of late, many studies showed advantages of this minimally invasive approach over the conventional one. These advantages are well established in the management of benign tumors. Tumor dissemination and inadequate margins are the two potential disadvantages as far as the malignant tumors are concerned.[25] But nevertheless, short term results are comparable to that of conventional surgery.[26] In managing malignant tumors, the oncological principles should not be violated.

Inspite of improvements in the technique and the availability of the modern gadgets, bleeding during the procedure is a common occurrence. In cases of associated cirrhosis, this complication is more exemplified. Hence patient selection becomes the critical determinant in the outcome of laparoscopic liver resection. Initially, one should choose a simple procedure like segmentectomy in a non cirrhotic patients. There should be low threshold for conversion to avoid undue complications.[27]

Table 2. English-language Reports of Laparoscopic Liver Surgery[35-44]

Author/Year	Proced-ures (N)	SolidN (%)	Maligna-nt N (%)	OR Time (Minutes) Mean*/Median (Range)	Pringle Time	Blood Loss	Length of Stay (Days) Mean*/Media-n (Range)	Conversion to Open	Complica-tions	Mortality
Lesurtel 2003	18	18 (100)	6 (33)	*202+48 (150-360)	*39+10(23-6-2)	*236+155 (100-600)	*8+3(4-21)	12.5%	11%	0%
Gigot 2002	37	37 (100)	37 (100)	NA	31 (15-50)	NA	6 (2-16)	13.5%	22%	0%
Farges 2002	21	21 (100)	0 (0)	*177+57 (50-270)	*33+12	*218+173 (50-800)	*5.1+1.3	0%	9.5%	0%
Descottes 2002	87	81 (93)	0 (0)	NA	50 (20-120)	NA	*5 (2-13)	10%	5%	0%
Mala 2002	15	15 (100)	15 (100)	187 (80-334)	Not performed	600 (100-3300)	4 (1-6)	0%	11.3%	0%
Cherqui 2000	30	26 (87)	12 (40)	180 (60-360)	*50 (10-117)	100 (0-1500)	7 (3-40)	6.6%	20%	0%
Descottes 2000	16	16 (100)	2 (13)	*232+130 (115-595)	NA	NA	*5.2+3.2(2-15)	6.3%	6.3%	0%
Fong 2000	11	10 (91)	10 (91)	248 (143-358)	NA	450 (20-5000)	5 (0)	54.5%	18.2%	0%
Katkhouda 1999	43	12 (28)	0 (0)	179 (45-325)	NA	156 (90-980)	4.7(1-17)	7%	14.1%	0%
Huscher 1998	38	35 (92)	32 (84)	*189 (110-285)	*44(20-80)	*380 (100-1200)	*10(2-25)	5.3%	43%	2.5%
Marks 1998	28	7 (25)	1 (4)	*179 (45-525)	NA	NA	*7.7(1-44)	11%	21%	0%

Venous embolism is a unique complication to laparoscopic surgery and it is better to avoid it that to treat it. Hence during bleeding the intraabdominal pressure should be lowered and the central venous pressure should be raised by fluid infusion.[28] Hypotensive anaesthesia is sometimes useful in this regard. Though debated earlier, recent studies have shown that there was no significant difference in hemodynamic changes because of pneumoperitoneum when compared to the open surgery.[32]

Technique wise, newer modalities are being employed by different authors. No single technique has been shown to be superior to others. It is author's preference to use two hand, single surgeon technique instead of widely practiced 4 hand, two surgeons method. Hand ports are occasionally used in our procedures especially in case of large tumors. Apart from few inaccessible areas like caudate lobe and segment VIII, most of the resectional procedures can be done laparoscopically. But this requires adequate experience and modern instruments.

Due to several improvements in laparoscopic instruments and operative technique, latest reports suggest reduced intraoperative blood loss, reduced fluid infusions and decreased loss of protein and electrolyes.[29,30,31] Moreover, recent animal studies have shown that laparoscopic approach results in diminished stress response and better preservation of immune function.[33] As a result, tumor growth may be slower and the infection rate may be decreased after laparoscopic liver surgery. The overall mortality rate is lower in laparoscopic liver resection when compared with the open approach. Post operative complications like subphrenic fluid collection, haemorrhage or wound related complication are much less in laparoscopic surgery.[34]

To date about 750 patients have been reported to have undergone laparoscopic liver resections, of which about 70% are for benign lesions and the remaining 30% for malignant tumors. Conversion to open surgery stood at 5% in the present scenario which can be reduced by proper patient selection. The overall morbidity was 12% wherein ascites and pleural effusion were the most frequent complications. Table 2 illustrates the reported series of 10 or more cases of laparoscopic liver resection.[35-45]

CONCLUSION

Laparoscopic liver resection has come here to stay. It needs adequate expertise in open liver resections, advanced laparoscopic skills and the availability of special instruments for hemostasis and parenchymal division. The results of the laparoscopic liver resection can be comparable to the open ones and in addition offers the benefits of minimally invasive approach. However long term results like tumor recurrences and survival rates remains to be seen with this newer technique.

References

1. Rau HG, Buttler E, Meyer G, Schardey HM, Schildberg FW. Laparoscopic liver resection compared with conventional partial hepatectomy - a prospective analysis. Hepatogastroenterology 1998;45:2333-8

2. Cherqui D, Husson E, Hammoud R, Malassagne B, Stephan F, Bensaid S, et al. Laparoscopic liver resections: a feasibility study in 30 pateints. Ann Surg 2000;232:753-62

3. Blumgart L.H., Liver resection for benign disease and for liver and biliary tumors, Surgery of the liver and Biliary Tract, Volume II, Liver and biliary diseases by Blumgart, p 1639

4. Couinaud Cl 1954 Bases anatomiques des hepatectomies gauche et droite reglees, Journal de Chirurgie 70:933-966

5. Couinaud Cl 1957 Etudes anatomiques et chirurgicales, Mason, p.400-409

6. Couinaud Cl 1995 Liver anatomy: a half century investigation. Selected topics of HPB Surgery and Medicine. IRCCS Pavia

7. Goldsmith NA, Woodburne RT 1957 The surgical anatomy pertaining to liver resection. Surgery, Gynecology and Obsterics 105:310-318

8. Palanivelu C, et al. Laparoscopic Surgery of the liver, Text Book of Surgical Laparoscopy, 2002;386-395

9. Joseph F Buell, Alan J Koffron et al : Laparoscopic Liver Resection, Surgeon at Work, vol.200, No.3, March 2005, p 472-480

10. Palanivelu C, et al. Laparoscopic Surgery of the liver, Text Book of Surgical Laparoscopy, 2002;387

11. Cherqui D, Sourbrane O et al : Laparoscopic living donor hepatectomy for liver transplantation in children. Lancet.2002 Feb 2;359(9304):392-6

12. Pinto PA, Montgomery RA, et al : Laparoscopic procurement model for living donor liver transplantation. Clin Transplant. 2003;17 Suppl 9:39-43

13. Lin E, Gonzalez R, Venkatesh KR et al : Can current technology be integrated to facilitate laparoscopic living donor hepatectomy, Surg Endosc 2003 May;17(5):750-3, Epub 2003 Mar6

14. Kurian MS, Gagner M, et al : Hand-assisted laparoscopic donor hepatectomy for living related transplantation in the porcine model. Surg Laparosc Endosc Percutan Tech.2002 Aug;12(4):232-7

15. Douard R, Ettorre GM, et al : A two-step strategy for enlargement of left arterial branch in a living relted liver graft with dual arterial supply. Transplantation. 2002 Mar 27;73(6):993-4

16. Cuomo O, Troisi R, et al : Living orthotopic liver transplant using right lobe: our experience in the first 19 donors. Transplant Proc. 2001 Nov-Dec;33(7-8):3801-2.

17. Romanelli JR, Kelly JJ, Hand-assisted laparoscopic surgery in the United States: an overview. Semin Laparosc Surg 2001 Jun;8(2):96-103

18. Yacoub OF, Cardona I, Coveler LA, Dodson MG. Carbon dioxide embolism during laparoscopy. Anesthesiology 1982;57:533-5

19. Takagi S. Hepatic and portal vein blood flow during carbondioxide pneumoperitoneum for laparoscopic hepatectomy. Surg Endosc 1998;12:427-31

20. Jakimowicz J, Stultiends G, Smulders F. Laparoscopic insufflation of the abdomen reduces portal venous flow. Surg Endosc, 1998;12:129-32

21. Belghiti J, Noun R, Malafosse R, Jagot P, Sauvanet A, Pierangeli F, et al. Continuous versus intermittent portal triad clamping for lvier resection: a controlled study. Ann Surg 1999;229:369-75

22. Gagner M, Rheault M, Dubue J. Laparoscopic partial hepatectomy for liver tumor. Surg Endosc 1992;6:99

23. Ferzli G. David A. Kiel T. Laparoscopic resection of a large hepatic tumor. Surg Endosc 1995;9:733-5

24. Azagra JS, Gowergen M, Gilbart E, Jacobs D. Laparoscopic anatomical left lateral segementectomy-technical aspects. Surg Endosc 1996;10:758-61

25. Kaneko H, Takagi S, Shiba T. Laparoscopic partial hepatectomyand left lateral segmentectomy: technique and results of a clinical series. Surgery 1996;120:468-75

26. Mala T, Edwin B, Gladhaug I, Fosse E, Soireide O, Bergan A, et al. A comparative study of the short term outcome following open and laparoscopic liver resection of colorectal metastases. Surg Endosc 2002;16(7):1059-63

27. Huscher CG, Lirici MM, Chiodini S. Laparoscopic liver resections. Seminars in Laparoscopic Surgery 1998;5:204-10

28. Jones RMCL, Moulton CE, Hardy KJ. Central venous pressure and its effect on blood loss during liver resection. Br J Surg 1998;85:1058-60

29. Lesurtel M, Cherqui D, Laurent A, Tayar C, Fagniez PL. Lapaoscopic versus open left lateral hepatic lobectomy: a case-control study. J Am Coll Surg 2003;196:236-42

30. Takanaka K. Kanematsu T, Fukuzawa K, Sugimachi K. Can hepatic failure after surgery for heaptocellular carcinoma in cirrhotic patients be prevented? World J Surg 1990;14:123-7

31. Abdel-Atty MY, Farges O, Jagot P, Belghiti J. Laparoscopy extends the indications for liver resections with cirrhosis. Br J Surg 1999;86:1397-400

32. Decailliot F, Cherqui D, Leroux B. Effects of portal triad clamping on hemodynamic conditions during laparoscopic liver resection. Br J Anaesth 2001;87:493-6

33. Burpee SE, Kurian M, Murakame Y, Benevides S, Gagner M. The metabolic and immune response to laparoscopic versus open liver resection. Surg Endosc 2002;16(6):899-904

34. Lesurtel M, Cherqui D, Laurent A, Tayar C, Fagniez PL. Laparoscopic versus open left lateal hepatic lobectomy: a case-control study. J Am Coll Surg 2003;196:236-42

35. Cherqui D, Husson E, Hammoud R, et al. Laparoscopic liver resections: a feasibility study in 30 patients. Ann Surg 2000;232:753-762

36. Descottes B, Glineur D, Lachachi F, et al. Laparoscopic liver resection of benign liver tumors (erratum appears in Surg Endosc 2003;17:668), Surg Endosc 2003;17:23-30

37. Descottes B, Lachachi F, Sodji M, et al. Early experience with laparoscopic approach for solid liver tumors: initial 16 cases. Ann Surg 2000;5:641-645

38. Farges O, Jagot P, Kirstetter P, et al. Prospective assessment of the safety and benefit of laparoscopic liver resections. J Hepatobiliary Pancreat Surg 2002;9:242-248

39. Fong Y, Jarnagin W, Conlon KC, et al. Hand assisted laparoscopic liver resection: lessons from an initial experience. Arch Surg 2000;135:854-859

40. Gigot JF, Glineur D, Santiago AJ, et al., for the Hepatobiliary and Pancreatic Section of the Royal Belgian Society of Surgery and the Belgian Group for Endoscopic Surgery. Laparoscopic liver resection for malignant liver tumors: preliminary results of a multicenter European study. Ann Surg 2002;236:90-97

41. Huscher C, Lirici M, Chiodini S. Laparoscopic liver resections. Sem Lapr Surg 1998;5:204-210

42. Katkhouda N, Hurwitz M, Gugenheim J, et al. Laparoscopic management of benign solid and cystic lesions of the liver. Ann Surg 1999;4:460-466

43. Mala T, Edwin B, Gladhaug I, et al. A comparative study of the short-term outcome following open and laparoscopic liver resection of colorectal metastases. Surg Endosc 2002;16:1059-1063

44. Marks J, Moueil J, Katkhouda N, et al. Laparoscopic liver surgery. Surg Endosc 1998;12:331-334

50

Laparoscopic Radiofrequency Ablation in Hepatic Malignancies

INTRODUCTION

Non surgical treatment of malignancies has been applied to a variety of organs and liver is one organ where this treatment modality is increasingly utilized. Radiofrequency (RF) ablation is one such thing that is gaining worldwide acceptance as the primary non surgical treatment for hepatic malignancies. It uses heat energy to destroy the tumor cells. However, the use of heat to induce tissue injury is not new. Edwin Smith Papyrus (1700 BC) contains the first written mention of the use of heat to treat tumors (Breasted 1930).[1] Since then varied modalities have been tried (eg.electrocautery, laser) to generate heat that will destroy the malignant cells. But unfortunately, electrocautery and laser tumor ablation which are useful to recannulate hollow organs have no clinical utility for most solid organs like liver. With recent technological advances, it is now possible to induce anatomically precise thermal injury within solid organs while avoiding injury to surrounding tissue.

D'Arsonval (1891)[2] performed the first experimental RF thermal ablation. But it took exactly a century for RF ablation to be used in hepatic malignancies, through it was used for other malignancies. Rossi et al (1990)[3] and Mc Gahan et al (1990)[4] were the first to use RF ablation for liver malignancies which paved the way for its wide applications. Recently several studies have shown RFA is the preferred method for ablating liver tumors. Initial experience with RFA has been via a percutaneous approach. Siperstein et al (1997)[5] was the first one to apply RFA via laparoscopic approach. Laparoscopic RFA offers many distinct advantages (Table) that is not possible with percutaneous approach. Moreover, it incorporates laparoscopic ultrasonography which improves intraoperative staging and better definition of the lesion. This section discusses the place of laparoscopic RFA in the management of hepatic malignancies.

Advantages of Laparoscopic RFA
Diagnostic Laparoscopy
Diagnoses extrahepatic involvement
Detects peritoneal deposits
Laparoscopic Intraoperative Ultrasound
Better assessment of lesions
Diagnoses occult lesions
Laparoscopic approach
Safe ablation of even superficial lesions
Avoids injury to adjacent viscera
Recognizes and treats bleeding from hepatic puncture site

WHY THE NEED FOR ABLATIVE THERAPIES?

Surgical resection still remains the gold standard in the treatment of both primary malignant tumors and metastatic disease. Unfortunately, less than 25% of patients with either primary hepatocellular cancer or metastatic colorectal cancer are candidates for surgical resection.[6] To add to the misery, none of the available systemic chemotherapeutic agents or radiotherapy prove to be significantly useful either as the primary modality of treatment or as an adjuvant therapy. Untreated, these patients have a poor prognosis with a median survival range of 4 to 21 months and virtually no 5 year survival. Though improvement in operative techniques and postoperative care had made resections possible in hitherto unresectable tumors, still three quarters of tumors are unresectable. The inability of the surgery to have an impact on the clinical course of most of the patients with malignant liver tumors has led to the development of multiple alternative treatments. The table lists the available non surgical minimally invasive techniques for the treatment of liver tumors.[7-9] Local ablation modalities like RFA aim to preserve residual normal functional tissue by ablating only the malignant lesions and a margin of normal tissue.[10-12] To extend the avenues of their uses, many of these modalities are used in conjunction with surgical resection. Of all the ablative therapies, RFA is a promising technique which will be discussed here.

Minimally Invasive Techniques for the treatment of liver tumors
Radiofrequency ablation
Microwave ablation
Laser ablation
Cryo ablation
Ethanol ablation
Chemoembolisation
Hepatic arterial embolisation

RADIOFREQUENCY ABLATION - PRINCIPLES

The underlying mechanism of RFA is the conversion of RF waves into heat.[19] A rapidly alternating current in the range of RF waves (460-500KHz) is applied from an RF generator and passed from an uninsulated electrode tip into the surrounding tissue. The current causes vibration as the ions attempt to follow changes in the direction of the rapidly alternating current. Heat is generated when the ionic agitation leads to localized frictional heating of the tissue surrounding the electrode.[13-16] By this, the temperature reaches above 50°C which results in thermal coagulation and protein denaturation ultimately leading to tissue necrosis.[17,18] In addition, local hyperthermia causes the secondary effects of recruiting peripheral blood effector cells, inducing cytotoxic cytokines, expressing heat shock proteins and inducing apoptosis.

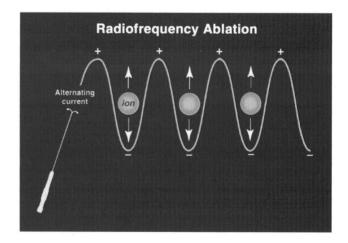

Figure 1: RFA Principles. Ionic agitation from alternating current causes tissue coagulation through frictional heating. Tissue desiccation increases impedance which eventually decreases current flow.

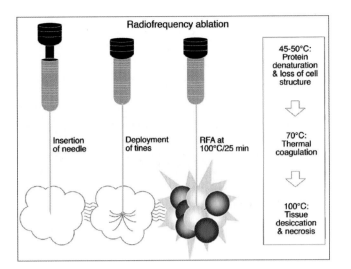

Figure 2: RFA Principles

RFA can be used to treat both primary and metastatic liver malignancies. RFA is feasible for tumors upto 5cms diameter. Similar to cryotherapy, RFA can be used to treat metastasis close to major intrahepatic vessels because the heat sink effect of blood flow protects the vascular endothelium. Bile ducts however do not tolerate heat well and may be injured, resulting in biliary fistula or abscess formation.

INSTRUMENTATION

There are three RF devices commercially available namely RITA Medical Systems (Mountain view, CA) Radiotherapeutics (Mountain view, CA, US) and Radionics (Burlington, MA, US). The most widely used device is RITA Medical Systems which will be described here. RITA (Radiofrequency Interstitial Thermal Ablation) consists of a RF generator operating at 480KHz frequency and supplied by 50RF Watt power output. The electrode is a 15 guage stainless needle insulated by thick plastic sheath with a 1cm active tip with multiple nickel titanium retractable hooks that deploy at equal angles to each other. This arrangement makes sure that the tissues are ablated uniformly without any residual lesion. The maximum deployment diameter for the hooks is 3cm and five prongs have individual thermistor to monitor the temperature in the surrounding tissue.

Recently two modifications to the RF electrodes have resulted in better ablation of tumors. One is the internally cooled needle electrode[20] which is believed to produce thermal tumor destruction with larger volumes necrosis. The other modification is the increase in number of hooks from four to ten[16] which are designed to produce large spherical thermal injuries.

INDICATIONS AND CONTRAINDICATIONS

RFA has now established itself as one of the primary ablative therapies for unresectable hepatic malignan-

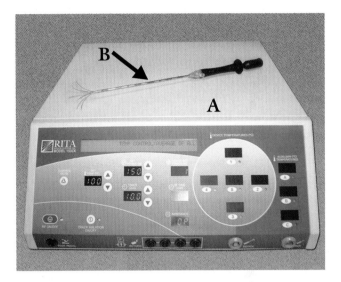

Figure 3: Radio frequency ablation equipment

A - Generator
B - Probe

cies. Recent studies have shown that RFA is safe and effective, even comparing favourably with that of the hepatic resections. To date, RFA is considered a reasonable alternative for patients with four or fewer tumors that are less than 5cm in diameter. However, cooled tip electrodes and multipronged electrodes may increase the cut off size further in the near future.

As with any other ablative technologies, the potential for complication increases as the number of lesions treated by RFA rises.[21] Moreover, patients with obvious extrahepatic disease and those with limited life expectancies (<6month) are unlikely to benefit from RFA and should not be treated. The general indications and contraindications for laparoscopic RFA are given in the following Table.

Indications for laparoscopic RFA
1. Patients with 4 or fewer tumors that are < 5cm and who are not candidates for surgical resection.
2. As an adjuvant ablative modality during laparoscopic hepatic resection to treat tumors that are not amenable for surgery
3. Patients with small (<5cm) HCC, awaiting orthotopic liver transplantation

Contraindications
1. Extrahepatic disease
2. Lift expectancy < 6 months
3. Cirrhosis - Child Pugh - C
4. Pregnancy
5. Active infection
6. Refractory coagulopathy
7. Tumor > 5cm in size
8. More than 4 hepatic tumors
9. Other active malignant diseases

TECHNIQUE

Position and Ports

Under general anaesthesia, patient is placed in supine position. If necessary, small left sided tilt can be given or else a small sand bag can be placed behind the right hypochondrium. This will make the right sided lesions more prominent. The surgeon and the camera assistant stand on the left side of the patient while the scrub nurse stands on the right side. The monitor is at the right shoulder of the patient. This arrangement is similar to the one used for laparoscopic cholecystectomy.

The first port is at the right midclavicular line, which is used for camera (10mm). Generally closed Veress needle technique is employed for creation of pneumoperitoneum, but if the liver is enlarged or multiple scars are present, then open Hasson's technique can be used. Right hand working port at the anterior axillary line (5mm) and left hand working port at the epigastrium slightly to the left (10mm) are then inserted under visual guidance.

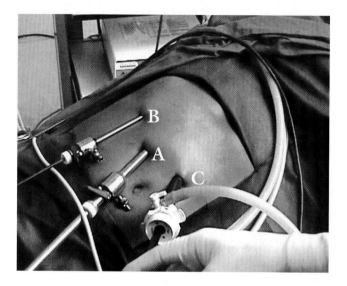

Figure 4: Port position for ablation of tumor in right lobe

A - Camera port
B - Working port
C - Laparoscopic ultrasound port

Diagnostic laparoscopy and intraoperative ultrasonography

Once the abdomen is entered, the adhesions if present, are divided and the abdomen is examined in a sequential manner. If the patient has gross evidence of disseminated carcinomatosis or extrahepatic disease, then a biopsy of the lesion is taken and the procedure is terminated. Otherwise, a formal assessment of the liver, parietal peritoneum, stomach, small bowel, colon, lesser sac and omentum is performed. Then the lesser omentum is divided and any pathology in the caudate lobe is looked for. The draining lymph nodes in the porta hepatis and celiac axis is checked for any gross abnormality and should be biopsied if doubts exist. The infra and the suprahepatic part of the IVC is visualized for any pathology.

Once direct visualization of the above mentioned areas is performed, then laparoscopic ultrasound probe is inserted through the working trocar and all segments of the liver are looked for any lesion. Note the size, number and location of the tumors, its relations to major blood vessels and the bile ducts. Even occult lesions of less than 5mm are picked up by the intraoperative ultrasound probe. But sometimes localising the lesions in segments 7 and 8 might be difficult.

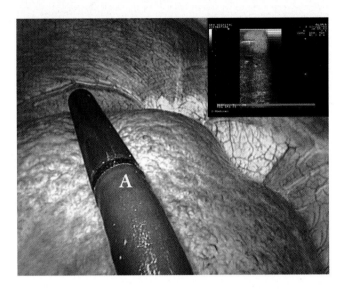

Figure 5: Location of tumor and identification of related major vessels using laparoscopic ultrasound

A - Laparoscopic ultrasound probe

Ablation of the tumor

After localizing the tumor, RITA probe is introduced into the abdomen via the percutaneous route. Then the electrode is visually and ultrasonographically guided into the tumor. RITA probe consists of a 15 gauge needle and curved electrode. The tract through which the probe passes should be the shortest one from the skin. During insertion, take care to avoid injury to hollow viscus, blood vessels and diaphragm. Once the needle position is confirmed, the prongs are deployed to approximately two thirds their maximum length and the ablation is started. 50W of alternating current is delivered to generate a target temperature of 90-110°C inside the tumor. Temperature can be measured using thermistor connected to the prongs. This temperature is maintained for 6-8 minutes. Overlapping ablations are completed to

encompass the entire lesion as necessary. In general, lesions larger than 3cm require multiple overlapping fields for complete ablation. During this procedure, a 1cm margin of normal tissue surrounding the tumor is ablated as well. The adequacy of ablation is checked by 3 factors. One is the appearance of micro bubbles within the lesion which is picked by the intraoperative ultrasound and the other is the temperature inside the lesion after 20 seconds. Tumor necrosis corresponds to a temperature greater than 60°C. Finally, loss of vascularity around the tumor suggests complete ablation. At the completion of the ablation process, the prongs are retracted and the needle tract is cauterized as it is removed. This is done specifically to prevent needle tract seedling with tumor cells. At one sitting, a maximum of four tumors are ablated. This procedure can be repeated many times either for recurrence or for the newer tumors.

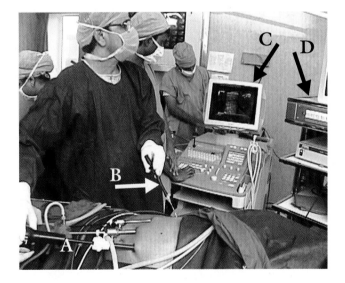

Figure 6: Insertion of RITA probe into the tumor under laparoscopic ultrasound guidence

A - Laparoscopic ultrasound probe
B - RITA probe
C - Ultrasound machine
D - Laparoscopic trolley

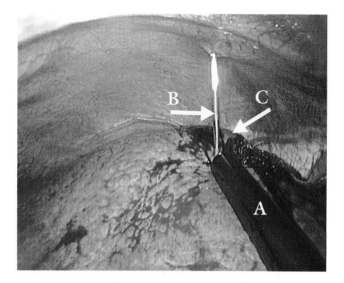

Figure 7: RITA probe is introduced into tumor under laparoscopic ultrasound guidance

A - Laparoscopic ultrasound probe
B - RITA probe
C - Liver Segment VIII

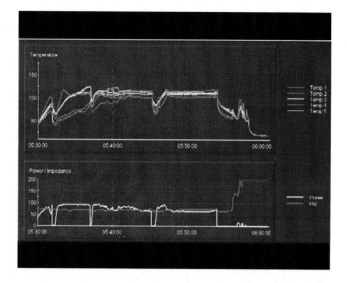

Figure 9: Final output graph shows the time and temperature during the entire process of ablation

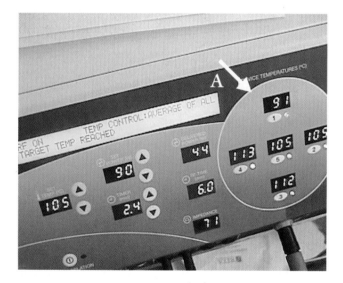

Figure 8: Completion of ablation. Target temperature is reached in all probes

A - Device temperature unit shows target temperature in all the 5 probes

POST OPERATIVE PERIOD AND FOLLOW UP

The postoperative period following laparoscopic RFA is generally uneventful. Due to systemic absorption of the necrosed tissue patients may have fever and pain. Other reported complications include haemorrhage, hemobilia, hemothorax, diaphragmatic injury, pleural effusion, cholecystitis, elevated transaminase levels and needle tract seeding. But fortunately, these complications are very rare.

Regarding completeness of the ablation, immediate postoperative CT or USG may not be appropriate as it may be difficult to distinguish between residual tumor and hyperemia induced by the ablation. Hence the current recommendation is to do CT scan one month after the ablation. If it shows tumor recurrence or incomplete ablation, then the procedure is repeated.

DISCUSSION

Although liver resection still remains the gold standard in the treatment of hepatic malignancies it is possible in only 25% of cases.[22] The reasons for such low operable rate include unresectable locations, multicentricity of the tumor, poor hepatic reserve as in cirrhosis and patient being unfit for major resections. As a result, ablative therapies have come into vogue which have the potential to destroy malignant tissues with minimal damage to the surrounding normal liver. Of all the ablative therapies available to date, radiofrequency offers the maximum advantage. Though radiofrequency was used in various fields of medicine, its use in liver tumors dates back only to a decade and half. It all began with the publications of Rossi et al 1990 and McGahan JP et al 1990. These initial reports are based on percutaneous route of ablation along with extensive use of intraoperative ultrasound. The first reported literature that uses laparoscopic route was from Sipenstein et al in 1997 who used laparoscopic probe to ablate hepatic neuroendocrine tumor metastases. Since then many authors[25-30] have published their initial experience with laparoscopic radiofrequency ablation of hepatic tumors. These results are promising and even offers an alternative approach for liver resection. Needle tract seedling[23] will sometimes be a problem which can be prevented by needle tract ablation Santambrogio et al[24] studied the survival and intrahepatic recurrences after laparoscopic radiofrequency ablation and showed that about 28% of the patients had new hepatic nodules diagnosed by the use of laparoscopic ultrasound. In his study about 50% patients had recurrences, most of which were treatable. This study proves that retreatment is possible with laparoscopic RFA. Moreover for hepatic metastasis from colorectal cancers, laparoscopic RFA can be combined with any colorectal procedures without any additional morbditiy.[25] Thus the technical feasibility[31] allows it to combine hepatic resections and colorectal procedures in a single sitting.

Laparoscopic RFA has a failure rate of about 12%.[32] The tumors which are at greater risk include larger adenocarcinoma and sarcoma. Failures occur early in follow up with most occurring by 6 months. These cases can be reablated if necessary provided the patient fits into the criteria for ablation as discussed previously. These parameters compare favourably with the published percutaneous or open radiofrequency ablation series.[33-41]

OUR EXPERIENCE

In our series, we ablated 25 patients using laparoscopic RFA. The age group is between 48 and 67 years. There were 18 males and 7 females. The mean size of the lesion was 3.5cm. 18 patients had cirrhosis of which 8 were hepatitis B and 4 were hepatitis C positive. Out of 25 patients, 16 had hepatocellular carcinoma, 7 had colorectal metastases and the remaining 2 patients had neuroendocrine tumors. 20 patients underwent successful tumor ablation while 5 underwent reablation later. Five patients had minor complications which were treated conservatively. Bleeding was the most common complication in our series. There was no procedure related mortality. Two patients died of hepatic failure due to advanced cirrhosis, after 30 and 45 days of ablation.

CONCLUSION

Laparoscopic radiofrequency ablation in selected cases provide a safe method to achieve local disease control in patients who are not candidates for liver resection. Combined with laparoscopic ultrasound many new lesions are diagnosed and treated using this approach. In addition, it can be combined with resectional procedures so that resection and ablation can at times be complimentary.

References

1. Breasted JH 1930 The Edwin Smith Surgical Papyrus. Vol 1. University of Chicago

2. d'Arsonval A 1891 Action physiologggique des courants alternatifs. Comp Rend Soc Biol 43:283

3. Rossi S, Fornari F, Pathies C et al 1990 Thermal lesions induced by 480 kHz localized current field in guinea pig and pig liver. Tumori 76:54-57

4. McGahan JP, browning P D, Brock J M et al 1990 hepatic ablation using radiofrequency electrocautery. Investigational Radiology 25:267-270

5. Allan E, Siperstein MD, Stanley J et al Laparoscopic thermal ablation of hepatic neuroendocrine tumor metastases, Surgery 1997, Vol.122(6) p1147-1155

6. Cady B, Jenkins RL, Steele GD, et al. Surgical margin in hepatic resection for colorectal metastasis-a critical and improvable determinant of outcome. Ann Surg 1998;227:566-571

7. Scudamore CH, Patterson EJ, Shapiro J, et al. Liver tumor ablation techniques. J Invest Surg 1997;10:157-164

8. Bilchik AJ, Sarantou T, Wardlaw JC, et al. Cryosurgery causes a profound reduction in tumor markers in hepatoma and noncolorectal hepatic metastases. Am Surg 1997;63:796-800

9. Bilchik AJ, Sarantou T, Foshag LJ, et al. Cryosurgical palliation of metastatic neuroendocrine tumors resistant to conventional therapy. Surgery 1997;122:1040-47

10. McGahan JP, Browning PD, Brock JM, et al. Hepatic ablation using radiofrequency electrocautery. Invest Radiol 1990;25:267

11. McGahan JP, Schneider P, Brock JM, et al. Tratment of liver tumors by percutaneous radiofrequency electrocautery. Semin Intervent Radiol 1993;10:143-149

12. Patterson EJ, Scudamore CH, Owen DA, et al. Radiofrquency ablation of porcine liver in vivo-effects of blood flow and treatment time on lesion size. Ann Surg 1998;227:559-565

13. Goldberg S N, Han P F, Tanabe K K et al 1998a Percutaneous radiofrequency tissue ablation: does perfusion-mediated tissue cooling limit coagulation necrosis? Journal of Vascular and Interventional Radiology 9:101-111

14. Goldberg S N, Solbiati L, Hahn P F et al 1998b Large-volume tissue ablation with radio frequency by using a clustered, internally cooled electrode technique: laboratory and clinical experience in liver metastases. Radiology 209:371-379

15. Goldberg S N, Gazelle G S, Dawson S L, et al 1995a Tissue ablation with radiofrequency using multiprobe arrays. Academic Radiology 2:670-674

16. Goldberg S N, Gazelle G S, Dawson S L, Rittman W J, Mueller P R, Rosenthal D I 1995b Tissue ablation with radiofrequency: effect of probe size, guage, duration, and temperature on lesion volume. Academic radiology 2:399-404

17. McGahan J P, Brock J M, Tesluk H et al 1992 Hepatic ablation with use of radio-frequency electrocautery in the animal model. Journal of Vascular and Interventional Radiology 3:291-297

18. McGahan J P, Gu W Z, Brock J M P et al 1996 hepatic ablation using bipolar radiofrequency electrocautery. Academic Radiology 3:418-422

19. Organ L W. Electrophysiologic principles of radiofrequency lesion making. Appl Neurophysiol 1976;39:69-76

20. Lorentzen T, Christensen NE, Nolsle CP, Torp-Pedersen ST. Radiofrequency tissue ablation with a cooled needle in vitro: US, dose response, and lesion temperature. Acad Radiol 1997;4:292-297

21. Livraghi T, Meloni F. Goldberg SN, et al. Hepatocellular carcinoma: radio-frequency ablation of medium and large lesions. Radiology 2000;214:761-768

22. Fong Y et al Liver resection for colorectal metastases. J Clin Oncol:1997;15:938-946

23. Jaskolka JD, Asch MR, et al Needle tract seeding after radiofrequency ablation of hepatic tumors. J Vasc Interv Radiol.2005 Apr;16(4):485-91

24. Santambrogio R, Opocher E, et al Survival and intra-hepatic recurrences after laparoscopic radiofrequency of hepatocellular carcinoma in patients with liver cirrhosis. J Surg Oncol. 2005 Mar 15;89(4):218-25; discussion 225-6

25. Berber E, Senagore A, et al Laparoscopic radiofrequency ablation of liver tumors combined with colorectal procedures. Surg Laparosc Endosc Percutan Tech. 2004 Aug;14(4):186-90

26. Berber E, Herceg NL, Casto KJ, Siperstein AE, Laparoscopic radiofrequency ablation of hepatic tumors: prospective clinical evaluation of ablation size comparing two treatment algorithms. Surg Endosc.2004 Mar:18(3):390-6

27. Salmi A, Metelli F, Laparoscopic ultrasound-guided radiofrequency thermal ablation of hepatic tumors: a new coaxial approach. Endoscopy. 2003 Sep;35(9):802

28. Topal B, Aerts R, Penninckx F, Laparoscopic radiofrequency ablation of unresectable liver malignancies: feasibility and clinical outcome. Surg Laparosc Endosc Percutan Tech. 2003 Feb;13(1):11-5

29. Isoda N, Ono K, Sato Y, et al Laparoscopic radiofrequency ablation for heaptocellular carcinomas, Nippon Rinsho 2001 Oct;59Suppl 6:596-600

30. Chung MH, Wood TF et al Laparoscopic radiofrequency ablation of unresectable hepatic malignancies. A phase 2 trial. Surg Endosc. 2001 Sep;15(9):1020-6 Epub 2001 Jun 12

31. Goleti O, Lencioni R, Armillotta N, Puglisi A et al Laparoscopic radiofrequency thermal ablation of hepatocarcinoma: preliminary experience. Surg Laparosc Endosc Percutan Tech.2000 Oct;10(5):284-90

32. Siperstein A, Garland A et al Laparoscopic radiofrequency ablation of primary and metastatic liver tumors. Technical considerations. Surg Endosc.2000 Apr;14(4):400-5

33. Siperstein A, Garland A, et al Local recurrence after laparoscopic radiofrquency thermal ablation of hepatic tumors. Ann Surg Oncol 2000 Mar:7(2):106-13

34. Rossi S, Di Stasi M, Buscarini E et al 1996 Percutaneous RF interstitial thermal ablation in the treatment of hepatic cancer. AJR American Journal of Roentgenology 167:759-768

35. Rossi S, Di Stasi M, Buscarini E et al 1995 Percutaneous radiofrquency interstitial thermal ablation on the treatment of small hepatocellular carcinoma. Cancer Journal from Scientific America 1:73

36. Solbiati L, Goldberg S N, Ierace T et al 1999 Radio-frequency ablation of hepatic metastases: postprocedural assessment with a US microbubble contrast agent-early experience. Radiology 211:643-649

37. Solbiati L, Ierace T, Goldberg S N et al 1997 Percutaneous US-guided radio-frequency tissue ablation of liver metastases: treatment and follow-up in 16 patients. Radiology 202:195-203

38. Livraghi T, Goldberg S N, Monti F et al 1997 Saline-enhanced radio-frequency tissue ablation in the treatment of liver metastases. Radiology 202:205-210

39. Allgaier H P, Deibert P, zuber I 1999 Percutaneous radiofrequency interstitial thermal ablation of small hepatocellular carcinoma. Lancet 353:1676-1677

40. Dodd G D, half GA, Rhim H 1999 thermal ablation of lvier tumors by radiofrquency, microwave, and laser therapy. In : Claveir (ed) Malignant Liver Tumors, 1st edn., Mosby, London: 170-180

41. Rhim H, Dodd G D 1999 Radiofrequency thermal ablation of liver tumors. Journal of Clinical Ultrasound 27:221-229

42. Bauer T, Spitz F, Nisenbaum H et al 1999 Radiofrequency ablation therapy for large complex hepatic metastases. Abstract 52nd Annual Cancer Symposium, Society of Surgical Oncology, Orlando, FL March 4-7

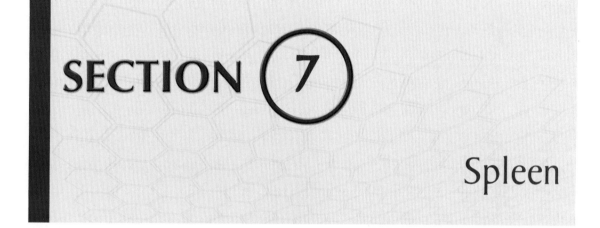

SECTION 7

Spleen

51

Laparoscopic Splenectomy

INTRODUCTION

The first case of laparoscopic splenectomy was described by Delaitre etal in 1991.[1,2] This was soon followed by the first case report of laparoscopic splenectomy in USA.[3] These reports were followed by numerous reports from all parts of the world indicating the growing popularity of laparoscopic splenectomy. As experience increased and technological advances took place, the indications and safety profile of this surgery laparoscopic splenectomy also rose. In the initial years, all laparoscopic surgeons adopted the traditional anterior approach with the patient in the semi-lithotomy position. The proponents of this approach cite several advantages. The lateral approach was first mooted by Delaitre again in 1995, the so called "hanged spleen" approach.[4] It was enthusiastically adopted by practitioners of this art, notably Park etal[5] Finally, the "leaning spleen" technique was adopted by Richardson etal which combined the advantages of both the previous approaches.[6]

ANATOMY [7]

The spleen is the second largest organ of the reticulo-endothelial system. It has two major ligaments the gastrosplenic ligament carrying the short gastric vessels and the splenorenal (lienorenal) ligament, which contains the splenic artery. It has several minor ligaments the splenophrenic, the splenocolic, the pancreaticosplenic, the presplenic fold, the phrenocolic, and the pancreaticolic ligaments. It is usually about 3 X 8 X 14 cm. and weighs about 200 gms. Its lateral surface is separated from the left ninth, tenth and eleventh ribs by the diaphragm. Its medial surface relates to the stomach, tail of pancreas and left kidney. It is entirely encapsulated by the peritoneum except at its hilum.

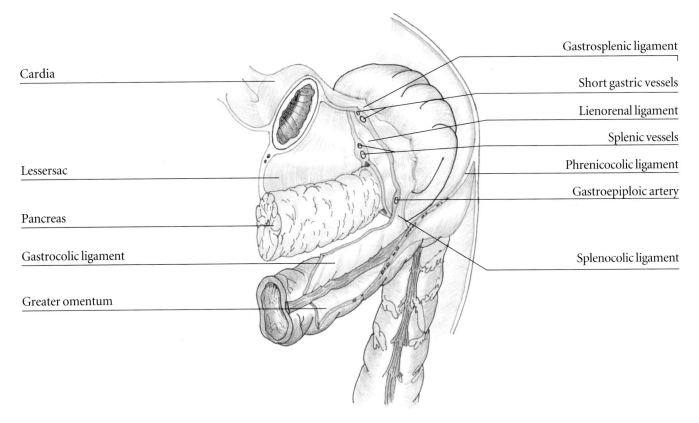

Cardia

Lessersac

Pancreas

Gastrocolic ligament

Greater omentum

Gastrosplenic ligament

Short gastric vessels

Lienorenal ligament

Splenic vessels

Phrenicocolic ligament

Gastroepiploic artery

Splenocolic ligament

Figure 1 : Suspensory ligaments of the spleen

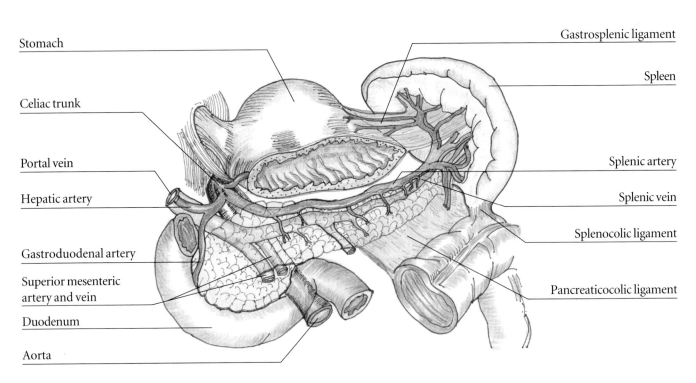

Stomach

Celiac trunk

Portal vein

Hepatic artery

Gastroduodenal artery

Superior mesenteric artery and vein

Duodenum

Aorta

Gastrosplenic ligament

Spleen

Splenic artery

Splenic vein

Splenocolic ligament

Pancreaticocolic ligament

Figure 2 : Relationship of splenic vessels and ligaments

The splenic artery arises as a branch of the celiac trunk in the majority of the cases or as a branch of the gastrosplenic or hepatosplenic trunk or directly from the aorta. It then runs along the superior border of the pancreas in the posterior leaf of the peritoneum, crosses the upper pole of the kidney, and enters the hilum. The splenic hilum most commonly divides into two major branches but occasionally into three branches. These further divide into 3 to 38 branches. Two or three vasa brevia or the short gastric arteries arise from the splenic artery or the left gastroepiploic artery.

There are two different types of splenic artery distribution:[8,9]

1. **Magistral type:** A long main splenic artery divides into short terminal branches, near the hilus, which enter over only one-third to one-fourth of the medial surface of the spleen.

2. **Distributed type:** The splenic trunk is short and numerous long branches enter over three-fourths of the medial surface of the spleen.

As a rule, notched spleens and those with tubercles or prominences have more entering arteries than do those with smooth borders. The cumulative blood flow through the spleen averages 300ml/min.

The tail of the pancreas lies in direct contact with the spleen in 30 percent of cadavers. The splenic vein is formed by joining of the intralobar veins near the splenic hilum and is usually joined by the left gastroepiploic vein but not the short gastric veins, which enter the upper part of the spleen in the majority of patients. It has a more direct course than the artery, passing through the splenorenal ligament to the right and usually inferior to the artery and posterior to the pancreas, ending by joining the superior mesenteric vein to form the portal vein.

The spleen can be divided into usually two or sometimes, three segments separated by avascular planes. In about a third of the cases, the plane separating the segments does not traverse the full thickness of the spleen and vascular communications exist between the segments.

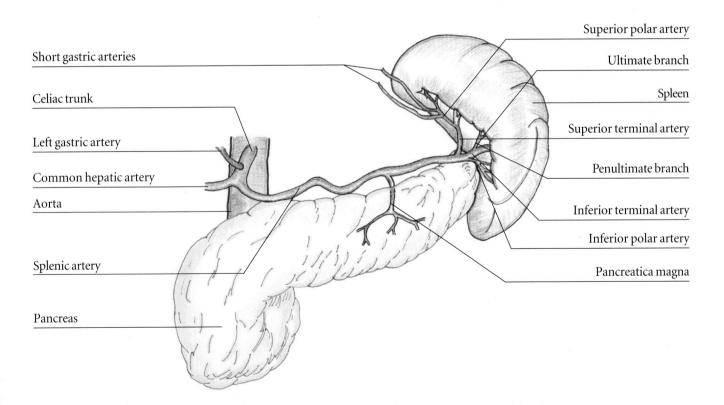

Figure 3 : Magistral (bundled) type of distribution of splenic artery

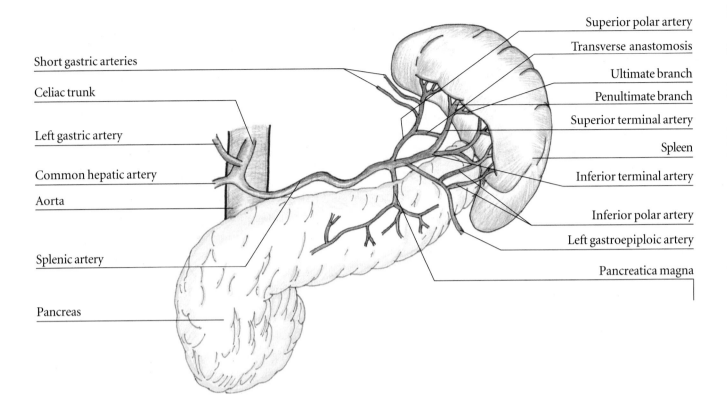

Figure 4 : Distributed Type of splenic artery distribution

ACCESSORY SPLEENS

Accessory spleens are found in about 10% of autopsy specimen and about 20% of surgical patients. They are more frequent in children and are thought to atrophy with age. The location of the accessory spleens varies from the commonest in the splenic hilum (54%) to the least common adjoining the left testes or ovary (0.5%) and includes along the splenic vessels, the tail of the pancreas, splenocolic ligament, greater omentum, perirenal regions, small intestinal mesentery and presacral regions. The clinical significance of accessory spleens lies in the fact that when splenectomy is done for hematologic conditions in which absence of the spleen is believed to be beneficial, missed accessory spleens have resulted in relapse. Hence, in such cases, care should be taken to include all the accessory spleens that can be identified.

EFFECTS OF SPLENECTOMY

Due to absence of pitting and culling of red cells, nuclear remnants remain in the form of Howell-Jolly bodies and absence of these remnants would suggest the presence of residual splenic tissue. It may be possible to assess residual splenic function after splenectomy followed by splenosis or after splenic auto-transplantation by measuring pitted red cell percentage. Leucocytosis, thrombocytosis, increase in CD8+ T-cells, decrease in opsonins, specifically properdin and tuftsin, decrease in serum IgM levels and impairment of immune response to circulating antigens and macrophage mobilization are the other important changes that take place.

After splenectomy for massive splenomegaly, there is a decrease in the blood volume and a decrease in the cardiac workload as the spleen was acting as an arteriovenous shunt. Finally, the risk of overwhelming post-splenectomy infection is increased, by about 60 times according to some investigators. The risk is greatest in children younger than 4 years of age and within 2 years of splenectomy.

Indications of Laparoscopic Splenectomy[10,11]

1. Hematological Disorders:
    i. Idiopathic Thrombocytopenic Purpura (ITP).
    ii. AIDS-associated ITP.
    iii. Thrombotic Thrombocytopenic Purpura.
    iv. Idiopathic autoimmune hemolytic anemia.
    v. Felty's syndrome.
    vi. Thalassemia.
    vii. Sickle cell disease.
    viii. Congenital and acquired hemolytic anemias.
2. Secondary hypersplenism systemic lupus erythematosus, leukemias, lymphomas, myeloid metaplasia, sarcoidosis, Gaucher's disease.
3. Splenic cysts.
4. Primary splenic neutropenia and pancytopenia.
5. "Wandering spleen".
6. Operative staging of Hodgkin's lymphoma St. IA or IIA.
7. Benign tumours of the spleen.
8. Splenic artery aneurysm.

Relative Contra-indications to Laparoscopic Splenectomy[10,12]

1. Splenic abscess (increased chance of perforation or leakage of abscess and spread of infection, dense peri-splenitis).
2. Ruptured spleen.
3. Malignant tumours of the spleen (potential of spread of disease).
4. Lymphoma (as above).
5. Secondary hypersplenism in portal hypertension (increased collateral formation and risk of hemorrhage).
6. Splenic vein thrombosis with left sided portal hypertension (as above).
7. Massive splenomegaly (visualization difficult).
8. Previous upper abdominal surgery (difficult dissection due to adhesions).
9. Pregnancy.
10. Calcified splenic artery.

The most common indication for laparoscopic splenectomy worldwide is ITP, constituting 40-100% of cases in most series. In ITP, the spleen is more or less normal in size, with the chances of hemorrhage being the same as in open splenectomy. However, some patients may require optimization by pre-operative administration of corticosteroids or IgG. To be on the safe side, a minimum platelet count of, 20,000 c.mm. is required pre-operatively, though successful laparoscopic splenectomy has been reported in patients with counts as low as 5000 c.mm.

Due to advances in radiographic staging, the need for surgical staging has decreased in Hodgkin's disease. Current indications include equivocal radiologic findings or when splenic tissue is required to clarify the disease status after therapy.

Laparoscopic splenectomy may be indicated for patients with NHL and other hematological malignancies for treatment of associated hypersplenism and cytopenias.

Obesity is not an absolute contra-indication for laparoscopic splenectomy though it considerably increases the difficulty of the surgery.

By a general consensus, it is deemed that spleen greater than 28-30 cms. in longitudinal dimension and 3000 gms. in weight should be managed by open surgery rather than laparoscopic surgery.

Whenever splenectomy is indicated, accessory spleen should be looked for and removed in the following locations: hilum of the spleen, ligamentous attachments of the spleen, small bowel mesentery, the omentum and adjacent to the structures of the pelvis.

Problems inherent to laparoscopic treatment of splenomegaly:

1. Structural friability of the spleen.
2. Increased risk of iatrogenic capsular trauma.

3. Increased propensity for hemorrhage.

4. Increased difficulties for manipulation of an enlarged spleen.

5. Difficulty in exposure and access of the splenic hilum.

SPLENIC ARTERY EMBOLISATION

Pre-operative splenic artery embolisation was already in vogue in open splenectomy for massive and difficult splenectomies. Its adoption for laparoscopic splenectomy was first advocated by Poulin etal in 1993.[19,20] They found that it helped to reduce operative blood loss and made the procedure easier to perform. Initially they recommended it liberally for elective removal of a normal sized or moderately enlarged spleen (< 20 cm long) when hematologic indications are present.[21,22] As more experience was gained with laparoscopic splenectomy, the indications of pre-operative splenic artery embolisation was restricted to massive splenomegaly, portal hypertension and splenic artery aneurysms[23-28] It has been adopted in pregnant patients while performing hand-assisted laparoscopic splenectomy[29] and post-operatively to control staple line bleeding from pedicle.[30] However, the major disadvantage of pre-operative splenic artery embolisation is that it induces an aseptic peri-splenitis which renders the subsequent dissection more difficult. Hence, we do not advocate this approach and this view is also supported by several workers.[31] Splenic artery ligation in continuity as a first step, through the lesser sac results in considerable shrinkage of the spleen. Thus, bleeding is minimized during dissection of the spleen.

PRE-OPERATIVE WORK-UP

Apart from the routine investigations including hematological work-up, ultrasonography and/or CT Scan, one special measure deserves mention immunization.

Immunization: Pre-operative immunization with pneumococcal vaccine is a must for all patients. The mortality rate for OPSI varies from 0.09 per 100 person-years[13] to 0.42 per 100 person-years.[14] The mortality is maximum in children less than 4 years and then gradually tapers off with increasing age.[15,16]

The mortality was also related to the indication of surgery, being higher in patients of hematologic malignancy than for non-malignancy indications.[16]

The commercially available vaccine covers 23 of the total 94 serotypes of pneumococci, which are responsible for around 90% of the illnesses caused by the organism. Most adults and children older than 2 years of age respond with a significant rise in antibody titre. The antibody response in variable with an overall response rate of around 61%.[17] The titre then falls off with time so that re-vaccination is recommended every six years.[11]

Recommendations for the treatment of asplenic pediatric patients include pneumococcal, Haemophilus influenzae type b, and meningococcal immunizations, antimicrobial prophylaxis for selected patients, and prompt evaluation and aggressive treatment of acute febrile illness.[18]

Advantages of Anterior Approach

1. Easier exploration of the entire peritoneal cavity for detection of accessory splenic tissue, staging of lymphoma and trauma.

2. Ability to perform concomitant surgical procedures.

3. Allows rapid performance of traditional midline incision if necessary.

4. Easy access to lesser sac for early splenic artery ligation or accessory spleen detection.

5. Improved exposure and less painful midline extraction incision in patients with massive splenomegaly.

Advantages of Lateral Approach

1. Enhanced Retraction
   i. The colon, stomach and small bowel are drawn out of the operative field by gravity.
   ii. Less manipulation of the spleen is required decreasing the chances of trauma and bleeding. Gentle elevation of the inferior pole is sufficient.

2. Enhances Exposure
   i. The tail of pancreas is well visualized, enabling dissection and avoidance of injury.
   ii. Lower pole splenic vessels are well visualized.

iii. After dividing the splenocolic ligament and elevating the lower pole of spleen, the splenogastric ligament and splenic pedicle is tented and easily divided.

iv. The splenic pedicle can be approached both anteriorly and posteriorly.

3. Enhanced Ease of operation

i. Trocar position entails superior operative ergonomics with less fatigue for the surgeon.

ii. Intra-operative bleeding is more easily managed as the splenic pedicle is hanging and exposed, can be approached anteriorly or posteriorly.

iii. Control of short gastric vessels does not require wide opening of the lesser sac.

LAPAROSCOPIC SPLENECTOMY - ANTERIOR APPROACH

Team set-up

The patient is placed in a 70-degree semi-right lateral position with a sandbag under the torso. With this, the surgeon enjoys all the advantages of the lateral position. If needed, e.g., for hemorrhage or for performance of another surgical procedure, the table can be tilted left side down to make the patient supine. The surgeon stands on the right of the patient. The camera surgeon stands to the left of the surgeon. The assistant surgeon stands at the head end of the patient for the epigastric retractor or on the left of the patient (opposite to the surgeon) for the left anterior axillary retractor.

Instruments

Apart from the standard laparoscopic instruments including a 30-degree telescope, the surgery is greatly facilitated by Harmonic scalpel (Ultracision). In addition, Babcock's forceps is needed for retraction of stomach and colon. Moreover, a three-prong retractor or fan-blade retractor is needed for the spleen and pedicle. Though we prefer to ligate the splenic artery, those who would like to apply endovascular staples will need an appropriate stapler and cartridge and a 12mm port.

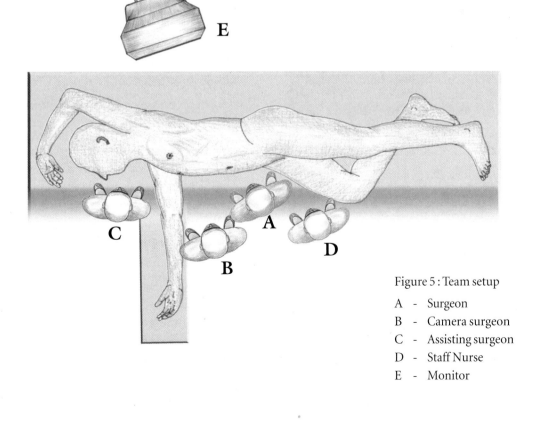

Figure 5 : Team setup

A - Surgeon
B - Camera surgeon
C - Assisting surgeon
D - Staff Nurse
E - Monitor

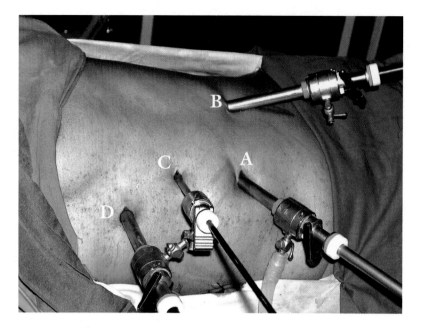

Figure 6 : Ports position

A - Camera port

B - Surgeon's right hand port

C - Surgeon's left hand port

D - Retraction port

Ports

10 mm   - Umbilical/Supraumbilical (depending on body habitus of the patient) - Camera/Telescope.

5 mm   - Midway between camera port and epigastrium - Surgeon's left hand working.

10 mm   - Left midclavicular line, supraumbilical - Surgeon's right hand working. (12 mm if endovascular stapler is to be used.

5 mm   - Epigastric - For retraction of stomach/spleen.

5 mm   - Left anterior axillary - for retraction of spleen (in selected cases).

Operative Technique[71,72]

The following points are to be kept in mind while performing laparoscopic splenectomy:

a. Three prong fan blade retractor, endoflex (Genzyme - USA) or blunt tipped holding forceps with ratchet mounted with rolled up gauze piece may be used for spleen retraction. Retracting instruments are used through subxiphoid or through left anterior axillary port depending on the stage of operation.

b. Babcock forceps is used for retraction of the stomach to the right.

c. If one prefers endolinear stapling device, then left midclavicular or left anterior axillary port should be 12mm.

d. 30 degree angled scope is preferred for its versatility of exposure.

e. Some surgeons prefer multiple 10mm ports, which allow flexibility in placement of the camera, instruments and stapling device. I prefer left midclavicular port 12mm as multifunctional port. The umbilical or supraumbilical camera port keeps the camera in the center of the field of vision all the time.

f. Splenic artery ligation as an initial step of the operation not only minimizes the bleeding during manipulation of the spleen, but also causes the spleen to shrink considerably before completion of splenectomy. It also obviates the need of preoperative splenic artery embolization.

g. Harmonic Scalpel facilitates control of the short gastric vessels and splenic attachments and decreases the operative time.

h. The operative table should be rotatable, right and left, up and down for better visualisation of important structures during various stages of the operation.

i. Accessory spleen should be looked before and at each stage of manipulation.

j. Two hand technique is considered important for isolation of vessels, ligamentous division, holding and for giving traction and counter traction.

Exposure of lesser sac

Gastrosplenic ligament is divided between the spleen and the stomach by clipping the vessels on either side or with bipolar cutting scissor, electrocautery or harmonic scalpel. Harmonic scalpel obviates the need for clipping and the division of short gastric vessels is carried out up to the fundus. Retraction of the stomach medially and anteriorly facilitates this maneuver.

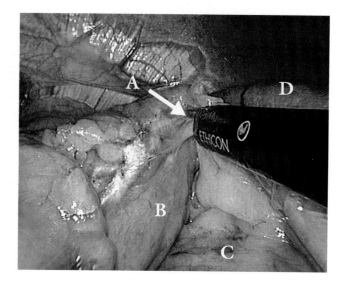

Figure 8 : Division of gastrosplenic omentum

A - Division of short gastric vessels using harmonic scalpel
B - Posterior wall of stomach
C - Pancreas
D - Spleen

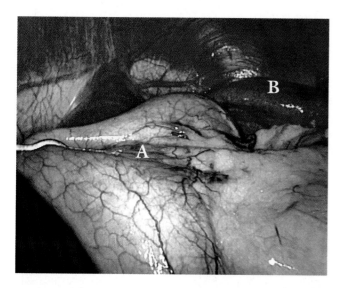

Figure 7 : Retraction of stomach medially to expose the gastro colic omentum

A - Stomach
B - Spleen

Control of splenic artery

The pancreas is retracted down and posteriorly with the use of fan blade retractor through left anterior axillary port. This maneuver pushes up the tortuous pulsating splenic artery. The peritoneum is lifted up by the left hand holding forceps and curved dissector is used to mobilize the artery all around. I perform this step by using a two hand technique and ligate the splenic artery with the silk ligatures. Some prefer clipping, but I feel the clip may slip out during mobilization. Ligation in continuity facilitates the entire procedure and makes it easy. Sometimes branches of the splenic artery distal to the ligature have to be divided particularly in distributed type of blood supply where the artery divides away from the splenic surface. In margistral type of blood supply, the distal splenic artery may be divided at the hilum after the entire spleen is mobilized. Some use vascular staples to divide the branches.

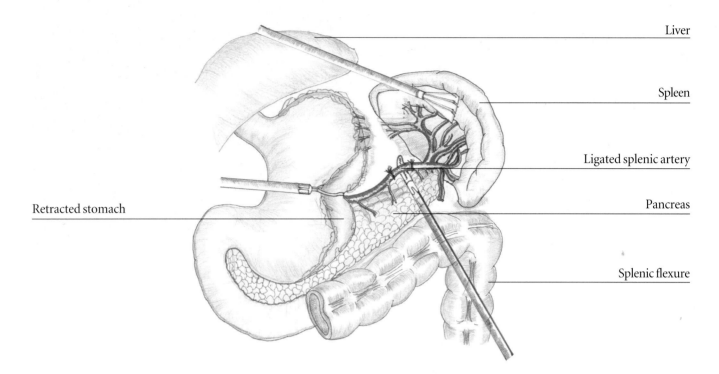

Liver

Spleen

Ligated splenic artery

Pancreas

Retracted stomach

Splenic flexure

Figure 9 : Ligation of splenic artery along the superior border of pancreas

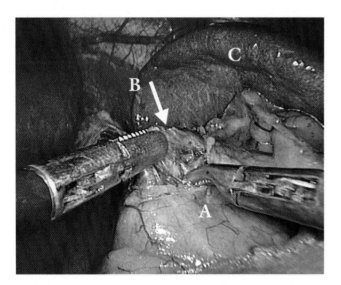

Figure 10 : Mobilization of splenic artery (Magistral type)

A - Pancreas
B - Splenic artery
C - Spleen

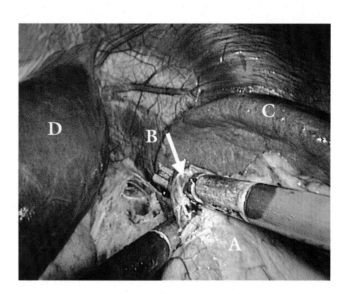

Figure 11 : Completely mobilised splenic artery

A - Pancreas
B - Splenic artery
C - Spleen
D - Left lobe of liver

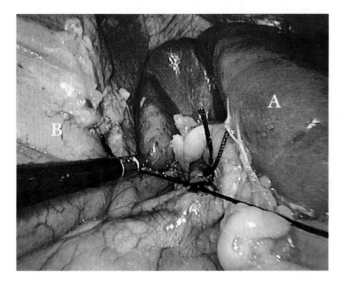

Figure 12 : Ligation of splenic artery using silk

A - Spleen
B - Posterior wall of stomach

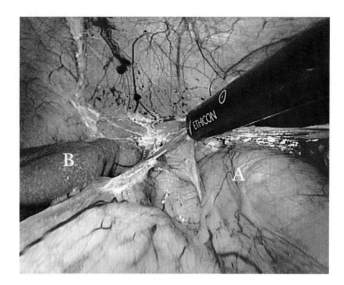

Figure 13 : Mobilization of splenic flexure of colon

A - Splenic flexure of colon
B - Spleen

Mobilization of splenic flexure

Splenic flexure of the colon is retracted downward and medially with Babcock through right midclavicular or subxiphoid port. Electro-cautery scissors or harmonic scalpel is used to divide the peritoneum lateral to the flexure and the ligamentous structure between the spleen and colon. Initial mobilization of splenic flexure prevents colonic injury.

Division of splenocolic ligament

The spleen is lifted upwards using fan shaped retractor through subxiphoid port and counter traction to the colon is given traction by the left hand holding forceps. The ligamentous attachments are divided by electrocautery scissors, hook dissection and clipping of prominent vessels if necessary. Inferior aspect of hilum is visualized by this maneuver.

Division of splenophrenic ligament

The fan shaped retractor on the inferior pole of the spleen is used to retract upwards and medially to give traction to the ligaments between spleen and

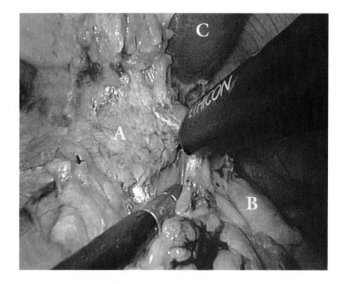

Figure 14 : Mobilization of colon from the tail of pancreas

A - Tail of pancreas
B - Colon
C - Spleen

diaphragm. Division of splenophrenic ligament exposes the splenorenal and retrosplenic ligaments, which can be divided. Division of these ligamentous attachments leaves the spleen hanging by the attachment of the upper pole to the diaphragm.

Hilar mobilization

Division of the above ligamentous attachment exposes the hilar vessels. Now, skeletonization of the hilar vessels is easier and even if bleeding occurs, it is easy to control in a fully mobilized spleen. Space is dissected in front and behind the splenic vein, keeping the distal pancreas in view. Most often, the main trunk of the splenic vein is seen and can be ligated with silk ligature. Sometimes inferior pole vessels are divided. The central vessels and superior pole vessels are then sequentially ligated and divided. Clipping alone may lead to bleeding by slipping of the clip during manipulation. Electrocautery or harmonic devices are also found to be ineffective in controlling the thin walled veins. Some surgeons prefer endo GIA stapling which also has been found to be not

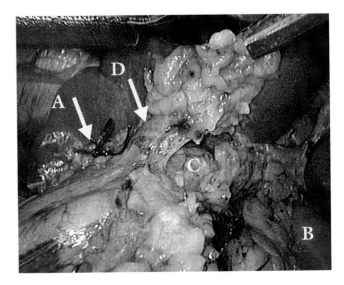

Figure 15 : Dissection of hilum

A - Ligated splenic artery
B - Separated colon
C - Tail of pancreas
D - Splenic hilum

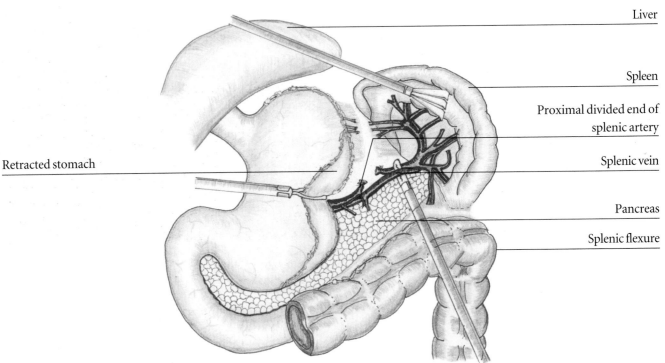

Figure 16 : Mobilization of splenic vein

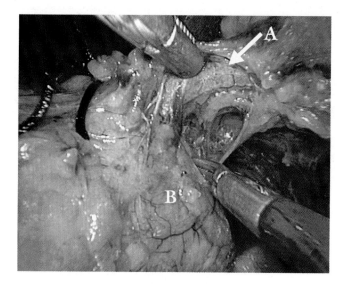

Figure 17 : Mobilization of splenic vein

A - Splenic vein

B - Tail of pancreas

effective at times and if necessary, the veins have to be ligated with endoloops. This is mainly due to inadequate mobilization of the hilar vessels and improper application of staplers. In my personal experience, ligature is not only effective in controlling the bleeding but also makes the procedure cost effective. It is dangerous to insert the endo vascular stapler blindly on the hilar vessels and removing it without firing since it may lead to bleeding of the thin walled splenic veins. Proper dissection of hilar "window" and proper application of the staplers is critical.

If the spleen has not been mobilized, control of hemorrhage is more difficult. Splenic artery is divided after ligation or with harmonic scalpel without ligation as already proximal ligature has been applied.

Mobilization of the upper pole of the spleen

After division of the hilar vessels, spleen can be rotated and retracted easily to visualize the remaining attachments. With use of electrocautery or harmonic scalpel, these attachments may be divided. Sometimes there may be vessels to the upper pole

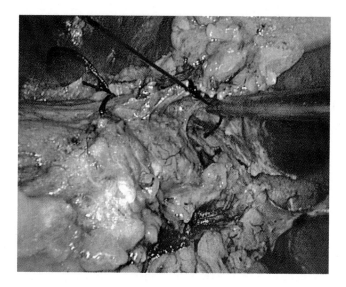

Figure 18 : Ligation of splenic vein with silk

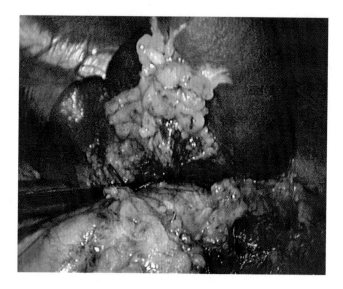

Figure 19 : Completely mobilized spleen

either from the retrogastric vessel or greater curvature of incompletely mobilized fundus, which needs to be divided carefully.

Removal of spleen

The spleen is placed in a large plastic impermeable bag and the bag is retrieved through the left midclavicular port. Kocher clamp or ring forceps is used to morcellate the splenic tissue to facilitate extraction. Lapsac (Cook urological) is the strongest and safest bag commercially available. Self made cheaper plastic bags can be used. Morcellation inside the bag can be performed by digital or instrumental fragmentation. Morcellation of the spleen with automatic morcellator is faster, but it is dangerous as it may damage the bag and spillage of spleen can occur.

If the procedure is for Hodgkin's lymphoma or any other tumor, the spleen is removed intact through minilaparotomy by extending the umbilical port. Surprisingly one needs a smaller incision than expected as the spleen is more often bean shaped.

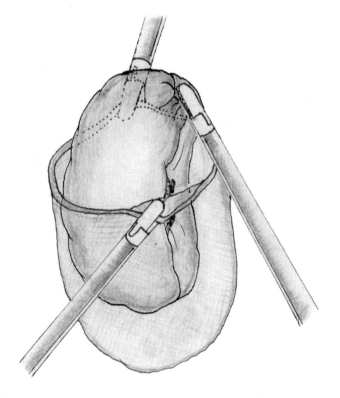

Figure 20 : Placement of spleen in the endobag. By keeping the endobag as shown above, even bigger size spleen can be slipped inside with the help of gravity

Before removal of the trocars, the splenic bed is always checked for hemostasis. It is better to place tube drainage in difficult laparoscopic splenectomy.

TECHNICAL CHALLENGES AND TIPS

1. In very large spleens, it is difficult to manipulate around the spleen and the hilum. With proper retraction, the hilum can be exposed. Control of splenic artery through the lesser sac approach initially minimizes the incidence of bleeding to large extent and also allows the spleen to shrink considerably, thereby enabling manipulation of spleen much better. Preoperative splenic artery embolisation has been suggested as a method to minimize intraoperative bleeding. Instead of facilitating surgery, the process of embolisation appears to incite a perisplenitis, rendering the dissection more difficult.

2. Perisplenitis often results in inflammatory changes around the spleen and envelopment of the spleen by the omentum and friable adhesions makes the mobilization difficult. Conditions such as splenic infarction, splenic abscess, splenic cyst and pancreatitis can be associated with splenitis. Meticulous dissection in these cases reduces the risk of bleeding.

3. Dense and vascular superior splenic polar adhesion can be difficult to approach. The lateral approach facilitates access in this situation with appropriate retraction.

4. Sometimes, when the proximal gastric fundus directly abuts the spleen, undue traction may avulse the short gastric vessels. The harmonic scalpel is very useful to divide the vessels and dissect the gastric fundus without much dissection.

5. Dilated, tortuous perisplenic veins present technical challenges. Meticulous dissection with use of harmonic scalpel or ligature may to a certain extent minimize bleeding. Preoperative splenic artery embolisation may help in these patients.

6. Specimen extraction, particularly large sized spleens, may turn out to be the most frustrating and challenging step of the operation. Even after

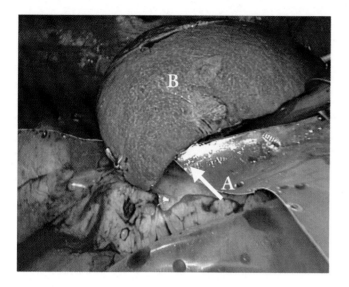

Figure 21 : Placement of spleen in the endobag

A - Endobag is tucked behind the spleen

B - Spleen

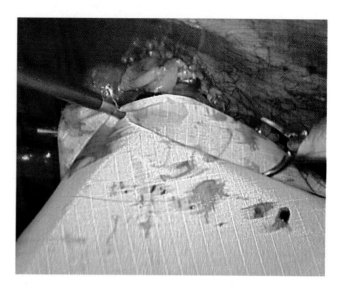

Figure 22 : Spleen is pushed into the endobag

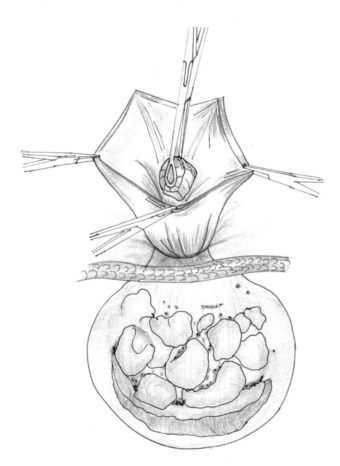

Figure 23 : Piece meal extraction of spleen

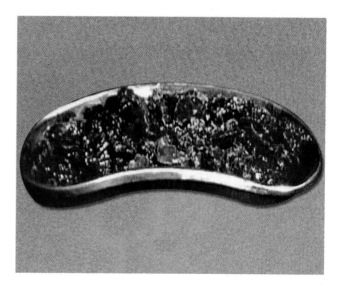

Figure 24 : Excised pieces of spleen

resection, the spleen must be gently and minimally manipulated to avoid the possibility of rupture and subsequent splenosis.

This can be solved by one of the following maneuvers :

i. Keeping the posterior limb of the mouth of the bag tucked under the spleen, the spleen is gently pushed into the bag at lower level than the specimen facilitates this maneuver.

ii. The final division of the attachment to the superior pole is not done to maintain it in position, which may help significantly in the "bagging process". In the hanging spleen approach, the bag is unfurled and advanced over a relatively stationary specimen.

Technical Challenges and tips

1. Large sized Spleens ligation of splenic artery as the initial step.

2. Perisplenitis ligation, meticulous dissection.

3. Dense adhesions of the superior pole lateral approach and appropriate retraction.

4. Gastric fundus abutting the spleen- Harmonic dissection or clipping and division.

5. Segmental portal hypertension
   i. Preoperative splenic artery embolisation.
   ii. Harmonic for haemostatic dissection.

6. Specimen extraction pushing technique, entrapment technique.

RESULTS

Total No. of Lap. Splenectomies: 120, ¾th Medium to Large Sized

Indications

Autoimmune Hemolytic Anemia	43
Idiopathic Thrombocytopenic Purpura	31
Tropical Splenomegaly	26
Hereditary Spherocytosis	18
Hydatid Cyst	2

Combined Lap. Chole. & Spleen.	10
Conversion	1*
Accessory Spleen	5
Average Hospital Stay (days)	3
Average Duration of Surgery (min)	85

* This patient had diffuse peri-splenitis and there was a lot of oozing during dissection, obscuring the field and necessitating conversion.

POST-OPERATIVE COMPLICATIONS

1. **Hemorrhage:** Hemorrhage is the most common cause for conversion to open surgery. The diseased spleen is a very friable organ and must be handled gently. Any coagulopathy must be corrected pre-operatively. In patients with refractory thrombocytopenia, platelet infusions should be given per-operatively after ligating the splenic artery and vein. Once it occurs, hemorrhage should be controlled rapidly with cautery, clips, sutures or conversion to open surgery.

2. **Overwhelming Post-Splenectomy Infection:** Abrupt onset with high fever followed by shock and frequently by disseminated intra-vascular coagulation. In some cases, this may be accompanied by the Waterhouse-Fredrichsen syndrome (adrenal hemorrhage and necrosis). All patients must be warned beforehand of this potential complication. They should be instructed to contact a physician immediately if they have fever. Only prompt recognition and aggressive treatment can avert the high percentage of morbidity and mortality associated with this complication.

3. **Failure to control the primary disease:** Careful selection of the patient after assessment of all risks and benefits is important. Patient with persistent disease requires evaluation for accessory spleen. A tagged RBC scan will detect accessory spleens, if present, which can be then removed laparoscopically. Though there was a fear initially, that laparoscopic splenectomy does not allow complete detection of accessory spleens,[32] this was later on proved to be unfounded with laparoscopic approach reporting the same incidence of

accessory spleens as detected during open splenectomies.[33,34]

4. **Injury to adjacent organs (Colon, stomach, pancreas):** Such injuries can occur due to excessive traction or instrumental laceration during dissection or improper application of clips. Chand B etal[38] reported a 16% incidence of pancreatic injury in laparoscopic splenectomy. They further suggested that post-operative hyperamylasemia can alert the surgeon to this condition.[35] If recognized during surgery, repair should be done laparoscopically or by conversion to open surgery. Late accumulation of pancreatic collection can be drained percutaneously. A gastric or colonic fistula will require a laparotomy.

5. **Subphrenic abscess:** Post-operative fever, leucocytosis and ileus indicate the development of a subphrenic abscess. Usually, it can be managed by antibiotics and USG or CT guided aspiration of pus. If above measures fail, laparotomy or laparoscopic evacuation is indicated.

6. **Some unusual complications:** like port site splenosis[36] and diaphragmatic perforation[37] have been reported.

DISCUSSION

Worldwide, the commonest indication for laparoscopic splenectomy is ITP. Patients with hemolytic anemias are prone to development of pigment stones in the gall-bladder and in such cases, laparoscopic cholecystectomy can be combined with laparoscopic splenectomy. Though trauma and ruptured spleen are relative contraindications for laparoscopic splenectomy, hand-assisted laparoscopic splenectomy,[38] laparoscopic partial splenectomy,[39] and total laparoscopic splenectomy[40] have been performed. Intraoperative blood loss is the commonest cause of conversion.[34] The conversion rates reported vary from 3.7% to 9% and decrease with increasing experience of the surgeon.[41] It has been established by several authorities that the rate of conversion is higher in patients with splenomegaly and when the operating surgeon is inexperienced with the technique.[42-46] A meta-analysis of 2490 patients comparing laparoscopic splenectomy with open splenectomy concluded that although operative times are longer for laparoscopic splenectomy than open splenectomy, laparoscopic splenectomy is associated with a significant reduction in splenectomy-related morbidity, primarily as a function of fewer pulmonary, wound and infectious complications.[33] Due to reduced hospital stay and less morbidity, laparoscopic splenectomy results in improved clinical outcomes and reduced costs for patients than open splenectomy.[47,48] We routinely use Ligasure and/or Harmonic Scalpel for dissection as they ensure a bloodless field. Both instruments are equally efficacious. However, Ligasure results in a greater reduction in operating time and blood loss as compared to other methods of dissection.[49] Early exposure of the splenic hilum and artery and its ligation increases the safety of the surgery and reduces blood loss[50,51] Hand-assisted laparoscopic splenectomy (HALS) was first reported by Meijer DW etal in 1999.[52] Thereafter, its use has been advocated for giant spleens,[53] trauma,[54] accessory splenectomy,[55] for advanced pregnancy[29] and for management of primary and secondary cancers of the spleen.[56] Though organ retrieval had been done using morcellator through the laparoscopic ports earlier,[57,58] concerns about splenosis and inadequacy of tissue for histological examination led to almost universal abandonment and removal of the specimen through a small midline incision. Laparoscopic splenectomy has also been done without pneumoperitoneum using a wall-lifting procedure.[59] Minilaparoscopic splenectomy using only one 12 mm port and three 2mm ports is also feasible but not recommended.[60] Other laparoscopic surgeries on the spleen include laparoscopic partial splenectomy for cyst, pseudocysts and benign lesions,[61-64] laparoscopic splenorrhaphy[65] and splenopexy for wandering spleen.[66-68]

The future of laparoscopic splenectomy lies in computer assisted surgery. Already reports are available of laparoscopic splenectomy being performed using the Da Vinci surgical robot.[69,70]

CONCLUSION

Laparoscopic splenectomy seems to be the "Gold Standard" treatment for normal or slightly enlarged spleens. With increasing clinical experience, the indications can be extended to even larger spleens. When laparoscopic splenectomy is successful, the post-operative functional benefits for the patients are comparable with those of laparoscopic cholecystectomy. Attention should be concentrated on cost saving for this technically demanding surgery, particularly in India.

References

1. Delaitre B, Maginien B. Splenectomy by the laparoscopic approach. Report of a case. Presse Med 1991; 20:2263.

2. Delaitre B, Maginien B. Laparoscopic splenectomy technical aspects. Surg Endosc. 1992 Nov-Dec; 6(6):305-8.

3. Carroll BJ, Phillips EH, Semel CJ, etal. Laparoscopic Splenectomy. Surg Endosc. 1992 Jul-Aug; 6(4):183-5.

4. Delaitre B. Laparoscopic splenectomy. The "hanged spleen" technique. Surg Endosc. 1995 May; 9(5): 528-9.

5. Park A, Gagner M, Pomp A. The lateral approach to laparoscopic splenectomy. Am J Surg. 1997; 173(2):126-30.

6. Richardson WS, Smith D. Branum GD etal. Leaning spleen: A new approach to laparoscopic splenectomy. JACS: 185 (4): 429-432.

7. Smith DL, Meyer AA. Anatomy, Immunology and Physiology of the spleen. In: Zuidema GD, Yeo CJ (eds). Shackleford's Surgery of the Alimentary Tract. W. B. Saunders Company, 5th edition, 2002,541-549.

8. Michel NA. The Variational Anatomy of the Spleen and Splenic Artery. Am. J. Anat 70:21, 1942.

9. Schwartz SI. The spleen anatomy and splenectomy. In Nyhus LM, Baker RJ, Fischer JE (Ed.) Mastery of surgery. Third edition. Chapter 114. Little, Brown and Company, Boston 1997;1267-1275.

10. Rege RV. Laparoscopic splenectomy. In: Scott-Conner, CEH (Ed). The Sages Manual: fundamentals of laparoscopy and GI endoscopy. Springer, 2003: 326-335.

11. Coon WW. Splenectomy for conditions other than trauma. In: Zuidema GD, Yeo CJ (eds). Shackleford's Surgery of the Alimentary Tract. W. B. Saunders Company, 5th edition, 2002, 550-561

12. Park AE. Lateral approach to laparoscopic splenectomy. In: Zucker KA (Ed.): Surgical Laparoscopy, 2nd edition, Philadelphia, Lippincott Williams & Wilkins: 2001:625-634.

13. Schwartz P, Sterioff S, Mucha P etal: Postsplenectomy sepsis and mortality in adults. JAMA 1982, 248:2279.

14. Cullingford G, Watkins D, Watts A etal. Severe late postsplenectomy infections. Br. J. Surg., 1991, 78:716.

15. Walker W. Splenectomy in childhood: A review in England and Wales 1960-6. Br. J. Surg., 1979, 63:36.

16. Konigswieser H. Incidence of serious infections after splenectomy in children. Prog. Pediatr. Surg. 1985, 18:173.

17. Shapiro E, Berg A, Austrian R etal. The protective efficacy of polyvalent pneumococcal polysaccharide vaccine. NEJM 1991, 325:1453.

18. Lane PA. The spleen in children. Curr Opin Pediatr. 1995 Feb;7(1):36-41.

19. Poulin E, Thibault C, Mamazza J, etal. Splenectomy by celioscopy. Experience of 20 casesAnn Chir. 1993;47 (9):832-7.

20. Poulin E, Thibault C, Mamazza J, etal. Laparoscopic splenectomy: clinical experience and the role of preoperative splenic artery embolization. Surg Laparosc Endosc. 1993 Dec;3(6):445-50.

21. Poulin E, Thibault C, Mamazza J, etal. Laparoscopic splenectomy: clinical experience and the role of preoperative splenic artery embolization. Surg Laparosc Endosc. 1993 Dec;3(6):445-50.

22. Poulin EC, Thibault C, Mamazza J. Laparoscopic splenectomy. Surg Endosc. 1995 Feb;9(2):172-6.

23. Poulin EC, Mamazza J, Schlachta CM. Splenic artery embolization before laparoscopic splenectomy. An update. Surg Endosc. 1998 Jun;12(6):870-5.

24. Poulin EC, Mamazza J. Laparoscopic splenectomy: lessons from the learning curve. Can J Surg. 1998 Feb;41(1): 28-36.

25. Totte E, Van Hee R, Kloeck I, etal. Laparoscopic splenectomy after arterial embolisation. Hepatogastroenterology. 1998 May-Jun;45(21):773-6.

26. Kobayashi S, Sekimoto M, Tomita N, Monden M. Laparoscopic splenectomy for a massive splenomegaly using a transcatheter technique Nippon Geka Gakkai Zasshi. 1998 Oct; 99(10):733-6.

27. Jaroszewski DE, Schlinkert RT, Gray RJ. Laparoscopic splenectomy for the treatment of gastric varices secondary to sinistral portal hypertension. Surg Endosc. 2000 Jan;14(1):87.

28. DeRoover A, Sudan D. Treatment of multiple aneurysms of the splenic artery after liver transplantation by percutaneous embolization and laparoscopic splenectomy. Transplantation. 2001 Sep 15;72(5):956-8.)

29. Iwase K, Higaki J, Yoon HE, etal. Hand-assisted laparoscopic splenectomy for idiopathic thrombocytopenic purpura during pregnancy. Surg Laparosc Endosc Percutan Tech. 2001 Feb; 11(1):53-6.

30. Kercher KW, Novitsky YW, Czerniach DR, Litwin DE. Staple line bleeding following laparoscopic splenectomy: intraoperative prevention and postoperative management with splenic artery embolization. Surg Laparosc Endosc Percutan Tech. 2003 Oct;13(5):353-6.

31. Caprotti R, Porta G, Franciosi C, etal. Laparoscopic splenectomy for hematological disorders. Our experience in adult and pediatric patients. Int Surg. 1998 Oct-Dec; 83(4):303-7.

32. Gigot JF, Jamar F, Ferrant A etal: Inadequate detection of accessory spleens and splenosis with laparoscopic splenectomy. A shortcoming of the laparoscopic approach in hematologic diseases. Surg Endosc. 1998 Feb; 12(2): 101-6.

33. Winslow ER, Brunt LM. Perioperative outcomes of laparoscopic versus open splenectomy: a meta-analysis with an emphasis on complications. Surgery. 2003 Oct; 134(4):647-53.

34. Baccarani U, Terrosu G, Donini A etal. Splenectomy in hematology. Current practice and new perspectives. Haematologica 1999; 84:431-6.

35. Chand B, Walsh RM, Ponsky J etal. Pancreatic complications following laparoscopic splenectomy. Surg Endosc. 2001 Nov; 15(11): 1273-6.

36. Kumar RJ, Borzi PA. Splenosis in a port site after laparoscopic splenectomy. Surg Endosc. 2001 Apr; 15(4):413-4.

37. Targarona EM, Espert JJ, Bombuy E etal. Complications of laparoscopic splenectomy. Arch Surg. 2000 Oct; 135(10):1137-40.

38. Ren CJ, Salky B, Reiner M. Hand-assisted laparoscopic splenectomy for ruptured spleen. Surg Endosc. 2001 Mar;15(3):324.

39. Poulin EC, Thibault C, DesCoteaux JG, Cote G. Partial laparoscopic splenectomy for trauma: technique and case report. Surg Laparosc Endosc. 1995 Aug;5(4):306-10.

40. Basso N, Silecchia G, Raparelli L, etal. Laparoscopic splenectomy for ruptured spleen: lessons learned from a case. J Laparoendosc Adv Surg Tech A. 2003 Apr;13(2):109-12.

41. Friedman RL, Hiatt JR, Korman JL. Laparoscopic or open splenectomy for hematologic disease: which approach is superior? JACS 1997;185(1):52-8.

42. Targarona EM, Espert JJ, Balague C etal. Splenomegaly should not be considered a contraindication for laparoscopic splenectomy. Ann. Surg.1988, 228:35.

43. Gigot JE, de Goyet JDV, van Beers BE etal. Laparoscopic splenectomy in adults and children: Experience with 31 patients. Surgery 1996, 119:384.

44. Flowers JL, Lefor AT, Steers J etal. Laparoscopic splenectomy in patients with hematologic diseases. Ann. Surg. 1996, 224:19.

45. Poulin EC, Mammaza J. Laparoscopic splenectomy: Lessons from the learning curve. Can J Surg 1998 41:28.

46. Katkhouda N, Huriwtz MB, Rivera RT etal. Laparoscopic splenectomy. Outcome and efficacy in 103 consecutive patients. Ann Surg 1998, 228:568.

47. Watson DI, Coventry BJ, Chin T etal. Laparoscopic versus open splenectomy for immune thrombocytopenic purpura. Surgery. 1997 Jan; 121(1):18-22.

48. Baccarani U, Donini A, Terrosu G etal. Laparoscopic splenectomy for haematological diseases: review of current concepts and opinions. Eur J Surg. 1999 Oct; 165(10): 917-23.

49. Romano F, Caprotti R, Franciosi C etal. The use of Ligasure during pediatric laparoscopic splenectomy: a preliminary report. Pediatr Surg Int. 2003 Dec;19(11): 721-4.

50. Asoglu O, Ozmen V, Gorgun E etal. Does early ligation of the splenic artery reduce hemorrhage during laparoscopic splenectomy? Surg Laparosc Endosc Percutan Tech. 2004 Jun; 14(3):118-21.

51. Machado MA, Makdissi FF, Herman P etal. Exposure of splenic hilum increases safety of laparoscopic splenectomy. Surg Laparosc Endosc Percutan Tech. 2004 Feb; 14(1):23-5.

52. Meijer DW, Gossot D, Jakimowicz JJ etal. Splenectomy revised: manually assisted splenectomy with the dexterity device a feasibility study in 22 patients. Laparoendosc Adv Surg Tech A. 1999 Dec; 9(6):507-10.

53. Borrazzo EC, Daly JM< Morrisey KP etal. Hand-assisted laparoscopic splenectomy for giant spleens. Surg Endosc. 2003 Jun; 17(6):918-20.

54. Taragarona EM, Balague C, Trias M. Hand-assisted laparoscopic splenectomy. Semin Laparosc Surg. 2001 Jun;8(2):126-34.Surg Endosc. 2004 Jun;18(6):1001.

55. Kaban GK, Czerniach DR, Perugini RA, etal. Use of a laparoscopic hand-assist device for accessory splenectomy. Surg Endosc. 2004 Jun;18(6):1001.

56. Takahashi H, Yano H, Monden T etal. Hand-assisted laparoscopic splenectomy for solitary splenic metastasis from uterine corpus carcinoma. Surg Endosc. 2004 Feb;18(2):346

57. Hebra A, Walker JD, Tagge EP, etal. A new technique for laparoscopic splenectomy with massively enlarged spleens. Am Surg. 1998 Dec;64(12):1161-4.

58. Hashizume M, Migo S, Tsugawa K, etal. Laparoscopic splenectomy with the newly devised morcellator. Hepatogastroenterology. 1998 Mar-Apr;45(20):554-7

59. Nishizaki T, Takahashi I, Onohara T, etal. Laparoscopic splenectomy using a wall-lifting procedure. Surg Endosc. 1999 Oct;13(10):1055-6.

60. Yuan RH, Yu SC. Minilaparoscopic splenectomy: a new minimally invasive approach. J Laparoendosc Adv Surg Tech A. 1998 Oct;8(5):269-72.

61. Seshadri PA, Poulin EC, Mamazza J, Schlachta CM. Technique for laparoscopic partial splenectomy. Surg Laparosc Endosc Percutan Tech. 2000 Apr;10(2):106-9.

62. Corcione F, Cuccurullo D, Caiazzo P, etal. Laparoscopic partial splenectomy for a splenic pseudocyst.Surg Endosc. 2003 Nov;17(11):1850.

63. Ho CM. Splenic cysts: a new approach to partial splenectomy. Surg Endosc. 2002 Apr;16(4):717

64. Kehila M, Abderrahim T. Partial splenectomy requiring ligation of splenic vesselaparoscopic splenectomy. Apropos of 40 cases Ann Chir. 1993;47(5):433-5.

65. Koehler RH, Smith RS, Fry WR. Successful laparoscopic splenorrhaphy using absorbable mesh for grade III splenic injury: report of a case. Surg Laparosc Endosc. 1994 Aug;4(4):311-5.

66. Cohen MS, Soper NJ, Underwood A, etal. Laparoscopic splenopexy for wandering (pelvic) spleen. Surg Laparosc Endosc. 1998 Aug;8(4):286-90.

67. Hirose R, Kitano S, Bando T, etal. Laparoscopic splenopexy for pediatric wandering spleen. J Pediatr Surg. 1998 Oct;33(10):1571-3.

68. Peitgen K, Majetschak M, Walz MK. Laparoscopic splenopexy by peritoneal and omental pouch construction for intermittent splenic torsion ("wandering spleen"). Surg Endosc. 2001 Apr;15(4):413.

69. Chapman WH 3rd, Albrecht RJ, Kim VB, Young JA, Chitwood WR Jr. Computer-assisted laparoscopic splenectomy with the da Vinci surgical robot.Laparoendosc Adv Surg Tech A. 2002 Jun;12(3):155-9.

70. Shimada M, Sugimachi K. Future aspect of robotic surgery Fukuoka Igaku Zasshi. 2002 Apr;93(4):57-63.

71. C. Palanivelu. Laparoscopic splenectomy. In: C. Palanivelu: CIGES Atlas of Surgical Laparoscopy. 2nd edition, Jaypee Brothers Medical Publishers (P) Ltd., 2003: 183-187

72. C. Palanivelu. Laparoscopic splenectomy. In: C. Palanivelu (ed). Textbook of Surgical Laparoscopy. Gem Digestive Diseases Foundation, 1st edition, 2002:337-348.

52

Laparoscopic Mesh Splenopexy

INTRODUCTION

Wandering spleen (splenoptosis) is a rare congenital disorder, fewer than 500 cases have been reported in the literature. The incidence, based on several large series of splenectomies, is less than 0.5%.[1] A review of the literature from 1960 to 1992 by Dawson and Roberts (1994), documented 148 cases, which included both pediatric and adult cases.[2] Brown et al reviewed the literature identified an additional 127 cases of wandering spleens in patients younger than 21 years of age and with very different clinical presentations.[3] The primary cause of splenoptosis is a fusion anomaly of the dorsal mesogastrium of the spleen that results in failure and laxity of its normal attachment to the diaphragm, retroperitoneum and colon. These include the gastrosplenic, splenorenal and phrenicocolic ligaments. With deficiency or laxity of these structures the spleen is not confined to its normal posterolateral position in the left upper quadrant and becomes essentially a totally intraperitoneal hyper-mobile organ. It is relatively more common in children than adults, and females outnumber males.

Clinical presentation can be acute or chronic. In an extensive review of 133 cases in the literature by Buehner and Baker, 76 presented with a mass and non-specific abdominal symptoms, 26 patients were asymptomatic, 25 presented with acute abdominal pain, and another six cases had an asymptomatic mass.[4] Mechanical factors resulting in urinary retention and constipation or symptoms due to pathological disturbances of the spleen such as thrombocytopenia, hypersplenism and lymphoma, have been described in the literature. The subacute gastrointestinal complaints are the result of torsion of the pedicle, ischemia and splenic sequestration. About 50% of spleens are lost to acute ischemia from torsion.[5]

Torsion of the spleen, whether acute or chronic, with infarction can lead to the development of an acute abdomen. Venous drainage is compromised by torsion and arterial ligation becomes difficult, so edema and ischemia of the spleen appears. This causes pain because the spleen capsule is stretched due to its enlargement.[5] Rarely, splenoptosis may be complicated by occlusion of the celiac axis, possibly by median arcuate ligament compression.[6] This can be picked up by angiography. Ballui et al reported a very rare case of a wandering spleen in a neonate that ruptured and presented as a perisplenic hematoma.[7] Another rare case of torsion of a wandering spleen following blunt abdominal trauma has been reported.[8] Other complications are pancreatitis,[9] hypersplenism, cyst formation and rarely gastric volvulus. An interesting case with multiple problems was reported - wandering spleen associated with a gastric volvulus, gastric outlet obstruction due to extrinsic compression of the duodenum and partial small bowel obstruction due to extrinsic compression of a mobile, distended cecum that lay under the right diaphragm.[9] Groszek-Terwei et al also reported a rare case where splenoptosis co-existed with gastric volvulus and torsion.[10] The clinical diagnosis may be quite difficult and haematological and biochemical investigations may be non-specific but may occasionally reveal evidence of hypersplenism or functional asplenia.

Diagnosis needs a high index of suspicion, and is achieved with imaging techniques and some of them, especially in combination, are able to suggest it strongly (ultrasonography, nuclear scintigraphy, enhanced CT scanning and magnetic resonance imaging). The gray-scale ultrasonograms will show a displaced spleen that appears as a homogeneous, hypoechoic mass suggestive of an enlarged, ectopic spleen.[11] Power Doppler sonograms will show no blood flow in the parenchyma or hilum of the spleen if there is torsion and infarction of the spleen.[12]

Plain radiogram of the abdomen is not very helpful.[13] Sulphur colloid scans can also show the abnormal location. CT shows displacement of the organ with enlargement if torsion with venous stasis is present. The diminished perfusion in arterial occlusive states is indicated by low density on contrast enhanced CT scan.[14]

Management consists of splenectomy for frank splenic infarct, or splenopexy for the viable spleens. Laparoscopic procedures have been used extensively for both splenectomy and splenopexy.[1] In the absence of infarction, thrombosis, hypersplenism and in patients presenting with an acute abdomen, detorsion and splenopexy is a recognised surgical option.[15,16,17] Different techniques for splenopexy have been described in the literature. Hirose, Kitano et al reported the first case of wandering spleen treated by laparoscopic mesh splenopexy in a 2 year old child in 1998.[18] Haj, Cohen et al reported laparoscopic splenopexy of a wandering spleen using an absorbable (Vicryl) mesh in an adult for the first time.[19,20] Splenopexy can be achieved by creating an extraperitoneal pocket, wrapping the spleen in absorbable mesh and anchoring to the retroperitoneum (laparoscopic pocket splenopexy).[10] The extraperitoneal space is created using an inflatable balloon device. Using a 3 ports approach, the spleen is introduced and fixated inside the created pocket. The ectopic spleen can also be inserted in a Vicryl mesh bag and fixed in the left upper quadrant.[21]

Nomura et al described a laparoscopic sandwich technique using two sheets of mesh to wrap the spleen in its normal position.[17] Peitgen et al successfully performed another modification of splenopexy by laparoscopic reposition and fixation of the spleen by omental pouch creation.[22] The spleen was repositioned and placed in the left phrenorenal angle. Splenopexy is achieved by suturing the left colophrenic ligament to the lateral diaphragm thus creating a pouch for the inferior part of the spleen and by suturing the gastrocolic ligament to the anterior diaphragm to create a pouch for the upper splenic pole.

Splenectomy has classically been the treatment of choice for symptomatic wandering spleen.[5] Nevertheless, the significant risk of post-splenectomy sepsis supports a conservative approach especially in children, asymptomatic patients or those with no splenic infarction.[23] Laparoscopic splenectomy is indicated in splenomegaly, hypersplenism and torsion of the vascular pedicle with splenic infarction to avoid future complications like recurrent organ torsion resulting from the long and twisted vascular pedicle.[24]

OUR EXPERIENCE

The patient was a 19-year old woman who presented with complaints of lower abdominal pain, dysuria and fever for 7 days. There was no history of vomiting, hematuria or increased frequency of micturition. Her bowel habits were normal. The vital signs were normal. Physical examination revealed a well-defined intraperitoneal mass in the left iliac fossa which was mobile. The size was 7x 8 cm, firm in consistency and tender.

Complete blood picture revealed mild anemia, normal red blood cell and white blood cell counts. The platelet count, bleeding and clotting times were normal. Peripheral smear study was normal. In other words, there was no evidence of hypersplenism. Urine analysis including culture and sensitivity were within normal limits. Ultrasonogram revealed an absence of spleen in its normal anatomical position, instead it was present in the left iliac fossa. Doppler study showed tortuous splenic vessels extending down into the left iliac fossa, there was no reduction in blood flow. Upper gastrointestinal endoscopy showed mild reflux esophagitis, chest radiogram and electrocardiogram were normal.

The patient was planned for laparoscopic mesh splenopexy with a possibility of splenectomy. She was prepared, anesthetic fitness obtained and posted for surgery.

Laparoscopic Splenopexy (Sandwich Technique)

Team Setup

Chief surgeon stands at the right of the patient; camera surgeon stands to the right of the chief surgeon; the assistant for liver elevation stands to the left of the chief surgeon; scrub nurse is behind the camera surgeon. There is one monitor on the left of the patient, diagonally opposite to the chief surgeon on the caudal side and one monitor on the cranial side. This setup is convenient in that we could use the caudal side monitor for mobilizing the ectopic spleen and the cranial side monitor for mesh fixation in the original position.

Patient Position

Patient was placed supine, with a 20⁰ right lateral and Trendelenburg tilt. Once the spleen was brought to its original position, reverse Trendelenburg position was given.

Port Position

The optical port was 10mm about 2 cm above the umbilicus; a 5mm port in the epigastrium for liver elevation initially and later left hand working; left midclavicular trocar in the left lumbar area for a working port. Midline between the umbilicus and suprapubic area, a 10mm port is inserted for initial working.

Procedure

Findings: At laparoscopy, a free-floating, macroscopically normal spleen attached to an abnormally long tortuous vascular pedicle with no gastrosplenic or phrenicosplenic ligaments was detected in the lower left quadrant There was 4½ clockwise torsion of the pedicle and mild congestion with darkish color change in the spleen. There was no splenic infarction. Adhesions to the transverse colon and greater omentum were present. The splenic flexure was pulled down with the spleen. The spleen was multilobulated and there were accessory spleens at the hilum.

The first step was to identify the exact location of the spleen and accessory spleens.

In this case, the spleen was found in the pelvis, on the left side. The dissection was started by releasing the adhesions between the spleen and transverse colon and omentum using Harmonic scalpel (Ethicon) The torsion of the splenic pedicle was untwisted 4½ turns in an anticlockwise direction. Up to this point, the monitor at the caudal end was used for visualization. For the rest of the procedure, the monitor at the cranial end was used. The spleen along with the splenic flexure were replaced in the left hypochondrium. The posterior peritoneum over the left kidney was opened and a flap including peritoneum over posterior abdominal wall was lifted up. A Parietex mesh of size 10 x 8 cm was placed in the defect which was created and fixed to the lateral wall and the diaphragm. The spleen was replaced cranially to the left hypochondrium and placed over the mesh, carefully looking at the pedicle for twisting. Another piece of Parietex mesh (10 x 8) was placed over the spleen, PTFE coated side towards the peritoneal cavity. The two meshes were sutured together caudal to the lower pole (inferior border of the mesh), medially and laterally. Both the meshes formed a pocket to hold the spleen - "Sandwich technique". The whole unit was fixed to the lateral abdominal wall and the diaphragm. The ports were closed with 3 0 Vicryl.

Oral liquids were allowed on the first postoperative day (POD) after her bowels had moved and normal diet on the second POD. Thereafter, she was discharged on the third POD. Analgesic requirement was by oral route from the second POD itself. Postoperative Doppler ultrasound follow-up can be done to confirm a well-fixated spleen in the left upper quadrant. Imaging studies after 3 and 6 months showed the spleen in the left hypochondrium.

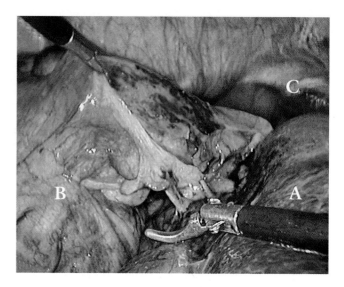

Figure 2 : Presence of spleen in the pelvis

A - Spleen
B - Colon
C - Medial umbilical ligament on left side

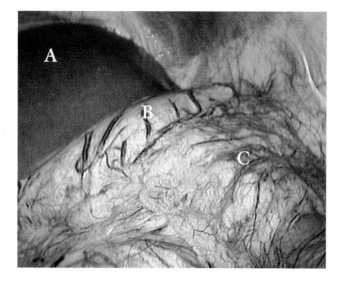

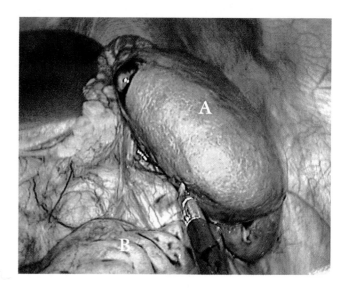

Figure 1 : Laparoscopic view of left hypochondrium. Spleen is absent

A - Left lobe of liver
B - Stomach
C - Left kidney

Figure 3 : Spleen is pushed up and replaced in the left hypochondrium

A - Spleen
B - Colon

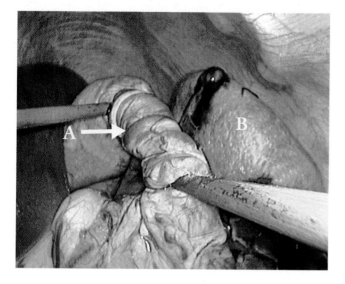

Figure 4 : After replacement twisting of the splenic pedicle is noted

A - Twisted splenic pedicle
B - Spleen

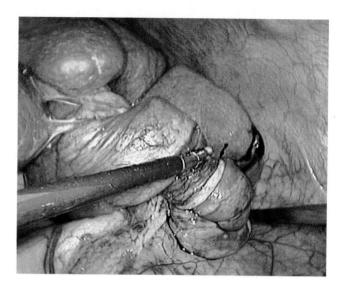

Figure 5 : Untwisting of the splenic pedicle was done

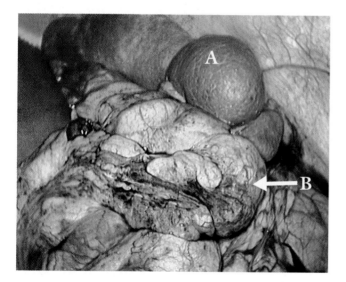

Figure 6 : Spleen was replaced in its original position

A - Untwisted splenic pedicle
B - Spleen

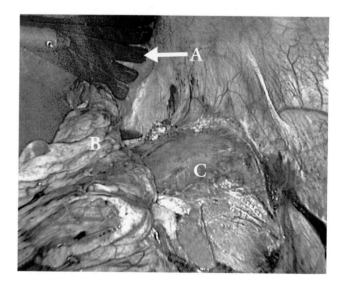

Figure 7 : Peritoneal covering of the left kidney was opened

A - Liver retractor was used to retract the spleen
B - Splenic pedicle
C - Left kidney

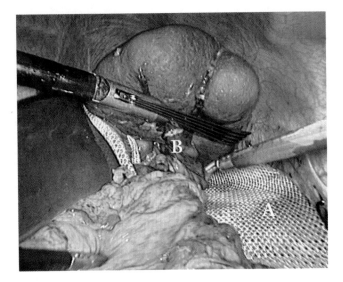

Figure 8 : Parietex mesh was placed over the dissected area and the spleen was placed over the mesh

A - Parietex mesh
B - Splenic hilum

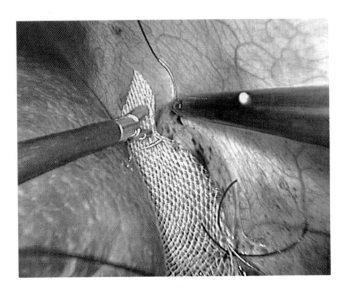

Figure 9 : Mesh was fixed to the lateral abdominal wall using prolene

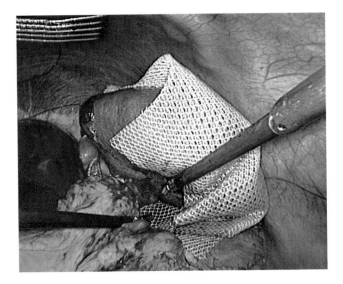

Figure 10 : Another mesh was placed over the spleen (smooth surface of parietex mesh was exposed to the peritoneal cavity)

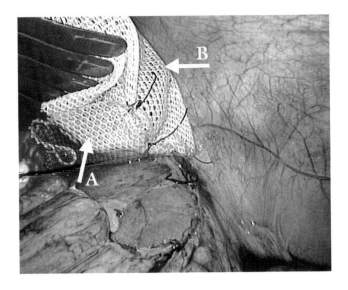

Figure 11 : Both the meshes were sutured together using interrupted prolene stitches

A - Mesh placed under the spleen
B - Mesh placed over the spleen

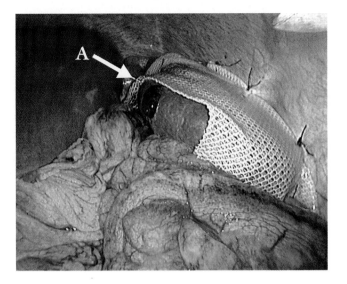

Figure 12 : Both the meshes were fixed to the lateral abdominal wall

A - Stitch on the medial side

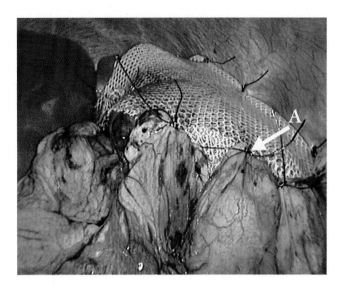

Figure 13 : Completion of splenopexy

A - Mesocolon was fixed to the mesh to keep the splenic flexure of colon in position

Table: Published case reports in the literature

Author	Year	Laparoscopic Procedure
Hirose R et al[18]	1998	Splenopexy
Cohen MS et al[20]	1998	Splenopexy
Haj M et al[19]	1999	Splenopexy
Nomura H et al[17]	2000	Splenopexy
Peitgen K et al[22]	2001	Splenopexy
Benevento A[23]	2002	Splenectomy
Ferro MM et al[16]	2002	Splenopexy
Rosin D[6]	2002	Splenectomy
Kim SS et al[15]	2003	Splenopexy
Cavazos S et al[21]	2004	Splenectomy
Corcione F[24]	2004	Splenectomy

DISCUSSION

Wandering spleen is a rare disease that can remain non-symptomatic for years. Torsion of its pedicle is what makes symptoms appear, but diagnosis is not easy to reach. Malignant involvement of a wandering spleen is even rarer and we could find only four reports in the literature - all four cases had malignant lymphomatous disease.[1,23] The dysuria was probably due to the irritation of the ectopic spleen on the ureter.

Image complementary examinations are very helpful and blood tests are usually non-specific, unless there is hypersplenism. Final confirmation is normally reached by laparoscopy. Laparotomy and laparoscopic approach are both perfectly valid options, although when a big specimen is found, laparoscopic extraction is done through a slightly extended port incision and fragmentation.

Surgery is the only definitive treatment for wandering spleen and the decision to perform splenopexy versus splenectomy depends on the pre- and intraoperative findings of a viable spleen. Splenopexy should only be done in asymptomatic, small specimen cases with no evidence of hyperpersplenism. According to our research, only 11 cases of wandering spleen treated laparoscopically have been reported in the literature until the year 2005.[23,24] Out of these reports, 7 cases underwent laparoscopic splenopexy and the other 4 underwent laparoscopic splenectomy. Ours was the eighth case of laparoscopic splenopexy.

CONCLUSION

Laparoscopic splenopexy is an effective procedure in the management of wandering spleen. Laparoscopic splenopexy is definitely better than open procedure in terms of less pain, better cosmesis, early ambulation, faster recovery, reduction of postoperative stay, wound complications, less overall morbidity and sooner return to work.

References

1. Kinori I, Rifkin MD.: A truly wandering spleen. J Ultrasound Med, 1988; 7: 101-5.

2. Dawson JH, Roberts NG: Management of the wandering spleen. Aust N Z J Surg, 1994; 64: 441-4.

3. Brown CVR, Virgilio GR, Vazquez VD, Vazquez WD.: Wandering spleen and its complications in children: a case series and review of the literature. J Pediatr Surg 2003; 38(11):1676-1679.

4. Buehner M, Baker MS.: The wandering spleen. Surg Gynecol Obstet. 1992;175:373-87.

5. Saayed S, Koniaris LG, Kovach SJ, Hirokawa T.: Torsion of a wandering spleen. Surgery. 2002; 132(3): 535-6.

6. Rosin D, Bank I, Gayer G, Rimon U, Gur D, Kuriansky Y, Morag B, Pras M, Ayalon A.: Laparoscopic splenectomy for torsion of wandering spleen associated with celiac axis occlusion. Surg Endosc. 2002 Jul;16(7):1110.

7. Balliu PR, Bregante J, Perez-Velasco MC, Fiol M, Galiana C, Herrera M, Mulet J.: Splenic haemorrhage in a newborn as the first manifestation of wandering spleen syndrome. J Pediatr Surg. 2004 Feb;39(2):240-2.

8. Horowitz JR, Black CT.: Traumatic rupture of a wandering spleen in a child: case report and literature review. J Trauma. Aug. 1996;41(2):348-50.

9. Choi YH, Menken FA, Jacobson IM, Lombardo F, Kazam E, Barie PS.: Recurrent acute pancreatitis: an additional manifestation of the "wandering spleen" syndrome". Am J Gastroenterol. 1996 May;91(5):1034-8.

10. Groszek-Terwei I, Saxena AK, Willital GH.: Torsion and volvulus of the stomach combined with a wandering spleen: creation of a extraperitoneal splenic pouch. Surgery. Feb. 2005;137(2):265.

11. Bollinger B, Lorentzen T.: Torsion of a wandering spleen: ultrasonographic findings. J Clin Ultrasound 1990;18 (6):510-1.

12. Danaci M, Belet U, Yalin T, Polat V, Nurol S.: Power Doppler sonographic diagnosis of torsion in a wandering spleen. J Clin Ultrasound. Jun. 2000;28(5):246-8.

13. Fasse A, Walgenbach S, Thelen M.: The wandering spleen - a rare differential diagnosis of acute abdomen. Rofo 1999 April;170(4):404-5.

14. Swischuk LE, Williams JB, John SD.: Torsion of wandering spleen: the whorled appearance of the splenic pedicle on CT. Pediatr Radiol. 1993;23(6):476-7.

15. Kim SS, Lee SL, Waldhausen JHT, Ledbetter DL.: Laparoscopic splenopexy for Wandering Spleen Syndrome. Pedriatic Endosurgery and Innovative Techniques, 2003; 7:237-241.

16. Ferro MM, Elmo G, Piaggio L.: Laparoscopic pocket splenopexy (LAPS) for wandering spleen: a new technique. Oral Abstracts, IPEG – 2002.

17. Nomura H, Haji S, Kuroda D, Yasuda K, Ohyanagi H, Kudo M.: Laparoscopic splenopexy for adult wandering spleen: Sandwich method with two sheets of absorbable knitted mesh. Surg Laparosc Endosc Percutan Tech. October 2000;10(5):332-334.

18. Hirose R, Kitano S, Bando T, Ueda Y, Sato K, Yoshida T, Suenobu S, Kawano T, Izumi T.: Laparoscopic splenopexy for pediatric wandering spleen. J Pediatr Surg. 1998 Oct;33(10):1571-3.

19. Haj M, Bickel A, Weiss M, Eitan A.: Laparoscopic splenopexy of a wandering spleen. J Laparoendosc Adv Surg Tech A. 1999 Aug;9(4):357-60.

20. Cohen MS, Soper NJ, Underwood RA, Quasebarth M, Brunt LM.: Laparoscopic splenopexy for wandering (pelvic) spleen. Surg Laparosc Endosc. 1998;8(4):286-90.

21. Cavazos S, Ratzer ER, Fenoglio ME.: Laparoscopic management of the wandering spleen. J Laparoendosc Adv Surg Tech A. 2004 Aug;14(4):227-9.

22. Peitgen K, Majetschak M, Walz MK.: Laparoscopic splenopexy by peritoneal and omental pouch construction for intermittent splenic torsion ("wandering spleen"). Surg Endosc. 2001 Apr;15(4):413.

23. Benevento A, Boni L, Dionigi G, et al.: Emergency laparoscopic splenectomy for wandering pelvic spleen: case report and review of the literature on laparoscopic approach to splenic diseases. Surg Endosc, 2002; 16(9): 1364-5.

24. Corcione F, Caiazzo P, Cuccurullo D, Miranda L, Settembre A, Pirozzi F, Bruzzese G.: Laparoscopic splenectomy for the treatment of wandering spleen. Surg Endosc, March 2004;18 (3):554-6.

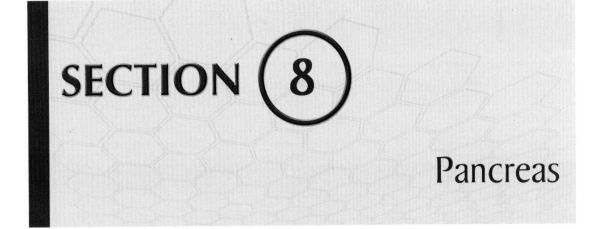

SECTION 8

Pancreas

53

Laparoscopic Pancreatic Surgery

INTRODUCTION

New technology has facilitated the application of minimally invasive procedures to their various open surgical equivalents. In recent years, technological advances and accumulated experience with laparoscopic procedures for the management of upper gastro intestinal tract and biliary tree diseases have made it possible to attempt laparoscopic pancreatic surgery. Since then, the minimal invasive approach is applied in the treatment of almost all pancreatic diseases, including even pancreatic carcinoma. These procedures range from the simplest diagnostic laparoscopy and biopsy to complex procedures such as lateral pancreaticojejunostomy or pancreaticoduodenectomy (Whipple's procedure). Different techniques were described and innovative approaches were developed. This development has been in part facilitated by advances in medical technology; the advent of mechanical endostaplers, ultrasonic dissectors, hand access devices, Endoscopic ultrasonogram and laparoscopic ultrasonography etc, all have contributed.

Compared with its open counter part, laparoscopic surgery is associated with less immune disturbance and more favourable short-term outcomes, notably better cosmesis and patients satisfaction. Despite these the penetration of the laparoscopic approach in the pancreatic surgery has not proceeded at a similar pace to laparoscopic cholecystectomy in general surgery. This might be due to the anatomic location of the pancreas, the particularity of pancreatic resection, the small number of indicative patients and the necessity of complicated techniques. Hence the associated steep learning curves and the recognized increase in morbidity associated with conversion. More importantly many surgeons claim the observed benefits in laparoscopic surgery are controversial, as many of the published comparative studies were not randomized and included hetrogenous groups of patients of different pathologies.

Laparoscopic pancreatic surgery was originally introduced for staging and palliative treatment of pancreatic cancer, but technologic advancement and accumulating experiences in laparoscopic procedures have led to attempt at more complicated surgeries. These include internal pseudocyst drainage, resection of pancreatic tumors including ennucleation, distal pancreatectomy (with or without spleen preserving), lateral pancreaticojejunostomy and even pancreaticoduodenectomy. The total number of laparoscopic pancreatic surgeries performed is still small, however and reports are often based on limited experience.

LAPAROSCOPIC PANCREATIC SURGERY - HISTORICAL PERSPECTIVE

In 1911, Bernheim[3] reported the use of diagnostic laparoscopy in a patient with a pancreatic mass and stated that the presence of liver metastasis precluded the possibility of any invasive surgical attempt. Cuschieri et al[6] in 1978 and Warshaw et al in 1986 also performed laparoscopic staging for the detection of metastases and tumor ingrowth.[47]

Pachter et al[27] in 1979, managed the transected pancreas following distal pancreatectomy with the aid of a stapling devise; followed by Fitzgibbons et al in 1982.[12] Using this technology, as well as vascular staplers, Soper et al,[36] were able to establish the safety and efficacy of laparoscopic distal pancreatectomy in an animal model, with no evidence of pancreatic leaks or fistula. Gagner and Pomp reported the first laparoscopic pancreatic resection for chronic pancreatitis in 1994.[16] They performed a pylorus preserving pancreaticoduodenectomy successfully in a 30 year old woman with chromic pancreatitis. Since then, laparoscopic pancreatic resections consisting of enucleation, distal pancreatectomy and pancreticoduodenectomy have been performed in fewer than 150 cases word wide excluding ours.

In 1996, Cuschieri et al[7] reported laparoscopic distal (70-80%) pancreatectomy with splenectomy in group of 7 patients. During the same period Gagner et al[13] attempted laparoscopic pancreatic distal resection with spleen preservation in 7 patients with islet cell tumor. Warshaw et al[46] is the first to describe the technique of spleen conservation distal pancreatectomy in open method during 1988. This technique has been adopted laparoscopically by Sussman[37] and Vezakis et al[44] in 1996.

In 1993, Pietrabissa et al, is the first to use laparoscopic ultrasonography for localization of insulinoma by laparoscopic infragastric inspection of the pancreas. In 1996, Gagner et al[15] did laparoscopic extirpation of insulinomas in 4 patients, followed by Bonjer et al and Cuschieri et al[8] during 1998.

The first laparoscopic cystogastrostomy was performed by J.Petilin in 1994. The first laparoscopic intraluminal cystogastrostomy was described by Gagner et al[14] and Way et al[48] in 1994.

GEM EXPERIENCE

The author has got more than a decade long experience in managing various pancreatic diseases by minimal access method. We started doing diagnostic laparoscopy for staging pancreatic malignancy and for tumor localization in case of neuroendocrine tumorus, as early in 1992. Next to Michael Gagner, we are the second in the world to do the totally laparoscopic pylorus preserving pancreatico duodenectomy in 1997 successfully. We started doing laparoscopic anterior cystogastrostomy since 1994 and have completed nearly 104 cases still to date. We did the first laparoscopic lateral pancreaticojejunsotomy (modified peustow) in 1997. The laparoscopic surgery video in Laparoscopic Whipples procedure and Laparoscopic lateral pancreaticojejunostomy were given SAGES video library award during 2000 and 2001 respectively and were included in the SAGES library catalogue. We performed our first laparoscopic spleen preserving distal pancreatectomy in 1999.

SURGICAL ANATOMY OF PANCREAS

The pancreas lies transversely in the retroperitoneal area between the duodenum on the right and the spleen on the left. It is related to the omental bursa above, the transverse mesocolon anteriorly, and the greater sac below and it is a fixed organ.

Parts of Pancreas

The pancreas may be arbitrarely divided into five parts : Head, Uncinate process, neck, body and tail.

Head

It is that portion lying to the right of the SMA and SMV. Its junction with the neck is marked anteriorly by an imaginary line from the portal vein above to the SMV below.

Uncinate Process

It is an extension of lower left posterior surface of the head, usually passing behind the PV and superior mesenteric vessels and infront of the aorta and IVC. In sagital section, it is located between the SMA and the aorta, having the left renal vein above and the 3rd or 4th part of the duodenum below. Short vessels from the SMA and vein supply the uncinate process and must be carefully ligated.

When distal pancreatectomy is performed, the presence or absence of the uncinate process finds to determine how much of the pancreas is removed. A well developed uncinate process most likely belongs to a pancreas with a small head. If the uncinate process in present, 60% to 65% pancreatectomy is performed; if the uncinate process in absent, 70% to 80% of the pancreas is removed. Carcinoma involving uncinate process is usually inseparable from aorta since it lies behind uncinate process.

Neck

It is 1.5 to 2cm in length, fixed between the celiac trunk above and the SM vessels below. On the right, the gastroduodenal artery gives off the anterior superior pancreaticoduodenal artery, its origin being at the upper part of the neck near its junction with the head. Posteriorly the PV is formed by the confluence of the SM and splenic vein.

Body

It lies to the left of the SM vessels and in relation to the 4th part of the duodenum, the ligament of Treitz some jejunal loops and the left side of the transverse

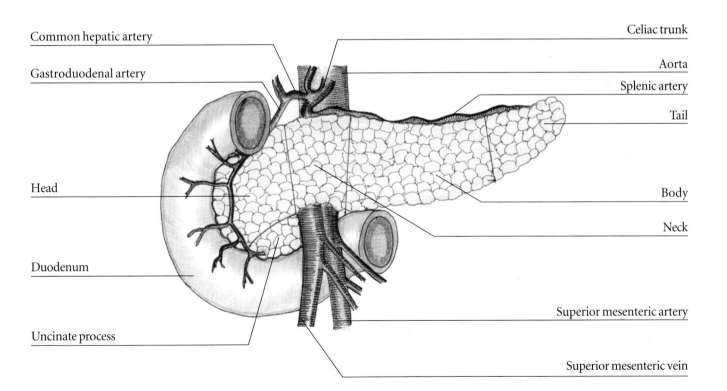

Figure 1 : Various parts of pancreas

colon. Anteriorly the body of the pancreas is covered by the double peritoneal layer of the posterior wall of the omental bursa, which separates the pancreas from the stomach. It is also related to the transverse mesocolon, which separates into two layers, one leaf covering the anterior surface and another covering the inferior surface. The middle colic artery travels between the leaves of the mesocolon.

Tail

It is mobile, at its tip reaches the visceral surface of the spleen. Together with the splenic artery and the beginning of the splenic vein, it is enveloped by the two layers of the splenorenal ligament. The outer layer of this ligament forms the posterior layer of the gastrosplenic ligament, so careless division may injure the short gastric vessels.

PANCREATIC DUCTS

The main pancreatic duct (of Wirsung) and the accessory duct (of Santorini) lie anterior to the major pancreatic vessels. The developmental variations may be as follows :

1. In 60% both ducts open into the duodenum

2. In 30% the duct of Wirsung carries the entire secretion, the duct of santorini ends blindly

3. In 10% the duct of santorini carries the entire secretion, the duct of wirsung is small or absent.

The greatest diameter of the PD is in the head of the pancreas, just before the duct enters the duodenal wall.

Major Duodenal Papilla (Papilla of Vater) and Ampulla of Vater

There is confusion in the literature about the correct definition and distinguishing points of the papilla of vater and ampulla of vater.

The papilla is a nipple like projection of duodenal mucosa. It constitutes the distal end of the ampulla of vater into the duodenum.

The ampulla is the common pancreaticobiliary channel, which can have several variations. If the septum

between the ducts extends to the orifice of the papilla, there is no ampulla. The papilla is on the posteriomedial wall of the 2nd portion of the duodenum, 7 to 10cm from the pylorus.

Minor Duodenal Papilla

It is situated approximately 2cm cranial and slightly anterior to the major papilla. An excellent land mark is the GDA, situated anterior to the accessory pancreatic duct (santorini) and the minor papilla. During gastrectomy, duodenal dissection should end proximal to or at this artery. It becomes important in those few patients in whom the accessory duct carries the major drainage of the pancreas.

ARTERIAL SUPPLY

The pancreas is supplied with blood from both celiac trunk and the SMA. The neck of the pancreas and the concave surface of the duodenum are supplied by two pancreaticoduodenal artrial arcades (anterior and posterior). Ligation of both vessels well result in duodenal ischaemia and necrosis. All major arteries lie posterior to the ducts. The anterior and posterior superior pancreaticoduodenal arteries arise from the GDA and the inferior branches of pancreaticoduodenal arteries arise from the SMA.

The splenic artery is located on the posterior surface of the body and tail of the pancreas. Around 2 to 10 branches of the splenic artery anastomosis with the transverse pancreatic artery. The largest of these, the great pancreatic artery (posterior) is the main blood supply to the tail of the pancreas. Ligation of the splenic artery does not require splenectomy but ligation of the splenic vein does.

VENOUS DRAINAGE

In general, the veins of the pancreas parallel the arteries and lie superficial to them. Both lie posterior to the ducts. The drainage is to the portal vein, splenic vein and superior and inferior mesenteric veins.

Four pancreatico duodenal veins form venous arcades draining the head of the pancreas and duodenum. The anterior superior pancreatico duodenal vein joins

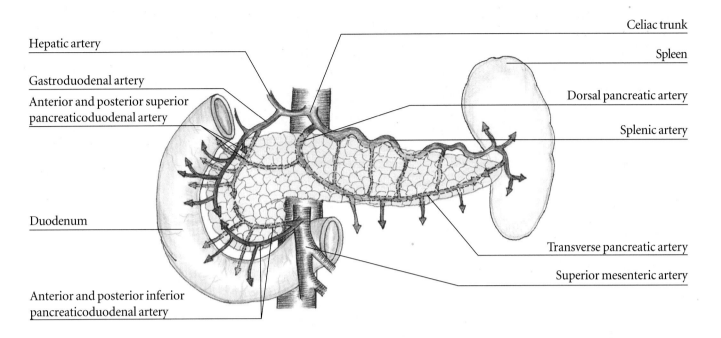

Figure 2 : Anterior view of major arterial supply to the pancreas

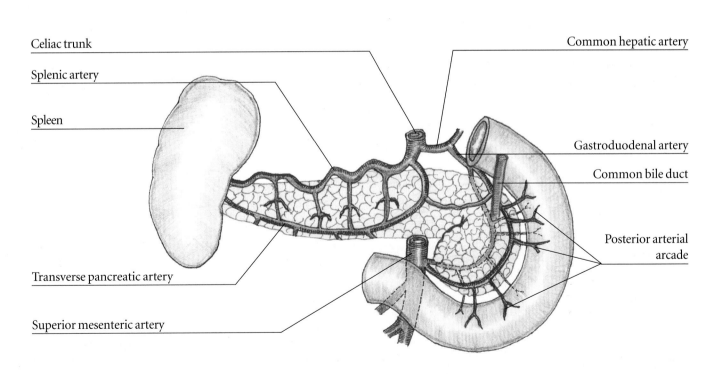

Figure 3 : Posterior view of major arterial supply to the pancreas

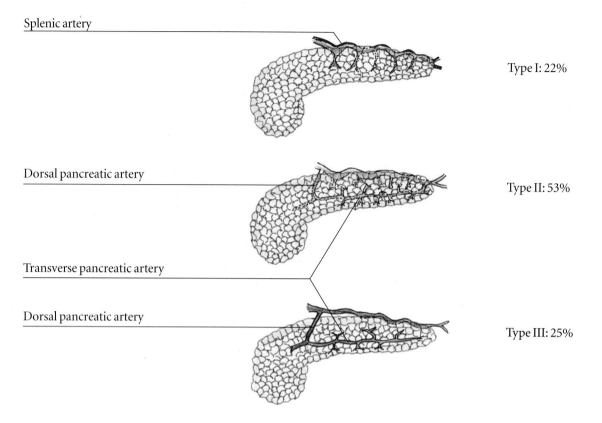

Splenic artery

Type I: 22%

Dorsal pancreatic artery

Type II: 53%

Transverse pancreatic artery

Dorsal pancreatic artery

Type III: 25%

Figure 4 : Diagram shows the possible configuration of the blood supply to the distal pancreas.
Type III blood supply is susceptible to infarction from emboli in the transverse artery

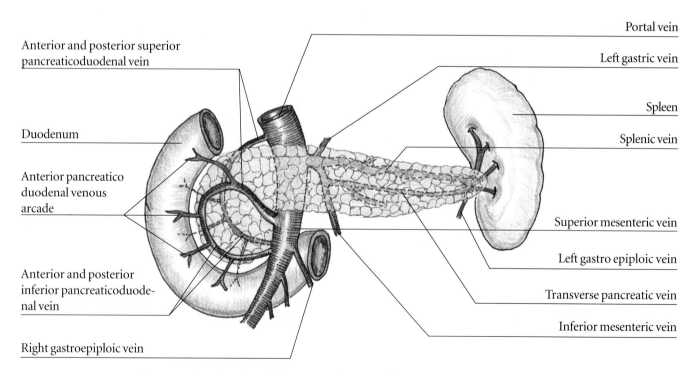

Anterior and posterior superior
pancreaticoduodenal vein

Portal vein

Left gastric vein

Spleen

Duodenum

Splenic vein

Anterior pancreatico
duodenal venous
arcade

Superior mesenteric vein

Anterior and posterior
inferior pancreaticoduodenal vein

Left gastro epiploic vein

Transverse pancreatic vein

Inferior mesenteric vein

Right gastroepiploic vein

Figure 5 : Anterior view of the venous drainage of the pancreas and the tributaries
of the hepatic portal vein

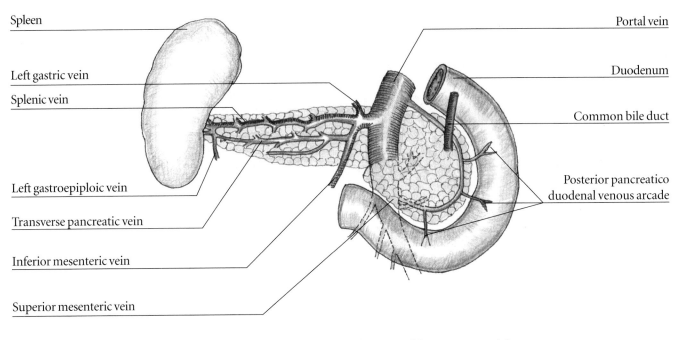

Figure 6 : Posterior view of the venous drainage of the pancreas and the tributaries of the hepatic portal vein

the right gastroepiploic vein. This vein receives a colic vein to form a short gastrocolic vein, which is a tributary to the SMV.

The veins of the left portion of the pancreas form two large venous channels, the splenic vein above and the transverse (inferior) pancreatic vein below.

The hepatic portal vein is formed behind the neck of the pancreas by the joining of the SMV and the splenic vein. The PV lies infron of the IVC with the CBD to the right and the hepatic artery to the left. The PV and SMV easily can be separated from the posterior surface of the pancreas in the absence of disease.

Lymphatic Drainage

It is a centrifugal drainage to the surrounding nodes. They drain into 5 main collecting trunks and lymphnode groups.

1. Superior Nodes

It drains the anterior and posterior superior half of the pancreas. Most end in the suprapancreatic lymphnodes located along the superior border of the pancreas

2. Inferior Nodes

The collection trunks drain the anterior and posterior lower half of the head and body of pancreas. They drain in to inferior pancreatic nodes. They may further extend to superior mesenteric and left lateral aortic nodes.

3. Anterior Nodes

Drains along the anterior surface of superior and inferior portions of the head of the pancreas.

4. Posterior nodes

Drain the posterior surface of the superior and inferior portions of the head of th pancreas. They drain into the posterior pancreatico duodenal nodes.

5. Splenic Nodes

Drain mainly from the tail of the pancreas. They drain into those at the hilum of spleen; splenophrenic ligament and inferior and superior lymphnodes of the tail of the pancreas.

No lymphatic communication exist between the pancreas and the lymphnodes of the greater and lesser curvatures of the stomach. The lymphatics of

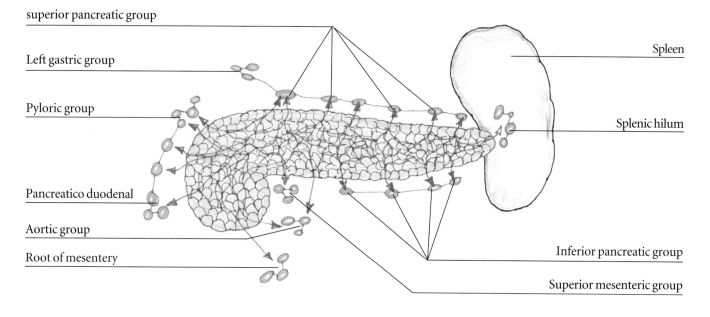

superior pancreatic group

Left gastric group

Pyloric group

Pancreatico duodenal

Aortic group

Root of mesentery

Spleen

Splenic hilum

Inferior pancreatic group

Superior mesenteric group

Figure 7 : Lymphatic drainage of the pancreas. Flow is toward the nearest margin of the pancreas

the head and body of the pancreas do not drain toward the tail of the pancreas or the splenic nodes.

Lymph moves from the pancreas to the duodenum, not from the duodenum to the pancreas and it is well known that pancreatic cancer disseminates rapidly because of the retroperitoneal position of the pancreas and its rich lymphatics and venous drainage with centifugel spread.

NERVE SUPPLY

The pancreas is innervated by sympathetic (splanchnic) parasympathetic (vagal) divisions. In general these nerves follow blood vessels to their destination. The celiac ganglion is the control station of both sympathetic and parasympathetic innervation. Extirpation, surgical or chemical of the celiac ganglion should interrupt afferent fibers of both sympathetic and parasympathetic systems.

The severe pain in pancreatic disease (ie chronic pancreatitis and tumor) may be due to (i) perineural inflammation (as in pancreatitis) or infiltration (in carcinoma) (2) Ductal hypertension due to obstruction leading to increased tissue and ductal pressure leading to severe pain.

DIAGNOSTIC IMAGING AND SPECIAL INSTRUMENTS

Diagnostic imaging modalities for patients undergoing laparoscopic pancreatic surgery includes, ulrasonography, dynamic contrast enhanced CT scan, magnetic resonance imaging (MRI), and magnetic resonance cholangiopancreatipancreatography (MRCP), Endoscopic Retrograde Cholangio Pancreatography (ERCP), Endoscopic Ultrasonography (EUS) and laparoscopic ultrasonography (LUS). Current technology allows accurate preoperative radiologic staging and assessment of resectability.

Detailed preoperative work up is essential before laparoscopic pancreatic resections because complete information of the pathological anatomy gained preoperatively compensates for certain limitations of laparoscopic approach. These limitations are lack of tactile feed back and restricted manipulation within the confined retrogastric/retroperitoneal space. In patients with presumed benign cystic lesions of the body and tail of the pancreas, as well in those suffering from chronic pancreatitis, the possibility of malignant disease must be excluded as far as possible. The delineations of the extent, nature and exact location of the pancreatic pathology combined with information on the relation of this major anatomic structures that require preservation is of crucial importance when assessing feasibility and in the planning of laparoscopic pancreatic resection. In this respect, each surgery has to be individualized.

Ultrasound, CT and MRI

Standard trascutaneous abdominal ultrasound remains the most sensitive test for the detection of gall stones and is useful in demonstrating a dilated intrahepatic and extrahepatic biliary tree in cases of obstructive jaundice. Ultrasound examination can provide information about liver metastasis, pancreatic masses, peripancratic adenopathy and ascites. It is however, highly operator dependent, and adequate examination of the retroperitoneal structures may be precluded by obesity and overlying bowel gas. Ultrasound scans reveal a pancreatic mass in 60 to 70% of patients with pancreatic cancers. However, the absence of a pancreatic mass on ultrasound scanning does not definitely rule out pancreatic cancer.

Currently high-quality, spiral or helical CT scanning appears to be the favoured investigation used to confirm the clinical suspicion of pancreatic cancer and for staging. It provides useful information not only about the tumor size but also about the extend of disease. Spread to the liver, peripancratic lymphnode or retroperitoneal structures may be demonstrated. In addition, the CT scan can be used to evaluate major vessels adjacent to the pancreas (SMA & SMV, PV, SV, HA) for tumor invasion, encasement or thrombosis, to give useful information regarding resectability. Tumors smaller than 1 cm can be missed and intrahepatic and extrahepatic ductal dilation may be the only finding on spiral CT.

Advances in MRI technology suggest that it may play an increasing role in pancreatic imaging. But MRI has not been shown to have a definitive advantage over modern CT scanning. MRCP holds promise as a noninvasive technique to image the biliary and pancreatic ductal systems in a fashion similar to ERCP. Likewise, magnetic resonance angiography (MRA) provides a non invasive technique to

evaluate major vascular involvement when CT is equivocal. This MRI or MRCP has the potential to provide information about tumor size and extent, biliary and pancreatic ductal anatomy and vascular involvement through a single, non invasive procedure.

ERCP - Endoscopic Retrograde Cholangio pancreatography

The role of ERCP in the diagnosis of lesions causing malignant biliary obstruction is well established. It provides not only high diagnostic accuracy (88-93%) for these tumors, but also the opportunity for the relief of jaundice by endoscopic sphincterotomy and endoprosthesis insertion and for pathological diagnosis by brush cytology. However this technique relies upon the interpretation of indirect tumor signs such as stricture and prestenotic dilation. It is therefore unable to provide information regarding the resectability of such tumors, and contributes little towards the staging of pancreatic cancer other than by identifying the presence of the mass favourable periampullary tumors.

With the current advances in CT and MRI, diagnostic ERCP is rarely necessary. It should be considered in patients with CBD or PD obstruction without the finding of pancreatic mass on CT or MRI. ERCP can also be useful in distinguishing chronic pancreatitis from pancreatic cancer. Chronic pancreatitis is usually characterized by multiple focal stenosis of the pancreatic duct, with involvement of secondary and tertiary radicles, where as pancreatic cancer is usually characterized by an abrupt cut off of the at a single location.

Visceral Angiography

Angiography plays no role in the primary diagnosis of pancreatic cancer, other then to differentiate it from rarer cystadenomatous tumors. By documenting, abnormal pancreatic vasculature can locate insulinomas in 35% to 75% of cases and should be considered preoperatively.

The portal venous phase is studied following selective celiac and mesenteric angiography, looking specifically for venous occlusion or displacement and arterial cuffing or encasement. The latter signs, however, may not occur without there first being evidence of venous involvement.

Endoscopic Ultrasonography (EUS)

The development of ultrasonic endoscopes, has been a significant development in overcoming some of the limitations associated with standard external ultrasound probes. The accuracy of EUS in the primary diagnoses of pancreatic cancer has been shown to be superior to ultrasound and CT scanning and at least as good as ERCP, especially with small tumors of <2cm in size.

There are limitations to the use of EUS, however including a restricted depth of tissue penetration, notably when scanning liver, making the reliable detection of distant metastases impossible. Difficulties with topographic orientation and a significant learning curve are well recognized. Another confounding factor is the inherent inability of this technique to detect the small peritoneal metastasis that are so typical of pancreatic cancer.

Laparoscopic Ultrasonography (LUS)

Invention of LUS replaces the tactile sensation of laparoscopic surgeon, as well as improved the localization of occult pancreatic tumors and liver metastasis. In experienced hands use of LUS may obviate extensive preoperative imaging techniques. Several authors concluded that LUS is a valuable addition to the staging laparoscopic procedure and the accuracy of staging is 98% with a positive predictive index of 100% and a negative predictive index of 98%. The advantages of LUS in that the probe can be placed in direct contact with the surface of the organ to be examined. This avoids the need for ultrasound signals to pass through media which would normally cause attenuation and degradation of the image, ie, the tissue of the abdominal wall and bowel gas. It is particularly helpful to identify small intra parenchymal liver metastases and to delineate resectability in patients with equivaocal findings at laparoscopy, such as retropancreatic vascular involvement. It also provides guidance during surgery (eg. Enucleation of insulinoma) and also useful in determining the optimal site of transection of the pancreas during laparoscopic distal pancreatectomy.

In 1963, Yamakawa et al[49] is the first surgeon who described A mode scanning of gallbladder cancer under laparoscopic guidance. The subsequent evolution of LUS over the last 10 years has seen the development of small versatile probes incorporating ultracompact ultrasound transducers which can be passed through 10-12mm laparoscopic ports. Refinements in equipment, in particular the development of laparoscopic probes incorporating linear array transducers, now provide for stable, good quality, high resolution, real time images of areas not normally amenable to inspection at laparoscopy, such as the head of pancreas, retroperitoneal vasculature, pancreatic lymphnodes and even the deepest regions of the hepatic parenchyma.

The ultrasound system in our setup has simultaneous imaging capability and employs pulsed and color flow Doppler for vascular assessment. The probes we use are all articulated varying from 5 MHz to 10MHz. The probes are equipped with linear and curved technology identifying lesions as small as 2mm. We follow a systematic examination of whole abdomen starting from liver. All the segments were examined starting from the segment I. After which, IVC, hepatic veins, PV, SMV, CBD, CHD, HA were examined. We use colour flow Doppler for examining the vascular structures. Then the aorta and origin of SMA were examined. The pancreas is examined by placing the transducer through the window in the gastrohepatic omentum directly on the surface of the gland. The tumor with its relation to the PD is noted. Gentle rotation of the probe at this stage allows for evaluation of the celiac axis and proximal hepatic artery. By collecting the data from laparoscopy and LUS a decision is made regarding the resectability of the tumor. We incorporate diagnostic laparoscopy and LUS into the investigative algorithm for all patients in our surgical unit with either suspected or established pancreatic or periampullary cancer.

Special Instrument

In the recent days more and more complicated gastro intestinal surgeries are attempted by laparoscopic method, because of the advance developments in hitech instrumentation for the purpose of resection and hemostasis. Few important instruments which should be mentioned at this juncture are laparoscopic ultrasonic shears, ligasure, Endo GI staplers and APC.

Laparoscopic Ultrasonic Shear : (Harmonic Scalpel)

Ultrasonically activated scissors and related instruments use high frequency (more than 20000 MHz) to induce mechanical vibration at the cellular level. The result is a localized heat generation from friction and shear producing a predictable pattern of thermal distinction. The heat and vibration together denature protein by disrupting hydrogen bonds, leading to the formation of a sticky coagulation in a very localized area around the instrument tip, at lower temperature. The ability to coagulate small blood vessels with minimum heat transmission causes less tissue trauma than electrocautery. Vibration of the edge results in a sawing action and cutting of the tissue and of blood vessels with a diameter of upto 2mm. The vibration of blunt instrument causes coagulation and control of larger vessels reliably upto 5mm.

Ultrasonically activated shears have been developed with function as combination grasper, coagulator, retractor and dissector in a single instrument. These sorts of instruments have the potential to reduce the number of instruments exchanges require to perform an operation and this reduces operative time and cost, especially when combined with other advanced technologies. As the temperature never exceeds beyond 80 degree the tissue charing effect is almost nil. Hence, operation is always clean and allows identification of tissue plan precisely in a bloodless field. It is extremely useful in advanced laparoscopic pancreatic surgeries, including dissection and division of greater omentum as well as transection of pancreas and enucleation of endocrine tumors of the pancreas.

Ligasure (Valley Lab)

Highly specialized version, where in even larger vessels upto 7mm can be sealed and divided. This can be used as an efficient coagulating device. For division and further dissection separate instruments should be used. This has been described in detailed in chapter 6.

Staplers

Experience with the state of art stapling instruments and techniques have elevated the operative strategy to higher level of sophistication and reduced the need for physically weaving for a long respective maneuvers. Manual sewing in laparoscopy is tedious and mechanical stapling anastomosis makes reconstruction phase of advanced procedure more effective.

Manufacturers of laparosopic instruments have greatly improved the versatility of endoscopic staplers. Currently, multiple types of stapling units such as straight versus roticulating in 2.0 to 4.8 mm in sizes are available. The length of the stapler jaw can vary from 30 to 45mm and upto 60mm, all via 12mm cannula. The most important is the advances in the development of the rotiaulating endoscopic stapling unit.

Endoscopic staplers have cartridges for normal thickness tissue, thick tissue, and vascular applications that can be used for dividing the mesentery. The multifire endo GIA 30 is for closure and transection of tissue. The instruments available 3.5mm (intestinal blue in colour) 2.5mm (vascular) white in colour and 4.1mm green in color. Each gun can be used according to the tissue. We use 2.5mm vascular staplers (white) for division of pancreas.

INDICATIONS AND PROCEDURES

Laparoscopy was initially introduced in the field of pancreatic surgery for the staging of pancreatic cancer. The increasing experience with minimal access surgery, particularly for advanced procedures such as Laparoscopic splenectomy, has lead to the performance of laparoscopic pancreatic surgeries including pancreatic resections. Advances in laparoscopic instrumentation and ancillary technology have facilitated the safe and efficient extention of these procedures by the laparoscopic approach. The indications for laparoscopic pancreatic surgeries in literature are discussed for benign and low grade malignant diseases. In particular, benign islet cell tumors (in insulinomas), cystic neoplasms of pancreas (body and tail) (serous cystadenoma, mucous cystadenoma, congenital cyst) etc, chronic pancreatitis, pseudocyst are suitable disease for laparoscopic pancreatic resection because they require no regional lymphadenectomy.

Surgical outcomes are acceptable for the laparoscopic procedure, with few complications such as pancreatic leakage or splenic infarction. A laparoscopic approach to the pancreas is anatomically complicated, with a high risk of pancreatic leakage. Therefore, it is necessary to perform laparoscopic pancreatic surgery carefully with gentle manipulation to prevent complication.

In dedicated advanced laparoscopic centers, where experienced laparoscopic GI surgeons, are available, the indications for laparoscopic surgery are extended further to pancreatic and periampullary malignancy as well as in treating the complications of acute pancreatitis.

Laparoscopic procedures for pancreatic diseases falls into one of the following categories.

I.   Pancreatic Resections

  a. Pancreaticoduodenectomy - Whipple's procedure - periampullary tumors

  b. Distal pancreatectomy with splenectomy - Cystic tumor of body and tail

  c. Distal pancreatectomy without splenectomy - Cystic tumor of body

  d. Median pancreatectomy

  e. Left pancreatectomy

II. Enucleation of tumors

  a. Insulinomas

  b. Benign cyst

III. Bilioenteric bypass procedure of pancreatic malignancy with obstructive jaundice

  a. Cholecysto jejunostomy

  b. Hepatico jejunostomy

  c. Choledocho jejunostomy

IV. Gastroenterostomy - for duodenal / gastric outlet obstruction in pancreatic malignancy

V.   Staging laparoscopy and biopsy in pancreatic malignancy

VI. Internal drainage of pseudocysts of pancreas

  a. Lap. Intraluminal cystogastrostomy

  b. Lap. anterior cystogastrostomy

  c. Lap. Posterior cystogastrostomy

VII. Decompression of pancreatic duct followed by pancreatico enteric bypass - (lateral pancreatico jejunostomy) modified Puestow procedure in chronic calcific obstructive pancreatitis

VIII. In the treatment of complication of acute pancreatitis

  a. Necrosectomy

  b. Drainage of abscess

  c. External drainage of infected pseudocyst

PANCREATIC RESECTION

Pancreaticoduodenectomy

In the literature the laparoscopic resection of the pancreas are divided into 4 types : enucleation, distal pancreatectomy with splenectomy, spleen preserving distal pancreatectomy and pancreaticoduodenectomy. The extensive review of literature of lap pancreatic resection, the total number was found to be around 150. Out of which 14 lap pancreaticoduodenectomy, 116 lap pancreatic resection, 41 enucleation, 4 left pancreatectomy and 2 hand assisted resection. Only few cases (14) of lap pylorus preserving pancreaticoduodenectomy have been reported excluding ours. Gagner[16] performed the first two procedures, one for chronic pancreatitis and the other for periampullary cancer. However, the procedure proved to be time consuming with prolonged hospital stay and Gagner concluded that although it was technically feasible the laparoscopic Whipples procedure did not promise to improve the post operative out come or shorten the post operative period. Cusheri et al[8] also agree with this appraisal, and have encountered both delayed gastric emptying and major pancreatic fistula in two patients under going laparoscopic assisted pancreaticoduodenectomy for perampullary cancer. He emphasized that this operation could be done via a laparoscopic approach only when the postoperative course of the patients showed a better outcome than could be obtained with the current open approach. We are proud to mention at this juncture that next to Michael Ganger, ours is the second laparoscopic centre in the world to perform total laparoscopic pylorus preserving pancreaticoduodenectomy in 1998. Till to date we have performed 35 cases in our centre with better outcome compared to our open counterpart. Though we have good outcome in our series compared to others, we still believe that it should be considered investigational and should be attempted by skilled laparoscopic surgeons only.

Local excision of the ampulla of vater was carried out laparoscopically by Letwin and Rossi for carcinoma of the ampulla. Still it has not found place in routine clinical practice and advisability is debatable.

Distalpancreatectomy with Splenectomy

In 1996 Cuschieri et al[9] described the technique they used to perform laparoscopic distal 70-80% pancreatectomy with enbloc splenectomy in a group of seven patients with intractable pain due to chronic pancreatitis. Tumors larger than 2cm in diameter, those located in the body or the tail of the pancreas, those connected to the pancreatic duct, or those involving malignancy were indications for distal pancreatectomy. In general, distal pancreatectomy is usually performed enbloc, along with resection of spleen. Most of the time the enbloc distal pancreatic spleen resection is performed for technical reasons since it makes the operation short and easy. We recommend gentle and careful traction of the pancreas, including the tumor, meticulous division of the transverse branches between the pancreas and splenic vein; and steady hemostasis to reduce intra operative blood loss. Further more, an endoscopic linear stapler is useful for distal pancreatectomy, resection of the distal pancreas and closure of the pancreatic stump without simultaneous pancreatic leakage or bleeding.

Distal pancreatectomy without splenectomy

Preservation of the spleen also is an immunology factor in pancreatic surgery. Over whelming sepsis after distal pancreatectomy and splenectomy has been reported. Spleen preserving distal pancreatectomy is technically demanding and more time consuming procedure. It is divided in two types. One type involved preservation of splenic vessels by meticulous division of small branches of splenic vessels between the splenic hilum and the pancreas. The other type involve transection of splenic vessels distally and proximally. In the latter case, the blood supply of the spleen is from the short gastric vessels. We believe the magnified view afforded by the laparoscopic approach facilitates the separation of the splenic artery and vein from the pancreatic parenchyma and the identification of the small arteries and veins, which are then easily controlled with the use of laparoscopic instruments such as the harmonic scalpel and the ligasure device.

Warshaw et al[46] first described the modified technique of spleen preserving pancreatectomy in 1988 in open method. This consists of ligation of both common splenic A & V proximal and distal to the proposed pancreatic resection. The residual blood supply to the spleen from the short gastric vessels seems to be sufficient for splenic survival. This technique has been adopted laparoscopically by Sussman[37] and Vesakis et al.[44] The largest experience with lap distal pancreatectomy has been reported by Kiely et al, who has done in 30 patients with cystic tumors out of which 82% where premalignant lesions. The most common post operative complications is pancreatic fistula. Suture ligation of the stapled transected duct and applications of fibrois glue to the residual pancreatic stump and administration of somatostatin may reduce this complication.

The procedure of spleen preserving is technically feasible and useful in lap pancreatic surgery. However, Warshaw[46] reported that spleen preservation is difficult in the case of tumor involving the hilum of the spleen and splenic hilar scarring from part of acute inflammation or abscess formation. In these cases, spleen preservation should be avoided because of several possible complications such as bleeding or splenic injury.

ENUCLEATION

Laparoscopic enucleation have been used for relatively small tumors (<2cm in dia) and for tumors located on the surface of the pancreas away from the pancreatic duct. Tumor location is an important factor in the success of lap pancreatic surgery. Enucleation is a safe and simple procedure using harmonic scalpel under the guidance of LUS. The use of LUS during lap pancreatic surgery is encouraged for the accurate enulceation of tumors. In our experience, harmonic scalpel is an effective tool for enucleation of the pancreatic parenchyma. Dissection of the pancreatic parenchyma should be performed with great care to prevent complications. Dissection of the pancreatic parenchyma must be performed carefully to prevent leakage resulting from the high incidence of pancreatic fistula. However, harmonic scalpel is useful in cases where it is possible to retain a sufficient margin of tissue near the pancreatic duct after resection. If there is not enough tissue, enucleation should be avoided. Enucleation or distal pancreatectomy is a suitable laparoscopic procedures for pancreatic diseases because neither requires reconstruction.

LAPAROSCOPIC PALLIATIVE BYPASS PROCEDURES

Bilioenteric and Gastroenteric bypass

Any discussion of pancreatic malignancy must include palliative options to provide patients relief from the ranges of the disease. Palliation for PC is directed at three primary problems; biliary obstruction, duodenal obstruction and pain. The aim is should to provide symptomatic relief with minimal morbidity and rapid return to function. The surgical options include creation of either a biliary or a gastric bypass, or both. The corresponding controversies include the effectiveness of endoscopic stenting versus surgical bypass of the bile duct for biliary obstruction, cholecystoenterostomy versus choledochoenterostomy and the need for gastric bypass in unresectable patients is supported by historical data as there is a 70% incidence of obstructive jaundice and 40% incidence of GOO. Though an ideal method of palliative biliary decompression is controversial, endoscopic stenting has become routine. Randomized trials comparing endoscopic stenting and surgery suggested that biliary stenting has less early morbidity and mortality, but recurrent jaundice and cholangitis occur in 13% to 60% of patients in the long term. By the time of death the length of hospitalization was similar, as a result of readmission due to stent obstruction/cholangitis and of duodenal obstruction. Patients who will not survive long enough to develop late complications (stent obstruction) or who are at high risk for surgery are best managed by stent. Surgical bypass is best for patients likely to survive more than four months. The mean time to stent obstruction and is certainly best if they survive more than 12 months.

Laparoscopic biliary bypass combines the advantages of minimal invasiveness and durability of surgical bypass, may be performed with a high success rate at the time of staging, if indicated. Choelcystojejunostomy is easier to perform but is inadvisable in patients with diseased gall bladder, a low insertion of the cystic duct, tumor with in 1 cm of the cystic common duct junction, and tumor encroachment of the cystic duct or gall bladder. We routinely perform triple bypass (cholecystojejunsotomy, gastrojejunostomy and jejunojejunsotomy) in all locally advance malignancy with biliary and duodenal obstruction whose suspected life expentancy is >6 months duration. But in selected cases (in low lying cystic duct - 20-30%) we perform hepaticojejunostomy to prevent recurrent biliary obstruction. In properly selected patients, the results of both cholecystoenteric and hepaticoenteric by passes are similar.

Gastric outlet obstruction (GOO) is a well known complication of pancreatic malignancy. Surgeons may vary in their approach to this problem, often reflecting different philosophies of tumor of pancreatic malignancy. It is interesting to note that gastroenterologists report lower rates of duodenal obstruction in pancreatic cancer (5%) than are found in surgical series (15-50%). Sarr and Cameron,[51] reviewed more than 8000 surgically managed patients with unresectable pancreatic malignancy and found that 33% of them suffered late sequale of GOO.

When compared to lap choledochojejunostomy, gastrojejunostomy is relatively straight forward.

Our preference is to place the jejunum antecolic to proximate the stomach. Though posterior can be done we routinely do anterior gastrojejunostomy. Previously we were doing hand sewn GJ and now changed to stapled GJ which is time consuming.

STAGING LAPAROSCOPY FOR PANCREATIC MALIGNANCY

Pancreatic malignancy is one of the most common cause of cancer death in the Western world as well as in India, and its incidence appears to be increasing. At the time of diagnosis, 50% of patients have distant metastasis and only 15-20% have resectable lesions, while the rest have locally advanced disease. Only patients with resectable disease should undergo exploratory laparotomy for resection with 100% predictive value. Therefore, accurate preoperative staging is essential. The aim of clinical staging for this group of patients should be to determine the extent of disease, allowing the appropriate therapy to be administered.

Accurate preoperative staging is gaining importance with continued progress in the multiplisciplinary approach to the tumors. Laparoscopy has long held a unique and well documented role in the assessment of pancreatic cancers. Staging laparoscopy with biopsy and LUS identified otherwise undetectable, unresectable disease such as small ulcer metastases, peritoneal and omental implants and regional node involvement. It therefore avoids unnecessary laparotomy with its added disadvantages. A number of recently published studies appear to support the use of staging laparoscopy as a valuable tool. One of the studies of laparoscopic staging identifies unresectability in 22% to 48% of patients who have resectable disease by CT scan.[45]

Meyer-Burg, in 1972,[24] first reported the technique of supragastric pancreascopy, which entails the laparoscopic visualization and probe palpation of the gland through the lesser omentum beneath the left lobe of the liver. This maneuver proved to be possible in 60% of patients in a subsequent report of Meyer-Brug et al.[25] Coupled with a positive cytological yield of 70% following needle aspiration. The presence of a pancreatic tumors mass, which is typically hard and incompressible, with adherent omentum and irregular vascular surface markings facilitates diagnosis and if necessary confirmatory laparoscopically guided biopsy.

Ishida and colleagues in 1983 described the techniques of supragastric bursascopy,[18] in which an incision is made in the lesser sac, allowing the surface of the body and tail of the pancreas to be observed directly and biopsied if desired. Using this approach, Ishida et al[19] reported a laparoscopic diagnostic success rate of 32% for cancer of the head of the pancreas and 88% for cancers of the pancreatic body and tail with a positive laparoscopically guided tissue diagnoses in 74.1% and 84.6% of cases respectively.

Stauch et al[52] in 1973 described an another method of lesser sac exploration by laparoscopy, which was later followed by Cuscheiri et al.[6] In this method the gastrocolic omentum is punctured, the telescope is inserted and the lesser sac insufflated, allowing the body and tail of the pancreas to be inspected. This procedure may be technically difficult and have to be combined with cholecystocholangiography to determine the level of bile duct obstruction and determining cystic duct patency in selecting patients for laparoscopic biliary enteric bypass procedures.

Small (<1cm) peritoneal and omental metastasis and small superficial liver metastasis are said to be a biological characteristic of pancreatic cancer at the time of presentation, and cannot usually be detected by CT scanning until they have reached a diameter of 2cm. Warshaw et al[46] initially reported 93% accuracy in 1985, which improved to 98% in recurrent series. Intraabdominal spread is more common in tumors of the body and tail (44%) than in tumors of the pancreatic head. Percutaneous needle biopsy increases possibility of peritoneal washings from 19% to 75%.

Laparoscopic ultrasound is performed to evaluate small intraparenchymal hepatic lesions, vascular invasion into the PV, SMA or SMV and peripancreatic extension of the tumor. Presence of any one of the following precludes resection.

1. Histologically confirmed hepatic, serosal, peritoneal or omental metastasis

2. Tumor extension outside the pancreas (i.e.) mesocolic involvement

3. Celiac or portal node involvement confirmed by frozen section

4. High portal vein involvement by tumor or invasion, encasement of celiac axis, HA or SMA

Portal or SMV involvement is not a contraindication and these patients can be explored.

INTERNAL DRAINAGE OF PSEUDOCYSTS OF PANCREAS

The management of patients with chronic pancreatic pseudocysts >6cm in diameter includes percutaneous drainage, surgical decompression by external or internal drainage (into the stomach or jejunum) and pancreatic resection. The success or failure of each of these therapeutic options is sometimes difficult to interpret in the current literature, especially when it is not clear whether the pseudocysts are the result of acute in chronic pancreatitis and whether there is a communication between the pseudocysts and the Wirsung duct.

For pancreatic pseudocysts that are symptomatic or don't shrink with conservative therapy, interventional internal drainage is recommended. We recommend laparoscopic internal drainage in all mature pseudocyst of > 6cm in size of > 6 weeks duration. The principle of both open and endoscopic drainage have been adopted by laparoscopic surgeons for the management of pancreatic pseudocysts. Since the first report of laparoscopic Cystogastrostomy in 1994 by J. Petelin, different techniques have been described for laparoscopic pseudocyst drainage.

Laparoscopic Intraluminal Cystogastrostomy

First, laparoscopic intraluminal cystogastrostomy was described by Gagner[14] and Way et al.[48] In this technique, radially expanding 5mm trocars are inserted into the stomach, allowing the introduction of 5mm laparoscopic instruments. A cystogastrostomy is created using electrocautery. The holes in the stomach are closed with intracorporeal sutures. Trias et al[42] used the same intraluminal approach, but they inserted 12mm cannulas with balloon, allowing the introduction of the endo stapler device and creating

a wide cystogastrostomy. After removing the cannulas both gastric holes were closed with staples.

Anterior Cystogastrostomy

Second, laparoscopic anterior cystogastrostomy was initially described by Meltzer and Amaral,[23] later reported by Holeczy and Danis[17] and more recently recommended by smadja et al.[35] We prefer this same method for all of our patients with mature pseudocyst. We started doing this procedure by laparoscopic method in 1994. Still todate with lot of modifications in our technique, we continue to follow the same technique with excellent results in our patients. An anterior gastrotomy is performed to allow easy access to the posterior wall of the stomach. Once the cystogastric interface is located, the pseudocyst cavity is penetrated using electrocautery or harmonic scalpel. Both cystogastrostomy and anterior gastric wall closure are done by intracorporeal suturing in our centre though endoscopic linear stapler may also be used.

Posterior Cystogastrostomy

Third, laparoscopic posterior cystogastrostomy was described by Morino et al[26] and more recently by Park et al.[28,29] This technique uses the "lesser sac" approach; the anastomosis is performed between pseudocyst and posterior wall using an endoscopic linear stapler.

We believe that patients with ductal strictures in the body of the pancreas and a distal pancreatic pseudocysts are best treated by distal pancreatectomy. The laparoscopic approach using the internal drainage of pseudocysts, should be reserved for pseudocysts >6cm that are located in the head or body of the pancreas. Communication with the main pancreatic duct does not exclude laparoscopic internal drainage, except in patients with obvious multiple pancreatic duct strictures.

Though endoscopic drainage into the stomach is the least invasive, compared to others, (open and laparoscopic methods), a considerable number of complications have been reported. Bleeding upon puncture of the cyst, leakage of gastric juice or cystic contents into the abdominal cavity, and dislodging of catheter are the major complications, all of which can lead to pan peritonitis or the need for emergency surgery. Even when endoscopic drainage is successful, the small catheter (usually <5mm in dia) can result in insufficient drainage; the recurrence rate is 15-18%. Open surgery is of course the most invasive approach. Minimally invasive laparoscopic cystogastrostomy, being simple and reliable with few complications, is now gaining much attention.

DECOMPRESSION OF PANCREATIC DUCT

Lateral pancreaticojejunostomy (modified puestow procedure) is performed to decompress the pancreatic duct with chronic obstructive calculous pancreatitis. Through lesser sac approach pancreatic surface can be visualized and pancreatic duct is identified with a probe or ultrasound guidance. The duct can be opened longitudinally extending from neck to tail of the pancreas. Roux en Y lateral pancreatojejunsotomy decompresses the PD as in conventional surgery. Michal Gagner[13] and myself reported our results in 1997 of the feasibility of this approach. Our video of this procedure has been included in the SAGES video library in the year 2001.

LAPAROSCOPIC TREATMENT OF COMPLICATION OF ACUTE PANCREATITIS

In severe infective necrotizing pancreatitis, a surgical intervention for drainage and debridement may be required for early recovery of the patient. The infected space may extend from the peripancreatic space to the retrogastric lesser sac area, right and left retrocolic, retromesentric (small bowel) and perinephric right and left space. According to the type and location of infected necrotizing pancreatitis seen in the CT scan, three operative approaches have been designed; retrogastric retrocolic debridement, retroperitoneal debridement and transgastric pancreatic necrosectomy.

We prefer retrogastric and transgastric approach. The indication for laparoscopic trans gastric pancreatic necrosectomy include late onset of infected pancreatic necrosis, pancreatic abscess or infected pseudocyst. Through the posterior wall of the stomach, debridement is performed with drainage into the stomach.

Thorough laparoscopic debridement of the cavity and closed tube drainage not only minimises morbidity with less or no pain, but also reduces the incidence of infection. For infected pseudocyst before the cyst wall matures, external drainage can be performed by laparoscopic approach, and later if the cyst still persist can undergo laparoscopic cystogastrostomy. We have performed laparoscopic internal drainage (anterior cystogastrostomy) for recurrent pseudocyst which formed (5-6 months) following external drainage in three patients.

CONCLUSION

The present experience with laparoscopic pancreatitic surgeries is minimal. With increasing clinical experience and new instrumentation laparoscopy will make an impact on the surgical approach to pancreatic diseases. Although some retrospective studies have shown that laparoscopic pancreatic surgery provides faster post operative recovery and comparable morbidity rates in comparison to those of open surgery, there has been no randomized controlled study confirming the actual reduced invasiveness or the superiority of endoscopic surgery. In addition, the learning curve is slow with the limited number of patients. However, outcomes to date, including ours are encouraging, and we conclude that with advanced instrumentation and improved skills, laparoscopic pancreatic surgery is feasible and desires further training and education. One must assess his own ability to carry out these procedures and determine whether short term and long term results meet the accepted standards.

References

1. Barthet M, Sahel J, Bodiou-Bertei C, Bernard JP (1995) Endoscopic transpapillary drainage of pancreatic pseudocysts. Gastrointest Endosc 42:208-213

2. Beckingham IJ, Krige JE, Bornman PC, Terblanche J (1997) Endoscopic management of pancreatic pseudocysts. Br J Surg 84: 1638-1645

3. Bernheim BM (1911) Organoscopy : cystoscopy of the abdominal cavity. Ann Surg 53:764-767

4. Chapuis Y, Bigourdan JM, Massault PP, Pitre J, Palazzo L (1998) video laparoscopic resection of insulinomas: report of five cases. Chirurgie 123: 461-467

5. Cuschieri A (2000) Laparoscopic hand-assisted surgery for hepatic and pancreatic disease. Surg Endosc 14: 1991-996

6. Cuschieri A, Hall AW, Clark J (1978) Value of laparoscopy in the diagnosis and management of pancreatic cancer. Gut 19:672-677

7. Cuschieri A, Jacomowics JJ, Van Spreeuwel J (1996) Laparoscopic distal 70% pancreatectomy and splenectomy for chronic pancreatitis. Ann Surg 223: 280-285

8. Cuschieri SA, Jakimowicz JJ (1998) Laparoscopic pancreatic resections. Semin Laparosc Surg 5: 168-179

9. Fabre JM, Dulucq JL, Vacher C, Lemoine MC, Wintringer P, Nocca D, Burgel JS, Donsergue J (2002) Is laparoscopic left pancreatic resection justified ? Surg Endosc 16: 1358-1361

10. Fernandez-Cruz L, Saenz A, Astudillo E, Martinez I, Hoyos S, Pantoja JP, Navarro S (2002) Outcome of laparoscopic pancreatic surgery: endocrine and nonendocrine tumors. World J Surg 26: 1057-1065

11. Fernandez-Cruz L, Saenz A, Astudillo E, Pantoja JP, Uzeategui E, Navarro S (2002) Laparoscopic pancreatic surgery in patients with chronic pancreatitis. Surg Endosc 16: 996-1003

12. Fitzgiobbons TJ, Yellin AE, Maruyama MM, Donovan AJ (1982) Management of the transected pancreas following distal pancreatectomy, Surg Gynecol Obstet 154:225-231

13. Gager M, Pomp A (1997) Laparoscopic pancreatic resection: is it worthwhile? J Gastrointest Surg 1: 20-26

14. Gagner M (1994) Laparoscopic transgastric cystogastrostomy for pancreatic pseudocyst. Surg Endosc 8:235 (Abstract)

15. Gagner M, Gentileschi P (2001) Laparoscopic enucleation of insulinoma in the pancreas. Surg Laparosc Endosc 11: 279-283

16. Gagner M, Pomp A (1994) Laparoscopic pylorus-preserving pancreaticoduodenectomy. Surg Endosc 8:408-410

17. Holeezy P. Danis J (1998) Laparoscopic transgastric pancreatic pseudocystogastrostomy – first experience with extraluminal approach. Hepatogastroenterology 45:2215-2218

18. Ishida H, Dohzono T, Furukawa Y, Kobayashi M, Tsuneoka K, 1984 Laparoscopy and biopsy in the diagnosis of malignant intra-abdominal tumors. Endoscopy 16:140-142

19. Ishida H, Furukawa Y, Kuroda H, Kobayashi M, Tsuneoka K 1981 Laparoscopic observation and biopsy of the pancreas. Endoscopy 13:68-73

20. Jimenez RE, Warshaw AL, Rattner DW, Willett CG, McGrath D, Fernandez-del Castillo C, 2000 Impact of laparoscopic staging in the treatment of pancreatic cancer, Arch Surg Apr; 135(4):409-14;

21. Luque-de leon E, Tsiotos GG, Balsiger B, Barnwell J, Burgart LJ, Sarr MG, 1999 Staging laparoscopy for pancreatic cancer should be used to select the best means of palliation and not only to maximize the respectability rate. J Gastrointest Surg, Mar-Apr;3(2):111-7

22. Mahon D, Allen E, Rhodes M (2002) Laparoscopic distal pancreatectomy. Surg Endosc 16: 700-702

23. Meltzer RC, Amaral JF (1994) Laparoscopic pancreatic cystogastrostomy, Minim Invas Ther 3:289-294

24. Meyer-Burg J 1972 The inspection, palpation and biopsy of the pancreas, Endoscopy 4:99

25. Meyer-Burg, Ziegler U, Kirstaedter HJ, Palme G 1973 Peritoneoscopy in carcinoma of the pancreas. Report of 20 cases. Endoscopy 5:86-90

26. Morino M, Garrone C, Locatelli L, Cavuoti G, Miglietta C (1995) Laparoscopic management of benign pancreatic cystic lesions, Surg Endosc 9:625 (Abstract)

27. Pacher HL, Pennington R, Chassin J, Spencer FC (1979) Simplified distal pancreatectomy with the Auto Suture Stapler : preliminary clinical observations. Surgery 85:166-170

28. Park A, Schwartz R, Tandian V, Anvari M (1999) Laparoscopic pancreatic surgery. Am J Surg 177:158-163

29. Park AE, Heniford BT (2002) Therapeutic laparoscopy of the pancreas, Ann Surg 236: 149-158

30. Patterson EJ, Gagner M, Salky B, Inabnet WB, Brower S, Edye M, Gurland B, Reiner M, Pertsemlides D (2001) Laparoscopic pancreatic resection: single-institution experience of 19 patients, J Am Coll Surg 193: 281-287

31. Rattner DW, Fernandez del, Castillo C, Warshaw AL (1996) Pitfalls of distal pancreatectomy for relief of pain in chronic pancreatitis. Am J Surg 171:142-146

32. Sakarofas GH, Farnell MB, Parley DR, Rowland CM, Sarr MG (2000) Long-term results after surgery for chronic pancreatitis. Int J Pancreat 27: 131-142

33. Salky BA, Edye M (1996) Laparoscopic pancreatectomy. Surg Clin North Am 76: 539-545

34. Shimizu S, Morisaki T, Noshiro H, Mizumoto K, Yamaguchi K, Chijiiwa K, Tanaka M (2000) Laparoscopic cystogastrostomy for pancreatic pseudocyst: a case report, JSLS 4: 309-312

35. Smadja C, Badaway A, Vons C, Giraud V, Franco D (1999) Laparoscopic cystogastrostomy for pancreatic pseudocyst is safe and effective. J Laparoendosc Adv Surg Tech 9: 401-403

36. Soper NJ, Brunt LM, Dunnegan DL, Meininger TA (1994) Laparoscopic distal pancreatectomy in the poreine model. Surg Endosc 8: 57-61

37. Sussman LA, Christie R, Whittle DE (1996) Laparoscopic excision of distal pancreas including insulinoma. Aust NZ J Surg 66: 414-416

38. Tagaya N, Ishikawa K, Kubota K (2002) Spleen-preserving laparoscopic distal pancreatectomy with conservation

of the splenic artery and vein for a large insulinoma. Surg Endosc 16: 217-218

39. Tagaya N, Kasama K, Suzuki N, Taketsuka S, Horie K, Furihata M, Kubota K (2003) Laparoscopic resection of the pancreas and review of the literature. Surg Endosc 17: 201-206

40. Takamatsu S, Teramoto K, Inoue H, Goseki N, Takahashi S, Baba H, Iwai T, Arii S (2002) Laparoscopic enucleation of an insulinoma of the pancreas tail. Surg Endosc 16: 217

41. Taylor AM, Roberts SA, Manson JM, Experience with laparoscopic ultrasonography for defining tumor respectability in carcinoma of the pancreatic head and periampullary region. 2001, Br J Surg Aug;88(8):1077-83

42. Trias M, Targarona EM, Balague C, Cifuentes A, Taur P (1995). Intraluminal stapled laparoscopic cystogastrostomy for treatment of pancreatic pseudocyst. Br J Surg 82:403

43. Uyama I, Ogiwara H, Iida S, Takahara T, Furuta T, Kiuchi K (1996) Laparoscopic minilaparotomy pancreatico-duodenectomy with lymphadenectomy using an abdominal wall-lift method. Surg Laparosc Endosc 6: 405-410

44. Vezakis A, Davides D, Larvin M, McMahon MJ (1999) Laparoscopic surgery combined with preservation of the spleen for distal pancreatic tumors, Surg Endosc 13: 26-29

45. Von Bubnoff AC, Schneider AR, breer H, Arnold JC, Riemann JF 2001 Significance of staging laparoscopy in pancreatic carcinoma: a case report Z Gastroenterol; Jan;39(1Suppl) : 35-40

46. Warshaw AL (1988) Conservation of the spleen with distal pancreatectomy, Arch Surg 123: 550-533

47. Warshaw AL, Tepper JE, Shipley WU (1986) Laparoscopy in the staging and planning of therapy for pancreatic cancer. Am J Surg 151 : 76-80

48. Way LW, Legha P. Mon T (1994) Laparoscopic pancreatic cystogastrostomy : the first operation in the new field of intraluminal laparoscopic surgery. Surg Endosc 8: 235 (Abstract)

49. Yamakawa K, Wagai T et al 1963 Proc Jap Soc Ultrasonics 5:41

50. Yoshida T, Bandoh T, Ninomiya K, Matsumoto T, Baatar D, Kitano S (1998) Laparoscopic enucleation of a pancreatic insulinoma : report of a case. Surg Today 28: 1188-1191

51. Sarr MG, Cameron JL, Surgical palliation of unresectable carcinoma of the pancreas. World.J.Surg. 1984; 8: 906-918

52. Strauch M. Lux G, Ottenjann R 1973 Infragastric pancreascopy. Endoscopy 5:30-32

53. Palanivelu's Text Book of Surgical Laparoscopy (2002). Laparoscopic Management of Pancreatic Surgery. VI:349-352

54. C.Palanivelu. CIGES Atlas of Laparoscopic Surgery. Spleen and Pancreas. Section 7:188-212

54

Role of Laparoscopy in Acute Pancreatitis

INTRODUCTION

Most patients have a mild; self limiting disease which requires only supportive treatment. Around 5 to 30% of patients have a severe form of disease; which requires aggressive treatment in the form of intensive care support. Various prognostic scoring systems allow the clinician to detect early possible life threatening complications. All those who survive the early phase of disease are at risk of developing complications like pancreatic pseudocyst, pancreatic abscess, pancreatic necrosis etc. Based on morphological, pathophysiologic, clinical, radiological and bacteriologic observations different entities of acute pancreatitis have been distinguished and all of them require different treatment approaches. These were classified as Ulm classification and later proposed at the Atlanta International Symposium in 1992.[1-3] According to it, the 4 entities are:

1. Interstitial edematous pancreatitis
2. Necrotising pancreatitis - Sterile / Infected
3. Pancreatic abscess
4. Pancreatic pseudocyst

1. **Interstitial edematous pancreatitis:** This type is characterised histo-morphologically by periacinar interstitial oedema and accumulation of inflammatory cells with intra and extra pancreatic fatty tissue calcification.

   There is usually no indication for surgery; even if complications develop. But at the same time patients with acute gall stone pancreatitis need to undergo a laparoscopic cholecystectomy during the same hospitalization. Studies have shown that there is a role for prophylactic ERCP within 24hrs in such cases.

2. **Necrotising pancreatitis:** This is characterized by an interstitial edematous inflammation combined with necrosis of the pancreatic exocrine and endocrine parenchyma and also with fat necrosis which includes the peripancreatic tissue compartment.

3. **Pancreatic abscess:** In this type, there is a circumscribed collection of pus containing little or no pancreatic necrosis caused by acute pancreatitis. It tends to occur late in the course of the disease process.[4]

4. **Pseudocyst:** These are collections of pancreatic secretion closed by a wall of fibrous granulation tissue, which arises as a result of sterile necrotizing pancreatitis. They lack an epithelial lining.

   Development of complications should be suspected in patients of severe pancreatitis, when there is clinical deterioration after a week; documented bacteremia and failure to resolve even after 1 to 2 weeks.

CLINICAL FEATURES

1. Pyrexia
2. Tachycardia
3. Abdominal pain
4. Abdominal distention etc.

INVESTIGATIONS

1. Hematological

i.   Hemoglobin + Hematocrit - early increase reflects loss of protein rich fluid (Retroperitoneal burn effect).

ii. LFT - Derangements most often seen in biliary pancreatitis.

iii. Serum Amylase - Persistent hyperamylasemia is seen in case of complications.

iv. Serum Calcium - level falls and value less than 2mmol/dl signifies severe pancreatitis.

v.   Serum Lipase - Elevated; specificity of 90%.

vi. C-reactive Protein - sharp rise indicates pancreatic necrosis and early marker of severity.

vii. Granulocyte Elastase - Potential marker of severity and peaks on days 1- 2.

2. Radiological

i. Plain abdominal X-rays - In case of pancreatic and peri pancreatic necrosis - Gaseous mottling is seen; ground glass appearance is seen when large amounts of free fluid accumulate in the retroperitoneum

ii. Barium or gastrograffin study - Not always required; but features like forward displacement of stomach; widening of duodenal loop with swelling of its folds; oedematous papilla of vater are seen.

3. Ultrasonography

i.   Most frequently used for diagnosis

ii. In 15-20% of cases there is poor acoustic window due to bowel gas

iii. Echogenecity increases in case of pancreatic necrosis; bleeding and saponification of fat.

iv. Pseudocysts and abscesses are readily detected

v.   Gall stones or CBD stones can be found in case of biliary pancreatitis

4. CT Scan

i.   Routinely done where necrosis and complications like abscess and pseudocyst are suspected.

ii. Dynamic contrast enhanced CT is helpful in defining the presence and extent of necrosis and other complications.[5]

iii. Air bubbles in the retroperitoneum are diagnostic but unfortunately they are absent in many cases.

iv. In cases of pseudocyst they appear as rounded or oval fluid collection with a wall or capsule which is thin and barely perceptible or at times thick and showing evidence of contrast enhancement.

v.   In cases of pancreatic abscess - presence of a focal low attenuation collection with a relatively thick wall which often contains gas bubbles. But these findings are nonspecific. Final diagnosis depends on clinical correlation.

5. MRI

i. Not routinely used, It is primarily used when ultrasonography or CT are equivocal. And in patients who cannot receive I.V. contrast safely because of allergy or reduced renal function.

ii. Heavily T1 weighted spin-echo sequence may be advantageous as compared to other pulse sequence for pancreatic imaging.

6. Endoscopic Ultrasound (EUS)

i. No definitive indication; but may be helpful in cases of biliary pancreatitis to pick up microlithiasis of CBD.

ii. Role of EUS has been expanding as its ability to diagnose and drain pseudocysts has been documented.[6-7]

OPERATIVE MANAGEMENT

Indications to intervene in general are

i. When there is uncertainity of clinical diagnosis

ii. Treatment of secondary infection

iii. Correcting the associated biliary tract pathology

iv. Progressive worsening inspite of optimum supportive care (>3days)

All the entities can be treated by either the conventional surgical techniques or by laparoscopic surgical techniques. The latter has better outcome in terms of early recovery, pain control, post operative sepsis etc.

With regard to pancreatic abscess; it can be drained by either percutaneous drainage under CT or USG guidance or by external drainage using laparoscopic technique.

LAPAROSCOPIC DRAINAGE OF PANCREATIC ABSCESS

Technique

Pneumoperitoneum is created using open Hasson technique followed by placement of a sub umbilical 10mm camera port. Subsequently, a 10mm left midclavicular port is placed for laparoscopic ultrasound so as to localize the abscess. Once localized, the same trocar is introduced into the abscess cavity and all the pus is drained out using suction cannula. A thorough wash is given to the cavity and an ICD tube drain of 20 or 24 F is placed into the cavity through the same port.[8]

With regard to necrotizing pancreatitis surgical intervention should be carried out to prevent life threatening local as well as systemic complications.

INDICATIONS FOR SURGICAL MANAGEMENT OF NECROTIZING PANCREATITIS

1. Clinical Criteria

i.   Sepsis syndrome

ii. Shock syndrome

iii. Acute surgical abdomen

iv. No response to intensive care treatment (>3days), persisting complications like pulmonary insufficiency; renal failure, cardio circulatory failure etc.

2. Bacteriological and Morphological criteria

i.   Infected necrosis

ii. Extensive pancreatic necrosis (>50%)

iii. Extensive intrapancreatic and retroperitoneal necrosis

iv. Stenosis of CBD, duodenum, large bowel etc.

Timing of surgery has been controversial with intervention can be performed as early as within a week or as late as during the post acute phase in 2nd week. Necrosectomy is performed in conventional surgery by opening the abdominal cavity; followed by exposure of pancreas. Debridment or necrosectomy is carried out using either digit or careful use of instruments. It has become increasingly clear that it is not necessary to remove every piece of necrotic or devitalised tissue. Remaining necrotic or tissue which is going to be necrotic may be thoroughly rinsed out later by the lavage fluid.[8-10]

Laparoscopic Necrosectomy

Technique

Pneumoperitoneum is created by open Hasson surgical technique in order to prevent injury to colon; small bowel etc., which may be adherent to the anterior abdominal wall. A 10mm subumbilical port is used for camera and 2 working ports are placed under vision, one right midclavicular (5mm) and the other left midclavicular (10mm). An optional 5mm or 10mm subxiphoid port may be used for left lobe liver or stomach retraction cranially. The gastro colic omentum is divided and the lesser sac entered. All necrotic pancreatic tissue is gently separated using bowel holding forceps and placed into a endo bag placed inside the abdomen priorly in order to prevent subsequent port site infection during extraction. It is always better to remove as less necrotic tissue as possible in order to prevent potential hemorrhage from splenic vessel injury. Thorough wash is given and 2 drains kept in the lesser sac through the port sites. These drain tubes may be used for subsequent lavage in the post operative period. The endobag containing necrotic material is brought out through the left midclavicular port.

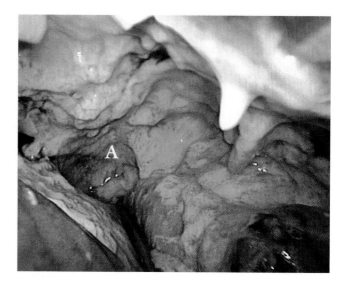

Figure 2 : Omental adhesions were separated and abscess cavity was opened

A - Pancreatic necrotic material

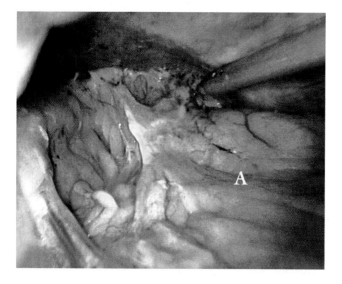

Figure 3 : separation of adherent stomach and omentum from the liver

A - Liver
B - Stomach

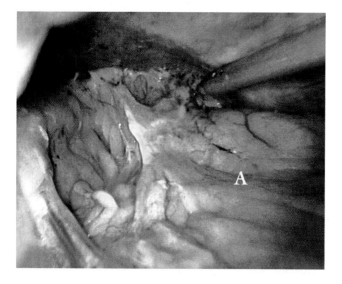

Figure 1 : Laparoscopy shows omental adhesion in the lesser sac area and midline

A - Stomach

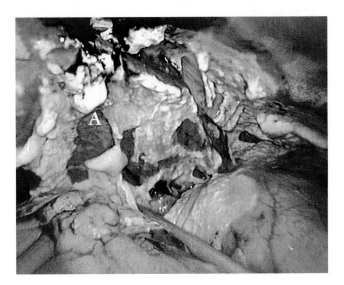

Figure 4 : Lesser sac was opened and all the necrotic tissue was sucked out

A - Inferior surface of left lobe of liver

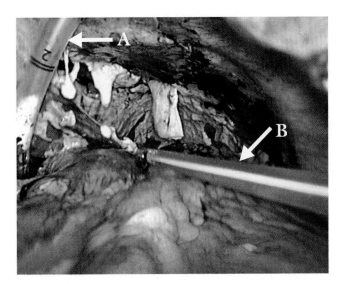

Figure 5 : After necrosectomy tube drains were kept

A - Drain in the lesser sac
B - Drain in the left subdiaphragmatic space

PANCREATIC PSEUDOCYST

This condition was first described by Morgagni. It accounts for over 75% of the cystic lesions of pancreas. It has been shown that some of the pseudocysts form as early as 2 to 3 weeks. Persistance of a pseudocyst implies an ongoing communication with the ductal system. Cysts larger than 5cm and presenting after 4 wks of acute pancreatitis are unlikely to resolve spontaneously and the incidence of complication also increases after this period. Hence, decompression is indicated in order to prevent complications. Diagnosis can be arrived at by either subjecting the patient to an abdominal ultrasonography or computed tomography. The prior is helpful and can be done repeatedly to assess the cysts during progression of pancreatitis at various stages. CT gives information regarding not only the fluid collection, but also the presence or absence of pancreatic necrosis. ERCP is performed selectively in patients with associated biochemical evidence of ampullary obstruction, all recurrent pseudocysts and pseudocysts that develop months after recovery from an acute episode of pancreatitis. MRI is helpful in selected cases to assess the ductal system; both biliary and pancreatic ductal disruption or dilatation. Prior to subjecting the patient to surgery all other differential diagnosis has to be excluded.

Various clinical conditions that simulate pseudocyst are

1. Pseudopseudocyst

2. Cystic neoplasms of pancreas - Cystadenomas - Mucinous; Serous

3. Cystadenocarcinoma
    i. Dermoid cyst
    ii. Cavitations of solid tumors - lymphoma, endocrine tumor, adenocarcinoma, leiomyosarcoma etc

4. True pancreatic cysts
    i. Unilocular cyst
    ii. Enterogenous cyst
    iii. Von Hippel Lindau disease
    iv. Retention cyst

5. Parasitic cyst - Echinococcal cyst; Taenia cyst

6. Extra pancreatic cyst - Duplication cyst, mesenteric cyst, splenic cyst, adrenal cyst

Guided fine needle aspiration of the cyst and fluid analysis is performed for differentiation of cystic lesions (cytology; CEA; CA - 175; viscosity).[11] An accurate differential diagnosis is mandatory in order to exclude possibility of over looking a treatable malignancy.

Pseudocyst presenting more than 4-6 weeks after the onset of pancreatitis with size more than 5cm with wall thickness of more than 5mm is treated by internal drainage into the stomach; duodenum or jejunum depending on the location of the cyst.

Internal drainage may be performed into some part of the gut; namely stomach, jejunum or duodenum depending on the location of the cyst. As majority of the cysts are situated retrogastric in lesser sac; cystogastrostomy is most commonly performed. This is easier to perform as compared to cystojejunostomy as it requires only a stoma; which is to be created between the posterior wall of stomach and the cyst where both are tethered together. Cystojejunostomy with Roux-en-Y loop of jejunum may be performed at any location of the cyst.[12-16]

Laparoscopic cystogastrostomy

Retrogastric pseudocyst is best treated by transgastric cystogastrostomy. The first laparoscopic cystogastrostomy was performed by J.Petelin; Kansas; USA

Patient position and team setup

Patient is placed in modified lithotomy position. The operating surgeon stands between the legs with camera surgeon on the right and 1st assistant on the left of the patient. The scrub nurse is to the right of operating surgeon.

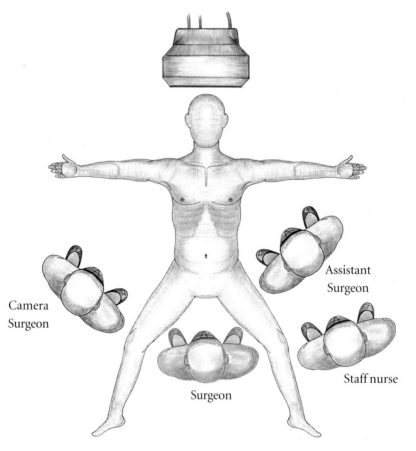

Figure 6 : Team setup

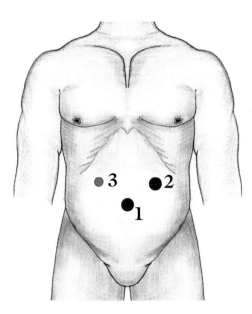

Figure 7 : Port position

No.	Instruments	Place
1	Camera	Umbilicus 10mm
2	Right hand working port	Left midclavicular 10mm
3	Left hand	Right midclavicular 5mm

Technique

Pneumoperitoneum is created by closed Veress needle technique. This technique should be avoided in severe acute necrotizing pancreatitis where open Hasson surgical technique is preferred as there may be adhesion between the colon; small bowel; omentum at the site due to previous inflammation. A subumbilical 10mm port is used for camera port; A 30 degree scope is preferred. Right (5mm) and left (10mm) midclavicular ports are used as working ports. Subxiphoid (5mm) port may be used for left lobe retraction in selected cases.

Anterior gastrotomy

Anterior gastrotomy is done longitudinally opening the anterior wall of the stomach over the most prominent part of the cyst. The opening of the stomach wall is performed by electrocautery with L shaped hook or harmonic scalpel or endolinear cutter. Self retracting sutures are placed to both edges of the stomach wall and the anterior wall of the greater and lesser curvature. This technique everts the divided edges of the stomach wall and allows adequate exposure of the posterior wall of the stomach even after decompression of the cyst. This is our preferred method of self retraction. Interior of the

stomach is adequately irrigated and washed prior to opening the cyst. Percutaneous aspiration of the cyst with a long Veress needle or a lumbar puncture needle introduced through the anterior wall of the abdomen and posterior wall of stomach is a must to know the exact nature of the fluid.[17] Sometimes pseudoaneurysm may masquerade as pseudocyst.

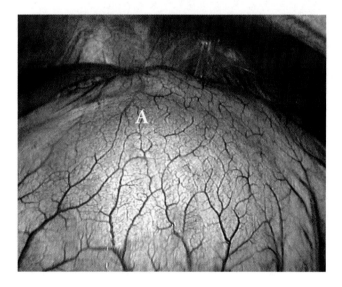

Figure 8 : Stomach is lifted up by the large pancreatic pseudocyst

A - Stomach

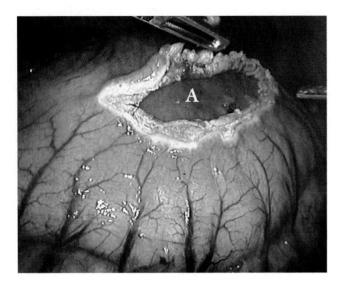

Figure 9 : Anterior gastrotomy using harmonic scalpel

A - Posterior wall of stomach

Premature opening may lead to profuse bleeding which is difficult to control. Intraoperative ultrasonography and Doppler study is helpful to assess the extension of the cyst and its proximity to vessels.

Cystogastrostomy stoma formation

A stay silk stitch is placed on the summit of the cyst. By holding the stay silk, a circumferential incision is made with electrocautery or harmonic scalpel. Circumferential full thickness of stomach wall is excised along with cyst wall.[18] Fluid is aspirated completely. Hemostatic stitches either continuous or interrupted are placed to approximate the stomach and cyst wall. This also prevents spread of infection into the lesser sac. Some surgeons prefer endolinear cutter to make adequate stoma. This technique is good for beginners; but we prefer excision and suture approximation for adequate stoma formation and there by making the procedure cost effective. Intracorporeal suturing is technically difficult to perform; endostapling makes the procedure simple. Creation of adequate internal conduit is pre-requisite for minimizing recurrence of pseudocysts which has been observed in open surgery in the past.[18-19]

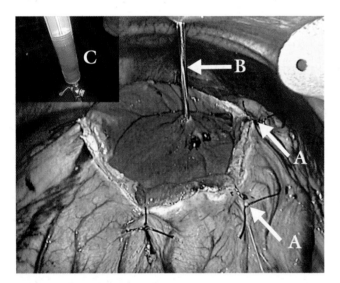

Figure 10 : Everting stitches are taken to expose the posterior wall and cyst contents aspirated to check the content

A - Everting stitch
B - Aspiration of cyst content by veress needle
C - Aspiration by syringe to confirm the cyst contents

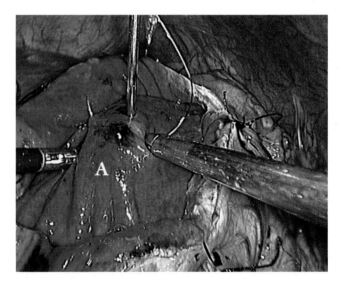

Figure 11 : Taking stay stitch in the summit of the cyst (including the cyst wall)

A - Posterior wall of the stomach

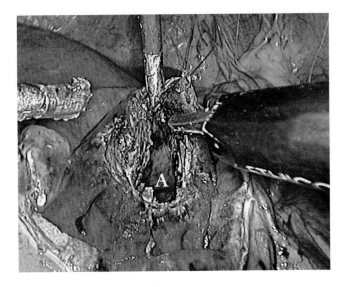

Figure 12 : Circumferential excision of the posterior stomach wall and cyst wall

A - Cyst cavity

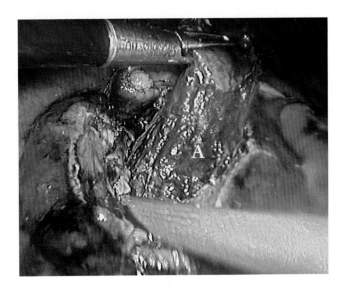

Figure 13 : Debridement of necrotic pancreatic tissues

A - Necrotic tissue

Debridement

Many pseudocysts contain necrotic pancreatic tissue within the cyst. This needs debridement which can be performed with a fenestrated bowel holding forceps. 30 degree scope is introduced into the cyst to facilitate the debridement completely. The cyst cavity is thoroughly rinsed with saline and sucked out. The nasogastric tube placed within the gastric lumen facilitates drainage of the fluid from the stomach. Unilocular matured cyst will collapse adequately as the pressure in the cyst is lower than the intragastric pressure. Adequate stoma between the cyst and the stomach is considered vital to prevent further fluid accumulation. Intracavitary tube should be avoided.

Closure of gastrostomy

After the operative field is checked for hemostasis the anterior stomach wall is closed by either continuous intracorporeal suturing or stapling technique. The peritoneal cavity is thoroughly irrigated and trocars are removed. Larger ports are closed using port closure devices.

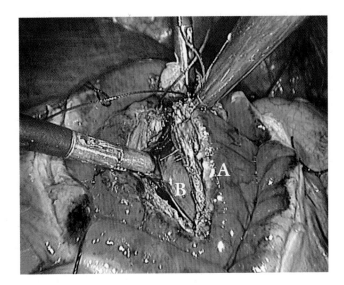

Figure 14 : Suturing of the cyst wall and posterior wall of stomach using continuous 2 0 vicryl stitches

A - Posterior wall of stomach
B - Cyst wall

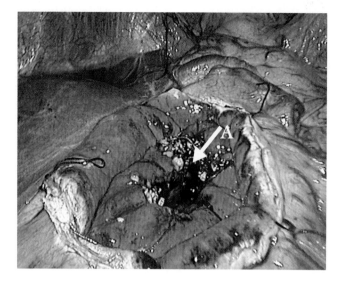

Figure 15 : Completion of suturing

A - Stoma between the stomach and the cyst

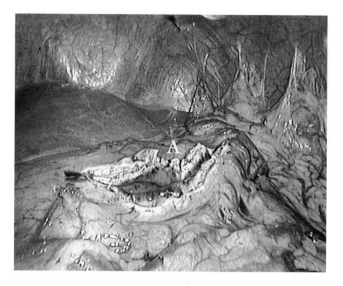

Figure 16 : Everting stitches are removed

A - Anterior wall of the stomach

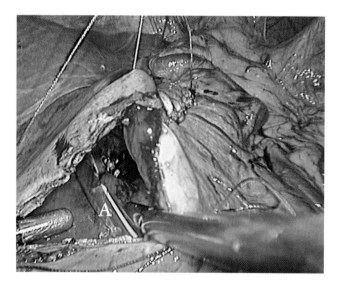

Figure 17 : Closure of the anterior gastrotomy using 2 0 vicryl continuous stitches

A - Placement of Ryle's tube

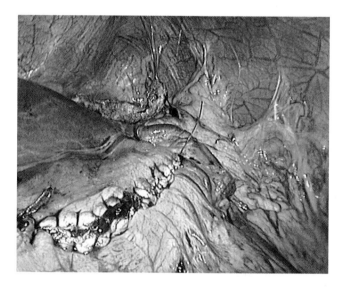

Figure 18 : Completion of gastrotomy closure

Laparoscopic Cystoduodenostomy

Patient is positioned in supine with left lateral tilt and operating surgeon stands on the left side. A 30 or 45 degree angled scope visualises the duodenum and head of pancreas well. Transverse colon is mobilized and retracted down by fan shaped retractor. Lateral wall of the duodenum is opened whenever the pseudocyst abuts the lateral wall of the duodenum. An incision is made on the medial wall avoiding the ampulla using electrocautery or harmonic scalpel. Cystoduodenostomy is performed through any intervening pancreatic tissue into the pseudocyst. Hemostatic interrupted stitches are made by vicryl. It is a rarely performed procedure today.

Laparoscopic Cystojejunostomy with Roux-en-Y loop

Infra and Supracolic approach

If the pseudocyst presents as a bulge at the base of the transverse colon; infracolic approach as described by Prof.Cuschieri may be performed. The cyst is opened longitudinally, fluid is aspirated and necrotic tissues are removed. Roux-en-Y limb of jejunum is anastomosed side to side and cystojejunostomy is performed with interrupted stitches. Laparoscopic suturing skill is very important for effective anastomosis. It may also be performed by a supra colic approach if the cyst does not bulge in the mesocolon or the mesocolon is very short to get adequate space for side to side anastomosis. Some surgeons prefer cystojejunostomy in place of cystogastrostomy as a routine. Large stoma formation is the main consideration in choosing the treatment. In our experience, we feel adequate stoma created by cystogastrostomy may be preferred as the first choice for retrogastric cyst location, unless the cyst projects more caudally and dependent drainage could not be effected by cystogastrostomy. Presence of mild infection in the cyst is not considered as contraindication for internal drainage. In the presence of signs of gross clinical infection such as inflammation and edema of the cyst wall; external drainage is considered since suture line dehiscence emerges as a significant risk in such a situation.

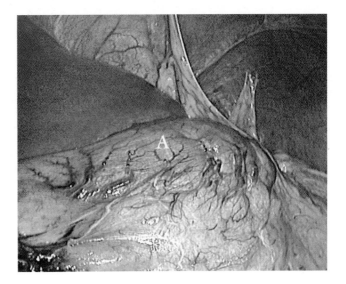

Figure 19 : Pancreatic pseudocyst buldges between the stomach and transverse colon

A - Stomach

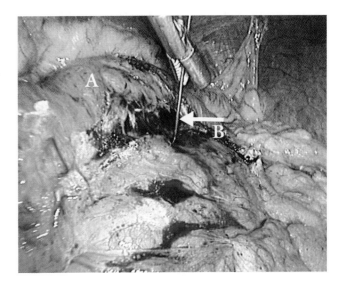

Figure 20 : Gastrocolic omentum is opened and the cyst contents are aspirated

A - Posterior wall of stomach
B - Aspiration of the cyst

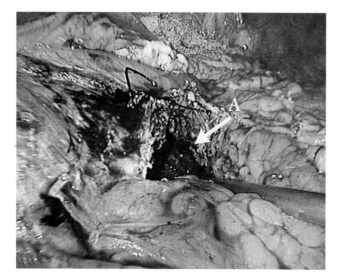

Figure 21 : Cyst is opened and the contents are suckedout

A - Cyst cavity

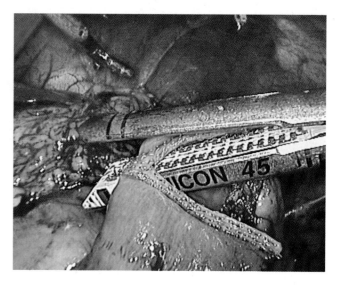

Figure 22 : Jejunum is divided using Endo GIA stapler for the Roux en Y loop formation

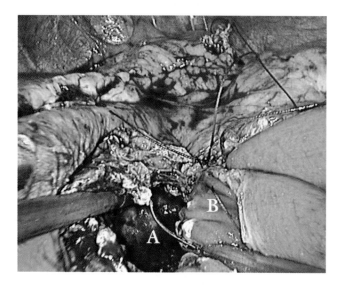

Figure 23 : Enterotomy is made in the long limb of Y loop and is being anastomosed to the cyst using vicryl stitches

A - Cyst
B - Jejunum

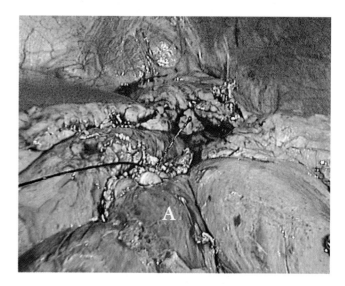

Figure 24 : Completion of cystojejunostomy

A - Long limb of jejunum

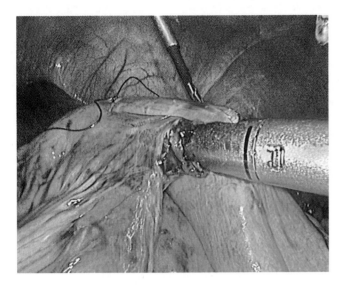

Figure 25 : Side to side jejunal anastomosis is done using Endo GIA stapler

Laparoscopic modified left paracolic approach[27-29]

Unusually some cyst presents in the left paracolic gutter as low down as to the left iliac fossa; shifting the descending colon medially. Approaching the lower limit of the cyst medial to the descending and sigmoid colon as described for infracolic approach is difficult to perform with risk of injury to the ureter; blood vessels and small bowel. Approaching the cyst as low down as possible; lateral to the colon is easier which can be done by mobilizing the sigmoid colon medially. No vital structures such as ureter or blood vessels are placed anterior to the cyst. We consider this approach allows most dependant anastomosis without increasing morbidity and mortality.

Decompression and Debirdment

The cyst is opened vertically starting from the lower limit. The fluid is sucked out and debridement performed. The preperitoneal fat need not be removed. It is difficult to remove the entire fat in the cavity of the cyst.

Roux-en-Y jejunal loop formation

Adequate length of jejunal loop is identified and held using a Babcock clamp. Umbilical port is extended by 2-3cms just sufficient to get the jejunal loop exteriorized. Roux-en-Y loop in fashioned; longitudinal opening in the Y limb is made for anastomosis. Jejunal loop is placed into the peritoneal cavity. Abdominal wound is closed. The trocar is reintroduced at the same site.

Side to Side Cystojejunostomy

The Y limb is placed side to side keeping the closed end on the cranial side. Side to side single layer suturing is performed by using either vicryl or silk. Till the anastomosis heals; it is ideal to keep the cyst decompressed by a tube passed percutaneously to keep as closed drainage system. The tube is removed on 4th or 5th post operative day and dressed with compression dressing or suturing of the skin to prevent leak from the cavity. Endo GIA stapler 30 or 45 mm cartridges may also be used for Roux-en-Y cystojejunostomy.

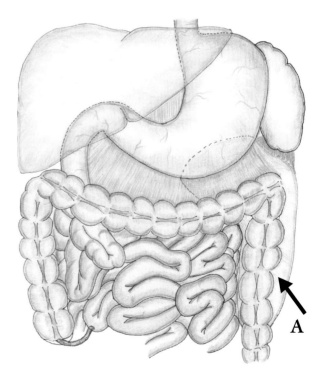

Figure 26 : Diagram shows left paracolic extension of the cyst

A - Left paracolic extension of cyst

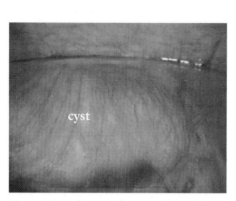

Figure 27 : Left paracolic extension of the cyst

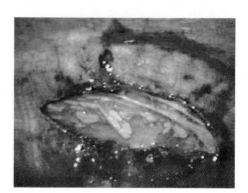

Figure 28 : Cyst was opened

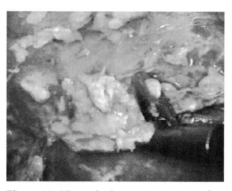

Figure 29 : Necrotic tissues were removed

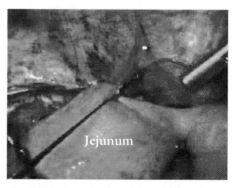

Figure 30 : Long limb of jejunal loop was anastomosed to the cyst wall

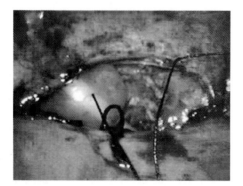

Figure 31 : Completion of posterior layer suturing and drain (Foley's catheter) is kept in the cyst

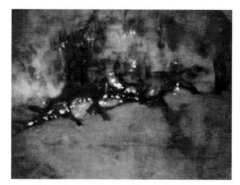

Figure 32 : Completion of cystojejuno-stomy

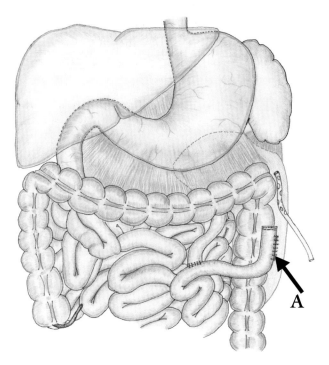

Figure 33 : Diagram shows Cystojejunostomy for left paracolic extension of the pancreatic pseudocyst

A - Jejunum is anastomosed to the cyst

Percutaneous Transgastric Drainage

Numerous anecdotal reports have appeared claiming advantages of guided percutaneous drainage for pancreatic pseudocysts. Many of these reports have no long term follow-up and often include a heterogenous group of patients with self-limiting acute pancreatic fluid collections, acute pseudocysts, chronic pseudocysts and even infected pseudocysts or pancreatic abscess. Significant number of patients treated by percutaneous drainage were smaller than 5cm in size.

Criado and associates reported 79% long term failure rate for continuous transcutaneous drainage in 42 patients with pseudocyst followed for an average period of 10 months. Complications such as hemorrhage, persistent pancreatic fistula and secondary infection occurred in 16%. Adaptation of percutaneous drainage as the standard method of cure for pseudocyst pancreas is debatable at this stage.[31]

COMPLICATED PSEUDOCYST

1. **Infection:** (a) Infected pseudocyst with inflammed oedematous wall. Percutaneous drainage often represents the preferred initial approach. If imaging investigations reveal presence of necrotic tissue, laparoscopic debridement followed by external closed drainage is preferred.

2. **Associated with gastric outlet obstruction:** Vomiting usually resolves once the cyst is decompressed. Laparoscopic transgastric cystogastrostomy and debridement resolves the cyst and relieves the obstruction. Rarely, DJ flexure is involved in the inflammatory mass with stricture due to extraneous fibrous tissue. In this situation gastrojejunostomy is indicated and may be performed by laparoscopic method.

3. **Pseudoaneurysm:** This is a true surgical emergency. In any patient with sudden catching pain in the epigastric region and increasing size of the cyst in a patient who had recent attack of pancreatitis; pseudoaneurysm should be suspected. If there is suspicion of this problem preoperative angiography for diagnosis and therapeutic emobilisation may be considered. 80% mortality occurs during surgery and it's due to hemorrhage. Urgent control of the involved artery by open surgery is mandatory if therapeutic embolisation fails.

POSTOPERATIVE COMPLICATIONS

1. Hemorrhage
2. Pancreatic fistula
3. Secondary infection
4. Recurrence - late complication

OUR RESULTS

Since 1994, 104 patients with pseudocysts have been treated successfully by laparoscopic transgastric cystogastrostomy. The results are excellent. The second patient in our series had recurrence after treatment of laparoscopic cystogastrostomy due to inadequate stoma size.[18] Reoperation was performed by conventional approach. In 86 of our patients out of the 104, debridement was performed. There was no evidence of infection or recurrence during the follow up of 10 years. One patient had bleeding from the edge of the stoma; readmitted and managed conservatively. Another patient had bleeding from the cavity in the immediate post operative period, but the bleeding stopped within 3 days. In over 20 patients, we assessed the obliteration of the pseudocystic cavity by regular endoscopy in the post operative period. Usually within 6-12 days, the entire cavity however big obliterates completely.

The first laparoscopic modified Roux-en-Y cystojejunostomy by left paracolic approach was performed in our institute in June 1996 and subsequently 3 more cases were done. All cases were treated by laparoscopic handsewn anastomosis. All patients recovered dramatically. One patient had infection in the cyst and had fever for a week due to previous external drainage. With the follow up period ranging from 4 months to 6½ years, there was no recurrence of pseudocyst.

DISCUSSION

Treatment of pancreatic pseudocyst has traditionally been surgical and it remains the principal method of treatment. However, during the last decade, with introduction and development of ultrasonography and computed tomography, new and innovative therapies like endoscopic internal fistula formation; percutaneous aspiration; percutaneous pancreatic cystogastrostomy by stenting have been developed competing with the traditional surgical treatment of chronic pancreatic pseudocyst. These new therapies have not attained popularity due to prolonged treatment period and higher incidence of recurrence.[20-22] Internal drainage of non-resolving pseudocyst can be effectively performed by laparoscopic cystogastrostomy so that an adequate surgical anastomosis can be carried out without laparotomy and need for external drainage.[20,23,24] The decreased morbidity and shorter duration of the therapy makes laparoscopic approach the preferred treatment at present.

The window between the stomach and cyst can be created in two ways.

i. By circumferential excision of the stomach and the cyst wall followed by suturing of the edges with absorbable interrupted intracorporeal knotting technique.[27,29]

ii. By Endo GIA staple cutting devices.[25]

Recently intraluminal stapled laparoscopic cystogastrostomy have been developed in which anterior gastrotomy can be avoided.[25,26] Though this procedure is less time consuming and easy to perform, it is too early to comment about recurrence. It is even difficult to apply in some, where the cyst wall is too thick.

Percutaneous transgastric drainage has been described under ultrasound and fluoroscopic guidance. It is best applied to pseudocysts complicated with secondary infection and in critically ill patients or those unfit for surgery.[20] Success rate is lesser than laparoscopic transgastric drainage with prolonged tube drainage (mean 31 days), drainage tract infection rate of 50% and overall failure rate of almost 47%.[21]

A potential advantage of operative drainage in post necrotic pseudocyst is its ability to clear the solid debris frequently present within the cavity. Adequate internal conduit is essential in the prevention of recurrence. In hand sewn group, a circumferential stomach and cyst wall are excised. Approximation is essential to prevent infection in the lesser sac and to avoid bleeding from the edge of the conduit. The cost of the procedure may be reduced considerably by using reusable trocars, instruments and intracorporeal hand sewn technique particularly in developing countries.

With regard to laparoscopic modified left paracolic approach in 4 patients since 1996;[27-29] who presented with pseudocyst in the left iliac fossa. This approach was for first time described by us and reported in 1996 at the 2nd World congress of HPB, Italy. All the cysts were opened vertically and decompressed. Roux-en-Y jejunal loop was anastomosed to the cyst by hand sewn technique, there were no recurrence. But we had one morbidity because of infection in the cyst. This cyst was previously subjected to external drainage. There are no case reports so far pertaining to this approach.

CONCLUSION

Laparoscopic technique offers new hope for treatment of complications of severe acute pancreatitis. It is recommended as a feasible, effective and less traumatic therapeutic means on condition that the strategy of individualization is followed.[8] A low mortality rate can be achieved in patients with necrotizing pancreatitis with early aggressive laparoscopic surgical technique. Persistence of pseudocyst for more than 4 to 6 weeks and the size is more than 5cms, all of them have been successfully treated by adequate internal drainage into the stomach, duodenum or jejunum depending on the location by laparoscopic method, with minimal morbidity and morality.[20,23,24] A randomized controlled trial that compares laparoscopic and endoscopic drainage techniques for retrogastric pseudocysts is required. Wide experience in laparoscopic surgery and skill of intracorporeal suturing is also essential for effective outcome. Laparoscopic cystogastrostomy also appears to be safe and effective approach for internal drainage and also facilitates debridement of necrotic pancreas.[26]

References

1. Beger HG, Krantzbugu, Bittner R, 1986 Bacterioal contamination of pancreatic necrosis. A prospective clinical study; gastroenterology 91;433

2. Bradly EL 1993 A clinically based classification system for acute pancreatitis. Archives of Surgery 128:586

3. Bittner : Block S, Buchler M 1987 pancreatic abscess and infected pancreatic necrosis different local septic complications in Acute pancreatitis; Digestive diseases and Sciences 32; 1082

4. William R Brugge, 2002 ; Pancreatic pseudocysts, diagnosis, imaging and treatment; VHJOE; Vol-1 Issue 2/1-2-154

5. Tzovaras G., Parks R.W.,et al; Early and long-term results after necrosectomy for necrotizing pancreatitis; 1999 British Journal of Surgery, Abstract p 417

6. Brugge, W.R., The role of EUS in the diagnosis of cystic lesions of the pancreas. Gastrointest Endosc, 2000. 52 (6 Suppl): p.S18-22

7. Soetikno, R.M. and K. Chang, Endoscopic ultrasound-guided diagnosis and therapy in pancreatic disease. Gastrointest Endosc Clin N Am, 1998.8(1):p.237-47

8. Zhou, Zong-Guang, et al; Laparoscopic management of severe acute pancreatitis. Pancreas.27(3):e46-e50, October 2003

9. Beger HG, Buchler M; Bittner R et al 1988; Necrosectomy and post operative local lavage in necrotizing pancreatitis; BJS 75; 207

10. Bradley El 1993; A 15 year experience with open drainage for infected pancreatic necrosis Surg; gynae and Obst 177;215

11. Hammel, P. Diagnostic value of cyst fluid analysis in cystic lesions of the pancreas: current data, limitations, and perspectives. J Radiol, 2000.81(5): p.487-90

12. Smadja C, Badawy A, Vons C, Giraud V, Franco D. Laparoscopic cystogastrostomy for pancreatic pseudocysts is safe and effective. J Laparoendosc Adv Surg Tech A 1999; 9:401-3

13. Mori T, Abe N, Sugiyama M, Atomi Y et al; Laparoscopic pancreatic cystgastrostomy. J Hepatobiliary Pancreat Surg 2000; 7:28-34

14. Ammori BJ, Bhattacharya D, Senapati PS. Laparoscopic endogastric pseudocyst gastrostomy: a report of three cases. Surg Laparosc Endosc Percutan Tech 2002; 12:437-40

15. Roth JS, Park AE. Laparoscopic pancreatic cystgastrostomy: the lesser sac technique. Surg Laparosc Endosc Percutan Tech 2001; 11:201-3

16. Hagopian EJ, Texeira JA et al : Pancreatic pseudocyst treated by laparoscopic Roux-en-Y cystojejunostomy. Report of a case and review of the literature. Surg Endosc 2000; 14:967

17. Brugge, W.R., EUS-guided pancreatic find needle aspiration : instrumentation, results, and complications. Techniques in Gastrointstinal Endoscopy, 2000.2:p.149-154

18. Michael Tarnoff, Fred Brody, et al; Comparison of laparoscopic and open management of pancreatic pseudocysts, 2001 Abstract, Clevelandclinic.org.misc /education

19. Cooperman, A.M., Surgical treatment of pancreatic pseudocysts. Surg Clin North Am, 2001.81(2):p.411-9,xii

20. Bhattacharya D, Ammori BJ, Minimally invasive approaches to the management of pancreatic pseudocysts: review of the literature, JOP. J Pancreas (Online) 2003

21. NG Bradley, Murrary Brendon et al : An audit of pancreatic pseudocyst management and the role of endoscopic pancreatography, ANZ Journal of Surgery, December 1998, vol68, No.12, pp.847-851(5)

22. Brugge, William R, Approaches to the drainage of pancreatic pseudocysts, Current opinion in gastroenterology 20(5):488-492, September 2004

23. Obermeyer, Robert J, et al, Laparoscopic Pancreatic Cystogastrostomy, Surgical Laparoscopy, Endoscopy & Percutaneous Techniques 13(4):250-253, August 2003

24. Steven Rosenblatt, et al, Laparoscopic Management of pancreatic pseudocysts; Cleveland clinicalg.misc/education/2001 abstract

25. Chowbey PK, Soni, Laparoscopic intragastric stapled cystogastrostomy for pancreatic pseudocyst. J Laparoendosc Adv Surg Tech A.2001;11:201-205

26. Ammori, B.J., Bhattacharya, Laparoscopic Endogastric Pseudocyst Gastrostomy : A report of three cases, Surgical Laparoscopy, Endoscopy and percutaneous techniques 12(6):437-440, December 2002

27. Palanivelu C, et al : Laparoscopic Cystogastrostomy for Chronic Pseudocyst of Pancreas - Totally Intracorporeal Hand Sutured , Second World Congress of International Hepato - Pancreato - Biliary Association, Bologna, Italy, 2-6, 1996-Abstract

28. Isla A, Griniatsos J, et al; Single-Stage definitive laparoscopic management in mild acute biliary pancreatitis; Journal of laparoendoscopic and advanced surgical techniques; April 2003, Vol.13, No.2, ;; 77-81

29. Palanivelu C et al; Pancreatic pseudocyst, Text Book of Surgical Laparoscopy, 2002, Edition 1:353-361

30. Giovannini M, Bernardini D et al : cystogastrotomy entirely performed under endosonography guidance for pancreatic pseudocyst: results in six patients, Gastrointest Endosc 1998 aug; 48:200-3

31. Adams DB, Srinivasan A, Failure of percutaneous catheter drainage of pancreatic pseudocyst, Am Surg 2000 Mar; 66:256-61

32. Fan ST, Lai EC, et al : Early treatment of acute biliary pancreatitis by endoscopic paillotomy, N Engl J Med 1993 Jan;328:228-32

33. Adams DB, Anderson MC, Percutaenous catheter drainage compared with internal drainage in the management of pancreatic pseudocyst; Ann Surg 1992 Jun;215:571-6

34. Mithofer K, Mueller PR, Interventional and surgical treatment of pancreatic abscess; World J Surg 1997 Feb; 21: 162-8

35. Bassi C, Falconi et al; The role of surgery in the major early complications of severe acute pancreatitis; Eur J Gastroenterol Hepatol 1997 Feb;9:131-6

55

Laparoscopic Pancreatico-jejunostomy

INTRODUCTION

Chronic pancreatitis is a condition characterized by irrecoverable distruction and fibrosis of exocrine parenchyma leading to pancreatic exocrine insufficiency and endocrine failure progressively. Zuidema reported a series of patient with pancreatic calculi in 1959.[1] From India Prof. M.G. Kini reported the first case of pancreatic calculi way back in 1937.[2] GeeVarghese documented one of the largest series in the world on tropical pancreatitis. Chronic obstructive calculous pancreatitis is at a higher incidence in South India.[3,4]

In tropical pancreatitis there are two types of chronic pancreatitis requiring active surgical treatment, one with dilated obstructive calculous pancreatitis and other is without dilatation of the pancreatic duct. In patients associated with dilatation of ducts, majority of them develop pain due to increased ductal pressure system with a stone obstructing the proximal duct. There may be multiple stones "chain of lake" appearance or a single stone. Decompression of the ductal system often relieves the pain. Some may continue to have pain due intraparenchymal calcification and perineural fibrosis.

In patients without dilatation of the pancreatic duct, pain is due to chronic inflammatory perineural fibrosis. It is often not related to food, unlike with dilated ducts where food induces pain.

INVESTIGATIONS

Investigations to assess morphological changes in the pancreas which forms the basis of surgical treatment.

X-ray abdomen - calcification at the level of L1-L2

Ultrasonography - ductal system, stones and parenchymal changes.[5]

CT scan - smaller stone, calcification, pancreatic duct - dilatation, vascular anomalies and parenchymal atrophy.[5,6]

ERCP - Structural changes in the secondary and tertiary branches as well as main pancreatic duct dilatation, stenosis obstruction, cyst formation and presence of calculi etc.[7-9]

MRI and MRCP - It can combine parenchymal imaging with pancreatography.[7,9-15]

EUS - ductal system and subtle change with in the parenchyma.[7, 15-19]

Ultrasonography / Computed Sonography Scan are the important investigations often performed before surgery in most of the centers and also ours.

INDICATIONS FOR OPERATION

1. Intractable pain - not relieved by narcotics
2. Biliary obstruction
3. Duodenal stenosis/colonic stricture
4. Pancreatic duct stenosis
5. Pseudocyst
6. Pancreatic ascitis
7. Portal venous compression (splenic/mesenteric venous thrombosis)
8. Pancreatic hemorrhage
9. Suspicion of pancreatic carcinoma

Surgical options

1. Denervation Procedures

   i. Splanchnicectomy + celiac ganglionectomy (percutaneous USG guided or EUS guided) [20,21]

   ii. Total denervation of pancreas

   iii. Denervated pancreatic flap

2. Drainage

   i. External cyst drainage

   ii. Internal cyst drainage (cystogastrostomy/ cystojejunostomy)

3. Prancreaticojejunsotomy

   i. Retrograde drainage with splenectomy

   ii. Lateral side to side

4. Resections

   i. Distal pancreatectomy

   ii. Pancreatoduodenectomy

     a. Whipple

     b. Pylorus preserving

   iii. Total pancreatectomy

   iv. Duodenum preserving resection

     a. Partial resection of head of pancreas[22]

     b. Total resection of pancreas

   v. Resection with autotransplantation

Therapy available

Pain associated with chronic pancreatitis without ductal obstruction may be treated by bilateral thoracic sympathetic ganglion denervation procedure or resections, which can be performed through laparoscopic approach. Pseudocyst requires internal drainage, either cystogastrostomy or cystojejuno stomy. In pancreatic ascitis if ERCP shows disruption of pancreatic duct, than pancreatico jejunostomy at the site of fistula is indicated.

Presence of malignancy is an indication for definitive resection by open method (i.e.) proximal, distal or total pancreatectomy. Laparoscopic decompression and lateral (modified Peustow Operation) pancreaticojejunostomy is the preferred procedure as in conventional open surgical approach. The surgeon must possess the experience and skill in intracorporeal knotting and suturing technique.[25] M. Gagner and myself (1997) were the first to perform laparoscopic pancreatico jejunostomy.[26]

LAPAROSCOPIC PANCREATICOJEJUNOSTOMY

Patient Position

Is placed in modified Trendelenburg semilithotomy position. A small sand bag is placed under the left side of the chest with 20 to 30 degree lateral tilt of the operating table which provides optimum position for adequate exposure.

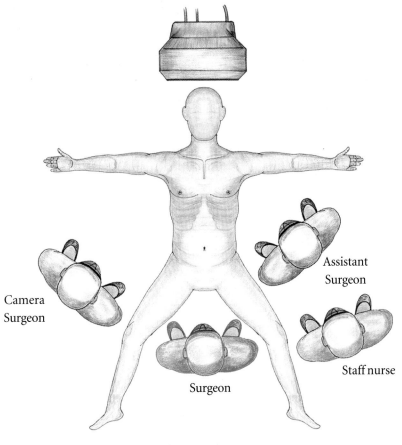

Figure 1 : Team setup

Camera
Surgeon

Assistant
Surgeon

Staff nurse

Surgeon

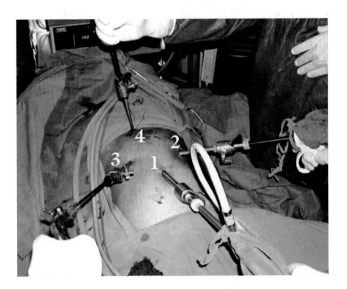

Figure 2 : Port position

No.	Instruments	Place
1	Camera	Umbilicus 10mm
2	Right hand working port	Left midclavicular 10mm
3	Left hand working port	Right midclavicular 5mm
4	Stomach retracting port	Subxiphoid 5mm

Ports

Normally 4 ports are used; umbilical (10mm) camera port; right Mid clavicular line (MCL) (5mm) and left MCL (10mm) surgeons working ports along with epigastric (5mm) for gastric retraction. Pneumoperitoneum is established with closed Veress needle technique or open Hasson method. Intraperitoneal pressure of 12mm of Hg is established.

Technique

1.Exposure of pancreas

The lesser sac is entered through gastrocolic omentum. Gastrocolic omentum is opened widely and the entire anterior surface of the pancreas is exposed from head to tail end. Adhesions of the posterior wall of stomach to the surface of the pancreas are released.

2. Identification and exploration of the pancreatic duct

Pancreatic duct can be identified by palpation with blunt probes and confirmed by percutaneous aspiration using a thin lumbar puncture needle. Laparoscopic ultrasound aids in identification of the main pancreatic duct. Electrocautery hook dissector or harmonic scalpel is used to open the pancreatic duct longitudinally and widely. The impacted stones in the proximal duct can be removed with right angled dissector. 2 to 3 stay stitches are applied to the cut edges of the duct for easy approximation of jejunum.

3. Roux-en-Y loop formation

Proximal jejunum is identified by the ligament of Treitz and inferior mesenteric vein. The site of Roux-en-Y formation is selected depending upon the vascular arcade and is held using a Babcock or a clip can be applied on the mesenteric border for identification. In case of laparoscopic assisted procedure a minilaparotomy is performed by extending the umbilical port by 2-3cm. The jejunal loop can be easily brought out and Roux en Y loop performed by anastomosing the short limb to the side of the long limb and distal end is closed. Now according to the length of the pancreatic duct; jejunum is opened longitudinally at its antimesenteric border. Minilaparotomy wound is closed and the umbilical

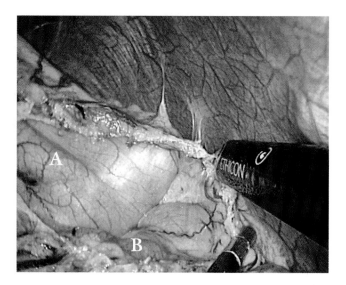

Figure 3 : Gastrocolic omentum is opened to expose the pancreas

A - Posterior wall of stomach

B - Pancreas

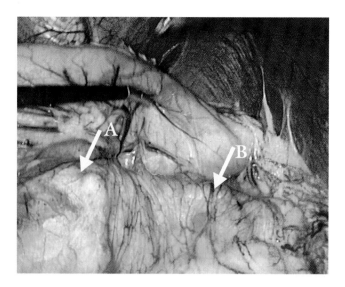

Figure 4 : Gastrocolic ligament is divided and whole pancreas is exposed. Dilated pancreatic duct is seen

A - Dilated pancreatic duct in head of pancreas

B - Dilated duct in body of pancreas

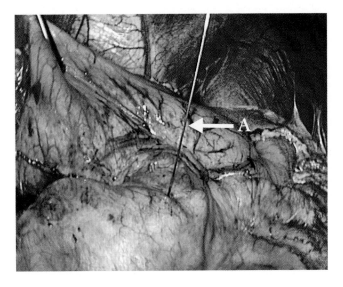

Figure 5 : Confirmation of pancreatic duct by needle aspiration

A - Lumbar puncture needle

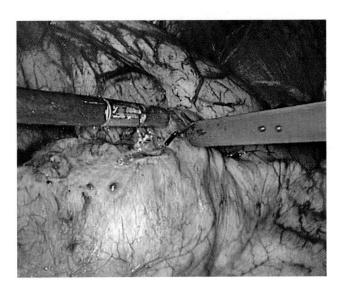

Figure 6 : After confirmation pancreatic duct is opened by electrocautery hook

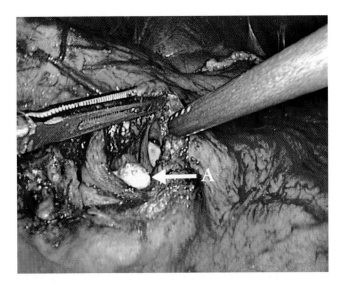

Figure 7 : Pancreatic duct is opened and impacted calculous seen in the head of pancreas

A - Stones with in the main duct

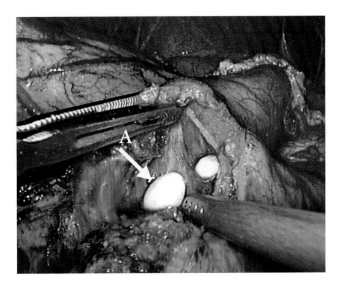

Figure 8 : Multiple Stones seen in the main pancreatic duct

A - Stone in the main duct

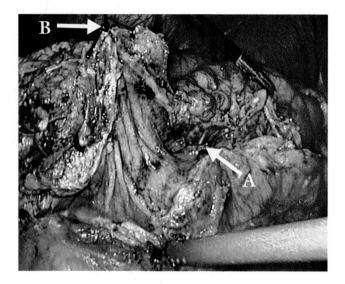

Figure 9 : Pancreatic duct opened completely from head to the tail end of pancreas

A - Pancreatic duct
B - Stay stitch

surface of the pancreas. A continuous mucosa to mucosa all coat stitching is performed using vicryl starting from left end and continued to the right. The anterior anastomosis is performed with interrupted stitches on either end first; then finally the central. Outer interrupted stitches are made for perfection of the anastomosis. Complete anastomosis is performed totally by intracorporeal knot tying technique. Anterior anastomosis also may be performed by continuous suturing.

In case of associated Gastric outlet obstruction due to stricture in the duodenum, may also be treated with loop gastrojejunostomy. Long segment CBD stenosis may also occur in small percentage of cases. In absence of duodenal obstruction choledocho duodenostomy side to side anastomosis may be done. If associated with duodenal obstruction, Roux-en-y choledochojejunostomy and gastrojejunostomy may be performed.

port can be refashioned for further continuation. Where as in case of total laparoscopic procedure this can be easily performed using Endo GIA stapler. 25-30cm distal to the DJF jejunal loop is selected for Roux loop formation.

The bowel is divided using white cartridge. The distal limb is taken to the lesser sac through a window in the meso colon. The proximal jejunum is anastomosed to the side of the long limb 40cms distal, side to side fashion using endo GIA 45 blue cartridge. The enterotomy is sutured with a layer of vicryl sutures.

4. Pancraticojejunostomy anastomosis

Long limb of the Roux en Y loop is taken to the supracolic compartment through a window in the mesocolon. The already made enterotomy is placed side to side of the laid open pancreatic duct. The enterotomy may be extended according to the length of pancreatic duct. Few interrupted stitches put between the seromuscular layer of jejunum and

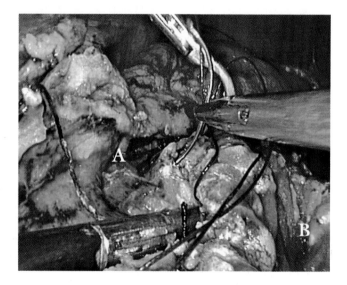

Figure 10 : Pancreatic duct is anastomosed to the long limb of jejunum

A - Pancreatic duct
B - Jejunum

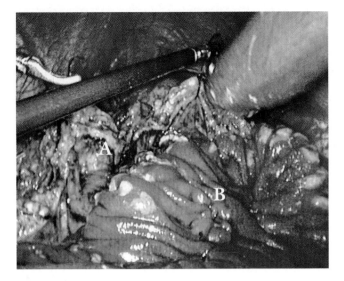

Figure 11 : Completion of posterior layer of anastomosis of
pancreas and jejunum

A - Pancreatic duct
B - Jejunum

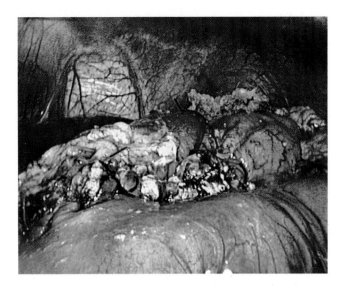

Figure 12 : Completion of side to side pancreaticojejunostomy

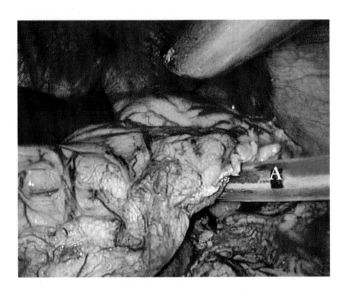

Figure 13 : Stomach is replaced after keeping the tube drain

A - Drainage tube

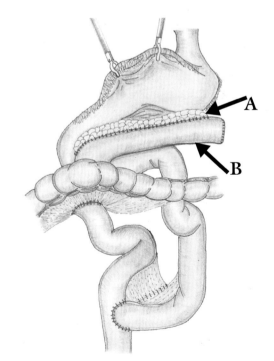

Figure 14 : Diagramatic representation of Roux en Y
pancreaticojejunostomy

A - Pancreas
B - Jejunum

RESULTS

So far we have performed around 12 cases since 1997; most were female patients hailing from Kerala where the incidence of chronic obstructive calculous pancreatitis is highest. Patients were in the age group of 6-50 years. Main pancreatic duct dilatation varied from 10 to 22mm. In all patients laparoscopic lateral pancraticojejunostomy was performed using the above mentioned technique; No conversions in our series, post operative pain was minimal with regard to analgesic requirements. There was no marked ileus in the post operative period and all patients tolerated oral fluids on 1st or 2nd day. Most of them were started on semisolid diet on third day. There were no anastomotic leak or any other morbidities. Hospital stay ranged from 5 to 7 days. Patient have been in followup from periods ranging shortest 6 months to 7 years. Relief from the previous pain is satisfactory in all of these cases.

DISCUSSION

Improved clinical experience and introduction of new technology has extended the indications of laparoscopic surgery. Gastrointestinal anastomosis such as gastro jejunostomy; cholecystojejunostomy, Transgastric cystogastrostomy etc can be performed entirely by laparoscopic method either using Endo GIA stapler or intracorporeal knot tying technique.[25] Chronic obstructive calculous pancreatitis and its complications is found quite commonly in the state of Kerala. Where incidence has been as high as 125 / 100000 population. But frequency may be probably much lower in other parts of India.[3-5]

Many of these patients present with dilated ducts and intraductal calculi not responding to other modalities of treatment. Lateral pancreticojejunostomy is the procedure of choice in conventional approach. Various studies have shown favourable intermediate and long term outcomes after performing LPJ alone or combining local Resection of the head of pancreas with LPJ for chronic pancreatitis.[22-25]

In our patients we have successfully performed the same procedure laparoscopically with equally good or even better results. But experience of intracorporeal knot tying is essential to perform such an anastomosis.[25-27]

In conventional surgery lateral pancreaticojejunostomy may be performed successfully in patients with pancreatic ducts of more than 7mm dilatation. Where as in our series smallest duct size was 10mm. Still a large number of cases should be performed to assess the routine use of laparoscopy for decompression of minimally dilated pancreatic duct.

CONCLUSION

Laparoscopic lateral pancreatico jejunostomy for chronic obstructive calculous pancreatitis is technically demanding; But possible and should be done selectively by surgeons who are expertised in intracorporeal suturing and knotting techniques. Early studies show a favourable outcome for this procedure in terms of recovery; shorter hospital stay; pain relief, significant increase in weight gain post operatively etc. Decompression of pancreatic duct can be combined with GJ or biliary bypass by forming Roux-en-Y loop for patients with associated duodenal and biliary obstruction.

References

1. Zuidema PJ. Cirrhosis and disseminated calcification of the pancreas in patients with malnutrition. Trop Geogr Med 1959;11:70-74

2. Kini MG, Multiple pancreatic calculi with chronic pancreatitis. Br J Surg 1937;25:705

3. Geevarghese PJ. Pancreatic diabetes. Bombay : Popular Prakashan, 1968:110-115

4. Geevarghese PJ. Calcific pancreatitis. Bombay : Varghese Publishing House, 1985

5. Barman K.K., Premalatha G, Mohan V; Tropical chronic pancreatitis; Postgrad.Med.J.2003;79;606-615

6. Joseph S. Imaging of pancreas in tropical pancreatitis : role of computerized tomographic scanning. In : Kumar N, Acharya SK, eds. Tropical calcific pancreatitis. Kerala : Roussel Scientific Institute, 1994:69-76

7. Robert H. Hawes, A clinician's Perspective on Chronic Pancreatitis-2002; Reviews Gastroenterological Disorders Vol2.No.2, 2002:57-65

8. Sarner M et al : Classification of pancreatitis; gut 1984;25:756-59

9. Czako L et al : Evaluation of pancreatic exocrine function by secretion enhanced MRCP. Pancreas 2001;23:323-328

10. Parada KS, Peng R, Erickson RA, et al : A resource utilization projection study of EUS. Gastrointest Endosc 2002, 55:328-334

11. Chowdhury RS, Bhutani MS, Mishra G, et al. : Comparative analysis of pancreatic function testing versus morphologic assessment (by EUS) for the evaluation of chronic unexplained abdominal pain. Gastroenterology 2001, 120:A-647

12. Hollerbach S, Klamann A, Topalidis T, et al : Endoscopic ultrasonography (EUS) and fine-needle aspiration (FNA) cytology for diagnosis of chronic pancreatitis. Endoscopy 2001, 33:824-831

13. Wiersema MJ, Hawes RH, Lehman GA, et al : Prospective evaluation of endoscopic ultrasonography and endoscopic retrograde cholangiopancreatography in patients with chronic abdominal pain of suspected pancreatic origin. Endoscopy 1992, 25:555-564

14. Wallace MB, Hawes RH, Durkalski V, et al.: The reliability of EUS for the diagnosis of chronic pancreatitis : interobserver agreement among experienced endosonographers, Gastrointest Endosc 2001, 53:294-299

15. Nattermann et al. Endosonography in chr panc : a comparison between ERCP & EUS; Endoscopy 1993;25:565-570

16. Lees WR et al : EUS of chronic pancreatitis and pancreatic pseudocysts. Scand J Gastroenterol 1986; 123 (Suppl) : 123-129

17. Wiersema MJ et al. Prospective evaluation of EUS & ERCP in patients with chronic abdominal pain of suspected pancreatic origin Endoscopy 1993;25:555-564

18. Zimmerman MJ et al : Comparison of EUS findings with HPE in chronic pancreatitis : Gastrointest Endosc 1997; 45:AB185

19. Zuccaro G et al : The role of EUS in the diagnosis of early and advanced chronic pancreatitis : Gastroenterology 2000; 188:A674

20. Gress F, Schmitt C, Sherman S, et al. : Endoscopic ultrasound-guided celiac plexus block for managing abdominal pain associated with chronic pancreatitis : a prospective single center experience. Am J Gastroenterol 2001, 96:409-416

21. Crus F et al. EUS guided celiac plexus block for managing abdominal pain associated with chronic pancreatitis : a prospective single center experience. Am J Gastroenterol 2001;96:409-416

22. Frey CF, Amikura K, focal resection of the head of pancreas combined with longitudinal pancreaticojejunostomy in management of patients with chronic pancreatitis, Ann Surg 1994 Oct;220(4);492-504

23. Schnelldorfar et al; Outcome after lateral pancreaticojejunostomy in patients with chronic pancreatitis associated with pancreatic divisum, Am Surg 2003 Dec;69(12):1041-4

24. Kalady MF et al ; Immediate and long term outcomes after lateral pancreaticojejunostomy for chronic pancreatitis, Am Surg 2001 May 67(5);478-83

25. Tantia O, et al; Lap. pancreaticojejunostomy : 17 cases; Surg Endosc 2004 July; 18(7) : 1054-7

26. Palanivelu .C, et al; Laparoscopic Pancreatico Jejunostomy for Chronic Pancreatitis, Text Book of Surgical Laparoscopy, 2002, Edition 1:363-366

27. Palanivelu C, et al; Laparoscopic Pancreato Jejunostomy for chronic obstructive calculous pancreatitis, Sixth World Congress of Endoscopic Surgery, Rome May 31-June 6,1998-Abstract

28. Rios GA et al : outcome of lateral PJ the management of chronic pancreatitis with nondilated ducts. J Gastro test Surg 1998;2:223-229

29. Augustine P. Discussion on epidemiology and clinical features of tropical calcific pancreatitis. In : Kumar N, Acharya SK, eds. Tropical calcific pancreatitis. Trivandrum : Roussel Scientific Institute, 1997 : 41-4

30. Kushno S et al : CT demonstration of fibrous stroma in chronic pancra : pathologic corrualtion. J Compart a Assist Tomogr 1999;23:297-300

31. Lin Y, Tamakashi A, Matsuna S, et al. Nation wide epidemiological survey of chronic pancreatitis in Japan. J Gastroenterol 2002;35:135-41

32. Copenhagen Pancreatic Study Group. An interim report from a prospective epidemiological multicentre study. Scand J Gastroenterol 1981;16:305-12

33. Robles-Diaz G, Vargas F, Uscanga L, et al. Chronic pancreatitis in Mexico city. Pancreas 1990;5:479-83

34. Narendranathan M. Chronic calcific pancreatitis in the tropics. Trop Gastroenterol 1981;2:40-5

35. Chari ST, Jayanthi V, Mohan V, et a. Radiological appearance of pancreatic calculi in tropical and alcoholic chronic pancreatitis. J Gastroenterol Hepatol 1992;7:42-4

36. Augustine P, Ramesh H. Is tropical pancreatitis pre-malignant ? AmJ Gastroenterol 1992;87:1005-8

37. Banks PA : Acute and chronic pancreatitis. In : Feldman M, Scharschmidt BF, Sleisenger MH, eds. Gastrointestinal and liver disease : pathophysiology / diagnosis / management, edn 6. Philadelphia : WB Saunders; 1998:809-862

38. Forsmark CE : The diagnosis of chronic pancreatitis. Gastrointest Endosc 2000, 52:293-298

39. Peter Draganov, Phillip P. Toskes ; Chronic pancreatitis, Current Opinion in Gastroenterology 2002, 18:558-562

40. Whitcom DC; Hereditary pancreatitis is caused by mutation the cationic trypsinogengener. Not cornet 1996;14:131-145

41. National Institution of Health Concerned development program. State of the science statement : ERCP for diagnosis and therapy. Available at : htp ://consuming.wih.gov/cons/116/166-statement.htm.accessed March 27;2002

56

Laparoscopic Distal Pancreatic Resections

INTRODUCTION

Over the last decade laparoscopic pancreatic surgery has advanced leaps and bounds in terms of improvements in instrumentation, advanced technology and also due to experience in other advanced laparoscopic procedures. The first description of a laparoscopic distal pancreatic resection was by Soper et al in 1994; where in he demonstrated that laparoscopic distal pancreatectomy was safe and feasible in a porcine model.[1] Laparoscopy is not universally accepted as the best approach for pancreatic tumours and cystic diseases. Even today these are rarely performed procedures and is considered an elite surgical approach especially because of the technical difficulties involved, long operating time and requiring highly trained surgeons.

But increasing experience, availability of laparoscopic ultrasound for localization of lesions and development of laparoscopic linear cutting stapler for perfect haemostatic pancreatic transection have all greatly facilitated laparoscopic pancreatic resections.

The extent of reported laparoscopic pancreatic resections varies from simple enucleation of benign insulinomas to pancreatico duodenectomy. In this chapter we will deal with the technical aspects of laparoscopic pancreatic resection particularly distal pancreatectomy with enbloc splenectomy as well as spleen preserving distal pancreatectomy. The experience with laparoscopic distal pancreatic resection has been entirely favourable with benefit to the patient in terms of postoperative recovery, minimal morbidity and short hospital stay in contrast to open surgical technique as well as laparoscopic pancreaticoduodenectomy.

INDICATIONS

1. Solid tumour - Carcinoma pancreatic tail, Neuroendocrine (Insulinoma, gastrinoma, nonfunctioning) tumors

2. Cystic tumours - Mucinous cystadenoma, serous cystadenoma, simple cysts, Echinocoecal cyst, unspecified etc (lymph cyst)

3. Isolated pseudocyst - Isolated left sided disease without evidence of malignancy

4. Chronic pancreatitis - Isolated left sided disease

Indications and Choice of Procedures

1.Distal tumours of pancreas

Patients with benign lesions located in the body and tail of the pancreas constitute the ideal indications for laparoscopic pancreatic resection

i.   Benign cystic lesions e.g. : cystadenoma

ii.   Pancreatic endocrine tumours eg. Insulinomas

In benign cystic tumours, spleen can be preserved.

Insulinomas can be treated by distal pancreatectomy or enucleation.[2-4]

Carcinoids are treated by enbloc pancreatico splenectomy as they are infiltrating in nature.

2.Intractable pain caused by chronic pancreatitis

Concept of near total pancreatectomy leaving a sufficient rim of pancreatic tissue close to the duodenal curve (Beger's procedure) is advisable over total pancreaticoduodenectomy due to higher incidence of post operative morbidity.

Contraindications

1. Obese patients are unsuitable for laparoscopic resections as exposure of pancreas is difficult and tedious.

2. Previous upper abdominal surgery is considered as relative contraindication for pancreatic resection

3. Lastly if the tumor is not located by laparoscopy; it is better to convert to open surgical technique.

PRE-OPERATIVE WORKUP

Prior to subjecting the patient to surgery the surgeon must take a detailed medical history and perform a thorough physical examination to confirm the diagnosis and also look for associated pathology.

A detailed pre-operative workup is essential for delineation of the extent, nature and exact location of the lesion and for information regarding the major anatomical structures that require preservation. This is crucial in assessing the feasibility of resection.

Investigations

Apart from the routine haematological and biochemical tests, Castillo and Warshaw support aspiration of cystic fluid pre operatively in a cystic lesion to distinguish pseudocysts from cystic tumours.[5] Various fluid indices are measured including viscosity, CEA, CA 15-3, CA19-9, CA72-4, Amylase and cytological examination of the aspirate is also performed.

Ultrasonography, contrast enhanced computed tomography scan and magnetic resonance imaging (MRI) will all usually provide sufficient diagnostic information. But in centers where Endoscopic ultrasound is available it is quite useful. It is an accurate tool that can be used to locate and define precisely the anatomy of a neuroendocrine tumour their relationship to surrounding structures especially the splenic vessels. Proye et al in 1998 reported a sensitivity in 79% for EUS[6] and also when combined with somatostatin receptor scintigraphy; the sensitivity increased to 89%.[7,8]

But nowadays the most sensitive localization test in intraoperative ultrasound with sensitivity ranging from 90 to 100%.[6]

ERCP is routinely done to assess the pancreatic ductal anatomy.[9] Visceral angiography is done in cases of suspected insulinomas; But most sensitive preoperative test is the portal venous sampling.

Computed Tomography Scan: ERCP or intraoperative findings showing isolated left sided ductal disease will help identifying patients who will benefit from distal pancreatic resections.

POSITIONING AND OPERATIVE TEAM

The patient is supine with sand bag under left side of the chest and right lateral tilt of about 30 degree. The surgeon and camera assistant stand to the right, the first assistant near the head end and the scrub nurse stands to the right of the operating surgeon.

Pneumoperitoneum is created by closed Veress needle technique. The ports are placed as shown in the figure similar to the description of Barry A Salky.[10]

INSTRUMENTATION

The following instruments and devices are recommended in laparoscopic pancreatic resection

1. 30 degree laparoscopic lens
2. 5 ports; 10mm-3, 5mm-2
3. Babcock forceps
4. Flat blade 3 prong retractor
5. Endo GIA / Endo TIA
6. Medium large clip applicator

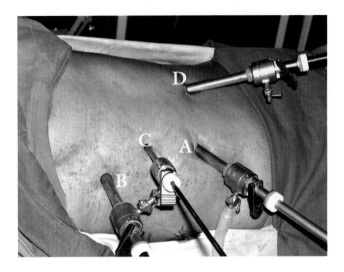

Figure 1 : Ports position

A - Supraumbilical camera port - 10mm
B - Epigastric retracting port - 10mm
C - Left midclavicular working port - 5mm
D - Left anterior axillary working port - 10mm

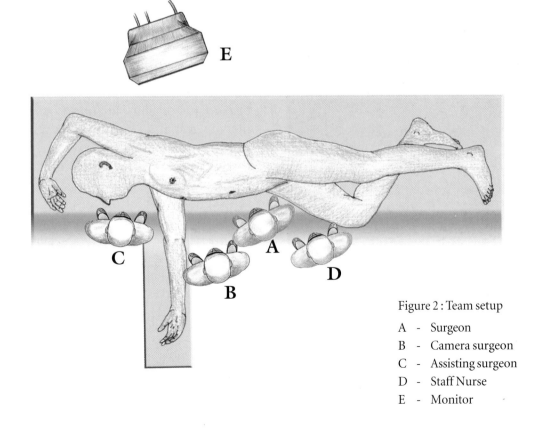

Figure 2 : Team setup

A - Surgeon
B - Camera surgeon
C - Assisting surgeon
D - Staff Nurse
E - Monitor

A 30 degree angled scope is used for multi angle visualization of pancreas. Endo GIA is kept for emergency use if necessary. I routinely do not prefer to use it. Disposable multi fire clip applicator is preferred by some. Reusable clip applicator may be of use for clipping with 11mm large clips. I prefer ligatures for large vessels and ultrasonic dissection (ultracision; Ethicon) which facilitates the entire procedure effectively without blood loss. I have not used stapler on any occasion for control of blood vessels or mobilisation of the greater omentum.

ENBLOC DISTAL PANCREATECTOMY

Operative Technique

Exposure of the pancreas

The first step is entry to the lesser sac by dividing the greater omentum below the gastro epiploic arcade starting half way along the greater curvature. The entire gastrocolic omentum from distal antrum upto the fundus of the stomach including the short gastric vessels is divided. Separation of the gastrocolic and gastrosplenic ligament are done by harmonic scalpel (ultracision, Ethicon). This is facilitated by retracting the stomach anteriorly with a Babcock.

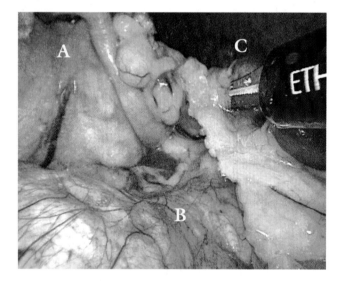

Figure 3 : Gastrocolic ligament is opened, body and tail of pancreas is exposed

A - Posterior wall of stomach

B - Pancreas

C - Spleen

Adhesions between the posterior wall of the stomach and fibrotic surface of the pancreas are released in case of chronic pancreatitis from head to tail including the hilum of the spleen.

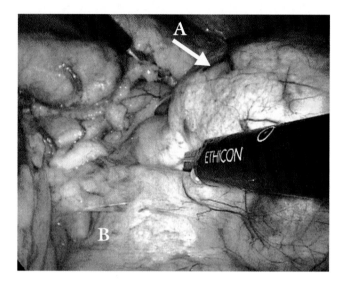

Figure 4 : Pancreatic tumor(Cyst adenoma) is seen

A - Tumor

B - Neck of pancreas

Splenic artery ligation in continuity

The artery is identified at the upper border of the body of the pancreas and dissected for an adequate distance proximal to the tumor and ligated in continuity by using silk ligature. This minimizes the risk of major bleeding during subsequent dissection. In case adequate length of splenic artery could be dissected distal to the ligature, it can be divided at this stage. In one of our cases splenic artery could not be identified due to bulky lesion in the body displacing the artery posteriorly. Splenic artery and vein are ligated posteriorly after complete mobilisation of the spleen, tail and body of the pancreas. In case of a benign cyst or tumor where the spleen is likely to be preserved; the short gastric vessels are not divided.

Dissection of the inferior border of the pancreas and mobilisation of its posterior surface

Splenic flexure of the colon is mobilized by dividing the lateral peritoneum, continuing upwards and medially. The transverse colon is retracted downwards, to visualize the inferior border of the pancreas. Division of the splenocolic ligament gives way to the inferior border at the tail end of the pancreas. The anterior layer of the transverse mesocolon is divided along the lower border of the pancreas. This opens the areolar tissue at the back of the pancreas. The pancreas is lifted up gently by the fan blade retractor through the epigastric port. Dissection is continued until the splenic vein is identified. The junction of the splenic and superior mesenteric vein is identified by opening the fascial layer using scissors. If the inferior mesenteric vein joins the splenic vein it is ligated and transected.

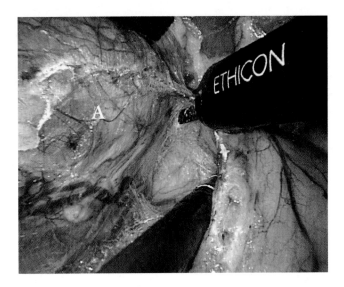

Figure 6 : Division of transverse mesocolon along the inferior border of pancreas using harmonic scalpel

A   -   Cystadenoma pancreas

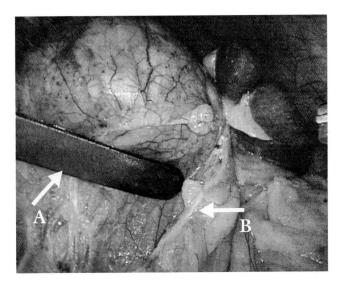

Figure 5 : Anterior layer of transverse mesocolon is divided from the inferior border of pancreas

A   -   Cyst adenoma is retracted by liver retractor
B   -   Transverse mesocolon

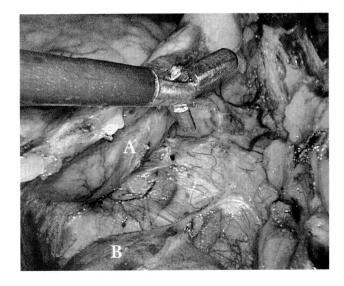

Figure 7 : After the division of transverse mesocolon, pancreas is mobilized

A   -   Inferior surface of pancreas
B   -   Duodenojejunal flexure

Division of the splenic artery

If the splenic artery had not been divided earlier, it can now be identified at the upper border of pancreas. It is clipped distal to the ligature and divided.

Ligation of splenic vein at the confluence with superior mesenteric vein

Splenic vein is doubly ligated with silk and divided. As there is insufficient space, Endo GIA should not be attempted. Splenic vessels are divided with scissors.

Mobilisation of body of the pancreas

After division of the splenic vessels, the body of the pancreas can be mobilized beyond the portal vein if necessary. Usually it is sufficient upto the neck of pancreas, keeping 2cms beyond the tumor margin.

Pancreatic transection

The site of transection is determined by the pathology in the individual case, Endo GIA with 48 mm staplers is used to transect the pancreas. [10,12] One or two cartridges may be needed to transect the pancreas. The pancreatic duct is ligated with vicryl stitches. This can also be divided with harmonic scalpel and the stump is sutured at the divided end using polypropylene.

Mobilisation of tail of pancreas and the spleen

The tail of the pancreas and the spleen is lifted by retractor and the spleno renal and spleno phrenic ligaments are divided. By retracting the pancreas down, the superior pole of the spleen and retrogastric vessels are divided.

Extraction of the specimen

The resected specimen of pancreas and spleen is placed into an impermeable bag. Umbilical port is extended sufficiently to enable extraction of the specimen without rupturing.

In case of splenic vein infiltration, where the spleen is likely to be big, the spleen may be separately removed by morcellation. Incision is made just for removal of the pancreatic tumor en-mass.

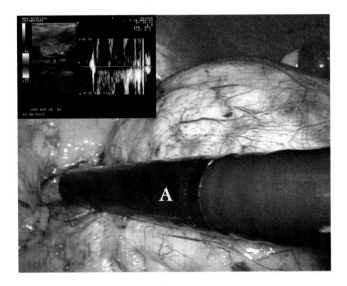

Figure 8 : Laparoscopic ultrasound examination of the tumor and color doppler study of splenic vessels

A - Laparoscopic ultrasound probe

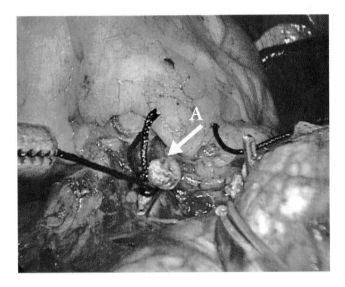

Figure 9 : Division of splenic artery after doubly ligated with silk

A - Divided end of splenic artery

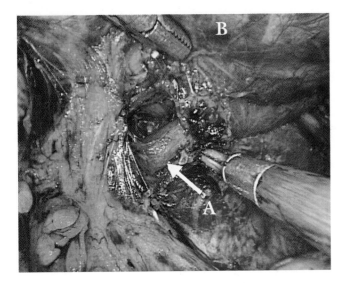

Figure 10 : Cystadenoma is lifted up and splenic vein is approached posteriorly

A - Splenic vein
B - Cystadenoma of pancreas

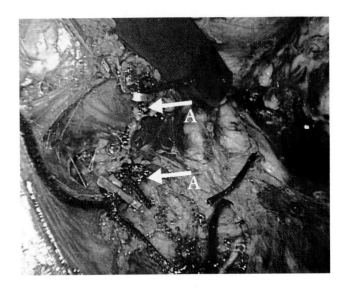

Figure 11 : Division of splenic vein after ligature

A - Divided end of splenic vein

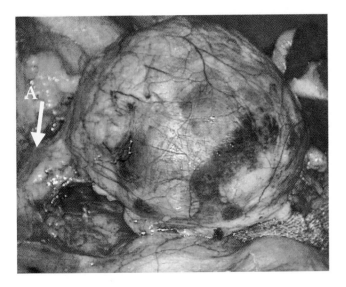

Figure 12 : Cystadenoma after complete mobilization

A - Neck of pancreas

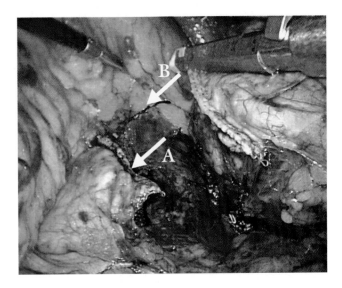

Figure 13 : Division of pancreas using Endo GIA stapler

A - Divided end of pancreas
B - Divided end of splenic artery

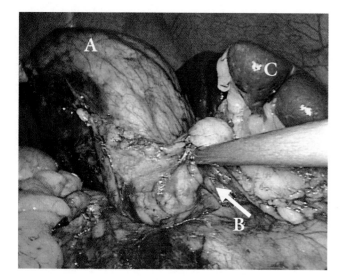

Figure 14 : Picture shows completely mobilized pancreas

A - Cystadenoma
B - Tail of pancreas
C - Spleen

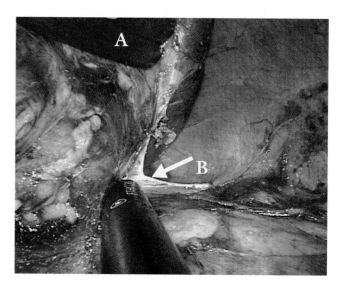

Figure 15 : Mobilization of spleen

A - Liver retractor is used to retract the spleen
B - Division of splenorenal ligament

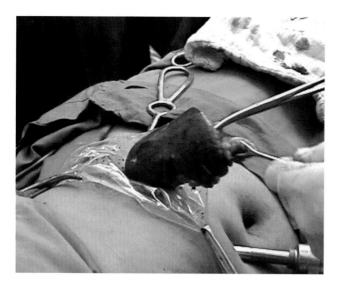

Figure 16 : Extraction of specimen by minilaparotomy

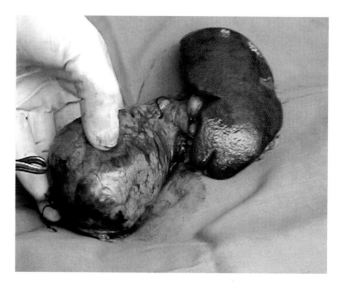

Figure 17 : Excised spleen and pancreas with cystadenoma

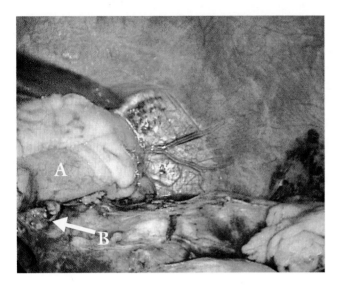

Figure 18 : Inspection of pancreas and splenic area after excision

A - Posterior wall of stomach
B - Divided end of splenic artery

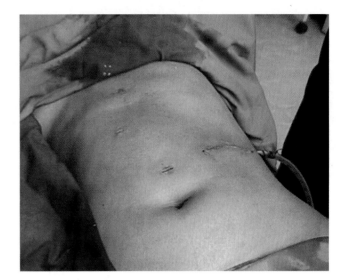

Figure 20 : Position of ports and minilaparotomy

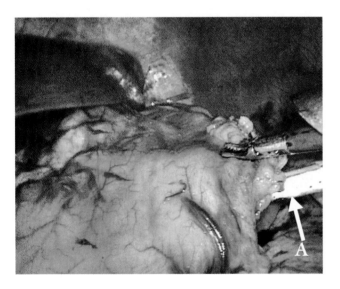

Figure 19 : Drainage tube in the pancreatic bed

A - Drainage tube

SPLEEN PRESERVING DISTAL PANCREATECTOMY

For known benign cyst of pancreas; spleen preserving distal pancreatectomy is an ideal procedure. For suspected or known malignant cyst of pancreas enbloc pancreatosplenectomy should be performed as already described earlier.

After lesser sac is thoroughly explored, intra operative laparoscopic ultra sonographic assessment of the tumor is performed and the level of division is assessed, particularly indicated for small intraparenchymal pancreatic lesions.[6] Splenic flexure is mobilized down and medially, mobilisation of the pancreas begins at inferior border of the body and tail. The pancreas is lifted up by the fan blade retractor, the posterior surface of the pancreas is dissected next by dividing the retroperitoneum and pancreatic plane, which is avascular. Mobilisation of the splenic flexure and splenocolic ligament exposes the tail of the pancreas. Dissection in this area must be done carefully in order to prevent injury to the splenic vein and artery.[10] If necessity arises, large vessels can be ligated in continuity. Harmonic scalpel is extremely useful in controlling smaller vascular communications to the pancreas.[12] One of the trocar is changed to 12mm preferably the left midclavicular for an Endo GIA stapler for pancreatic transection. Few sutures are placed on the anterior surface for control of vessels. The jaws are placed across the pancreas 2-3cms proximal to the lesion, particularly when malignant cysts are suspected. The specimen is always placed in a bag and extracted through mini laparotomy incision.

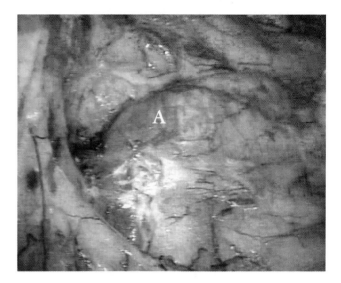

Figure 22 : Gastrocolic omentum was opened and Pancreatic tumor was exposed

A - Tumor in the body of pancreas

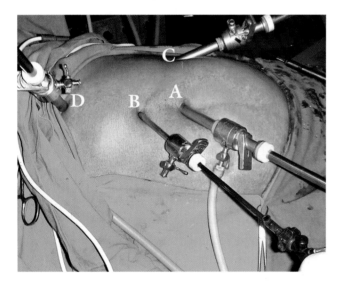

Figure 21 : Position of ports

A - Camera port
B - Left Working port
C - Right hand working port
D - Rectracting port

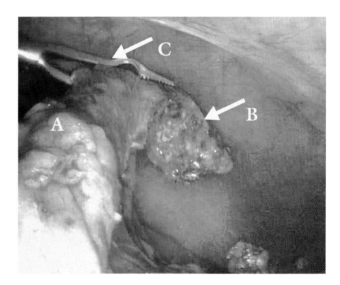

Figure 23 : Pancreas is mobilised completely

A - Body of pancreas
B - Tail of pancreas
C - 10 mm babcock is used to hold the pancreas

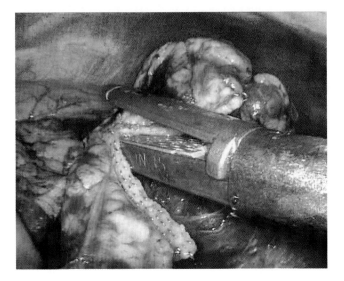

Figure 24 : Division of proximal pancreas using Endo GIA stapler

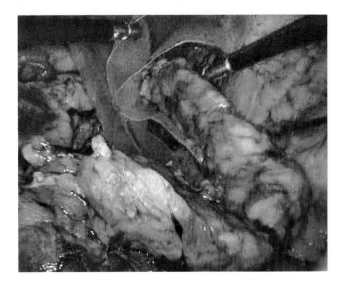

Figure 25 : Excised pancreas placed in the endobag

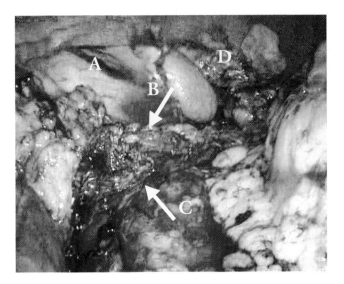

Figure 26 : Inspection of the area after excision

A - Posterior wall of stomach
B - Splenic artery
C - Splenic vein
D - Excised pancreas

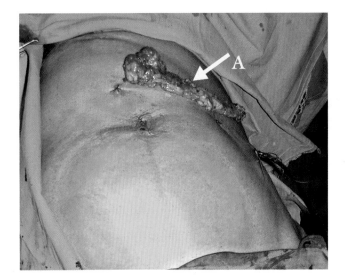

Figure 27 : position of ports and drainage tube

A - Excised pancreas

MEDIAN PANCREATECTOMY

Exposure of the pancreas

Lesser sac is entered by dividing the gastrocolic omentum from distal antrum upto the fundus of stomach including the short gastric vessels so as expose the tail of pancreas. Gastrocolic and gastrosplenic ligament are divided to facilitate retraction of the stomach anteriorly with a babcock. Adhesions between the posterior wall of stomach and pancreas are released. Intraoperative laparoscopic ultrasonographic assessment of the tumor is performed and the level of division and vascular relation is assessed.

Dissection of the inferior border of pancreas and mobilisation of its posterior surface is similar to that of distal pancreatectomy with spleen preservation. Care taken not to injure the splenic vein and splenic artery at the upper border.

Mobilisation of body of the pancreas done beyond the portal vein if necessary. But it is usually sufficient if mobilisation is done upto the neck of pancreas, keeping 2 to 3 cms of tumor free margin. pancreatic transection at the neck is done using Endo GIA 48mm stapler. The stapled line can be reinforced with interrupted vicryl stitches if necessary.

Division of pancreas distal to the tumor is done using harmonic scalpel. Pancreaticogastrostomy is done by invaginating the pancreatic stump to the posterior wall of stomach in two layers. Pancreaticogastrostomy is done in end to side fashion.

Specimen Extraction

Resected specimen is extracted through a small minilaparotomy wound after placing in a non permeable endobag.

Drain placed in the pancreatic bed posterior to the stomach through the left lateral port.

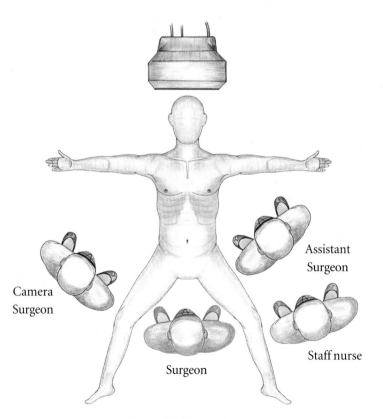

Figure 28 : Team setup

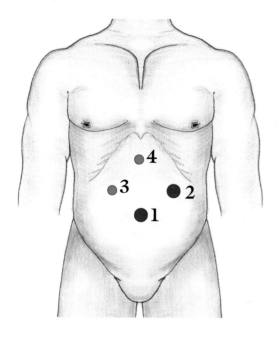

Figure 29 : Port position

No.	Instruments	Place
1	Camera	Umbilicus 10mm
2	Right hand working port	Left midclavicular 10mm
3	Left hand working port	Right midclavicular 5mm
4	Stomach retracting port	Subxiphoid 5mm

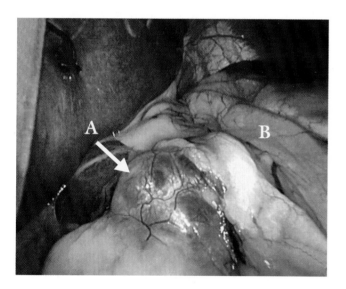

Figure 30 : Tumor in the body of pancreas seen through the lesser sac

A - Pancreatic tumor
B - Stomach

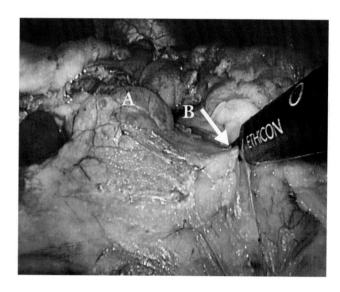

Figure 31 : Gastrocolic omentum is opened and pancreas exposed

A - Pancreatic tumor
B - Division of transverse mesocolon from the inferior border of pancreas

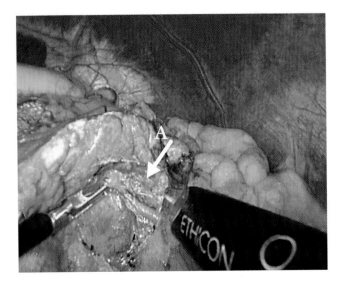

Figure 32 : Mobilization of pancreas

A - Pancreas is lifted up and posterior surface is dissected

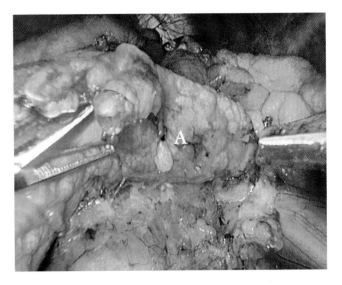

Figure 33 : Completion of pancreatic mobilization

A - Posterior surface of pancreas

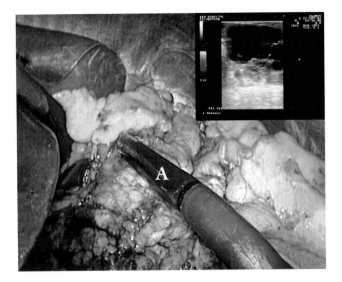

Figure 34 : Laparoscopic ultrasound examination of the pancreas before the division

A - Laparoscopic ultrasound probe

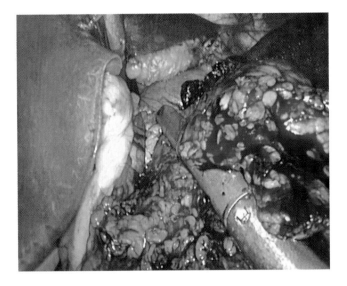

Figure 35 : Division of the proximal pancreas using Endo GIA stapler

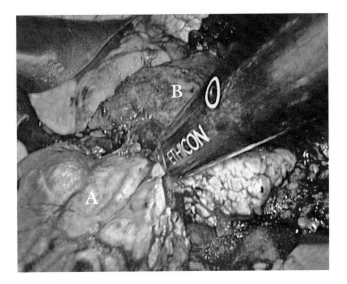

Figure 36 : Division of the pancreas distal to the tumor using harmonic scalpel

A - Pancreas with cyst
B - Distal pancreas

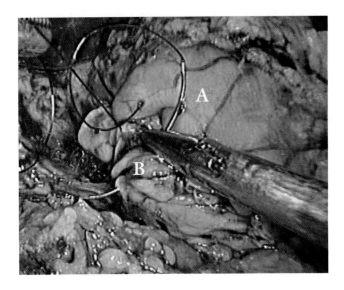

Figure 38 : End to side anastomosis of stomach to the distal end of pancreas

A - Posterior wall of stomach
B - Pancreas

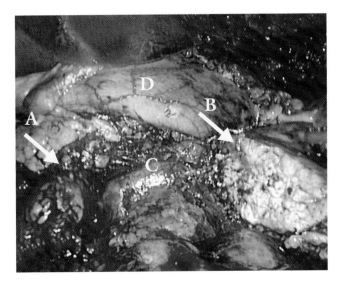

Figure 37 : Proximal and distal end of pancreas after the excision of the middle portion

A - Proximal end
B - Distal end
C - Splenic vein
D - Posterior wall of stomach

OUR EXPERIENCE AND RESULTS

Since 1998 to 2005, we have performed laparoscopic distal pancreatic resections in 23 patients aged between 12 to 69 years. Male to female ratio was 4:18; with most of them presenting as asymptomatic and accidentally found to have cystic lesions on routine abdominal evaluation. After thorough workup of these patients, following exclusion criteria were used.

1. Size of tumor Max - 8 to 10cm,

2. Pre-op biopsy (FNAC) - suspicion or confirmation of malignancy

3. Extensive adhesions with previous upper abdominal surgery

All the patients according to the criteria were subjected to laparoscopic distal pancreatic resection, we were able to conserve spleen in 7 of our cases and the remaining 15 patients had a pancreatosplenectomy. One patient underwent laparoscopic median pancreatectomy for a 4cm cystic lesion in the body of pancreas in our series. The patient had an uneventful postoperative period.

Indication for Lap. Pancreatic Resection and Final pathological diagnosis in our series

Indications	No.of patients	Pathology	No.
Cystic pancreatic lesions	23	Mucinous cystadenoma	3 (malignant)
		Ductal papillary hyperplasia	1
		Serous cystadenoma	16
		Inflammatory cyst	2
		Unspecified cyst (?lymph)	1

Average operating time in our series is around 215 mins with no blood transfusions either perioperative or in the post operative period. Patients were started on liquid on the 1st POD and normal diet on the 2nd day (2-3 days) and discharged from the hospital between 3rd and 4th day.

DISCUSSION

The experience with distal pancreatic resection has been entirely favorable; with benefit to the patient in terms of post operative recovery with minimal morbidity and shorter hospital stay. The reported experiences are all limited and the follow up is also short and very little is known about the long term outcome. Laparoscopic distal pancreatectomy should be considered in patients with chronic pancreatitis; islet cell tumours including insulinomas and patients with benign cystadenomas. Laparoscopic distal pancreatectomy with preservation of spleen is indicated for treatment of neuroendocrine tumors, provided these are benign and well localized. Infiltrative lesions require a distal pancreaticosplenectomy. Spleen preservation is feasible in benign tumors; But not in chronic pancreatitis due to retroperitoneal fibrosis. Warshaw described a modified technique of ligation of the splenic artery and preservation of the spleen with intact short gastric vessels.[21] This technique has been adopted laparoscopically by Vezakis and Sussman et al.[18,23]

Laparoscopic distal pancreatectomy for cystic tumors of the pancreas remain controversial because some benign cystadenomas are found malignant on histological examination of the excised specimen

Kiely et al described 30 patients with asymptomatic cystic pancreatic neoplasm and found 82% of enucleated lesions were premalignant. In our series, out of the 23 cases 3 were more than 5 cms and showed evidence of malignancey after resection. Since tumors were resected with intact capsule, it is unlikely to alter the prognosis. If any tumor on laparoscopy is more than 5cms, solid in nature and has invasive vascularity, then malignancy should be suspected. Laparoscopy may be applied for tumors with intact capsule only. Open surgery should be performed in all cases of proved malignancy.

Cystadenoma of the pancreas is one of the few pancreatic tumors with reasonably good long term prognosis provided radical resection is performed. The most common post operative complication is a pancreatic fistula.[11-14,18,20] Suture ligations of the stapled transected duct and application of fibrin glue to the residual pancreatic stump and administration of somatostatin may reduce this complication. One of our patients had pancreatic duct leakage, treated conservatively.

Laparoscopic contact ultrasonography is extremely useful during laparoscopic surgery which helps in the selection of the optimal transection site and can be used to guide enucleation.[6] Laparoscopic approach has added advantages of Hand Assisted technique (HALS) which helps during management of perioperative complications.[12,16,17] But there is still a need for prospective randomized trials to confirm all the benefits of laparoscopic distal pancreatic resection.

Comparison of intra operative variably and post operative results with other studies

Variables	John Hopkins (1999)[11]	Mount Sinai (2001)[12]	Gem Hospital (2005)
Open / Laparoscopic	Open	Lap	Lap
Total No.	235	19	23
Operative time	4.3 hrs (270mins)	4.4 hrs (280 mins)	3.4 hrs (215mins)
Blood loss	450ml	200ml	185ml
Type of Resection			
DP with SP	16%	16%	30.4%
DP with splenectomy	84%	64%	65.2%
Enucleation	Nil	20%	Nil
Median pancreatectomy	Nil	Nil	4.4%
Technique			
Complete lap		16 (84%)	100%
Hand asst	NA	1 (5%)	Nil
Conversion		2 (11%)	Nil

Comparison of results of open Vs laparoscopic distal pancreatectomy

Author	No	Stay (days)	Op time (hrs)	Complication Major (%)	Pan fistula/ I.A. collection	30 days mortality
Laparoscopic						
Palanivelu (2005)	23	4	3.4	1 (4.3%)	1	0
Shimizu (2004)[13]	15	-	5	14	14	0
B.Edwin (2004)[14]	17	5.5	4	38	6	8.3
Patterson(2001)[12]	19	7	4.3	16	16	0
Salky (2000)[10]	7	4	3.7	0	0	0
Vezakis (1999)[18]	6	34.5	5.0	33	33	0
Gagner (1997)[19]	9	5	4.5	-	-	-
Open						
Lillemoe (1999)[11]	235	10	4.3	31	5	0.9
Benoist (1999)[20]	40	15	-	98	23	-

Comparison of Post Operative Results with other open and laparoscopic series

Variables	John Hopkins[11] (1999)	Mt Sinai[12] (2001)	Kyushu Unv[13] (2004)	U.U.Hosp Norway[14] (2004)	GEM (2005)
Mortality (within 30 days)	0.9%	0	0	8.3%	0
Reoperation	14(6%)	0	0	0	0
Complication (Major)					
Pancreat Fistula / I.A. collection	12 (5%)	3 (16%)	1 (14%)	1 (6%)	1 (4.3%)
Haemorrhage	10 (4%)	Nil	Nil	2 (12%)	Nil
Hospital Stay	10 days	6 days	-	5.5 days	4 days

CONCLUSION

The experience of laparoscopic distal pancreatectomy has been entirely favourable; But still the indications have to be defined. The morbidity and mortality rates are same or even less than that of open series. Laparoscopic distal pancreatectomy has almost same operating time as compared to open with advantages of shorter hospital stay and reduced post operative pain. In case of laparoscopic median pan cratectomy, it can be performed safely as in conventional surgery and is an effective alternative to major pancreatic resection. It also allows for preservation of pancreatic endocrine and exocrine function without disruption of enteric continuity.[41-48] Finally it is important that all surgeons performing laparoscopic distal pancreatectomy be proficient with open pancreatic surgery. Moreover surgeons should be proficient with advanced laparoscopic techniques such as intracorporeal suturing and knotting. As surgeons gain more experience, laparoscopic distal pancreatectomy will become the choice of approach for pancreatic resections in carefully selected patients.

References

1. Soperas NJ, Brunt LM, Dunnegan DL, et al. Laparoscopic distal pancreatectomy in the porcine model. Surgical Endoscopy, 1994;8:57-61

2. Yeo JY, Wang BH, Anthone GJ, et al. Surgical Experience with pancreatic-islet cell tumors. Achieves of Surgery, 1993;128:1143-1148

3. Yeo CJ, Neoplasms of the endocrine pancreas. In:Greenfield LJ, ed. Surgery Scientific Principles and Practice, 2nd ed. Philadelphia: Lippincott - Raven, 1997;918-927

4. Broughan TA, Leslie JD, Soto, JM, et al. Pancreatic islet cell tumors. Surgery, 1986;99(6):671-678

5. Fernandez-del Castillo C, Warshaw AL. Cystic tumors of the pancreas. Surgical Clinics of North America, 1995;75(5):1001-1016

6. Boukhman MP, Koram JM, Shawa JS et al; Localisation of insulinoma, Archives of Surgery 1999, 134;818-23

7. Proye C, Malvaux P, Patton F et al, Non invasive imaging of insulinomas and gastrinoms with EUS and somatostatin receptor scintigraphy. Surgery 1998;121:1134-44

8. Cuschieri A, Jakinowicz JJ, van Spreeuwel J. Laparoscopic distal 70% pancreatectomy and splenectomy for chronic pancreatitis. Annals of Surgery, 1996;233(3):280-285

9. Rattner WR, Fernandez-del Castillo, Warshaw AL, Pitfalls of distal pancreatectomy for relief of pain in chronic pancreatitis, American journal of Surgery 1996;171:142-46

10. Salky BA, Edye, M. Laparoscopic pancreatectomy. Surgical Clinics of North America, 1996;76(3):539-545

11. Lillemoe KD, Kaushal S, Cameron JL, Distal Pancreatectomy: Indications and outcomes in 235 patients. Annals of Surgery, 1999;229(5)693-700

12. Patterson EJ, Gagner M, Salky B, et al, Laparoscopic pancreatic resection : single-institution experience of 19 patients, J am coll Surg.(2001) Sep;193(3):281-7

13. Shimizu S, Tanaka M, et al, Laparoscopic pancreatic Surgery, Surg Endosc (2004) 18:402-406

14. Edwin B, Mala T, et al, Laparoscopic resection of the pancreas, Surg Endosc (2004) 18:407-411

15. Mahon D, Allen E, Rhodes M, Laparoscopic distal pancreatectomy, Surg Endosc (2002) 16: 700-702

16. Shinchi, Hiroyuki MD, et al, Hand-Assisted Laparoscopic Distal Pancreatectomy With Minilaparotomy for Distal Pancreatic Cystadenoma, Surgical Laparoscopy, Endoscopy & Percutaneous Techniques. 11(2):139-143, April 2001

17. Klingler, Paul J. M.D. et al, Hand-Assisted Laparoscopic Distal Pancreatectomy for Pancreatic cystadenoma, Surgical Laparoscopy & Endoscopy 8(3):180-184, June 1998

18. Vezakis A, Davides D, Larvin M, et al. Laparoscopic surgery combined with preservation of the spleen for distal pancreatic tumors. Surgical Endoscopy, 1999;13:26-29

19. Gagner M, Pomp A. Laparoscopic Pancreatic Resection: Is it worthwhile? Journal of gastrointestinal Surgery, 1997;1:20-26

20. Benoist S, Dugue L, Sauvaner A, et al; Is there a role of preservation of the spleen in distal pancreatectomy ?; J Am Coll Surg 1999;188:255-260

21. Warshaw AL. Conservation of the spleen with distal pancreatectomy. Archives of Surgery, 1988;123:550-553

22. Palanivelu C, et al; Laparoscopic Pancreatic Resection, Text Book of Surgical Laparoscopy, 2002:367-372

23. Sussman LA, Christie R, Whittle DE. Laparoscopic excision of distal pancreas including insulinoma. Aust N Z J Surg 1996;66;414-416

24. Cuschieri A, Jakimowicz JJ. Laparoscopic Pancreatic Resections. Seminars in Laparoscopic Surgery, 1998;5(3):168-179

25. Gagner M, Pomp A., Herrera MF. Early experience with laparoscopic rsections of islet cell tumors. Surgery 1996;120:1051-4

26. William B Inabnet, Mount Sinai Medical Center, New York, Laparoscopic Distal Pancreatectomy: Overview. http://endocrinesearch.com

27. Park, Adrian E., Heniford, B. Todd, Therapeutic Laparoscopy of the Pancreas, Annals of Surgery. 236(2):149-158, August 2002

28. Cuschieri A., Laparoscopic Pancreatic Resections, Semin Laparosc Surg. 1996 Mar;3(1):15-20

29. Doi, Ryuichiro, Komoto, Izumi, Nakamura, et al Pancreatic Endocrine Tumor in Japan, Pancreas 28(3):247-252, April 2004

30. E.Barlehner, S. Anders, R. Schwetling, Laparoscopic Resection of the Left Pancreas : Technique and Indication, Digestive Surgery 2002;19:507-510

31. Piccoli M, Bassi C, Butturini G, Distal Pancreatic Neoplasms: Is there a role for Minimally-Invasive Surgical Procedures? Indications, Technique and Results on 32 Consecutive Patients Treated by the Same Surgical Team, JOP.J Pancreas (Online) 2004; 5(5 Suppl):424

32. Fernandez-Cruz L., Saenz A, et al, Outcome of Laparoscopic pancreatic surgery : endocrine and nonendocrine tumors, World J. Surg26, 2002, 1057-1065

33. Barlehner E, Anders S, Laparoscopic Resection of the left pancreas : Technique and Indication, Dig Surg 2002; 19:507-510

34. Johannes H.W., et al, Laparoscopic spleen preserving distal pancreatectomy after blunt abdominal trauma, Injury, Int. J.Care Injured 34(2003)233-234

35. Pinhas P. Schachter, et al, The role of laparoscopy and laparoscopic ultrasound in the diagnosis of cystic lesions of the pancreas, Gastrointest Endoscopy Clin N Am12 (2002) 759-767

36. Gramatica Jr, et al, Videolaparoscopic Resection of Insulinomas : Experience in Two Institutions, World J.Surg.26, 1297-1300, 2002

37. Pinhas P., Schachter et al, The impact of laparoscopy and laparoscopic ultrasound on the management of pancreatic cystic lesions, Arch Surg, Vol135, mar 2000, 260

57

Laparoscopic Whipple's Procedure

INTRODUCTION

In this fast growing laparoscopic era, more and more complex challenging surgeries have been performed by laparoscopic method. Whipple's procedure is one of the most challenging among all. Very few papers have been published in medical literature describing this procedure. The aim of this chapter is to emphasis the technical feasibility of laparoscopic Whipple's procedure and its added advantages over the conventional open method.

Laparoscopic pancreaticoduodenectomy and reconstruction for periampullary carcinoma, though time consuming is technically possible. Large series of cases have to be studied before any consensus is developed.[6]

Laparoscopic approach to the pancreas is more difficult due to retroperitoneal location and complex vascular relationship. Adequate experience in conventional Whipple's operation and laparoscopic operative skill are prerequisites for performing a laparoscopic Whipple's operation. Preoperative workup, particularly accurate staging is very important. Early periampullary tumors (<2cms) are ideal cases for laparoscopic approach. Larger lesions with involvement of major vessels are considered as a contraindication.

Pancreatic adenocarcinoma is the most common of the periampullary neoplasms. It accounts for more than 75% of all non-endocrine tumors arising in this region, which includes pancreas, the ampulla of vater, the distal CBD and the duodenum. The others account for 15 to 20% of all periampullary malignant disease.[11]

HISTORICAL ASPECT

In 1900, it was William James Mayo[25] who successfully removed the papilla (ampulla) for a papillary cancer. Later, advances in the surgical technique lead to the first successful removal of periampullary tumor with a sleeve of duodenum by William Halsted in 1898.[12] In the same year the Italian surgeon Alessardon Codivilla performed the first unsuccessful enbloc resection of pancreas for a periampullary carcinoma.[13] In 1907, Walter Kausch, a German Surgeon performed the first successful pancreatico-duodenectomy as a two stage procedure.[14] Later, in 1940, Whipple, the father of modern pancreatic surgery, performed pancreatico-duodenectomy as a single stage procedure and it is called as "Whipple's procedure" after him.[15] The concept of pylorus preservation was popularized by Traverso and Longmire in 1978.[16] Pylorus preserving pancreaticoduo-denectomy is now the favoured procedure because the gastric reservoir and the pyloric mechanism are kept intact, thus minimizing the nutritional and digestive upset associated with the conventional resection.

Till today, only a few cases of laparoscopic pancreaticoduodenectomy have been reported in English literature excluding ours. In 1994, Michel Gagner reported the first laparoscopic pylorus preserving pancreaticoduodenectomy in a 30 year old woman with chronic pancreatitis.[17] Delayed gastric emptying (DGE) complicated her post operative course and required nasogastric tube drainage for more than 30 days. The second patient was a 72 year old woman operated, for periampullary carcinoma, who developed a pancreatic leak and fistula. Consequently her hospital stay was prolonged for 62 days. With this, he concluded that, although it is technically feasible, laparoscopic Whipple's procedure did not improve the postoperative outcome or shorten the postoperative hospitalization period. After that, he started using hand port for pancreaticoduode-nectomy and he has done so in more than 9 cases till date.[23]

Next to M. Gagner, we were the second and performed the laparoscopic pylorus preserving pancreaticoduodenectomy in April 1998.[6] The first case was a 31 year old gentleman with early ampullary carcinoma. We did the entire reconstruction by laparoscopic method. He was discharged on the 9th POD without any complication. His wife conceived after the operation, fathered a child, and he is still alive. One of our videos of this procedure was selected in 2000 SAGES as one of the best videos and was included in SAGES Library catalogue. These early encouraging results, both from patients and forum, stimulated us to do further procedures. Till today we have performed 35 cases of pancreaticoduodenectomy by totally laparoscopic method with excellent results.

During the same period in 1998, Cuscheri et al reported two cases of laparoscopically assisted pancreaticoduodenectomy for periampullary carcinomas.[18] He also encountered both, DGE and pancreatic fistula, similar to M.Gagner, and he agreed with his appraisal that there was no role of laparoscopy in Whipple's procedure.

Next to ours, Prof. J.L. Dulucq from France has performed laparoscopic pylorus preserving pancreaticoduodenectomy in 7 cases with good results. He is one of the fastest laparoscopic surgeon who could finish laparoscopic Whipple's in 4 ½ hours (personal communication). Prof. Cristiano G.S Huscher (Italy) has done over 34 cases. He blocks the pancreatic duct instead of anastomosis. The leak rate is high in his series Prof. Cristoforo Guilionotti of Italy did the first robotic assisted laparoscopic Whipple's procedure. He also used to block the pancreatic duct with glue.

INDICATIONS

Selection of patient is extremely important for successful laparoscopic procedure, decreased post operative complication and delayed hospital stay. Early periampullary carcinomas without nodal metastasis in non obese individuals with ASA grade I & II are good candidates. The indications include

1. Ampullary tumors
2. Distal CBD tumors
3. Early carcinoma head of pancreas
4. Duodenal carcinoma

CONTRAINDICATIONS

1. Liver, peritoneal and (or) positive regional lymph nodes
2. Inability to localize the lesion

3. Vascular invasion of SMV/SMA

4. Obesity

5. Extensive adhesions due to previous surgery

PREOPERATIVE DIAGNOSTIC IMAGING AND STAGING

Current technology allows accurate pre-operative radiological staging and assessment of resectability. Our preoperative evaluation includes a careful physical examination, chest radiography, abdominal ultrasonography and contrast enhanced helical CT scan of abdomen.

Ultrasound

Ultrasound reveals a pancreatic mass in 60 to 70% of patients with pancreatic cancer. However, the absence of a pancreatic mass on ultrasound scanning does not definitively rule out pancreatic cancer. If a pancreatic mass is identified, spiral CT is often indicated, because CT provides more complete and accurate imaging of the pancreatic head and surrounding structures.

CT Scan Abdomen

Currently, we prefer high quality contrast enhanced helical CT is preferred for diagnosis of carcinoma pancreas. Pancreatic cancer usually appears as an area of enlargement in the pancreas, as a hypodence, focal lesion. CT scan provides information regarding the tumor size, extent of the disease, spread to liver and peripancreatic lymph nodes and retroperitoneal lymph nodes. In addition, it can be used to evaluate major vessels adjacent to the pancreas (SMA, SMV, PV, SV, HA for tumor invasion, encasement or thrombosis). For patients with a mass in the pancreatic head, the CT scan findings for tumor resectability include (1) absence of extrapancreatic disease. (2) A patent SMV/PV confluence and (3) no direct tumor extension to the hepatic artery or SMA. Patients who not meet these CT criteria are not considered candidates for resection.

Tumors smaller than 1cm can be missed and intrahepatic, or extrahepatic ductal dilatation may be the only finding on spiral CT. For such patients, we do MRCP/MRI or ERCP. MRI has not been shown to have a definite advantage over modern CT scanning. MRCP is a non invasive technique to image the biliary and pancreatic ductal system in a fashion similar to ERCP. Likewise, MRA - Magnetic resonance angiography - provides a non invasive technique to evaluate major vascular involvement when CT is equivocal.

ERCP

With the current advances in CT and MRI technology, diagnostic ERCP is unnecessary. It is a sensitive diagnostic test for periampullary carcinoma with sensitivity as high as 90%. The findings of a long, irregular stricture in an otherwise normal pancreatic duct or "double duct sign" (cut off of both the pancreatic and distal bile duct at the left of the genus of the PD) with an appropriate history is nearly pathognomonic for periampullary carcinoma.

ERCP should be considered in patients with CBD or PD obstruction without the finding of pancreatic mass on CT or MRI. It can also be useful in distinguishing chronic pancreatitis from pancreatic cancers. Beyond its use in diagnosis, ERCP can be used therapeutically in patients with significant jaundice, because endoscopic stent (endoprothesis) can be placed for decompression of the biliary tree.

CLINICAL FINDINGS

Approximately 65 to 75% of patient with periampullary carcinoma seek treatment when they develop obstructive jaundice secondary to obstruction of the intrapancreatic portion of the CBD. Jaundice is often associated with vomiting, dark coloured urine and pale stools. Early in the course, the pain is often described as vague upper abdominal, epigastric, or back discomfort. Then, it can progress to unremitting epigastric pain, fatigue and change in bowel habits in majority of patients. Nausea and vomiting usually indicate duodenal/gastric outlet obstruction due to locally advanced disease.

In some patients, acute pancreatitis may be the clinical presentation of pancreatic neoplasm, resulting from partial or complete obstruction of the pancreatic duct.

At the time of diagnosis, common findings on physical examination include jaundice, hepatomegaly and palpable gall bladder (Courvoisier's law). Many patients will show scratch marks on the skin due to severe pruritus. Cachexia and muscle wasting are often signs of advanced disease. Presence of left supraclavicular lymph adenopathy (Virchow's node), periumbilical adenopathy (Sister Mary Joseph's nodule) and pelvic metastases encircling the perirectal region (Blumer's shelf) on clinical examination indicates metastatic disease.

The blood investigations may reveal altered liver function tests including, elevated serum bilirubin, alkaline phosphatase and hepatic transaminases. In patients with marked elevated bilirubing levels, coagulation parameters including prothrombin time (PT) should be checked. Decreased enterohepatic circulation of bile salts leads to malabsorption of fat soluble vitamins and subsequent decrease hepatic production of vitamin K dependent clotting factors. Hypoalbuminemia and normochromic anaemia are often seen as reflection of poor nutritional status as a result of the underlying malignant process.

Tumor marker CA 19-9 (carbohydrate antigen) is elevated in more than 75% of patients with pancreatic cancer. Increased CA19-9 level has an accuracy of 80% in identifying patients with pancreatic cancer. In addition to diagnosis, CA 19-9 has been useful in following the patients after resection of disease and during adjuvant and neoadjuvant regimens. Increasing levels of CA 19-9 reflect progression of disease, while steady levels suggest presence of residual disease.

STAGING

Primary tumor (T)

Tx - Primary tumor cannot be assessed

To - No evidence of primary tumor

Tis - Carcinoma in situ

T1 - Tumor limited to the pancreas, 2cm or less in greatest dimension

T2 - Tumor limited to the pancreas, more than 2cm in greatest dimension

T3 - Tumour extends beyond the pancreas but without involvement of the celiac axis or the SMA

T4 - Tumor involves the celiac axis or the SMA (unresectable primary tumor)

Regional lymph nodes (N)

Nx - Regional lymph nodes cannot be assessed

N0 - No regional lymph node metastasis

N1 - Regional lymph node metastasis

Distant Metastasis (M)

Mx - Distant metastasis cannot be assessed

M0 - No distant metastasis

M1 - Distant metastasis

TNM Staging			
Stage 0	Tis	N0	M0
Stage I	T1	N0	M0
	T2	N0	M0
Stage II	T3	N0	M0
Stage III	T1	N1	M0
	T2	N1	M0
	T3	N1	M0
Stage IV A	T4	Any N	M0
Stage IV B	Any T	Any N	M1

PREOPERATIVE PREPARATION

Selection of suitable patients is extremely important for a successful completion of laparoscopic Whipple's procedure with good outcome. Patients are admitted few days before surgery and we are happy if we have a tissue diagnosis before starting the procedure. When the side viewing endoscope shows an obstructive ampullary lesion, even the negative histology of the same does not preclude surgery. In case of obstructive jaundice with abnormal liver function test (LFT) and coagulation profile, we always do an ERCP and stenting and obtain brush cytology and biopsy for confirmation. After doing so, we operate within 5 to 7 days in all operable cases.

All patients posted for this procedure undergo mechanical bowel preparation. Informed consent was obtained after explaining the complications and outcome of the proposed procedure to the relatives. A third generation cephalosporin along with metronidasole are given before induction of anesthesia in all cases.

TECHNIQUE

Anaesthesia, patient positioning and instrumentations

The procedure is undertaken under general endotracheal anesthesia with standard intraoperative monitoring. Patients are positioned in the semilithotomy position with both legs abducted and with a left lateral tilt. The surgeon stands between the legs of the patient to gain access for suturing and assistants stand on either side of the patient.

Bladder catheterization is done. Nasogastric tube, central venous line and arterial line are essential in all cases. CO_2 pneumoperitoneum is created by closed Veress needle technique and a 30° angled scope is used.

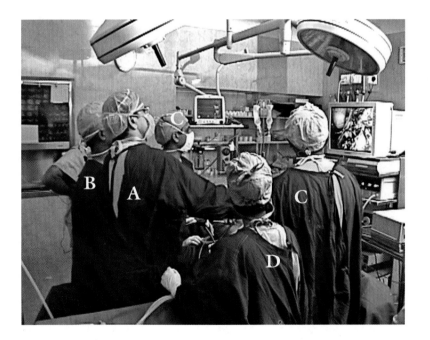

Figure 1 : Team setup. Patient placed in lithotomy position

A - Surgeon
B - Camera surgeon
C - Assisting surgeon
D - Staff nurse

Instrumentation

High quality imaging system preferably with 3 chip digital camera should be used apart from routine hand instruments. Other special instruments which are very useful are,

1. Harmonic Scalpel, 5mm and 10mm
2. Bipolar coagulation probe
3. Endo GIA and Endo TIA stapler
4. Laparoscopic ultrasonography probe (LUS) - 5mm, 7.5mm, 10mm

Ports

Ports are placed under video guidance. Subxiphoid port is used for retraction of the stomach and the duodenum. Cranial retraction of the fundus of the gall bladder gives adequate exposure of the subhepatic region.

Umbilical 10mm port - Camera

Subxiphoid 10mm port - Traction

Left epigastric 10mm port
    - Right hand working port and traction

Right midclavicular supraumbilical 5mm port
    - Left hand working port

Right anterior axillary 5mm port
    - Fundus traction

Left midclavicular at the level of umbilicus 5mm port - Traction

Operative Details

We confirm the preoperative findings before proceeding to resection with the help of laparoscopic ultrasonogram and colour Doppler system.

The technique of laparoscopic pylorus preserving pancreaticoduodenectomy is similar to that of open surgery. It involves 4 phases.

1. Assessment of resectability and laparoscopic staging
2. Resection
3. Reconstruction
4. Extraction

Resection as such involves dissection, ligation and division of vessels and transection of tubular structures. Reconstruction involves duodenojejunostomy, pancreaticojejunostomy/gastrostomy and hepatico or choledochojejunostomy. It is easy to remember the procedure by the number 3 and 4. The dissection involves 3 planes and reconstruction involves 3 structures. Whereas, 4 named vessels are ligated and 4 named structures are transected. The 4 named vessels that are ligated and divided during this procedure are:

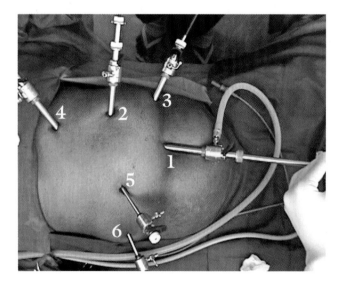

Figure 2 : Port position

No.	Instruments	Place
1	Camera	Umbilicus 10mm
2	Right hand working port	Left epigastrium 10mm
3	Working port	Left midclavicular 10mm
4	Retracting port	Subxiphoid 10mm
5	Left hand working port	Right mid clavicular 5mm
6	Retracting port	Right anterior axillary port 5mm

1. Gastrocolic trunk / vein of Henle

2. Gastroduodenal artery (GDA)

3. Right gastroepiploic vessels

4. Inferior pancreatic duodenal artery

The 4 structures which are divided during this procedure are

1. Duodenum or antrum of stomach

2. Jejunum beyond DJ flexure

3. Common bile duct (above the junction of cystic duct)

4. Pancreas (at the junction of neck and body)

PHASE I

Assessment of Resectability and Laparoscopic Staging

Patients thought to be resectable following dynamic CT scan proceed to laparoscopy with possible resection. Laparoscopic staging of periampullary and pancreatic lesions is entirely different from the conventional method. The tactile sensation of open method has been replaced by laparascopic ultrasound and Doppler study.

Initially any ascites is aspirated and sent for cytology. Then a systematic examination of peritoneum is performed and any serosal metastasis is biopsied. The extent, size and mobility of the primary tumor are noted. Then a systematic inspection of liver is performed on all surfaces, which is facilitated by head up and left lateral tilt of the table. The gastro hepatic omentum overlying the caudate lobe of the liver is opened using Harmonic Scalpel, exposing the caudate lobe, celiac axis and vena cava. The HA in its course to the porta is visualized. Portal, perigastric and celiac lymphnodes are biopsied if enlarged. Inspection of body and tail of pancreas is performed by opening the gastro colic omentum using the Harmonic Scalpel and the primary tumor is assessed.

LUS is performed to evaluate small intraperitoneal hepatic lesions (<1cm) which are not usually picked up by conventional spiral CT. All the segments of the liver are examined sequentially by moving and rotating the probe slowly. The hepatoduodenal ligament is evaluated by placing the probe transversely. The PV and SMV are examined. The CBD, CHD and HA are identified using probe and color flow Doppler. The transducer is placed transversely on the gastro colic omentum, and the SMA is identified at its origin on the aorta and followed distally. The confluence of the PV with the SMV is identified, and the relationship of tumor to this structure is assessed. The pancreas is examined by placing the transducer through the window in the gastrohepatic omentum directly on the surface of the gland. The tumor with its relation to the PV is noted. Gentle rotation of the probe at this stage allows for evaluation of the celiac axis and proximal HA.

Gastrocolic vein/trunk, which opens on the anterior aspect of the SMV, is divided to approach the SMV and PV. Looking from below, it can be assessed using blunt irrigation/suction probe. Resectability can be easily assessed in early periampullary lesions but it is difficult in case of cancer of head of pancreas, particularly in association with chronic pancreatitis, where the LUS with Doppler cannot accurately assess and stage the disease.

PHASE II - Resection

Mobilisation of Head of Pancreas

To start with, Cattle's maneuver is done followed by extended Kocher's maneuver. Colohepatic peritoneum is incised and the hepatic flexure and transverse colon are mobilized down, exposing the entire second and third part of duodenum upto the neck of pancreas. Kocherisation is facilitated by retracting the duodenum anteriorly and medially by a 10mm Babcock through the subxiphoid port.

Division of gastrocolic trunk vein facilitates separation of the neck of the pancreas from the superior mesenteric vein. Right gastroepiploic vein and artery are clipped, divided and the first part of duodenum is divided using endo GIA stapler, 1-2cm distal to the pyloric ring in case of early ampullary cancer. Resection of the antrum is performed for pancreatic head malignancy. While doing so 2 or 3 are transverse branches of right gastro epiploic arcade are divided.

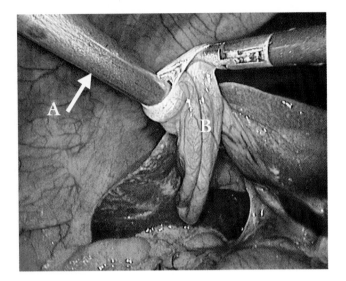

Figure 3 : Decompression of gallbladder using right midclavicular 5mm trocar

A - 5 mm trocar
B - Gall bladder

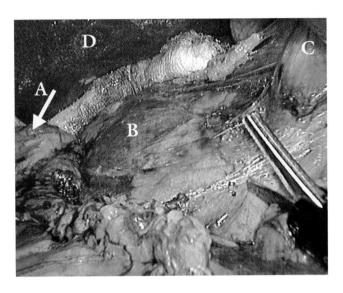

Figure 4 : Mobilisation of hepatic flexure and transverse colon

A - Hepatic flexure
B - Right kidney
C - Duodenum
D - Inferior surface of right lobe of liver

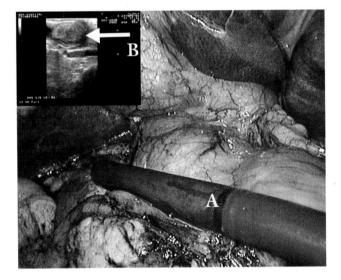

Figure 5 : Laparoscopic ultrasonographic examination over the head of pancreas

A - Laparoscopic ultrasound probe
B - Periampullary growth

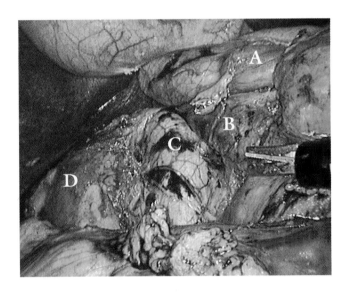

Figure 6 : Mobilisation of second part of duodenum and uncinate process of pancreas medially

A - Second part of duodenum
B - Pancreas
C - Inferior vena cava (IVC)
D - Right kidney

The peritoneum covering the CBD is opened anteriorly and laterally and it is then dissected free from the portal vein and common hepatic artery. Lymphnodes identified at this stage, are removed for HPE. Metastasis are most likely to occur in these lymph nodes.

The gastro duodenal artery is identified at the groove between the neck and head of pancreas, which is ligated and divided. The CBD is divided 2cm above the pancreatic border. A chromic catgut loop is applied to the divided proximal common duct after the decompression of the intrahepatic biliary system as temporary control of bile leakage. Nowdays, we have been using bulldog clamp for the same.

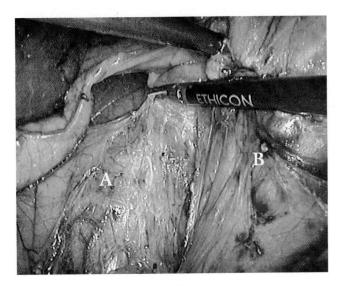

Figure 7 : Dissection continued above along the course of IVC

A - IVC

B - Second part of duodenum

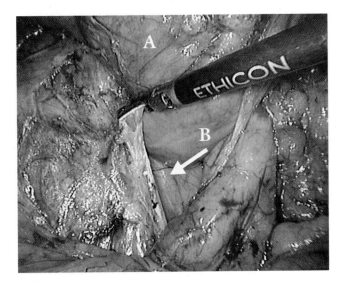

Figure 8 : Dissection continued upto the third part of duodenum and infracolic compartment reached

A - Third part of duodenum

B - Inferior mesenteric vessels

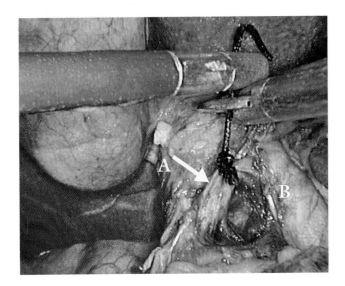

Figure 9 : Ligation of gastroduodenal artery

A - Gastroduodenal artery

B - Common hepatic artery

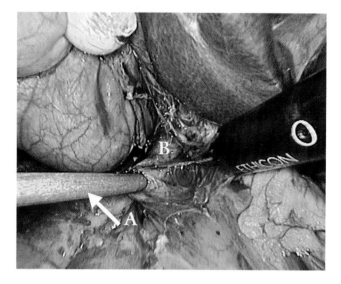

Figure 10 : Decompression of Common bile duct

A - Suction cannula
B - Common bile duct

Mobilisation of Duodeno Jejunal Flexure (DJF)

The peritoneum lateral to the DJF is incised while carefully retracting the inferior mesenteric vein to the left and the ligamenum of Treitz is divided. Jejunum distal to the DJF is divided using endo GIA. Jejunal vessels of the proximal jejunum and duodenum are freed from the mesenteric vessels using Harmonic Scalpel. Care should be taken, while dividing the proximal jejunal tributaries that drain to the SMV-PV confluence, which goes posterior to SMA. The same jejunal branches also receive small tributaries from the uncinate process. So extreme care should be taken in delineating these SMV branches to avoid bleeding. After the addition of Harmonic ace (5mm) instrument in our theatre setup, we are comfortable in dealing with these vessels. The free end of the duodenum and jejunum is displaced under the route of mesentery to the supracolic compartment.

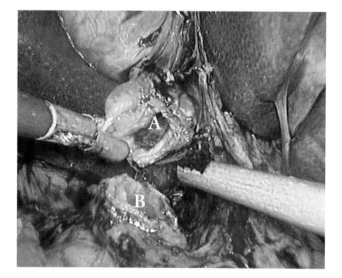

Figure 11 : Division of common bile duct

A - Proximal end
B - Distal end

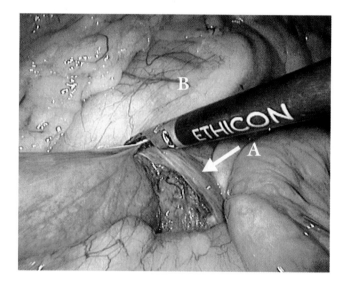

Figure 12 : Division of Ligament of Treitz

A - Inferior mesenteric vein
B - Inferior border of pancreas

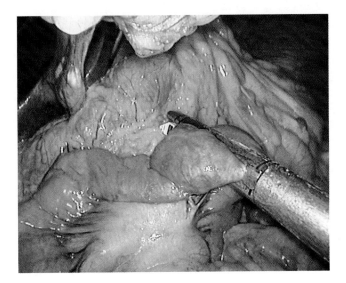

Figure 13 : Division of Proximal jejunum using Endo GIA stapler

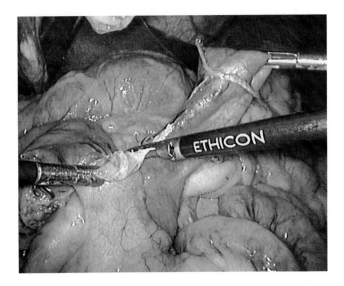

Figure 14 : Division of mesenteric vessels using harmonic scalpel

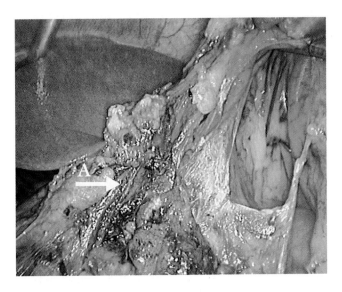

Figure 15 : Mobilisation of part I duodenum

A - Right gastroepiploic vessel

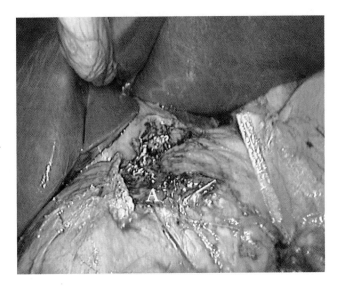

Figure 16 : Division of first part of duodenum using Endo GIA stapler

A - Pancreas

Resection of Pancreas

Patient is tilted to the left with head up position which facilitates exposure of pancreas. Neck of pancreas is carefully divided using Harmonic Scalpel. The lateral tributaries of the superior mesenteric vein from the head of pancreas are divided by clipping the individual vessels or with Harmonic Scalpel. I found division of pancreas at the neck using the blunt edge of 10mm ultrashear at level 3 is appropriate and totally bloodless. Inferior pancreaticoduodenal artery is controlled and clipped by retracting the mesenteric vein medially. Mobilisation of the uncinate processmay require division of small vessels as mentioned earlier.

Resection of Uncinate Process

A hook retractor or an umbilical tape is applied across the root of the mesentery to give traction anteriorly and to the left. This maneuver clearly exposes the uncinate process for further careful dissection. Initially by blunt dissection using suction nozzle it is separated from the root of the mesentery. All the venous tributaries from uncinate process and the small arteries suppling it where identified separately and clipped or divided using 5mm harmonic scalpel. Great care is taken not to injure the portal vein or superior mesenteric vein at this stage.

Similarly, the vein draining the pancreas that joins the portal vein at its upper border can be controlled between the common bile duct and portal vein. After this, the specimen is free and kept aside.

Nodal Clearance

All the lymphofatty tissues, including the lymph nodes, are dissected out from the Inferior vena cava, common hepatic artery (CHA), aorta, superior mesenteric vein and portal vein, skeletonising the structures individually upto porta hepatis and are placed into an endobag, which is removed later through the extended umbilical port site.

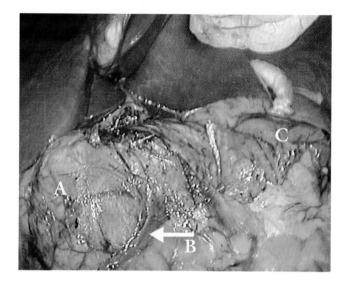

Figure 17 : Idenfication of gastrocolic trunk for the division of neck of pancreas

A - Head of pancreas
B - Gastocolic trunk
C - Stomach

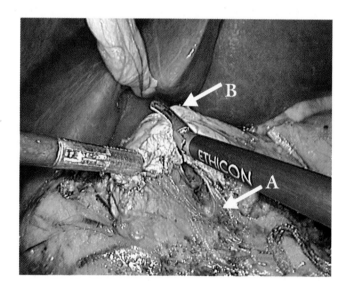

Figure 18 : Division of neck of pancreas using 5mm harmonic scalpel

A - Superior mesenteric vein
B - Pancreas

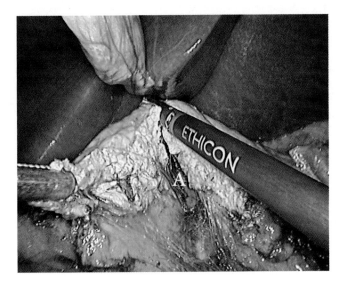

Figure 19 : Division of the neck of pancreas

A - Portal vein

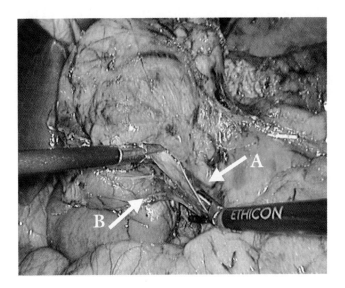

Figure 20 : Dissection of uncinate process anteriorly

A - Uncinate process

B - Third part of duodenum pulled into the supracolic compartment after the division of proximal jejunum

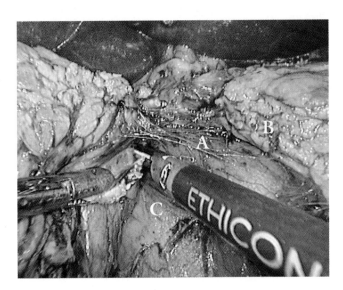

Figure 21 : Dissection of uncinate process using harmonic scalpel

A - Portal vein

B - Divided end of neck of pancreas

C - IVC

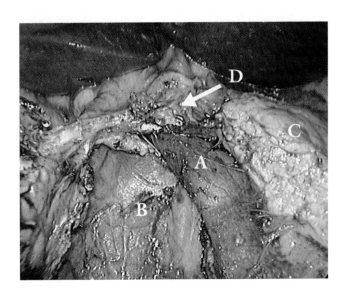

Figure 22 : Completion of uncinate dissection

A - Portal vein

B - IVC

C - Pancreas

D - Divided end of gastroduodenal artery

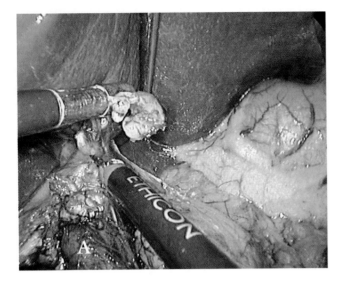

Figure 23 : Lymphonodal clearence along the course of common hepatic artery

A - Portal vein

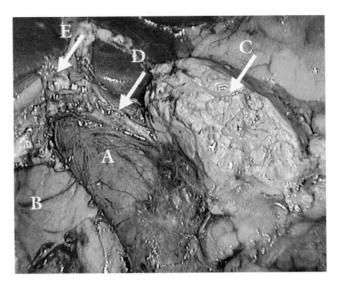

Figure 25 : Completion of pancreatoduodenectomy

A - Portal vein
B - IVC
C - Neck of pancreas
D - Common hepatic artery
E - Divided end of gastroduodenal artery

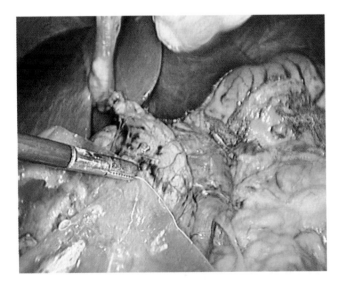

Figure 24 : Placement of the specimen (C loop of duodenum and head of pancreas) in the endobag

PHASE III

Choledochojejunal Anastomosis

Once the resection is completed, the specimen is kept aside and preparation starts for reconstruction. First, a window is made in the mesocolon to the right of the middle colic artery. The proximal jejunum is placed into the supracolic compartment through the mesocolon window. End of the CBD is trimmed freshly and end to side choledochojejunsotomy is performed with single layer interrupted 2-0 vicryl suture. Corner sutures are made in 'U' fashion. 2-0 vicryl is preferred in the presence of dilated thick walled common bile duct. We found it easy to make biliary enteric anastomosis before pancreatic anastomosis.

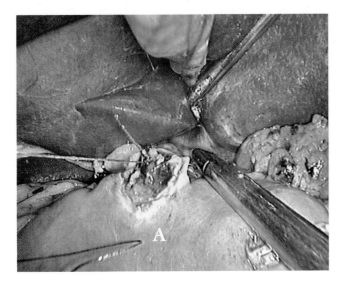

Figure 26 : Posterior layer of end to side choledochojejunal anastomosis

A - Jejunum

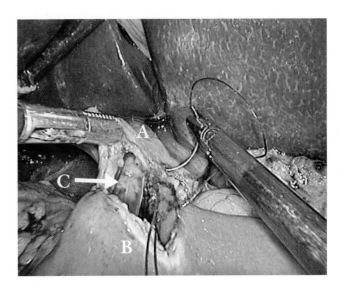

Figure 27 : Anterior layer of choledochojejunal anastomosis

A - Common bile duct
B - Jejunum
C - Decompression tube

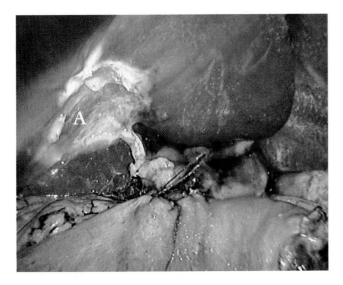

Figure 28 : Completion of end to side choledochojejunal anastomosis

A - Gallbladder bed

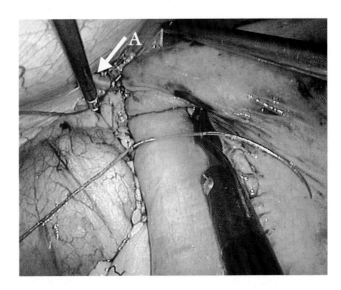

Figure 29 : Fixation of jejunal loop to the lateral wall

A - Jejunal decompression tube

Pancreaticojejunal Anastomosis

The proximal jejunum is traced, keeping an adequate length from the choledochojejunal anastomosis to the pancreatic stump. Suturing begins from the cranial edge. Few silk stitches are placed from sero-muscular layer of jejunum to the posterior side of the pancreas. Stitches posterior to the pancreatic duct should be avoided since the pancreatic tissue is too thin posteriorly that it could injure the duct. I have found that thin 3-0 prolene is better for approximating the edge of the pancreatic stump to the end of jejunum. At the level of pancreatic duct, the mucosa is approximated with mucosa of the jejunum. At the completion of the posterior anastomosis, a 5F or 7F stent is placed and there is no need to bring the stent outside for drainage. Chromic stitch holds temporarily for 2-3 weeks after which the stent passes away. If the surgeon wants to drain it outside, an infant feeding tube of 5F or 7F size or according to the size of the pancreatic duct can be placed in the duct and brought beyond the choledochojejunal anastomosis through a separate stab wound in the jejunum and sutured with purse string suture and this is exteriorized through a separate stab wound. A jejunal drain of 12-14F side is placed in the Roux loop through a lateral stab incision intracorporeally used as a stent across the

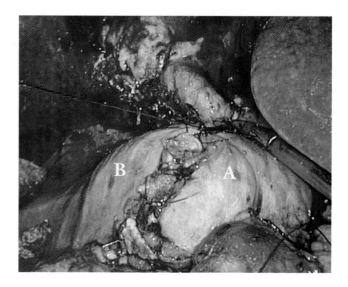

Figure 31 : Completion of pancreticojejunostomy

A - Pancreas
B - Jejunum

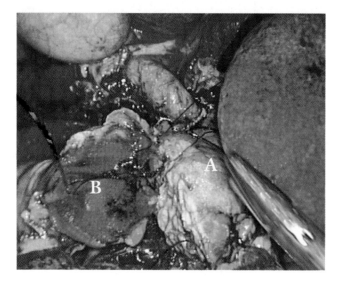

Figure 30 : Posterior layer of end to end pancreaticojejuno-stomy

A - Pancreas
B - Jejunum

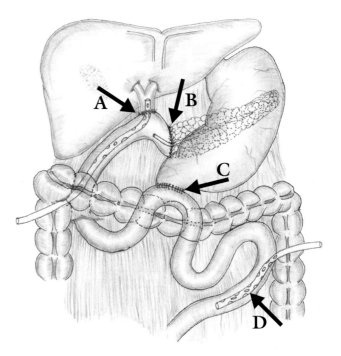

Figure 32 : Diagram shows the anastomosis after whipple's procedure

A - Choledochojejunal anastomosis
B - Pancreaticojejunal anastomosis
C - Duodenojejunal anastomosis
D - Feeding jejunostomy tube

choledochojejunal anastomosis, and fixed with purse string suture. This drain is brought out through one of the trocar entry sites. A tube drain is kept in the flank separately. Finally the entire port site wound is closed with subcuticular vicryl.

Pancreaticogastric Anastomosis

Initially we used to do pancreaticojejunostomy in the reconstructive procedure. But in the last 10 cases we have done pancreaticogastrostomy instead of pancreaticojejunostomy. Though it is technically difficult compared to pancreaticojejunostomy, the leak rate is numerically less in our series. In this reconstructive step, first we use to mobilize the proximal 2-3 cm of the cut end of pancreas from the splenic vessels and retroperitoneum. Then pancreaticogastrostomy is performed by invaginating the pancreatic stump into the posterior wall of lower part of stomach in two layers. The outer layer of the anastomosis is done by approximating the seromuscular layer of the posterior wall of stomach to the pancreatic surface using 3-0 prolene continuous sutures. The inner layer is done by approximating the full thickness of stomach wall with transected pancreatic parenchyma using 2-0 vicryl continuous suture. We keep pancreatic stent routinely in the laparoscopic group, unless the pancreatic duct is not dilated.

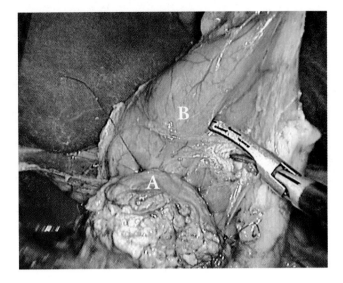

Figure 34 : Completion of seromuscular prolene suture. Gastrotomy using harmonic scalpel

A - Pancreas

B - Posterior layer of stomach

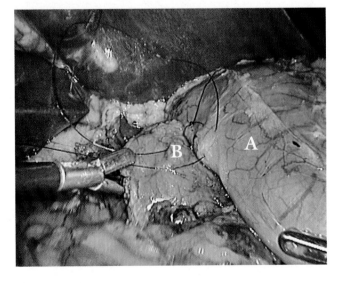

Figure 33 : Posterior layer of pancreaticogastric anastomosis

A - Pancreas

B - Posterior layer of stomach

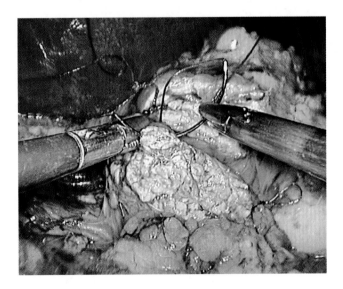

Figure 35 : performing posterior layer of end to side pancreatico gastric anastomosis

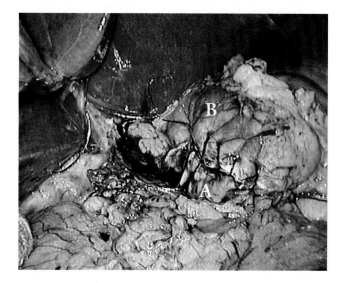

Figure 36 : Completion of pancreaticogastric anastomosis

A - Pancreas
B - Posterior layer of stomach

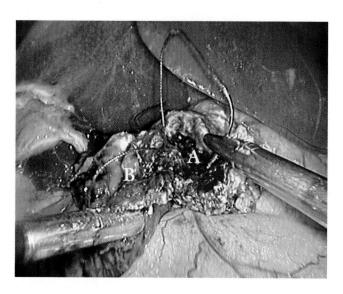

Figure 37 : Performing posterior layer of end to end duodenojejunostomy using 2 0 vicryl

A - Duodenum
B - Jejunum

PHASE IV

Extraction and Duodeno Jejunal Anastomosis

The camera port is vertically extended by 4-6 cm and the endobag with the specimen is removed. This facilitates the construction of gastro intestinal continuity by extracorporeal approach. First pyloromyotomy is performed which prevents prolonged gastric stasis in the postoperative period. The edges of the duodenum are trimmed freshly and end to side anastomosis is performed, 30-40cm distal to the divided end of the jejunum. After replacing the bowel inside the peritoneal cavity the wound is closed and camera trocar is reintroduced. Gastrointestinal continuity may be performed intracorporeally by hand sewn technique, which we did in a small series of our cases.

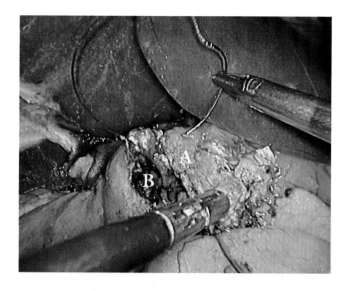

Figure 38 : Anterior layer of duodenojejunostomy

A - Duodenum
B - Jejunum

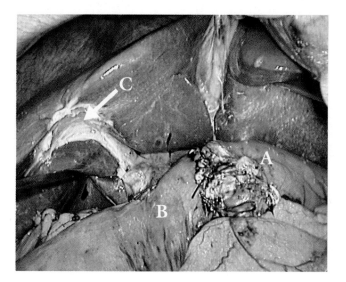

Figure 39 : Completion of hand sewn end to end duodenojejunal anastomosis

A - Duodenum
B - Jejunum
C - Gall bladder bed

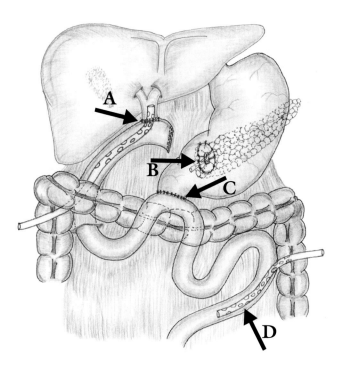

Figure 40 : Diagram shows the anastomosis after whipple's procedure

A - Choledochojejunal anastomosis
B - Pancreaticogastric anastomosis
C - Duodenojejunal anastomosis
D - Feeding jejunostomy tube

RESULTS

The total number of cases is 35 of which 19 male and 16 female. The age varies from 28 to 63 years. Mean age is 48.7 years. The indications were ampullary growth (23), carcinoma head of pancreas (7) lower CBD growth (3) and duodenal carcinoma (2). Mean duration of surgery is 6.4 hours (400 mt). The first case took 680 minutes (11½ hours) to finish and the last case we could manage to complete in 310 minutes (5 hrs 10 min). The average blood loss was 395ml. The mean post operative high dependency unit (HDU) stay was 3.2 days and the average hospital stay was 10.2 days. Table shows the demographic profile and compare various parameters of laparoscopic and open Whipple's procedure during 1998-2005 at GEM hospital, Coimbatore, India. The mortality and morbidity comparision between open and laparoscopic Whipple's procedure during 1998-2005 is shown in Table 2.

All the patients had excellent recovery except for one who had prolonged gastric stasis. Post operative pain was very minimal and all were mobilized on the 1st or 2nd post operative day. Most of them passed flatus after 48 hours, the mean being 2.2 days. Jejunal enteral tube feeding was started on the 2nd or 3rd post operative day. Wound infection was virtually absent. None of them had post operative pulmonary complications like atelectasis or pneumonia. There were two pancreatic leak in our series so far. One of the patients developed features of cholangitis which was subsided with change of antibiotics. I personally feel that placing the gastroenteric anastomosis in the infracolic compartment, 30-40 cm distal to the biliary and pancreatic anastomosis will help in early recovery of gastro intestinal function.

One of the patients had prolonged gastric stasis, for which we did laparotomy on the 12th post operative day. Oesophago Gastro Duodenoscopy (OGD) revealed stomal edema and stenosis. This was due to the ischaemic damage caused by the temporary endoloop applied at the gastric stump to prevent the spillage of gastric contents after the transection. Failure to trim the edges had lead to ischaemic changes at the anastomotic site leading to stenosis. The stoma was incised and widened as we do in pyloroplasty. Insufflation of the stomach showed free

Table 1: Demographic profile of Laparoscopic Vs Open Whipple's Group between 1998 - 2005 at GEM hospital

Description	Laparoscopy	Open
Total No. of patients	35	124
Male	19	68
Female	16	56
Age group in years	28-63	27-66
(Mean)	(48.7)	(44.8)
ASA Grade	I & II	I, II & III
Indications		
Ampullary tumors	23	61
Distal CBD tumours	3	22
Early CA head of pancreas	7	26
Duodenal carcinoma	2	6
Others	-	9
Procedure		
Pancreatico jejunostomy	25	90
Pancreaticogastostomy	10	34
Operative time in hours	5.1 - 11½	2½ - 6½
(Mean)	(6.4)	(4.12)
Mean blood loss	395ml	435ml
HDU stay in days	2 - 6	3 - 8
(Mean)	(3.2)	(4.4)
Total hospital stay in days	10.2	13.3
(Mean)	(8 - 14)	(11 - 22)
Mobilisation started on	1st POD	3rd POD
Jejunostomy feed started	3rd POD	4th POD
Passed Flatus (Mean)	2.2	4.4
Passed stool (Mean)	4.8	7.3

Table 2 : Mortality and Morbidity comparison between open and laparoscopic Whipple's procedure during 1998 - 2005 at GEM hospital

Description	Laparoscopy	Open
Total No.	35	124
30 day mortality	Nil	5 (4%)
Complications		
Nil	25	79
Delayed Gastric Emptying	3	8
Pancreatic leak	1	12
Bile leak	2	11
Hemorrhage	1	4
Intra abdominal abscess	1	3
ARDS-SEPSIS	1	5
DJ stomal edema	1	Nil
Wound dehesence	Nil	2
Wound infection	Nil	15
Incisional hernia	Nil	4
Follow up (mean)	3month - 7yrs (3 ½ yr)	1 month - 7 yrs (4 yr)
3yr survival rate for periampullary adenocarcinoma	62.25%	52.02%

entry of air into the jejunum. Post operative recovery was so quick that the patient was started on oral fluids on the 2nd day of reexploration. After this, we have been using Endo GIA stapler in all cases to divide the duodenum. We routinely administer somastostatin analogue (Octride) 8 hourly to suppress the pancreatic function for 3 days post operatively. In case of dilated pancreatic duct and satisfactory anastomosis with a stent, pancreatic suppression may not be required. Fibrin glue on the anastomotic surface prevents leakage. We usually insert feeding jejunostomy in all cases so that enteral feeding can be started early. It is our routine practice to remove the pancreatic and jejunostomy tubes as outpatient when they come for follow up after a week to 10 days of discharge. We have used erythromycin tablet 500mg tid in few of our open surgery patients who had prolonged stasis but not in any of the laparoscopic group.

In this small series we don't have any mortality. Morbidity has been well reduced to 10-20% when compared to 30-40% of open method. The percentage of pancreatic and biliary leak may be similar or less to that of open method, wound infection and post operative pulmonary complications are virtually absent in laparoscopic group.

CONCLUSION

When compared to open method, laparoscopic procedure clearly emphasizes the better outcome with less morbidity of the patient. Proper selection of patient is mandatory in order to assure a successful operation. It should be performed by an experienced team of surgeons in both advanced laparoscopic surgeries and heaptopancreatico biliary surgeries. To prove that it is oncologically sound, a large number of patients have to be randomized for longer duration. Whether in future this complex laparoscopic procedure with extensive gastro intestinal anastomosis should be allowed in routine practice is still debatable. With the new inventions of high-tech instrumentation and with greater experience and knowledge, experienced surgeons in dedicated gastro intestinal institutions will be able to practice this procedure.

References

1. Gagner M. Laparoscopic duodenopancreatectomy. In : Steichen F, Welter R, eds. Minimally invasive surgery and technology. St. Louis : Quality Medical Publishing, 1994:192-199

2. Gagner M, Pomp A. Laparoscopic pylorus-preserving pancreatoduodenectomy, Surg Endosc 1994 May;8(5):408-10

3. Genitileschi P, Gagner M. Laparoscopic pancreatic resection, Chir Ital 2001 May-Jun;53(3):279-89

4. Jones DB, Wu JS, Soper NJ. Laparoscopic pancreaticoduodenectomy in the porcine model, Surg Endosc 1997 Apr;11(4):326-30

5. Palanivelu C. Laparoscopic Pylorus preserving pancreatoduodenectomy, SAGES meet in Atlanda 2000, SAGES Video Library 2000 (Catalog).

6. Palanivelu C, Laparoscopic Pylorus preserving pancreatoduodenectomy, In the Text book of Laparoscopy Ed Palanivelu C, Gem Digestive Diseases Foundation 2002, 373-382

7. Palanivelu C, Laparoscopic Whipple's Operation, In CIGES Atlas of Laparoscopic Surgery Ed Palanivelu, JAYPEE publishers 2003, Lippincott Williams Wilkinson, 201-209

8. Palanivelu C. Laparoscopic Pylorus preserving pancreatoduodenectomy. 7th World Congress of Endoscopic Surgery abstract book 2000, Singapore

9. Palanivelu C. Laparoscopic pancreatic surgery. Journal of international medical science academy, Vol.14 No.3;2001:137-139

10. Uyama I, Ogiwara H, Iida S, Takahara T, Laparoscopic minilaparotomy pancreaticoduodenectomy with lymphadenectomy using an abdominal wall-lift method. Surg Laparosc Endosc 1996 Oct;6(5):405-10

11. Wilentz, R.E. and Hruban, R.H : pathology of cancer of the pancreas. Surg.Oncol.Clin. North Am., 7:43, 1998

12. Halsted, W.S. : Contributions to the surgery of the bile passages, especially of the common bile duct. Boston Med. Surg J., 141:645, 1899

13. Sauve, L : Des Pancreatectomies et specialement de la pancreatectomie cephalique. Rev. Chir (Chir) 37:335, 1908

14. Kausch, W.: Das carcinom der Papilla duodeni and seine radikale enfeinung. Beitr Z. Clin. Chir., 78:439, 1912

15. Whipple, A.O., Parson, W.B., and Mullins, C.R. : Treatment of carcinoma of the ampulla of Vater. Ann. Surg.102:763, 1935

16. Traverso, L.W., Longmire, W.P : Preservation of the pylorus in pancreaticoduodenectomy. Surg. Gynecol. Obster., 146:959, 1978

17. Gagner M, Pomp A. Laparoscopic pylorus-preserving pancreatoduodenectomy. Surg Endosc 1994;8:408-10

18. Cuschieri A, Jakimowicz JJ. Laparoscopic pancreatic resection. Semin Laparosc Surg 1998;5:168-79

19. Milone L., Turner P., Gagner M., Laparoscopic surgery for pancreatic tumours, an update. Minerva Chirugica. 59:165-73, 2004

20. Cuschieri A. Laparoscopic pancreatic resections. Semin Laparosc Surg 1996;3:15-20

21. Patterson EJ, Gagner M, Salky B, Inabnet WB, Brower S, Edye M et al. Laparoscopic pancreatic resection: single-institution experience of 19 patients. J Am Coll Surg 2001;193:281-7

22. Tagaya N, Kasama K, Suzuki N, Taketsuka S, Horie K, Kubota K et al. Laparoscopic resection of the pancreas and review of the literature. Surg Endosc 2003; 17:201-6

23. Gentileschi P, Gagner M. Laparoscopic pancreatic resection. In: Cueto-Garcia J, Jacobs M, Gagner M editors. Laparoscopic surgery. New York: McGraw-Hill; 2003. p.385-92

24. Menack MJ, Splitz JD, Aregui ME. Staging of pancreatic and ampullary cancer for respectability using laparoscopy with laparoscopic ultrasound. Surg Endosc 2001;15:1129-34

25. Mayo W 1901; Cancer of common bile duct. Report of a case of carcinima of the duodenal end of the common bile duct with successful excision: St. Paul Medical Journal 3;374

26. C. Palanivelu, CIGES Atlas of Laparoscopic Surgery (2003). Laparoscopic Whipple's Operation; 7:34, p 201-212

27. Palanivelu's Text Book of Surgical Laparoscopy. Laparoscopic pancreatico duodenectomy - Whipple's operation. 2002; VI : 373-384

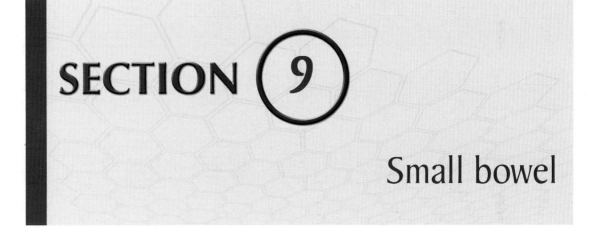

SECTION ⑨

Small bowel

58

Laparoscopic Appendectomy

INTRODUCTION

Appendectomy continues to be one of the commonest procedures in general surgery. Reginald Fitz coined the term "Appendectomy" for removal of inflamed appendix as a cure in 1886. McBurney popularized the concept of early surgery and the muscle splitting incision technique.[9] Even though modern diagnostic facilities, surgical skill, fluids and antibiotic therapy have brought down the mortality from 50% (before 1925) to less than 1 per 1,00,000 persons, still the morbidity is more than 5-8% mainly due to wound infection and delayed diagnosis and treatment. Laparoscopy has so much to offer for the early diagnosis and treatment of appendicitis with least morbidity.

In 1982, Kurt Semm performed the first successful laparoscopic appendectomy.[11] Schreiber, another German gynaecologist reported his small series of laparoscopic appendectomy for acute appendici-tis. Only after the report of 625 cases of laparoscopic appendectomy with superb results by Pier & associates in 1991, the role of laparoscopy for appendciitis became popular.[7] Still laparoscopic appendectomy has not attained the popularity of laparoscopic cholecystectomy, since many have described different techniques with varied results. There is no uniformity in placement of trocars and techniques of laparoscopic appendectomy. After the experience of over 6500 laparoscopic appendectomies in my department since 1991, I consider laparoscopic appendectomy should be the standard approach for removal of the diseased appendix, irrespective of its anatomical and pathological types. The highest success rate and least complications are due to the two hand technique of my own which I continue to practice since 1991. Surgeons trained in this technique are all producing excellent results.

The advantages of laparoscopic appendectomy includes diminished post operative pain, early return to work, decreased wound infection, better cosmesis, ability to explore the entire peritoneal cavity for diagnosis of other conditions and effective peritoneal toilet without the need for extending the incision.

Potential Advantages of Laparoscopic Appendectomy

1. Allows thorough exploration of peritoneal cavity.
2. Allows definitive treatment for non-appendiceal lesions.
3. Reduced hospital stay.
4. Avoids negative or unnecessary laparotomy.
5. No need for extension of incision for abnormal location of appendix.
6. Minimum postoperative discomfort and narcotic requirement.
7. Early resumption of routine work.
8. Reduced incidence of complications - wound infection, post-operative adhesions, incisional hernia, infertility.
9. Improved cosmetic result.
10. Allows thorough peritoneal toilet in case of appendicular perforation.

INDICATIONS

The indications for laparoscopic appendectomy are almost the same as in conventional appendectomy. There are specific indications for those who follow the selective applications of laparoscopic approach.

1. Appendicitis in obese patient and young women.
2. When the diagnosis is in doubt.
3. Diagnosis of appendicitis at unusual positions.
4. Normal looking appendix on laparoscopy in the absence of other pathology.
5. Incidental appendectomy along with other laparoscopic procedures should be considered when the appendix is found to be diseased or highly prone for inflammation e.g. long, kinked with faecolith and narrow base, etc.

RELATIVE CONTRAINDICATIONS

The following relative contra-indications should be considered in choosing the approach:

1. Inexperience with the technique, difficult anatomical position, severely inflamed appendix, perforated appendicitis with or without peritonitis and appendicular abscess should be considered as relative contraindications.
2. Prior lower abdominal surgery.
3. Pelvic inflammatory disease and endometriosis.
4. Pregnancy.

ABSOLUTE CONTRAINDICATIONS

1. Suspicion of malignancy.
2. Severe co-morbid illness pulmonary / cardiac disorders
3. Patient on radiotherapy and immuno-compromised pateints

The surgeon should be ready for conversion in case of difficulty and this should not be considered as a complication or failure, instead it represents a sound clinical judgement for safe removal of appendix.

Incidence

Acute appendicitis is a very common abdominal emergency, accounting for 1% of all surgical operations.[8] Common age group affected is 5-30 years and it is sometimes encountered in infants as well. Below the age of 25 years, males are affected more and above 25 years the incidence is equal in both the sexes.

Symptoms

Initially, the pain of appendicitis is periumbilical and moves to the right iliac fossa in about 7 hours. 75% of patients present within 24 hours of occurrence of pain.[1] Anorexia, nausea, vomiting and altered bowels are the other common symptoms. In case of appendicular abscess, a tender mass is palpable in the right iliac fossa. There will also be fever, tachycardia, local guarding, diarrhea (irritation of rectum) and frequency of micturition (irritation of bladder). In pelvic appendicitis and in obese patients, abdominal symptoms are minimal. Perforated appendix presents as peritonitis localized or generalized.

Signs

The physical signs of acute appendicitis are due to local peritoneal irritation in the right iliac fossa.

Tenderness and localized guarding are most common at the McBurney's point. In retrocecal position, tenderness is over a larger area without guarding. In pelvic appendicitis, neither pain nor guarding is present. Rebound tenderness, Rovsing sign (pain in right iliac fossa on pressing in left iliac fossa) and pain on coughing are the classical signs. Mass in the right iliac fossa is caused by adherence of omentum, ileum, cecum and in females, adnexa. Abscess will also form a mass. Psoas sign-raising the right leg while supine elicits pain is due to irritation of psoas muscle by the inflamed appendix. Ruptured appendix will give rise to generalized peritonitis. If it is localized, appendicular abscess is formed.

Incidence of appendicular perforation in infants is high and the mortality is high due to delayed diagnosis. Early surgery should be done in presence of appendicitis increased infant mortality is due to delay in diagnosis. Appendectomy should be done if it is suspected in all trimesters of pregnancy, general anaesthesia may be avoided during the 1st trimester.

COMPLICATIONS OF APPENDICITIS

It is mostly due to perforation of a gangrenous appendicitis.[10]

1. Wound infection (10-12% in appendicitis and 35-75% in perforation).[8]
2. Septicemia.
3. Generalised peritonitis.
4. Localised peritonitis.
5. Abscess.
6. Fecal fistula (giving way of the stump).
7. Recurrent intestinal obstruction (due to adhesions).
8. Pylephlebitis (due to portal pyemia).
9. Hemorrhage (slipping of ligature of pedicle).
10. Appendicovesical fistula (very rare).
11. Death (overall mortality rate in non-perforated appendicitis is 0.5%, in the perforated group, it is 1.18%. Above 60 years of age it is 6-14% and is mainly due to the high incidence of perforation).[8]

Differential Diagnosis

Children: Gastroenteritis, mesenteric lymphadenitis, Meckels diverticulitis (incidence is 0.3-0.4%),[10] pyelitis, small bowel intussusception, enteric duplication, basal pneumonia and sickle cell crisis.

Young Men: Acute regional enteritis, right renal or ureteric calculi, torsion testis, acute epididymoorchitis, infective hepatitis and Munchausen syndrome.

Young Women: Ruptured ectopic pregnancy, Mittelschmerz, endometriosis, salpingitis, regional enteritis and chronic constipation.

Elderly: Diverticulitis, perforated peptic ulcer, acute cholecystitis, acute pancreatitis, intestinal obstruction, perforated caecal carcinoma, mesenteric vascular occlusion, ruptured aortic aneurysm, right renal and ureteric calculi, diabetic ketoacidosis and coronary thrombosis.

Investigations and Diagnosis

It must be remembered that acute appendicitis is essentially a clinical diagnosis, there is no laboratory or radiological test yet that is 100% diagnostic. In the early stages, laboratory tests are of little value. Almost 1/3 patients will have normal total WBC count. More than half will have mild elevation. There is evidence to suggest that total and differential counts do not correlate well with the degree of inflammation. Clinical diagnosis should take precedence over laboratory tests. Other tests like C-reactive protein estimation are of limited use. Urinalysis is helpful for differential diagnosis.

X-Ray in general, cannot be used for confirming the diagnosis. Findings which suggest appendicitis are cecal distension, sentinel loop of small bowel in right iliac fossa and mass outside the cecum.

USG and CT scan-USG done by a good sonologist has an accuracy greater than 90%.[2] The diagnosis is made by: a maximal cross-sectional diameter of more than 6mm, noncompressibility, fecolith, mass, abscess and periappendicular fluid. Many studies have proved CT scan as having more accuracy than USG.[8] Recent developments include radionuclide imaging studies that are supposed to be highly accurate in diagnosis. Diagnostic laparoscopy has a sensitivity and specificity of 100%, as evidenced by many studies.[5]

SURGICAL ANATOMY

Appendix is a vestigeal organ situated on the posteromedial aspect of the cecum 2.5cm below the ileocecal valve. It is the only organ in the body that has no constant position. The base arises from where the three tenia coli meet. Length varies from 1cm to 25cm. The various positions are retrocecal (65.28%), pelvic (31%), subcecal (2.26%), preileal (1%) and postileal (0.4%).[7] Subhepatic and lateral pouch are very rare sites.[25] Unusually, the appendix may be present in the right hypochondrium (inflammation can mimic cholecystitis), in the left iliac fossa or in the epigastrium (in malrotation of gut).

Embryologically, appendix is part of the cecum and histologically they resemble each other except for the abundance of lymphoid tissue in the submucous layer of the appendix. The mesoappendix is continuous with the lower leaf of the small bowel mesentery as it passes behind the terminal ileum. The appendicular artery runs on the free border of the mesoappendix and is a branch of the ileocolic artery. The artery runs parallel to the appendix and ends at the tip. It gives off small branches that run perpendicular to the organ. This pattern is important during dissection of mesoappendix and ligation of the pedicle. This is the only arterial supply to the organ, which is why thrombosis (due to appendicitis) can cause gangrene and perforation. Rarely, an accessory appendicular artery is present.

PRINCIPLES

The treatment of appendicitis is very important because it is the most common major abdominal emergency requiring surgery. The basic rule is - 'Sooner the better'.[9]

ROLE OF LAPAROSCOPY

Suspected Appendicitis

The incidence of negative laparotomy in patients suspected to have appendicitis is 20%. Diagnostic laparoscopy has reduced this rate to 10%. It is especially useful in fertile women and obese patients. The rate of perforation has also reduced. The earlier dictum was 'when in doubt, take it out'. This has now changed to 'when in doubt, check it out'.[9]

Laparoscopy is a very valuable tool in the situation where diagnosis is in doubt.[5] Not only can the appendix be visualized, other organs can be inspected as well. It is far superior access than a McBurney incision gives. If there is appendicitis, laparoscopic appendectomy offers all the benefits of minimally invasive therapy like less pain, shorter hospital stay, early return to work and physical activity and better cosmesis.[14] Obese patients benefit more from laparoscopy because they would need a larger incision than thin patients, whereas in laparoscopy the trocars are the same for both. Infection rate is probably lower as the pelvis can be irrigated thoroughly which is not possible in open method.

Some centers prefer a dual approach open appendectomy for thin, young men with classical appendicitis and laparoscopic approach for suspected appendicitis, obese patients and premenopausal women.[9] We perform laparoscopic approach for all pathological or anatomical type of appendicitis.

Accuracy of Diagnosis (Open vs Laparoscopy-175 cases)				
	PPV (%)	FP (%)	NPV (%)	FN (%)
Open	91	1	74	26
Laparoscopy	96.5	0	95	5

PPV - Positive Predictive Value, FP - False Positive

NPV - Negative Predictive Value, FN - False Negative

Indications for appendectomy during diagnostic laparoscopy and incidental appendectomy as part of other procedure:

1. Acute appendicitis
2. Normal examination (No other pathology)
3. Large fecolith
4. Recurring pathology
5. Long kinked appendix

Even if the examination is normal, appendectomy is to be done to simplify the future differential diagnosis of pelvic pain and to treat early mucosal (catarrhal) appendicitis which may not be obvious macroscopically. If some other surgical pathology is identified, it should be treated laparoscopically if possible.

INSTRUMENTATION

Basic equipment is enough for the procedure but it is wise to use good quality for this or any procedure. A 30^0 telescope, xenon light source, 3-chip camera, medical monitor, electronic CO_2 insufflator, bipolar forceps, ligaclips with applicator, suction/irrigation device, scissors, atraumatic graspers, endoloop ligatures and tissue extraction bag are the usual equipments used. Harmonic shears is highly useful in removing difficult appendix, either due to anatomical position (retrocecal) or pathological condition (mass).

PATIENT PREPARATION

Prophylactic antibiotics are given perioperatively, patient made to pass urine before induction of anesthesia. Indwelling Foley's catheter and nasogastric tube are placed if there is gaseous distension of stomach imperforated appendix. The beginner is advised to do so in all cases.

PRINCIPLES

1. Primary trocar placement open/close technique.
2. In case of previous surgery, place trocar away from scar site (open technique is preferable).
3. In blunt dissection, keeping close to lateral abdominal wall.
4. Avoid unnecessary handling of bowel.
5. Minimize contamination.
6. Avoid peritoneal spillage.

TECHNIQUE OF LAPAROSCOPIC APPENDECTOMY

Patient position and room setup

As with all laparoscopic procedures, basic principles of exposure, retraction, and ligation or coagulation of the blood vessels should be considered in positioning the patient and placing the trocars. Patients are usually placed in the supine position with left lateral tilt, reverse Trendelenburg's in high-placed appendix and Trendelenburg's in low-placed appendix. Split leg position is indicated for pelvic exploration in female patient.

Port Position

The pneumoperitoneum is created with closed Veress needle or open Hasson cannula technique. I prefer closed needle technique in all except in patients with perforative peritonitis or with distended bowel loops. The first 10mm trocar is inserted blindly at the umbilicus. Two additional trocars are placed under video guidance. The second suprapubic port (10, 5 or 3 mm - depending upon the telescope size available) is made 2-3 cm cranial to the pubic symphysis to protect injury to the dome of urinary bladder. Before entering the peritoneal cavity, facing the tip of the trocar towards the right lower quadrant the avoids injury to the major vessels. The telescope is then shifted from the umbilicus to the suprapubic port and it continues to be the camera port till the end of the procedure. The third port (3mm or 5mm) is placed in the right iliac fossa, at a level slightly caudal to the base of the appendix for the working left hand. I have adopted this approach in over 6500 cases and it appears to be simple and effective. The camera at the suprapubic port gives perfect triangulation and any anatomical type of appendix can be easily approached. It also allows direct exposure of the base of appendix and ileocaecal junction. The right iliac fossa port helps in manipulation of the appendix according to the need with the left hand of the surgeon for two hand manipulation. Fourth cannula is occasionally placed for retraction of the distended ileum or caecum. Though 0 degree is sufficient, 30 degree angled scope is preferred in difficult situations. Umbilical port is used as right hand working port for dissection, coagulation and division of meso-appendix and for extraction of the appendix.

Division of Mesoappendix

The appendix is held with a grasper by the left hand to mobilize the appendix from the caecum. A clip is applied at the base of the mesoappendix which minimizes bleeding during division and adhesiolysis is performed. Monopolar cautery with scissors is used to divide the mesoappendix distal to the clip. The

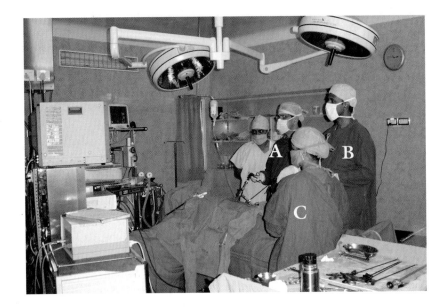

Figure 1 : Team setup

A - Surgeon
B - Camera surgeon
C - Staff nurse

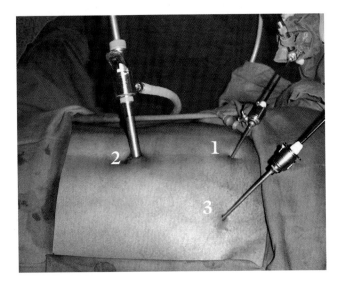

Figure 2 : Port position

No.	Instruments	Site
1	Camera	Suprapubic 5 mm
2	Right hand working port	Umbilicus 10mm
3	Left hand working port	Right iliac fossa 3mm

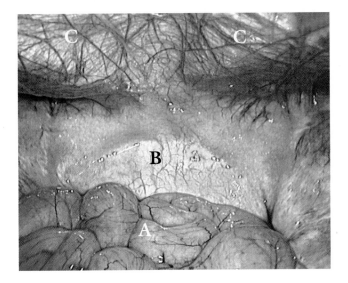

Figure 3 : Laparoscopic view of pelvis

A - Small bowel

B - Urinary bladder

C - Rectus muscle

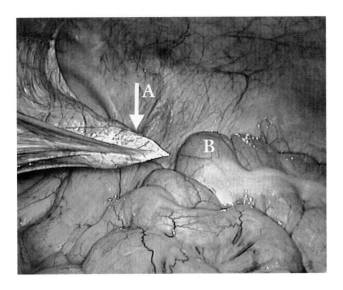

Figure 4 : Suprapubic port placement under laparoscopic guidance

A - 5mm trocar introduced vertically just above the bladder dome and directed towards the caecum before piercing the peritoneum

B - Cecum

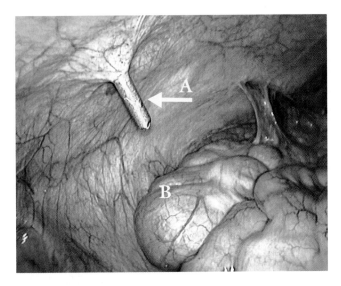

Figure 5 : Placement of left hand working port at the level of ileocaecal junction

A - Left hand working port

B - Cecum

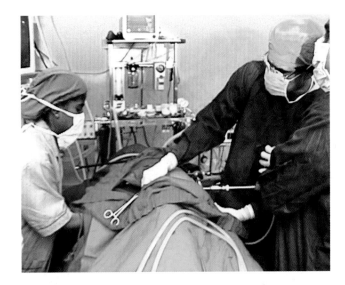

Figure 6 : Placing the sand bag below the level of the ileocecal junction. It displaces the small bowel to the left side and exposes the cecum and the base of the appendix

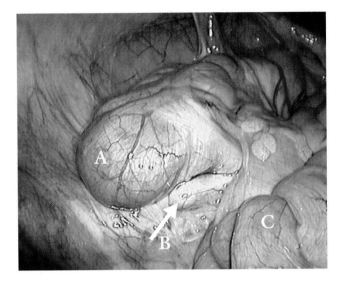

Figure 7 : Displacement of small bowel after placing the sand bag

A - Cecum
B - Appendix
C - Small bowel

remaining mesoappendix is stripped bit by bit by using curved dissector and haemostasis is achieved using electrocautery applied carefully keeping the tissue away from the appendico-caecal junction. Excessive use of electrocautery may cause thermal injury. During the skeletonization of the appendix, the level of the base has to be repeated to avoid cecal injury. In case of harmonic scalpel or bipolar diathermy use, there is no need for proximal clipping of the mesoappendix. If the appendix is not visible by simple retraction of the caecum, the peritoneum along the lateral border is divided and the caecum is retracted medially and cranially to expose the posterior surface of cecum. The retrocaecal appendix is thus identified. In case of retroileal, appendix patient is placed in Trendelenburg's position and all the small bowel loops are displaced cranially. In addition to lateral division of peritoneum, the peritoneal incision is extended medially caudal to the mesenteric attachment and the avascular tissue lateral to the appendix is stripped by blunt dissection till the tip of the appendix is reached. In these types there may be multiple branches of the appendicular artery which need to be clipped before dividing , because it is difficult to approach them after

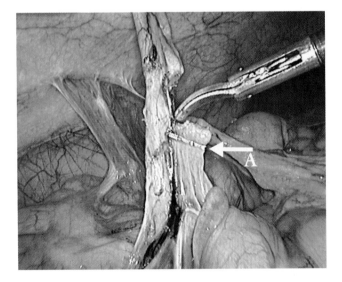

Figure 8 : Division of mesoappendix using scissors with monopolar electrocautery after clipping

A - Clip on the mesoappendix

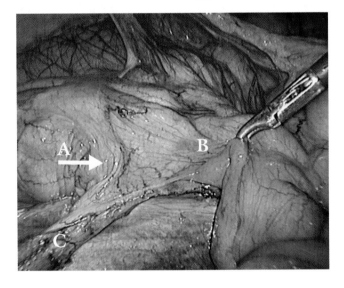

Figure 9 : Identify the base of the appendix by tracing the tenia coli

A - Tenia coli on the anterior surface of cecum
B - Ileocecal junction
C - Appendix

division. Sometimes it may be required to mobilise the peritoneum along the lateral border till the hepatic flexure for complete exposure. In 25 of our cases, the caecum was subhepatic and the appendix was lying between the liver, gallbladder and the cecum. In 7 patients, the appendix was lying close to the second part of the duodenum under cover of the peritoneum.

Ligation and division of appendix

Two self made pre-tied endoloops (2-0 chromic catgut) are applied at the base using a plastic knot. The distance between these 2 loops should be less than 5 mm. The first loop should not be too tight. In case of acutely inflamed appendix care must be taken to avoid cut through of the appendix while applying the loop. A third optional loop is applied about 1 cm distal to the second to enable cutting in between the two. If the appendix contains pus or faecolith, curved dissector is used to milk it upto the body from the base. The thread is kept long without cutting to control the appendix from outside to prevent contamination of the peritoneal cavity and also to enable extraction of appendix through the umbilical trocar.

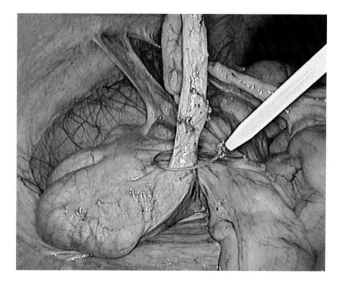

Figure 11 : Application of endoloop to the base of the appendix

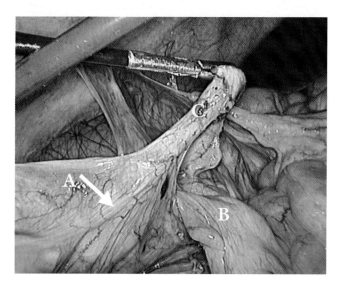

Figure 10 : Identify the base of the appendix

A - Tenia coli on the posterior surface of caecum

B - Terminal ileum

C - Appendix

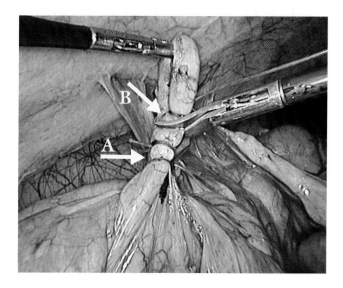

Figure 12 : Division of the appendix after applying endoloop

A - Two endoloops on the base

B - Third loop to prevent the spillage and to hold the appendix after division

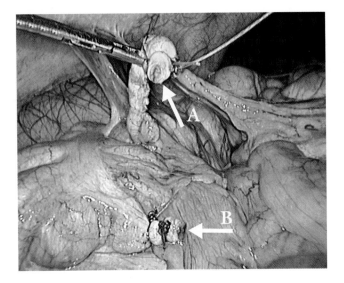

Figure 13 : Appendix after division

A - Divided appendix

B - Base of the appendix

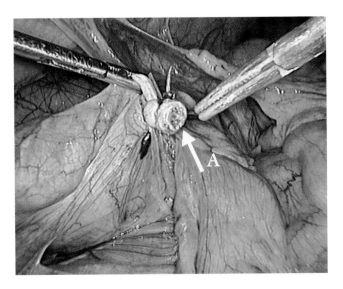

Figure 14 : Cauterising the mucosa of the base

A - Judicial application of caurtery to the mucosa using curved dissector

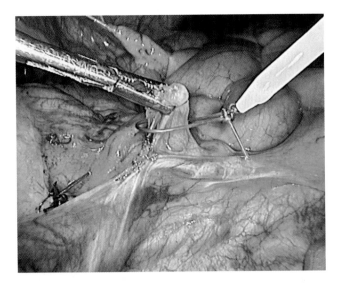

Figure 15 : Application of endoloop to the divided mesoappendix

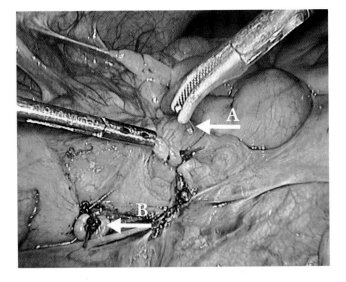

Figure 16 : Clip is removed after applying the endoloop

A - Clip

B - Base of the appendix

Peritoneal toilet and drainage tube

The operative area is thoroughly irrigated in the following order: pelvis, paracolic gutters and both subdiaphragmatic areas. In the presence of generalized peritonitis, peritoneal cavity can be effectively cleared of the infected fluid by repeated irrigation

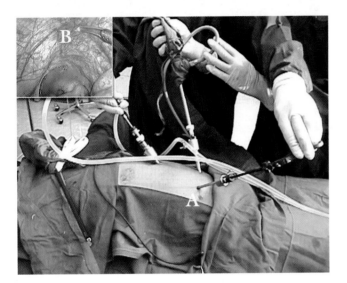

Figure 17 : Peritoneal toileting of the pelvis. All the trocars are facing the pelvis, left hand instrument retracting the small bowel and pouch of Douglas is exposed

A - Left hand instrument
B - Washing of pelvis

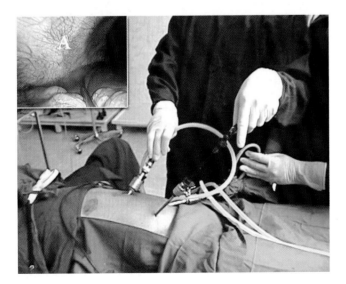

Figure 18 : Peritoneal toileting on the sub diaphragmatic area, all the trocars are facing the right hypochondrium

A - Washing of right subdiaphragmatic space

and suction. Drainage tube is kept through the lateral trocar into the pelvis.

APPENDECTOMY IN SPECIAL SITUATIONS : COMPLICATED APPENDICITIS

Appendicular Mass

In the presence of large inflammatory phlegmon, identifying the appendix sometimes becomes very difficult. In those cases omental attachment is freed first. Then small and large bowels are freed by dividing inflammatory adhesions by blunt dissection. Some prefer blunt dissection using a cylindrical gauze. I do not practice any gauze dissection.

Extraction of the Appendix

After separating the appendix from the cecum, it can be removed by keeping it in an impermeable bag. This prevents contamination of the abdominal wall. The appendix can also be removed by bringing it first into the reducing sleeve and the appendix along with the sleeve is brought out through the umbilical port. After delivery, the appendicular stump is sterilised in two ways: (i) touching it with a small povidine gauze or (ii) cauterising the mucosa with a forceps using electrocautery. One should be very

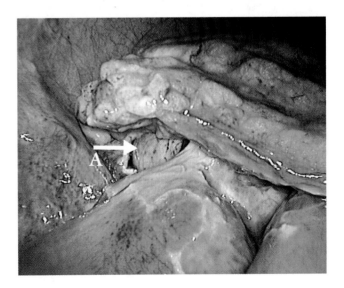

Figure 19 : Appendicular mass, the gangrenous appendix is covered by the omentum

A - Gangrenous appendix

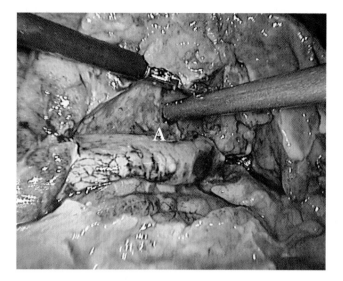

Figure 20 : Ometal covering and small bowel were separated and appendix is exposed

A - Gangrenous appendix

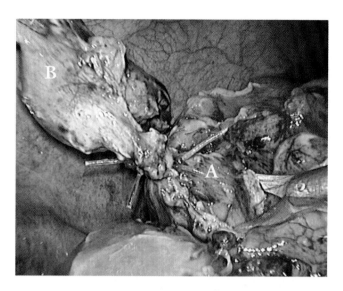

Figure 21 : Endoloop is applied after completion of dissection

A - Base of caecum

B - Appendix

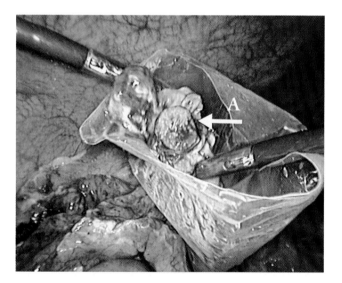

Figure 22 : Excised appendix is placed into the endobag

A - Hard stone like faecolith in the base of the appendix

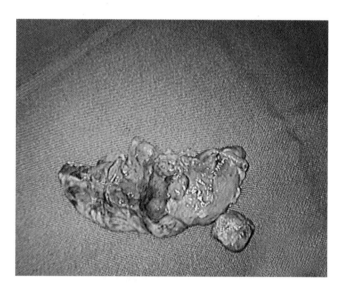

Figure 23 : Excised gangrenous appendix with faecolith

careful while applying cautery, since too much of centerisation causes thermal spread to the base which may cause necrosis of the base of the caecum (cecal burn).

Appendicular Abscess

In certain cases, there may be abscess around the perforated appendix, which can be aspirated instantaneously with the same suction cannula.

In over 325 cases, where there was abscess cavity, appendix could be removed completely. In five patients, the whole appendix was necrotic and the necrotic slough was sucked out along with the pus. In 34 cases the perforation was at the base with faecolith lying within a confined abscess cavity. Appendix could be removed in all cases, but the endoloop application was not possible. In these cases, suturing of the stump with 2-0 vicryl could be

performed in all except 12 cases. All the abscess cavities, including the ones sutured at the base were drained with large drainage tubes. Suturing of the base should not be attempted in friable tissue; either suture through the normal caecal tissue or leave it unsutured and keep a drainage tube which usually heals without problems.

I prefer a tube drainage for post operative irrigation. In two cases we required irrigation for 3 to 5 days as there was leakage of intestinal fluids. In both the cases, the leak was controlled once the bowel started functioning. In the third patient, there was a big retrocaecal abscess cavity, the appendix could not be identified and the patient continued to have drainage for more than 4 weeks in spite of taking normal diet and normal bowel movements. Laparotomy was done through loin incision and limited colectomy was performed. Histology showed evidence of

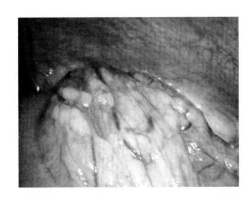

Figure 24 : Appendicular abscess is covered by ometum

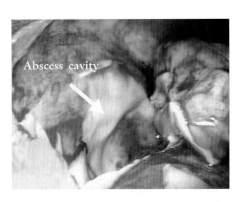

Figure 25 : Cavity was opened and all the pus was sucked out

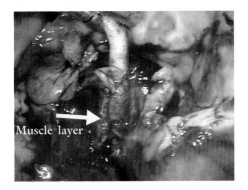

Figure 26 : Mucosal tube of the appendix is dissected

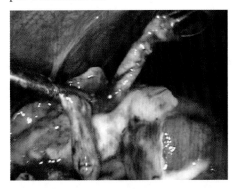

Figure 27 : Excised mucosa of the appendix

tuberculosis in the resected specimen. I feel, unless there is some specific infection, appendico-cecal junction heals normally with the usual closure of the base. In high risk patients, caecal fistula may be prevented by avoiding placing sutures in the friable cecum. Technique of mother and baby tube drainage enables faster healing of the uncontrolled appendicular stump and the abscess cavity.

Appendicular Perforation

The important step is to copiously irrigate the entire peritoneal cavity with saline after removing the entire purulent fluid & debris. The next step is to work on the infected appendix, which can be usually identified. The perforation may be found in the tip, body or at the base. The technique is same as described earlier, except care is taken in holding the friable appendix. In case of early perforation (within 12 hours) and when the base can be ligated, there may not be a need for a drainage at all because thorough peritoneal toilet is adequate. In delayed perforation, it is ideal to drain the peritoneal cavity.

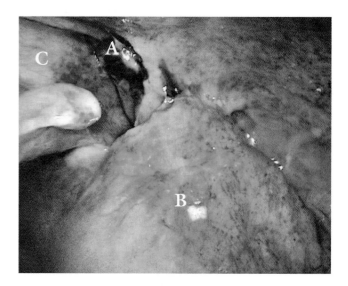

Figure 29 : Perforated appendix is adherent to the right inguinal region and covered by the omentum

A - Tip of the appendix
B - Omentum
C - Median umbilical ligament

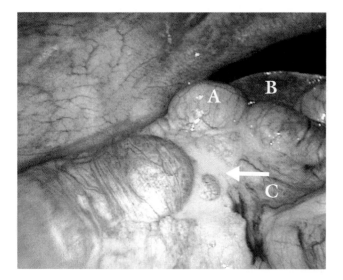

Figure 28 : Pus in the peritoneal cavity

A - Hepatic flexure of colon
B - Liver
C - Frank pus

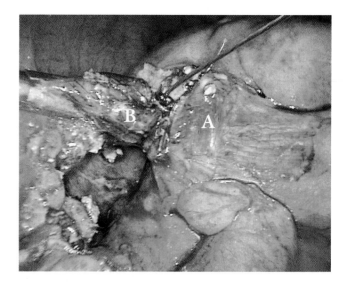

Figure 30 : Endoloop to the base of appendix after complete mobilization

A - Base of the cecum
B - Appendix

Difficult Cases - From 1991 to 2004	
Perforated Appendix	
Localised peritonitis	240
Generalised peritonitis	86
Non-perforated Appendix	
Phlegmon	176
Severely inflamed	412

Retrograde Removal of the Appendix

Occasionally the appendix is involved in a phlegmon or associated with dense adhesions of the distal portion of the appendix to the greater omentum, colon, ileum etc., particularly in paracolic, retrocaecal or retro-ileal types. Initial dissection of the appendix as mentioned in standard method is difficult here. In these circumstances, it is technically easier and safer to mobilize and dissect the proximal part of the appendix at its base. Clips are applied to the base, keeping sufficient distance for application of endoloops at the end of the procedure. The cut

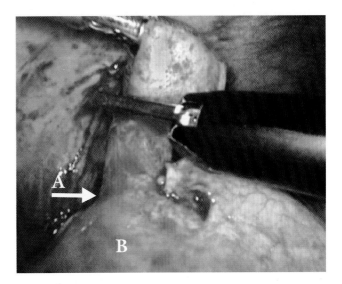

Figure 32 : Division of the appendix 1cm above the base of the appendix using Harmonic Scalpel

A - Base of the appendix
B - Cecum

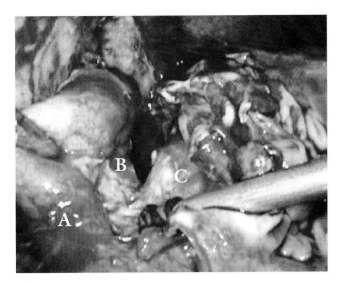

Figure 31 : Paracolic position of inflamed appendix

A - Appendix
B - Mesoappendix
C - Ascending colon

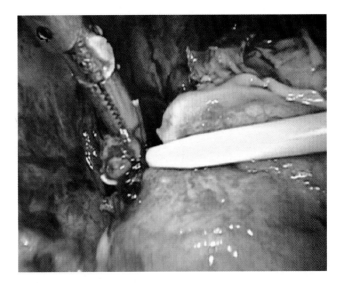

Figure 33 : After appendectomy endoloop is being applied to the base and excess of the stump is excised

end of the appendix is ligated with endoloop and held with left hand forceps to give adequate traction and manipulation. The appendix may be easily separated from the mesoappendix by dividing it with cautery or harmonic scalpel. This provides opportunity to safely separate the appendix from the dense adhesions and inflammatory mass without injuring the bowel or mesentery. In less than 3% of my cases retrograde technique was utilised for removal of appendix.

Sub-mucosal Appendectomy

In case of dense fibrous adhesions of mesoappendix, particularly when it is short, it is difficult to dissect the appendix from the mesentery, ileum, caecum and control of mesoappendix may be difficult or dangerous and may even result in injury to the adjoining bowel or mesentery. In 52 cases, I found this situation and adopted the modified technique to remove the appendix. There is always a lucid zone between the muscular wall and the mucosa. When the muscle is divided longitudinally on the lateral aspect, the entire mucosa can be removed as a tube. The entire dissection is performed by blunt dissection in the lucid zone using suction tip as a blunt dissector. It is easy to identify and dissect in this plane, simultaneously with suction, the entire mucosa up to base of the appendix. In half of the

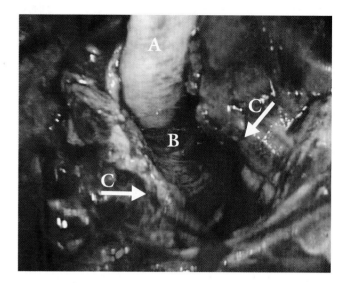

Figure 35 : The mucosal tube of the appendix is dissected

A - Mucosa of the appendix

B - Mucosa of the base of the caecum

C - Divided muscle layer of the appendix

cases, this was necessary at the distal end and half at the proximal end for safe removal. I successfully utilized sub mucosal appendectomy in 52 cases without complications. This prevents immediate complications. Late complications are also unlikely as the entire diseased mucosa is removed. Even in the open technique, the same problem will occur and similar technique has to be performed for safe removal of the appendix.

Stump Appendectomy

There are situations where a long stump is left out either due to anatomical, not recognized, a surgeon with less experience or pathological reasons could not be identified in a severely inflammatory appendicitis associated with phlegmon or abscess. In 8 occasions, patients operated elsewhere presented to us with repeated attacks of symptoms suggestive of appendicitis. Radiological imaging showed evidence of stump inflammation. 3 cases occured following open appendectomy few years ago and the remaining five were operated by laparoscopic method. Laparoscopy confirmed the presence of long stump with inflammation and stump appendectomy was performed successfully.

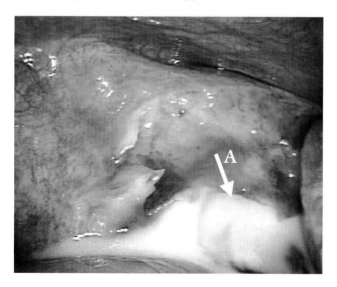

Figure 34 : Abscess cavity was opened and pus was sucked out

A - Pus

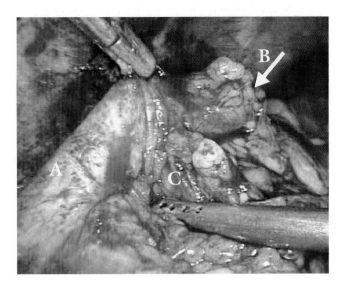

Figure 36 : Appendicular stump is identified

A - Base of the stump appendix

B - Tip of the stump

C - Mesoappendix

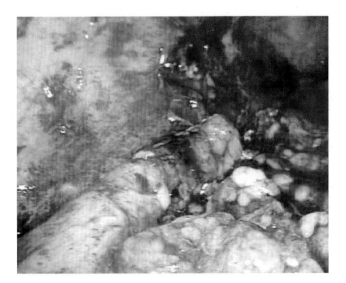

Figure 37 : Appendicular stump after dissection

TECHNIQUES ACCORDING TO ANATOMICAL TYPES

1. Pelvis, Subcaecal or Pre ileal Type

Appendix is freely mobile in these types and is dealt by the classical method.

2. Paracaecal Type

In this type, only the proximal part of the appendix is covered by peritoneum and the remaining portion of the appendix is lying free in the paracaecal or paracolic gutter. Division of the lateral peritoneal fold makes the appendectomy simple as in classical method.

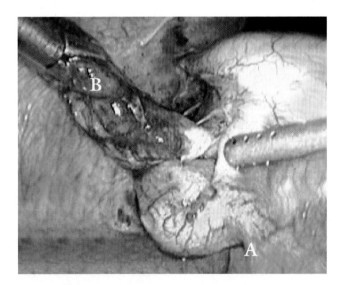

Figure 38 : Paracaecal position of the appendix

A - Base of the appendix

B - Gangrene of the tip

3. Retrocaecal Type

Here the appendix is totally covered by caecum and ascending colon. Base of the appendix is identified by tracing the taenia coli and the peritoneum is divided along the gutter, and the caecum is mobilized medially. In most of the cases, left hand of the surgeon is enough to retract the caecum to the left keeping the patient in left lateral tilt and if necessary, another port may be utilized for retraction. The whole appendix will be exposed and is dealt as in classical method. Retrograde technique may be utilized in some difficult situations.

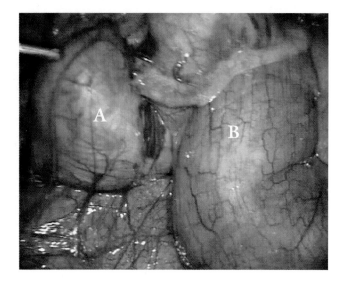

Figure 39 : Ileo cecal juntion

A - Cecum
B - Terminal ileum

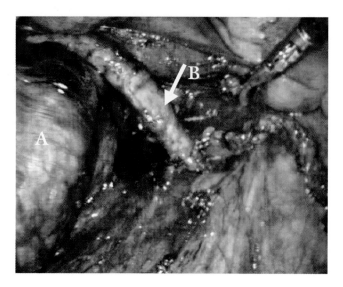

Figure 41 : Retrocecal appendix is mobilised completely

A - Cecum
B - Appendix

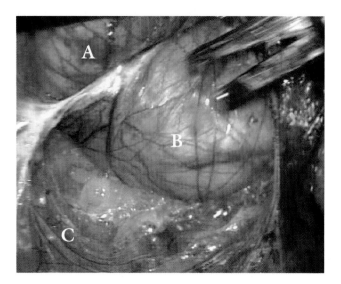

Figure 40 : Cecum is mobilised after dividing the peritoneum

A - Anterior wall of the cecum
B - Posterior wall of the cecum
C - Retro peritoneal space

4. Retroileal Type

The cecum is mobilized as above to a limited extent. The tip of the appendix is difficult to identify in this type. The avascular retroperitoneal tissue on its lateral and caudal aspect may be stripped by blunt dissection till the tip of the appendix. Usually, mesoappendix is absent. The appendicular artery is divided after clipping the individual branches or using Harmonic Scalpel. Again retrograde technique may be utilized in some, if difficulty arises.

5. Subhepatic Type

The same method as in retrocaecal approach may be utilized for subhepatic type with 30 degree angled scope. In this particular type, I prefer umbilical port for camera and epigastric port is used as surgeon's right hand working port. It makes the procedure simple. In 5 patients, hepatic flexure was mobilized down and medially. The appendix was lying retroperitoneally lateral to the second part of the duodenum.

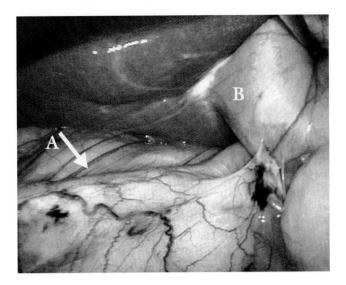

Figure 42 : Subhepatic position of the appendix, tip is going behind the gallbladder

A - Appendix
B - Gall bladder

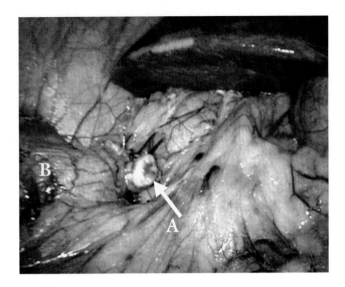

Figure 44 : Completion of Appendectomy

A - Base of the appendix
B - Cecum

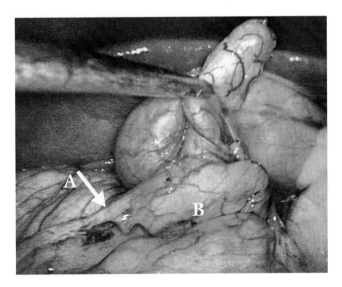

Figure 43 : Subhepatic position of the appendix. Tip was held with left hand instrument

A - Appendix
B - Mesoappendix

6. Lateral Pouch

This is a rare type of anatomical position as described in anatomical books but considered insignificant in conventional approach when looking down from anterior aspect. The appendix is found in a cavity in the lateral abdominal wall due to a developmental peritoneal fold from the lateral wall towards the ileocaecal junction as a septum. The caecum and appendix lie above and lateral to the septum which blocks the camera as well as the instruments for manipulation. Here a 30-degree telescope in the umbilicus, right midclavicular 10mm as working port and suprapubic 5mm as assisting port ease the procedure.

7. Situs Inversus and malrotation of gut

The appendix and caecum lie in the left iliac fossa usually associated with situs inversus totalis where there is mirror image displacement of bowels. Surgeon operates standing on the right side of the patient, patient positioned supine with left side up. Three ports are placed as a mirror image of the

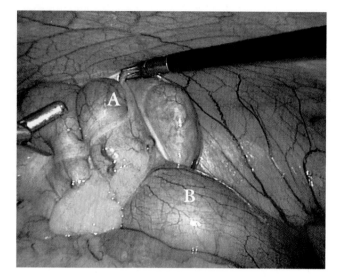

Figure 45 : Ileocecal junction in the left iliac fossa (Situs inversus)

A - Cecum
B - Terminal ileum

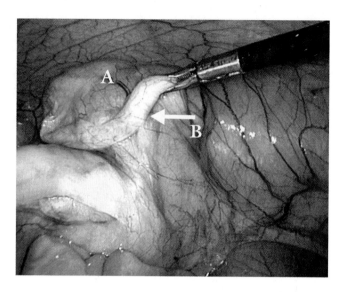

Figure 46 : Paracecal position of the situs inversus appendix

A - Cecum
B - Appendix

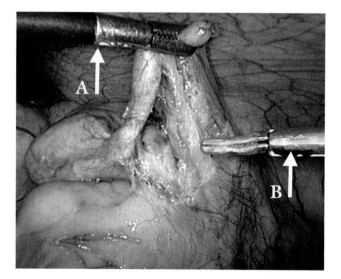

Figure 47 : Mobilization of appendix

A - Left hand instrument from the umbilical port
B - Right hand instrument from left iliac fossa port

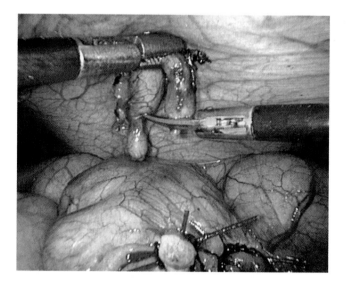

Figure 48 : Division of the appendix after applying endoloop to the base

conventional port placement. The difference is the supra pubic port is always 10mm used as working port instead of the umbilicus. The umbilicus 10 or 5mm is used as camera port. Some difficulties can be overcome by using 30 degree angled scope.

The other situation is the left sided or centrally placed appendix. Most often the caecum and proximal colon are mobile, associated with malrotation of gut. We did appendectomy as a part of correction of malrotation of gut in 2 adults and 4 children. Here we cannot follow a definite pattern of port placement.

OUR EXPERIENCE

We started doing laparoscopic appendectomy in 1991. The total number of cases from 1991-2004 is 6500. The age incidence varied from 3-88 years. Sex ratio showed that females had a slightly higher incidence (3367 females and 3133 males). The two hand technique was used in all cases. All the patients suspected with appendicitis were submitted for laparoscopic approach. CO_2 pneumo-peritoneum with closed Veress needle technique was the standard procedure. In 20 patients, gasless laparoscopy with Plan lift system under spinal anaesthesia was adopted. 271 patients had different pathology, diagnosed by laparoscopy for whom appendectomy was done combined with other procedures, according to the need.

In the first 250 cases (from 1991-1995), conversion rate was 6% (15 cases). Duration of surgery in straight forward cases (90%) was 10-20 minutes, hospitalization was 12-24 hours and in difficult cases (10%) operating time was 40-50 minutes with hospitalization of 3-4 days.

In the next nine years (1996-2004), 6250 cases of laparoscopic appendectomy were done. The incidence of acute appendicitis was 67% (4355 cases), perforated appendix with peritonitis was 5.4% (351 cases) and phlegmon was found in 2.2% (143 cases). There were abscess cavities in 6% (390 patients), 9 of which had complete necrosis of appendix and 36 cases had the perforation at the base with fecolith lying in the abscess cavity. In 22 cases, suturing of the stump with 2-0 vicryl was done. The appendix could be removed in all cases. Conversion rate was 0%.

	First 250 cases	Next 6250 cases
Operation time	30 min.	25 min.
Conversion rate	6%	0%
Hospital stay	2.5 days	2.5 days
Return to work	14 days	12 days
Wound complications	8.6%	6%
Postoperative complications	2.5%	1.8%
Intraoperative complications	1.4%	0.7%
Incisional hernias	4.2%	2.9%

As indicated by the above table, we have improved over the years. These statistics are comparable to international figures, though we observed faster operating times and reduced incidence of incisional hernias. In our centre, appendicular perforation, abscess and peritonitis are not contraindictions for laparoscopy. We had to modify our technique according to the individual patient. As is evident by our statistics, the conversion rate from 6% initially has come down to 0% in the last 12 years.

Intraoperative bleeding from the branches of the appendicular vessels near the base of the appendix was controlled by additional clipping, cauterization or loop application. There were no bowel or bladder injuries. Drainage tube was kept in all patients with perforated appendicitis. In five adult patients, there was leakage of stump of which, four were treated conservatively and in one relaparoscopy was performed for paracaecal pus collection.

Relaparoscopy was performed in 4 children who had severe pain at the umbilical region to rule out omental adhesion or Richter's type of hernia. Laparoscopy revealed nothing abnormal and surprisingly all the children were free from symptoms subsequently. Hospitalization ranged between 12 to 24 hours in 97% of patients and 23% of patients with severe infiction were hospitalized for 2-3 days mainly for intravenous antibiotic coverage. One patient had urachal ligament injury and he continued to have urinary leak which was treated by suturing on 3rd post operative day.

Duration of surgery was 10-20 minutes for straightforward cases (90%) and 40 - 50 minutes for the difficult group (10%).

DISCUSSION

Although laparoscopic appendectomy has several advantages over open surgery, many centers remain reluctant to adopt this approach routinely because of lack of standardization of the technique, inadequate trained personnel in emergency situation and increased cost. Cost is not a factor with the use of reusable trocars and instruments and self made pretied endoloops. If the diagnosis is in doubt, early laparoscopy is indicated by which complications related to appendix may be minimized to a great extent.

INTERNATIONAL RESULTS

There are several reports comparing open versus laparoscopic appendicectomies.[16,17,19,20] The parameters used are cost, pain, length of hospital stay, return to work, incidence of incisional hernias, adhesions, postoperative leak, postoperative abscess and morbidity. Some studies show that the rate of wound infection is much lower and post-operative deep abscess formation is more in laparoscopic appendicitis.

After analyzing a nationwide database of more than 43,000 patients, Duke University Medical Center researchers have determined that laparoscopic approach for appendectomy has significant advantages over the traditional open surgical approach.[6] Patients who received laparoscopic surgery were discharged from the hospital sooner, were more likely to be discharged home as opposed to further medical care and had fewer complications while in the hospital. Also, the laparoscopic approach was as effective as the open approach in appendicular abscess and perforated appendix.

The median hospital stay for patients who underwent laparoscopic appendectomy was 2.06 days, compared to 2.88 days for the open approach - a statistically significant and clinically relevant difference. There was no significant difference in complications between the laparoscopic and open procedure in patients with perforated appendix and appendicular abscess, suggesting that surgeons should consider using the laparoscopic approach for these patients as well.

Another study shows the following:

	Open	Laparoscopy
Wound complications (706 cases)	5.7%	3.65%
Postoperative sepsis (528 cases)	3%	13%
Analysis of other studies:	232 cases	219 cases
Operation time	51 min.	61.8 min.
Conversion rate		8.4%
Hospital stay	3.84 days	3.08 days
Return to work	31 days	17.3 days
Wound infection	9.25%	3.5%
Complications	10.75%	7.25%

European studies of large series of patients that compare open and laparoscopic appendicectomies favour laparoscopic approach. 583 patients were analysed, 301 patients were allocated to open appendectomy and 282 patients to laparoscopy, 65 required conversion to open appendectomy. Analysis revealed an equally short hospital stay in the two groups (median 2 days). The median time to return to normal activity (7 versus 10 days) and work (10 versus 16 days) was significantly shorter following laparoscopy. Laparoscopy was associated with fewer wound infections and improved cosmesis, but the operating time was longer (60 versus 40 min). Laparoscopy was associated with more intraperitoneal abscesses (5 versus 1 per cent) but, adjusted for a greater number of gangrenous or perforated appendices in this group, the difference failed to reach statistical significance. Hospital stay was equally short, whereas laparoscopic appendectomy was associated with fewer wound infections, faster recovery, earlier return to work and improved cosmesis.

The Italian Society of Young Surgeons analysed 26863 cases of laparoscopic appendectomy in a multicenteric study.[26] Their main aim was to determine the diffusion of the practice of laparoscopic appendectomy in their country among surgeons less than 40 years of age. Laparoscopic appendectomy is being performed in 95% of institutions in Italy, which shows that it is widely accepted.

Their statistics

Wound complications	13.6%
Postoperative complications	1.2%
Intraoperative complications	0.32%
Conversion rate	2.1%
Hospital stay	2.5 days
Incisional hernias	8.8%

TWO HAND TECHNIQUE OF LAPAROSCOPIC APPENDECTOMY

Patients are usually placed in the supine position. Modified lithotomy position is preferred in female patients with suspicion of pelvic pathology for the use of a blunt transvaginal probe for manipulation of the uterus and adnexa. In the initial phases both Foley's catheter and nasogastric catheter are placed routinely, later in clear cut cases, these catheters are not necessary unless it is perforated appendicitis. The placement of ports have been described differently by different authors. All these authors have described umbilicus as the camera port. None of these approaches give direct view of the base of the appendix and allows to work with both hands simultaneously. In 1991 when I started my first appendectomy by laparoscopic method, I placed the camera port in the suprapubic region. Through the suprapubic port appendix at any anatomical location can be visualised. As I am accustomed to work with right hand, standing on the left side for laparoscopic cholecystectomy, I am comfortable to work with my right hand through the umbilical port. By keeping left hand instruments in the right iliac fossa, I can manipulate the appendix in all directions. Since over 6500 appendix have been completed in my institute, I personally feel this two hand technique is much easier to learn and practice by any general surgeon. I presented this two hand technique of laparoscopic appendectomy during the 3rd International congress of New technology and advanced technique at Luxemberg in 1995 which was appreciated by all. In the last 12 years I have not converted any laparoscopic appendectomy to open

approach. Kollmar et al have also found this technique useful in a study.[24]

The meso-appendix is first divided along the length of appendix. In North America, this is done by placing surgical clips on each branch of the appendiceal artery, whereas in Europe many surgeons routinely cauterise these small vessels with bipolar electrical energy. In the first few years, I used clips for the main appendicular vessels at the base of mesoappendix and divided the artery distal to the clip using monopolar cautery. A single or occasionally two or three clips are used to control bleeding during division. After I started using Harmonic Scalpel, I found that there was no need for clipping the appendicular vessel. Bipolar coagulation and cutting is equally effective and can be used routinely if Harmonic Scalpel is not available.

Many surgeons in the west use Endo GIA stapler for controlling the appendix and meso-appendix. I personally don't recommend stapler, since it is not cost effective and patient requires a 12mm trocar introduction which is cosmetically unacceptable. Also in many occasions, stapling of meso appendix may not be possible even after mobilisation.

Control of Appendicular Stump

With either the ligature or stapled technique the result is an everted appendiceal stump. Most contemporary surgeons were trained to invert the remnant into the wall of the caecum, despite trials comparing everted versus inverted appendiceal stump closure showing no difference in clinical outcome.[23] There have been no problems reported to date with leaving an everted appendiceal remnant.

Two methods of ligating and dividing the appendix are in common use. The most common method of controlling the appendicular stump is with the use of multiple pre-tied endoloops. Two ligatures are placed at the appendico-caecal junction and third loop to the specimen side and the appendix divided with scissors between the second and third loops. The third loop is not divided which helps in prevention of contamination and accidental slippage of appendix.

Tips to Minimize Contamination During Laparoscopic Appendectomy

1. Patient should be placed in supine position to prevent spread of infectious material due to gravity.

2. Use short bursts of cautery to sterilize the stump after resecting.

3. Remove the specimen with a pouch device.

4. Do not reinsert trocar used for extracting the appendix.

5. Always irrigate the field and suck all the fluid out.

MUCOCELE OF THE APPENDIX

It occurs in obstructive and neoplastic situations. In the obstructive type, there is accumulation of mucus in the lumen due to proximal obstruction in the absence of infection. Simple appendectomy is the treatment.[4]

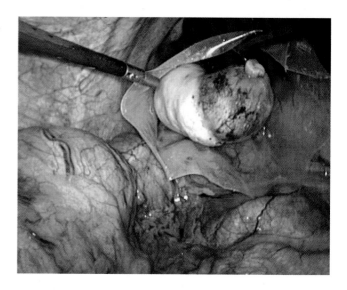

Figure 50 : Placement of excised appendix into the endobag for extraction

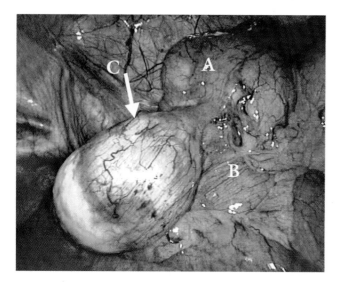

Figure 49: Mucocele of the appendix

A - Cecum
B - Terminal ileum
C - Appendix

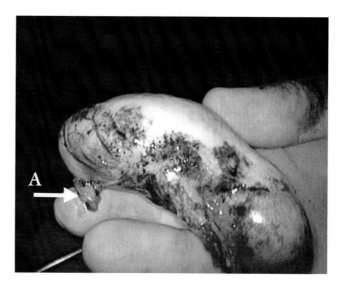

Figure 51 : Excised mucocele of the appendix. Compared to the size of the finger, appendix is dilated grossly

A - Base of the appendix

The neoplastic variety may be benign or malignant. The benign type is called mucinous cystadenoma and the malignant type is called mucinous cystadenocarcinoma.[3] Here, mucocele occurs due to distension of the lumen by mucus secreted by multiplying tumor cells. Malignant neoplasms are rare. The two most common types are argentaffinoma (carcinoid tumor) and adenocarcinoma. Carcinoid tumor is the most common tumor of the appendix and appendix is the most common site of this tumor.[10] It occurs in 0.1% of all removed appendices. Usually, the diagnosis is made during or after surgery. Treatment is by right hemicolectomy in tumors >2 cm, musoappendix involvement, and base of appendix.

TUBERCULOSIS OF THE APPENDIX

In developing countries since the incidence of abdominal tuberculosis is more, histology of the specimen should always be done. Six patients operated elsewhere presented to us with sinuses of the ports following appendectomy between 4th week and 22nd week. Radialogical imaging revealed communications of the sinuses to the site of appendectomy.

In 4 cases scrapping of the sinus tract showed evidence of tubercles. In the other 2 cases, the fistulous tract in the lateral abdominal was excised which confirmed the presence of tuberculosis. Full course of antitubercular therapy was given in all cases. In all the patients the port sinuses healed completely with no recurrence till date.

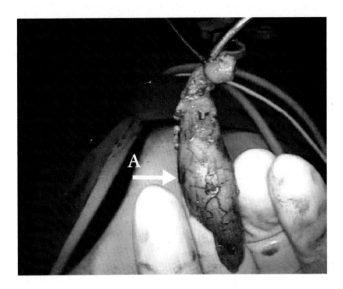

Figure 53 : Excised appendix

A - Dilated segment in the body of the appendix

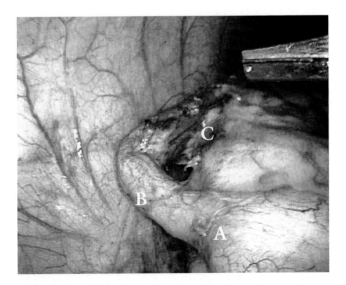

Figure 52 : Paracecal position of the appendix

A - Cecum
B - Appendix
C - Divided mesoappendix

ALTERNATIVE TECHNIQUES

Bipolar Appendectomy

Laparoscopic appendectomy by bipolar coagulation is simple and economical. This was first popularized by Pier, Got and Baker in their large series of 625 cases.[7] The technique consisted of identifying the appendix and coagulating the appendicular stump with bipolar coagulation. The base of the appendix is cut at this point and removed. Duration of surgery is less, no clip applicators, needle holders or knot pushers are required, and no foreign materials like ligatures or clips are needed.

Stapler-Assisted Appendectomy

Laparoscopic staple assisted appendectomy claims to make laparoscopic appendectomy technically easier to perform.[21] The ENDO GIA passes through a 12-mm trocar and allows placement of two triple-staggered lines of titanium staples with a simultaneous cut. Using this technique, operating time for laparoscopic appendectomy was reduced from an average of 30 minutes to a minimum of 5 minutes. With this technique, no appendiceal contents leaked intraperitoneally. The larger trocar allowed easier removal of the separated appendix with minimal dissection of the mesoappendix. Preliminary experience by several surgeons with the ENDO GIA 30/45 stapler suggests that it is a safe, easy and rapid (although expensive) method of removing the appendix laparoscopically.[7]

In practice, there is no need for endolinear stapler in any case and the cost may be minimized to a great extent by avoiding stapler. In certain situations, it is difficult or impossible for stapler application.

COMPLICATIONS ASSOCIATED WITH LAPAROSCOPIC APPENDECTOMY

For the most part, any complication associated with open appendectomy can also occur during laparoscopy, such as post operative abscess formations, appendiceal stump leak/blow out, wound infection and early or late intestinal obstruction.

1. Large retrospective clinical series have shown reduced incidence of wound infection and post operative abscess formation

2. Visceral and vascular injury related to Veress needle or trocar placement.

3. Iatrogenic injuries to small bowel and colon due to laparoscopic instruments.

4. Caecal burn. Excessive use of cautery on the stump can result in thermal injury to the caecum. This is due to conduction of electricity through narrowed base, producing intense heat and thermal injury to the adjoining caecum.

5. Douglas syndrome: Few patients develop post-operative pain and tenderness over the site of appendectomy between 5-7 days. Investigations such as ultrasound and CT do not reveal any abnormalities. Total and differential counts may be raised. In the absence of intraperitoenal collection, it is called Douglas syndrome (named after Douglas who described it in the early part of the laparoscopic appendectomy experience). I also had 1-2% of patients with this syndrome in the earlier period of my experience. All of them responded to antibiotics and analgesic on an out-patient basis. Necrosis of the long distal stump may be the cause for this pain, so less than 0.5cm lone stump is preferred. In between the two ligatures, we should leave only less than 0.5cm. In one of my cases, scan revealed a localized collection 1-2cm at the site of appendectomy. Relaparoscopy was done after 3 weeks and the collection was aspirated and the cavity irrigated. The patient recovered well. This happened following a straight forward appendectomy.

NORMAL - LOOKING APPENDIX : TO REMOVE OR NOT ?

Normal looking appendix in absence of other pathology should be removed for two reasons, one the appendix may appear grossly normal but subsequent histological examinations may reveal early or mucosal appendicitis. Secondly , failure to remove

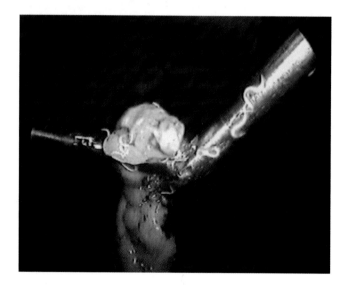

Figure 54 : Worms (Enterobius) from the appendix lumen coming out and climbing over the scissors

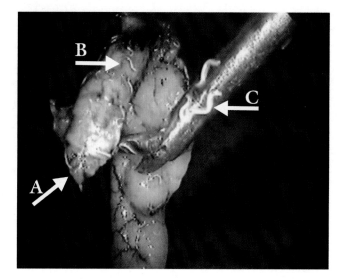

Figure 55 : Worms from the appendix (enterobius). This is one of the causes of apppendiates of developing cautery. Macro surgically   normal, divided appendix shows worms.

A - Divided end of appendix

B - Worms over the appendix

C - Worms over the instrument

the appendix may result in confusion if the patient continues to have right iliac fossa pain. Most surgeons have adopted a policy of removing normal appearing appendix in order to avoid any such confusion that could potentially result in a delay of appropriate treatment.[12]

CONCLUSION

At present, there is overwhelming evidence that laparoscopic approach is superior to open method in treatment of appendicitis.[18] The benefits have to be balanced with the marginal increase in costs. The international consensus and certainly my personal opinion seems to be leaning towards laparoscopic appendectomy as the treatment of choice for appendicitis, even though it is not popular in the West.

In conclusion, I feel laparoscopic appendectomy is the gold standard for appendicitis which will become universally allogated in the near future.

References

1. Lewis FR, Holcroft JW, Boey J, Dunphy JE.: Appendicitis: A critical review of diagnosis and treatment in 1000 cases. Arch Surg, 1975; 110:667.

2. Rioux M.: Sonographic detection of the normal and abnormal appendix. Am J Radiol, 1992, 158:773.

3. Andersson A, Bergdahl L, Boquist L.: Primary carcinoma of appendix. Ann Surg, 1976; 183: 53.

4. Broders CW, Miranda R.: Mucocele of appendix: Review of eleven cases and report of two cases. Am Surg, 1971; 37:434.

5. Moberg AC, Ahlberg G, Leijonmarck CE, et al.: Diagnostic laparoscopy in 1043 patients with suspected acute appendicitis. Eur J Surg, 1998; 164:833.

6. Guller U, Hervey S, Purves H, Muhlbaier LH, Peterson ED et al.: Laparoscopic versus open appendectomy: out comes comparison based on a large administrative database. Ann Surg. Jan., 2004:239(1):43-52.

7. Ellis H, Nathanson KL. Appendix and Appendectomy. In Zinner MJ, Schwarts SI, Ellis H eds., Maingots Abdominal Operations, 10 ed., Vol.2, Chapt 39. Connecticut:: Appleton & Lange, 1997: 1191-1227.

8. Telford GL, Wallace JR. Appendix. In Zuidema GD, Yeo CJ eds., Shackelfords Surgery of the Alimentary Tract, 5 ed., Vol.4, Chapt 13. Philadelphia: W.B.Saunders Company, 2002: 180-190.

9. Fitzgibbons RJ, Ulualp KM. Laparoscopic Appendectomy. In Nyhus LM, Baker RJ, Fischer JE eds., Mastery of Surgery, 3 ed., Vol.2, Chapt. 130. Boston: Little, Brown and Company Inc., 1997: 1412-19.

10. Cuschieri A. The Small Intestine and Vermiform Appendix. In Cuschieri A., Giles G.R., Moossa A.R eds., Essential Surgical Practice, 2 ed. Chapt. 72. Bucks (England): Butterworth International Edition, 1988: 1136-63.

11. Semms K. Endoscopic Appendectomy. Endoscopy 1983;15:59-64.

12. Grunewald B, Keating J.: Should the normal appendix be removed at operation for appendicitis? J R Coll Edinb, 1993;38:158-160.

13. Cox MR, McCall JL, Wilson TG, et al.: Laparoscopic appendectomy: a prospective analysis. Aust NZ J Surg, 1993;63:840-847.

14. Schirmer BD, Schmieg RE Jr, Dix J, et al.: Laparoscopic versus traditional appendecectomy for suspected appendecectomy. Am J Surg, 1993;165:670-675.

15. Gilchrist BF, Lobe TE, Schopp KP, et al.: Is there a role for Laparoscopic appendecectomy in pediatric surgery.: J Pediatric Surg,1992; 27:209-214.

16. Kum CK, Ngoi SS, Goh PMY, et al.: Randomised controlled trial comparing laparoscopic appendecectomy and open appendecectomy. Br J Surg, 1993.

17. Tate JJT, Ching SCS, Dawson J, et al. Conventional versus laparoscopic surgery for acute appendicitis. Br J Surg, 1993:80:761-764.

18. Nowzaradan Y, Barnes JP, Westmoreland J, et al.: Laparascopic appendecectomy: treatment of choice for sus-

pected appendicitis. Surg Laparosc Endosc,1993 ;5:411-416.

19. Attwood SEA, Hill ADK, Murphy PG, et al.: A prospective randomized trial of laparoscopic versus open appendecectomy. SURGRY, 1992:112;497-501.

20. Pedersen AG, Petersen OB, Wara P, Rønning H, Qvist N, Laurberg S.: Randomized clinical trial of laparoscopic versus open appendectomy. Br J Surg, Feb.2001; 88(2):200-205.

21. Klaiber C, Wagner M, Metzger A.: Various stapling techniques in laparoscopic appendectomy: 40 consecutive cases. Surg Laparosc Endosc, 1994 Jun;4(3):205-9.

22. Houben F, Willmen HR.: Simplified appendectomy without stump embedding. Experiences of 20 years conventional and 5 years laparoscopic application. Chirurg, 1998 Jan;69(1):66-70.

23. Lavonius MI, Liesjarvi S, Niskanen RO, Ristkari SK, Korkala O, Mokka RE.: Simple ligation vs stump inversion in appendectomy. Ann Chir Gynaecol, 1996; 85(3):222-4.

24. Kollmar O, Z'graggen K, Schilling MK, Buchholz BM.: The suprapubic approach for laparoscopic appendectomy. Surg Endosc March 2002;16(3):504-508.

25. PalaniveluC. Laparoscopic Appendectomy. In: Text Book of Surgical Laparoscopy, 1 ed., Chapt. 53. Coimbatore (India): GEM Foundation, 2004:411-24.

26. Agresta F, Leone L, Arezzo A, Biondi A, Bottero L.: Laparoscopic appendectomy in Italy: an appraisal of 26863 cases. J Laparoendosc Adv Surg Tech A, 2004, 14(1):1-8.

27. Pier A, Got F, Backer C. Laparoscopic appendectomy in 625 cases: from innovation to routine. Surg Laparoendosc Endosc. 1991; 1:8-13.

59

Laparoscopy in Small Bowel Obstruction

INTRODUCTION

Small bowel obstruction (SBO) is a common surgical problem and is associated with significant morbidity and mortality (5.5%).[1] Description of patients with small bowel obstruction probably dates back to the 3rd century. Patients were managed with attempted reduction of hernia, laxatives, ingestion of heavy metals and leeches to remove toxic agents from the blood. Creation of an enterocutaneous fistula to relieve bowel obstruction is also recorded in history.[2] It was only in late 1800s when antisepsis and antiseptic surgical techniques made operative intervention safer, surgery became accepted as a treatment modality. Management of SBO still has major problems like difficulty in accurate diagnosis and the cause, lack of sensitive tests to identify presence of strangulation and difference in opinion regarding the appropriate management.

Laparoscopy was considered an absolute contraindication in the presence of intestinal obstruction till recently. Successful laparoscopic management of SBO was first reported by Bastug in 1991,[3] and after that there has been several reports of laparoscopic management of SBO. Now we know that laparoscopy is effective in selected patients with SBO.

ADHESIONS

Intestinal obstruction is responsible for approximately 20% of surgical admissions for acute abdominal conditions.[4] The small bowel is a site of obstruction in 60-80% of these cases. The commonest cause of small bowel obstruction is adhesions, usually secondary to prior abdominal operations. The other common causes are neoplasms and incarceration in hernia. All three combined, account for 70-80% of all cases of small bowel obstruction. Adhesions can

Etiology

Extrinsic causes

Adhesions

Hernias

Neoplasm (extra intestinal or carcinomatosis)

Volvulus

Intra abdominal abscess

Superior mesenteric artery syndrome

Tight fascial opening of stoma

Intra luminal causes

Gall stone ileus

Bezoars

Swallowed foreign body

Worms

Balloons of intestinal tubes

Enterolith

Intrinsic causes (intramural)

i. Congenital

Malrotation

Duplications and cysts

ii. Inflammatory

Crohn's disease

Tuberculosis

Actinomycosis

Diverticulitis

iii. Neoplastic

Primary

Metastatic

iv. Traumatic

Haematoma

Ischaemic stricture

v. Miscellaneous

Intussusception

Endometriosis

Radiation enteropathy/stricture

also occur as a result of intraabdominal inflammatory process. In a smaller percentage adhesions/bands are congenital.

Intraabdominal adhesions	
Previous surgery	79%
Peritoneal infection	18%
Congenital bands	11%

Perry Jr JF (1955)[5]

Approximately 4-5% of patients with previous abdominal surgery will develop SBO.[6] In general, surgery in the infracolic compartment is associated with more risk of SBO. Previous appendicectomy, gynaecological surgery and colorectal surgery are common causes of adhesive SBO. This may partly reflect the high frequency of these operations. The higher risk of lower abdominal procedures to produce adhesive obstruction may be due to the fact that the bowel are more mobile in the pelvis and it is more tethered in the upper abdomen.

In patients who have undergone previous surgery it is difficult to differentiate between recurrent disease (malignancy, inflammatory bowel disease, TB) and adhesions as the cause of SBO. In those with a previous history of surgery for malignancy, a significant proportion will have adhesive small bowel obstruction (30-39%).[7, 8] Following colorectal surgery for cancer, in those presenting with SBO, the cause is mostly adhesions and not recurrent malignancy. Whereas in those following surgery for gastric or ovarian cancer it is commonly due to malignancy.[7,8]

NEOPLASMS

Approximately 20% of SBO are caused by neoplasms. Of this, majority are metastatic lesions (peritoneal deposits) causing obstruction by external compression (commonly from ovary, pancreas, gastric and colonic primary). It may be also be from distant sites like breast, lung or melanoma. Large intraabdominal tumors may cause SBO through extrinsic compression of the bowel lumen.[2] Primary small bowel tumors can cause intraluminal obstruction but are rare.

INCARCERATED HERNIA

Approximately 10% of SBO are caused by hernias. Routine elective repair of external hernias has caused a drop in the incidence of small bowel obstruction caused by hernias. Still it is a leading cause of intestinal obstruction in developing countries.

Ventral and inguinal hernias are common causes of SBO. Internal hernias can also result in SBO. Internal hernia may be congenital (para duodenal, diaphragmatic, paracaecal, foramen of Winslow) or acquired (post operative mesenteric defects).

POSTOPERATIVE INTERNAL HERNIA

Small bowel may herniate through post operative defects in the mesentry or omentum and cause SBO. Following reconstructive gastrointestinal surgery, there are potential areas for small bowel to herniate. Follwing Roux-en-Y reconstruction three potential areas for internal hernia are created. These are the Roux-en-Y anastomosis, the opening in the transverse mesocolon through which the Roux loop is brought up and behind the Roux limb before it passes through the mesocolon (Paterson Hernia). These are particularly common after gastric bypass surgery for morbid obesity. Colostomy, ileostomy and vascular bypass procedures may also create potential spaces for small bowel herniation. These patients are at risk for developing closed loop obstruction and bowel strangulation. Intermesenteric defect is another potential site for herniation. Intermesenteric defect is another potential site for herniation.

PORT-SITE HERNIAS

Incisional hernia occurring at trocar sites following abdominal laparoscopy has an incidence of around 1%.[9-14] They commonly present as small bowel obstruction in the early post operative period. In majority of cases the hernial content is small intestine or omentum. Several cases of port site hernias have been reported and most of them are with 10mm or larger trocar sites. Most of the hernias are Richter's type hernias without peritoneal lining and contain small bowel. Most of the surgeons do not routinely close 5mm port sites. Few cases of small bowel herniation through 5mm trocar site has also been reported, particularly following lengthy procedures if the port is used for active operative instruments. Repetitive motions may cause the 5mm defect to enlarge significantly allowing hernia to develop.[9-14]

OTHERS

Tuberculosis is an important cause of intestinal obstruction in developing countries. Crohn's disease can cause obstruction secondary to acute inflammation during a flare or from chronic stricture. Strictures secondary to ischaemia, inflammation, radiation injury or surgical trauma can cause SBO. A Meckels diverticulum may produce SBO by volvulus, intussusception or inflammation. Volvulus is often caused by adhesions or intestinal malrotation. Intraluminal obstruction may be caused by gall stones, bezoars or foreign bodies. Intussusception of small bowel in adults is usually initiated by lead points like tumors, polyps or enlarged mesenteric nodes.

CLASSIFICATION

Partial or Complete

Simple or Strangulated

Proximal or Distal

Acute or Subacute

Chronic or Acute on chronic

Closed loop obstruction

Intestinal obstruction can be classified according to the degree of obstruction of the flow of intestinal contents into partial or complete, the absence or presence of vascular compromise into simple or strangulated, and the site of obstruction into proximal or distal. These distinctions have prognostic and therapeutic relevance. For example, complete or strangulated obstruction requires urgent surgical intervention, whereas a partial obstruction may, in selected cases, be successfully managed conservatively.

A closed loop obstruction refers to a mechanical obstruction in which both the proximal and distal parts of the involved intestinal segment are occluded.

Examples included torsion of a loop of bowel around a band, incarcerated loop of bowel in a hernia, volvulus of sigmoid colon or caecum and colonic obstruction with a competent ileoceacal valve. This condition has a particularly high risk of strangulation, necrosis, and perforation. Depending on the rate of progression of obstruction it can be classified as acute (hours), sub acute (days), chronic (weeks) or acute on chronic.

PATHOPHYSIOLOGY

The duration and degree of obstruction, presence and severity of ischemia determine the local and systemic consequences of intestinal obstruction. Initially, the intestinal motility and contractility is increased in an attempt to propel intestinal contents past the obstruction. This increased peristalsis is found both above and below the point of obstruction, hence diarrohea may be present in the early stages of SBO. Later in the course of obstruction intestine becomes fatigued and dilates, the contractions become less frequent and less intense. Intestinal obstruction causes profound accumulation of fluid and swallowed air within the intestinal lumen proximal to the obstruction. The intestinal tract secretes upto 8.5 L of fluid every 24 hours, and the majority of this fluid is reabsorbed in the small intestine. Impaired water and electrolyte absorption and enhanced secretion result in the net movement of isotonic fluid from the intravascular space into the intestinal lumen. This massive third space fluid loss accounts for the dehydration and hypovolaemia. The accumulation of swallowed air, and to a much lesser extent gas generated by bacterial overgrowth within the obstructed lumen, also contributes to intestinal distention. The intestinal distension causes increased intraabdominal pressure, decreased venous return and elevation of diaphragm, compromising ventilation. These factors potentiate the effect of hypovolaemia.

The failure of normal intestinal motility results in the bacterial overgrowth within the small intestine. Disruption of the ecologic balance of the normal enteric microflora is associated with the translocation of bacteria to mesenteric lymph nodes and systemic organs. This is important in the production of sepsis associated with intestinal obstruction.

The systemic manifestations of intestinal obstruction are related, to hypovolemia and the inflammatory response initiated by ischaemia or gangrenous intestine. Hypovolemia is primarily due to the loss of fluid into the third space. When this is combined with anorexia and vomiting, a marked reduction in the intravascular volume results. Intestinal infarction markedly exacerbates the loss of intravascular fluid both locally into the bowel and systemically through a generalized microvascular damage mediated by proinflammtory agents like neutrophils, complement, cytokines, eicosanoids, and oxygen-derived free radicals. These are implicated in the production of remote organ failure associated with intestinal ischemia and infarction.

CLINICAL FEATURES

The classical symptoms of SBO are colicky abdominal pain with nausea and vomiting, obstipation and abdominal distension. The magnitude of symptoms depends on the degree, site and duration of obstruction. The more proximal the obstruction, the earlier and more prominent are the symptoms. In distal obstructions, the symptoms take time to manifest.

Pain is typically peri-umbilical and colicky, occurring at 4-5 minute intervals for proximal obstruction and less frequently for more distal obstructions. Pain may be absent in proximal intestinal obstructions like gastric outlet obstruction, duodenal obstruction or high intestinal obstruction. Nausea and vomiting may be the only symptoms. In contrast, with more distal obstruction the initial and most prominent symptom is colicky abdominal pain. The development of a continuous severe pain, particularly localized, strongly suggests the presence of strangulation.

Vomiting occurs early in high small bowel obstruction. It may be absent or late in distal small bowel obstruction. Initially the vomitus may contain altered food, but later it becomes bile stained. Further with dilatation and stasis in the intestine, there is bacterial proliferation and the vomitus turns faeculent and foul smelling.

Obstipation is a late phenomenon. Patients may continue to have bowel movements and pass flatus as the distal, unobstructed intestine empties. Patients with partial obstruction may continue to pass flatus and have diarrhoea intermittently.

Abdominal distention develops progressively later in the course of the obstruction as the proximal intestine becomes dilated. It is prominent in mid gut and low gut obstructions and usually absent in patients with high obstruction.

Patients with closed loop obstruction, a relentless reflex vomiting may be the initial symptom. This is due to acute, unrelieved intestinal distension and irritation. These patients may experience a constant, visceral pain rather than a colic. The pain may be out of proportion to the physical findings.

PHYSICAL EXAMINATION

Peristaltic waves are some times visible through the abdominal wall in thin patients. Surgical scars should be noted and indicates the possible presence of adhesions or previous disease like malignancy or crohn's disease.

Auscultation may reveal periods of increasing bowel sounds and abnormal borborygmi that corresponds with the abdominal colic. Patients in early high intestinal obstruction may have normal bowel sounds. Mild generalized tenderness occurs in patients with intestinal obstruction related to intestinal and abdominal distention. Presence of localized tenderness, rebound and guarding indicates presence of strangulation. Thorough search of all the possible hernial orifices should be performed. An obstructed external hernia may produce little local pain or tenderness and the central abdominal colic may distract the attention away from the causative lesion.

Digital rectal examination is essential. Faecal impaction, low rectal cancer and a mass in the rectovesical pouch can be felt. Presence of faeces should be noted. Hematochezia may occur with cancer, intussusception or strangulation.

Presence of fever, tachycardia, tachypnoea, altered mental status, oliguria and hypotension suggests strangulation.

DIAGNOSIS

A meticulous history and physical examination complemented by plain abdominal radiography are all that is required to diagnose SBO in majority of patients (>60%). Other investigations may be necessary when diagnosis and cause are uncertain.

Plain abdominal radiographs

They usually confirm the clinical diagnosis of intestinal obstruction. They are also useful in determining the cause and site of obstruction. A supine film will show dilated loops of bowel without evidence of colonic dilatation and an erect view will show multiple air fluid levels. Some times it demonstrates the cause of obstruction like foreign bodies or gall stones. Plain abdominal radiographs are unreliable if the obstructed loops are completely filled with fluid or if performed at a relatively early stage. Paucity of gas in the colon and rectum is an important finding of SBO.

Finding of air in the biliary tree and a radio opaque gall stone in right lower quadrant are suggestive of gall stone ileus. Perforation can be detected by the presence of free intraabdominal air (erect or right lateral decubitus film).

Contrast Radiology

Small bowel follow through or enteroclysis is indicated in patients with a history of recurrent obstruction or low grade mechanical obstruction to precisely define the obstructed segment and degree of obstruction.

Ultrasound

Presence of abundant gas in the bowel limits its use in small bowel obstruction. It can delineate, fluid filled loops, extraluminal solid lesions causing obstruction and free peritoneal fluid. It is helpful in differentiating mechanical SBO from paralytic ileus by detection of peristalsis[15]. It is useful in pregnant women since there is no risk of radiation exposure.

Computed Tomography (CT)

It is highly sensitive (81-96%) in complete or high grade obstruction of the small bowel and for determining the cause and location of obstruction. It is also helpful in extrinsic causes of intestinal obstruction like abdominal tumors, inflammatory disease or abscess. Even small quantities of free intraperitoneal gas is visualized on CT.[16] CT is also useful in determining bowel strangulation, but the findings are those of irreversible ischemia and necrosis. Hence it is useful only in detecting late stages of irreversible ischemia.

Computer Aided Diagnosis (CAD)

CAD appears to be superior to a clinical diagnosis, in predicting presence of strangulation. Pain et al (1987) did a retrospective analysis of 310 cases of SBO.[17]

Type	CAD	Clinical
Simple SBO	85%	-
Viable strangulation	82%	66%
Non viable strangulation	97%	46%

Laboratory Investigations

Laboratory investigations are important in assessing the degree of dehydration; serial determination of serum electrolytes should be performed to assess the adequacy of fluid resuscitation. Leucocytosis may be found in patients with strangulation, though its absence does not eliminate strangulation.

Strangulation is associated with increased morbidity and mortality and therefore recognition of strangulation early is important. Signs of strangulation described include raised temperature, tachycardia, abdominal tenderness, absence of bowel sounds, leukocytosis and a constant noncramping abdominal pain. But significant proportion of cases are unsuspected preoperatively or do not show all the clinical features. Various laboratory tests have been studied to predict the presence or absence of strangulation. Serum lactic dehydrogenase, serum amylase, alkaline phosphatase and ammonia levels have been assessed but found to have no clear value. Initial reports have shown limited usefulness with serum D-lactate, creatine phosphokinase iso enzyme (BB) and intestinal fatty acid binding protein. Noninvasive

methods which detect mesenteric ischemia using SQUID (super conducting quantum interference device) have been described.[18]

TREATMENT

Prompt recognition of cases requiring immediate surgery is the key to successful management of SBO. Initial management involves fluid resuscitation and nasogastric decompression in all cases. Mortality rate for intestinal obstruction with strangulation ranges from 5-30% whereas for simple obstruction relieved within 24 hrs, it is 1%.[19-21]

1. **Situations requiring emergency operation**

   Incarcerated, strangulated hernias

   Peritonitis

   Pneumoperitoneum

   Suspected or proven intestinal strangulation

   Closed-loop obstruction

   Complete bowel obstruction

2. **Situations in which an initial non-operative management is usually safe**

   Immediate postoperative obstruction

   Acute exacerbation of Crohn disease, diverticulitis, or radiation enteritis

   Chronic, recurrent partial obstruction

   Gastric outlet obstruction

   Postoperative adhesions

   Metastatic malignant disease

   Poor general condition of the patient

3. **Indications for Surgery in patients under observation**

   Rapidly progressing constant, noncrampy abdominal pain or distension with or without peritoneal signs

   Peritoneal signs, fever, tachycardia, leucocytosis and metabolic acidosis

   Failure of complete obstruction to resolve within 12 to 24 hrs even in the absence of signs

More than 50% of cases are directly related to post-operative adhesions. In these cases an initial non operative management is acceptable with a success rate of 50 to 85%. However if symptoms and signs indicate bowel ischaemia, immediate surgical intervention is required. The major problem in managing these patients is the difficulty in differentiating simple from strangulating obstruction. Aggressive, early surgical intervention to avoid ischaemic bowel must be balanced against the significant morbidity (30%) associated with it. 70-80% of patients with adhesive partial obstruction resolve with conservative measures.[20,21]

LAPAROSCOPY IN SMALL BOWEL OBSTRUCTION

Initially acute small bowel obstruction was considered an absolute contraindication for laparoscopy because of the risk of injuring the distended bowel. However with increased laparoscopic experience and better surgical instrumentation, there has been a change towards laparoscopic surgery. In 1991, Bastug reported successful laparoscopic adhesiolysis in a patient with partial small bowel obstruction and showed that in selected patients laparoscopy is viable.[3] Many case reports and case series of successful laparoscopic management of small bowel obstruction have been reported[22-43]. These reports show that laparoscopy is safe and feasible and is a useful technique in the management of selected cases of small bowel obstruction. Laparoscopy has been used for confirming the diagnosis, finding the cause of obstruction and relieving obstruction by division of single or multiple bands, reducing and repairing obstructed hernias, for bowel resection and for enterotomy in intra luminal obstruction (gall stone ileus).[25]

Indications

1. Non resolving partial small bowel obstruction
2. Early acute small bowel obstruction
   i. With mild abdominal distension
   ii. Proximal obstruction
   iii. Patient less than 2 previous laparotomies
   iv. Anticipated single band obstruction
   v. Children with malrotation without critical bowel ischemia

Contraindications

1. General contraindications – coagulopathies / inability to tolerate general anesthesia
2. Severe abdominal distention
3. Presence of peritonitis
4. Presence of dense adhesions and fixed loops of bowel – it is safe to convert to open procedure.

The stomach and bladder needs to the decompressed prior to the procedure. When the preoperative evaluation is inconclusive of the cause of obstruction, intra operative colonoscopy or enteroscopy should be considered and the patient is placed in modified lithotomy position. This is also helpful for laparoscopic assisted hydrostatic reduction of intussusception, if encountered.

Surgical Technique

The site for placement of the first trocar should be away from previous scars and an open technique is used for insertion of the blunt tipped Hasson trocar. In selected cases with minimal distension, Veress needle placed away from scars can be used to create pneumoperitoneum. Additional ports are placed according to the intraperitoneal findings. Entry sites should be planned to provide adequate working distance from the area of interest. According to the findings laparoscopic or laparoscopic assisted procedures like resection of bowel and anastomosis, hernia reduction and repair, reduction of intussusception, release of adhesions or bands, diverticulectomy can be performed.

The dilated bowel should be handled gently to avoid iatrogenic perforation. Only atraumatic instruments should be used. Small bowel is inspected from distal collapsed segment to proximal dilated part to decrease manipulation of the dilated bowel. Small bowel is inspected by a hand over hand technique using atraumatic instruments. Angled lens laparoscopes are better for visualization in the presence of distended loops. Fan blade retractors are useful to get into the site of obstruction.

Table tilt should be fully utilized to facilitate exposure. If a loop of bowel needs to be resected, the bowel is exteriorized through a small protected incision and anastomosis is performed extracorporeally. After adhesiolysis, those sites should be inspected carefully for any bowel injury. Doubtful areas can be tested by submersion in saline or instillation of air through nasogastric tube or endoscopes.

Following division of band, adhesiolysis or reduction of hernia, if the viability of an ischemic segment of bowel is doubtful, a planned relook laparoscopy after 24-48 hrs is indicated - "second look laparoscopy".

Laparoscopic assisted small bowel resection can be performed for lesions like stricture, diverticula, ischaemic segment of bowel and neoplasms. After a thorough exploration of entire small bowel, the segment to be resected is identified and grasped with an atraumatic grasper. The mesentry to be divided can be marked with ultrasonic scalpel. Enlarge the umbilical or adjacent trocar site to 3-4 cms. CO_2 is let out and the segment of bowel with its mesentry is pulled out through the incision. If neoplasm is suspected, the wound should be protected. The segment of bowel is resected and anastomosis performed by suturing or with a stapler. Small bowel resection can also be performed by a totally laparoscopic technique. Bowel is resected using a laparoscopic stapler (3.5 mm Staples). Proximal and distal ends of the bowel are anastomosed in a side-to-side manner using endoscopic gastrointestinal stapler. The defect from the stapler and the mesenteric defect are closed by interrupted intra corporeal sutures.

SBO following laparoscopy due to incarceration of small bowel in the trocar site has been reported. These port site hernias can be prevented by fascial closure when 10mm or larger trocars are used. Another precaution to be taken is, the trocar sheath be opened to room air during its removal to avoid creating a vacuum and pulling of bowel loop into the incision. 5mm trocar site incisions where there has been extensive manipulation are also better closed. Also during laparoscopy, umbilical hernias must be ruled out and if found repaired. Laparoscopy can confirm the diagnosis and treat port site hernias effectively.[9-14]

OUR EXPERIENCE

Since 1991, 143 patients of acute small intestinal obstruction, etiology either doubtful or unknown were treated by laparoscopic method. The age group ranged between 12 years and 74 years. 80 patients were male and 63 were female. 38 patients had previous operations. 49 gave history of recurrent episodes. Pneumoperitoneum was created by closed technique in 41 and open surgical technique in 102.

1. Adhesions and Bands

There was adhesive obstruction in 47, developmental band in 4 and Cocoon in 3 patients. Majority of the adhesive obstructions were surprisingly due to single band causing the obstruction at the distal ileum. Just simple division relieved the obstruction. Patients were tilted to the opposite side and fan blade retractor was used to get into the site of obstruction. In four patients, the segment of compressed ileum with doubtful viability was resected. Lysis of small bowel adhesion to the anterior abdominal wall was performed using monopolar scissor dissection in the early cases. Ultrasonic shears and bi-polar scissors are preferred now for adhesiolysis.

One patient developed re-obstruction 12 months later with stricture ileum probably due to ischaemia at the site of band compression. Relaparoscopy was performed and the diseased bowel was resected. Three patients had matted loops of distal ileum entirely lying in a bag of peritoneal covering. Incidentally, there was a loop proximal to the Cocoon adherent to the anterior abdominal wall at the site of previous scar. The entire segment of ileum was separated and the peritoneal coat was excised.

One patient who had laparoscopic anterior resection for carcinoma rectum developed SBO in the postoperative period. After a period of observation, he was explored and was found to have a loop of ileum densely adherent in the pelvis. Laparoscopic assisted by-pass of the obstructing segment was performed.

2. Inflammatory Stricture

In 30 patients, obstruction was due to stricture either in the ileum or in the ileoceacal junction. Resection of ileum in 23 patients and limited colectomy in 7 patients were performed. In 26 patients it was due to tuberculosis and in 4, it was due to non-specific stricture.

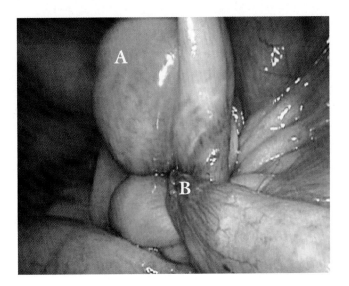

Figure 1 : Obstruction due to band

A - Dilated small bowel

B - Band

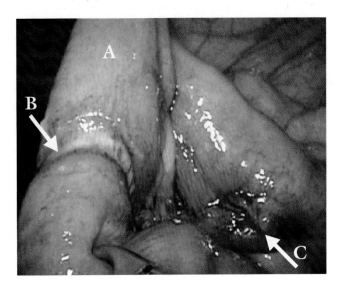

Figure 2 : Band is divided

A - Dilated segment

B - Constricted area

C - The area of mesenteric attachment of the band

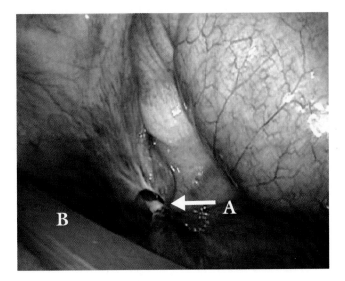

Figure 3 : Attachment of the band to the lateral abdominal wall

A - Band

B - Liver retractor is used to retract the dilated loop of the small bowel

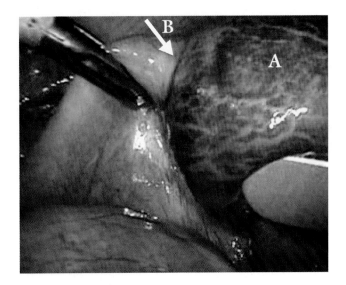

Figure 4 : Inspection of the bowel to assess the viability after the division of band

A - Dilated segment

B - Constricted area

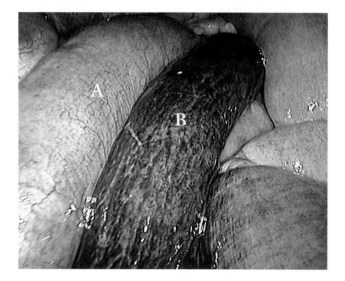

Figure 5 : Small bowel obstruction due to band.Edematous congested bowel with doubtful viability

A - Dilated segment
B - Bowel loop with doubtful viability

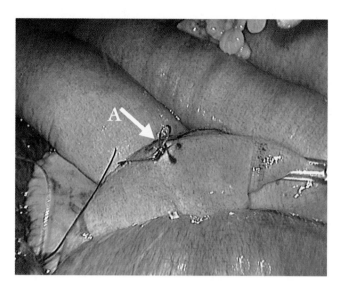

Figure 6 : Band was released. During the time of checking the bowel, injury occured in the dilated portion which was sutured using vicryl

A - Sutured site

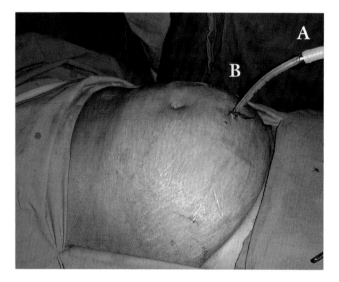

Figure 7 : Relaparoscopy was performed after 48 hrs to check the viability of the bowel loop. Pneumoperitoneum was created using the drainage tube which was kept during the first laparoscopy

A - Insufflation tube
B - Drainage tube

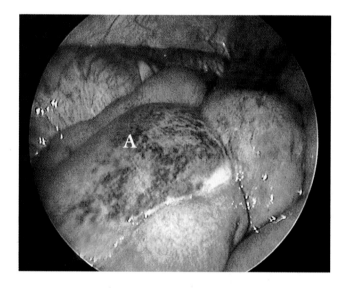

Figure 8 : Second look laparoscopy shows the viable bowel loop

A - Viable Bowel

3. Intussusception

Eleven patients with intestinal intussusception were treated laparoscopically. The etiology and discussion is given in chapter 60.

4. Meckel's Diverticulum

In 4 patients, obstruction was due to Meckel's diverticulitis with adhesions to the lateral pelvic wall. 5 patients had obstruction due to vitello intestinal bands and 4 due to intussusception. Diverticulectomy was performed laparoscopically by endoloop ligation in 1 and endo stapler in others. In 7 patients, ileum was resected and anastomosed extracorporeally by extending the umbilical port.

Diverticulitis with adhesions/kinking	4
Vitello intestinal band	2
Intussusception	4
Band with volvulus	3

5. Hernial Obstructions

In five patients, incarcerated inguinal hernia presented with intestinal obstruction. Successful reduction and hernioplasty was performed by laparoscopic method in three patients and in two laparoscopic assisted resection was performed for strangulated ileum.

Inguinal (5)

Incisional (5)

Diaphragmatic-congenital posterolateral (1)

Femoral (4)

Internal (Paraduodenal) (2)

Return of gastrointestinal function was much faster with laparoscopy or laparoscopic assisted procedures. Wound infection was not noticed in any of the patients. Requirement of analgesia was comparatively less. In all the patients, obstruction got relieved.

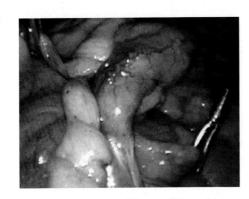

Figure 9 : Knotting of the small bowel loop with obstruction

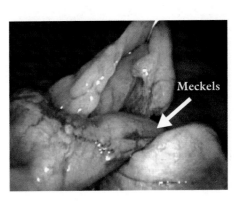

Figure 10 : Meckel's diverticulum producing obstruction

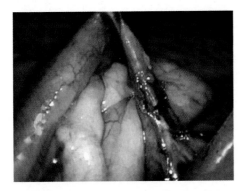

Figure 11 : Meckel's diverticulum is being mobilised

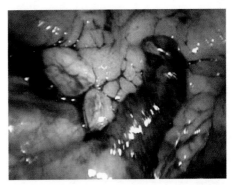

Figure 12 : Mobilised Meckel's diverticulum (can be resected using Endo GIA stapler)

RICHTER'S HERNIA WITH OBSTRUCTION

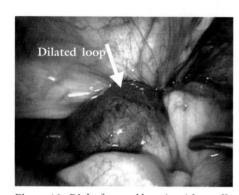

Figure 13 : Right femoral hernia with small bowel obstruction

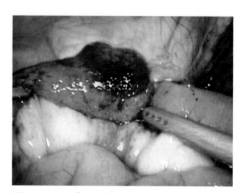

Figure 14 : After reduction

PARADUODENAL HERNIA WITH OBSTRUCTION

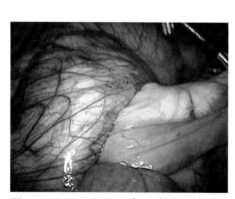

Figure 15 : Herniation of small bowel through the mesenteric

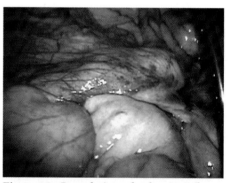

Figure 16 : Completion of reduction of small bowel

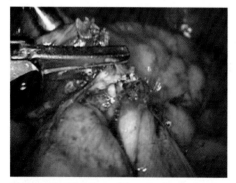

Figure 17 : Division of the attachment to the bowel

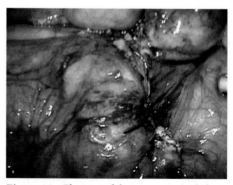

Figure 18 : Closure of the mesenteric defect using 1 - 0 prolene

With mean follow-up of 48 months, four patients had recurrence of small bowel obstruction in whom relaparoscopic enterolysis was performed in three (four times over a period of 5 years in one patient) and ileal resection anastomosis due to ischaemic stricture in one patient.

The average operative time for the entire series was 1 hour and 30 minutes. Mean length of hospitalization was 3.5 days. Major morbidity in the series was small bowel perforations. In 5 patients, repair was performed by laparoscopy using intracorporeal suturing technique. In one patient, laparotomy was performed on 3rd post operative day for localized peritonitis due to failure of identifying ileal perforation during adhesiolysis.

6. Tumor

Nine patients with intestinal obstruction due to tumor in ileum were treated as shown in Table 1.

DISCUSSION

Laparoscopy in the setting of small bowel obstruction has the obvious limitations of access and visualization. Most of the researchers advocate an open technique for the initial access. The distended bowel is much more fragile than normal bowel, hence one

Table 1.

Cause	Number	Treatment
Carcinoid ileum	2	Ileal resection-2
Metastatic deposit in ileum	3	Resection-1, By pass-2
Lymphoma of small bowel	3	Bypass-1
		Biopsy & chemotherapy -1
		Right hemicolectomy-1
Adeno carcinoma ileum	1	Ileal Resection

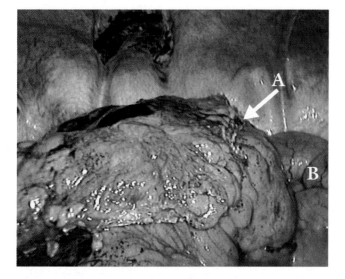

Figure 19 : Small bowel mass with obstruction

A - Small bowel mass
B - Normal bowel

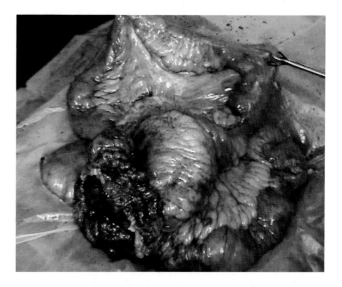

Figure 20 : By mini laparotomy small bowel with mass was exteriorised with wound protection for resection and anastomosis

Table 2.

Type	Cause	Number of Patients
1. Adhesion / band	Postoperative adhesion	47
	Developmental band	4
	Cocoon	3
2. Stricture	Tuberculosis	26
	Non specific	4
3. Tumor	Carcinoid	2
	Lymphoma	3
	Secondary deposits	3
	Adenocarcinoma ileum	1
4. Meckel's diverticulum	Diverticulitis with adhesions	4
	Band with volvulus	3
	Vitello-intestinal band	2
5. Intussusception	Round worms	1
	Submucus polyp	2
	Inverted Meckel's diverticulum	4
	Mucocele of appendix	1
	Adenocarcinoma	1
	Lipoma of ileum	1
	Lymphoma of ileum	1
6. Intra Abdominal Abscess	Appendicular Abscess	8
7. Hernial Obstructions	Inguinal	5
	Incisional	5
	Femoral	4
	Diaphragmatic-postero lateral	1
	Internal (Paraduodenal)	2
8. Malrotation		3

must be very careful in manipulating them. The reported incidence of iatrogenic enterotomy ranges from 6 to 16%.[24,27,32-35]

In most of the studies successful laparoscopic treatment was possible in around 50% of cases (35% to 60% of patients).[32,33,35,39,42]

In a prospective trial by Chosidow D, 134 patients admitted for acute small bowel obstruction secondary to adhesions were studied. 39 had emergency laparoscopy and 95 had laparoscopic adhesiolysis shortly after resolution of the obstruction with nasogastric decompression. 36% of patients who had emergency laparoscopy had to be converted to open surgery, where as only 7% of patients who had elective laparoscopy needed to be converted. Successful laparoscopic treatment was possible in 80% of patients who had elective laparoscopy and 59% in patients who had emergency laparoscopy. A limited work area and fragile small bowel make emergency laparoscopy in acute small bowel obstruction difficult. They opinion that laparoscopic adhesiolysis after the crisis has passed away may give better results but the role of elective adhesiolysis after successful conservative management is successful, is controversial.[39]

The reasons for conversions in the studies included, inadequate visualization, infarcted bowel, iatrogenic enterotomy, neoplasia, dense adhesions, inability to find the cause and inability to relieve the obstruction laparoscopically. In a retrospective study by Bailey I S[31], he found that the risk of early unplanned reoperation was increased in patients managed laparoscopically. Almost all the studies show that patients who had effective laparoscopic surgery had a shorter hospital stay. Some studies have shown good long term results also.[33] Laparoscopy also appears to result in an earlier return of bowel function.[29,35]

By laparoscopy an accurate diagnosis was possible in over 90% of cases, in most of the studies. Laparoscopy has a definite role in establishing an early diagnosis in patients with SBO. It can help in avoiding laparotomy and allow therapeutic laparoscopy in suitable cases.

In a multi-centre retrospective study (Levard H, 2001) 308 patients with acute small bowel obstruction treated laparoscopically in 35 centres were reviewed.[42] Successful laparoscopic treatment was possible in 54.6% of patients. Conversion was required in 45.5% of patients. Laparoscopy was significantly more successful in patients with a history of one or two surgical interventions than in those with more than two. It was significantly more successful in patients who had undergone appendectomy only than in patients who had no previous surgery or underwent other surgery. Success was significantly higher in patients operated on early (<24hr) and in patients with bands, than in those with adhesions or with other causes of obstruction. Duration of post operative ileus were significantly shorter following laparoscopic treatment, so was the postoperative hospital stay. Immediate wound complications were fewer after laparoscopy. The mortality rate and number of recurrent obstructions did not differ significantly. Successful laparoscopic treatment of small bowel obstruction can be expected in patients who are seen early, have one or two previous surgeries (particularly appendectomy, especially if bands are found).[42]

Manipulation of gangrenous bowel without rapid vascular control may lead to systemic spread of toxins. The pneumoperitoneum may compromise the mesenteric blood flow by increasing the already raised intra abdominal pressure. An experimental study in rabbits showed that laparoscopy (CO_2 hyper pressure) causes increased bacterial access to the blood following peroperative perforation of occluded small bowel. Hence great care should be taken to avoid perforation of bowel during laparoscopy.[52] Because of these problems, the laparoscopic surgeon should have a low threshold for conversion if bowel compromise is suspected or dense adhesions are encountered.

There are also few reports of successful laparoscopic treatment of acute small intestinal obstruction in children.[34,36,43] In children with chronic intermittent obstructive symptoms and an upper gastrointestinal xray series suggestive of malrotation, laparoscopy is useful in confirming the diagnosis and treat them by laparoscopic Ladd's procedure. It can also be safely performed in children with midgut volvulus without critical bowel ischaemia. The morbidity of open laparotomy can be avoided in these children. Laparoscopic Ladd's procedure involves division of Ladd's bands from the pylorus along the length of the duodenum, division of the intermesenteric bands and appendectomy.[44-51]

CONCLUSION

The role of laparoscopy in the management of small bowel obstruction is not yet fully defined. Currently patients with early obstruction, mild distension and partial obstruction are candidates for laparoscopic surgery. In selected patients, laparoscopy has been proved to be safe and feasible. Long term studies are required to prove that laparoscopic adhesiolysis is associated with less recurrence when compared with conventional surgery.

Table 3. Results of Laparoscopic Management of Small Bowel Obstruction

Sl. No.	Author	Year	No. of patients	Correct Diagnosis	Laparoscopic Treatment	Conversion	Morbidity	Mortality
1	Bastug DF	1991	1	1	1	0	0	0
2	Keating J	1992	5	5	5	0	0	0
3	Adams S	1993	3	3	3	0	0	0
4	Levard H	1993	25		9	16	2	1
5	Franklin ME Jr	1994	23	23	20	3	4	0
6	Federmann G	1995	25	23	15	3+5	-	-
7	Parent S	1995	35	30	21(70%)	9	5	0
8	Ibrahim IM	1996	33	100%	22 (4 assisted)	5	1	1
9	Benoist S	1996	31		16 (51.6%)	15	19%	0
10	Chevre F	1997	20		60%			
11	Bailey IS	1998	55		31 (15 assisted)	9	4	1
12	Navez B	1998	68	66%	31 (40%) +4	31+2	-	2
13	Leon EL	1998	40	-	14 (35%) + 12(30%)	14 (35%)	3	-
14	Becmeur F*	1998	86	-	66	-	3	0
15	Strickland P	1999	40	-	24 (60%)	13	10	
16	DC Van der Zee*	1999	9	-	6	3		
17	Kyzer S	1999	14		13(93%)	1	0	0
18	El Dahha AA	1999	14	14	12 (85.7%)	2 (14.3%)	7.1%	0
19	Chosidow D	2000	39 (emergency) 95 (after resolution)	-	59% 80%	36% 7%	-	0
20	Agresta F	2000	63	58 (92%)	52 (82.5%)	11 (17.4%)		
21	A.A. Al.Mulhim	2000	19	17 (90%)	13 (68%)	6	0	0
22	Levard H	2001	308		168 (54.6%)	140(45.4%)		
23	Shalaby R*	2001	30		20 (66.7%)	10 (33.3%)	0	0

*Pediatric patients

References

1. Landercasper J, Coghill T H, Merry W H 1993 Long-term outcome after hospitalization for small bowel obstruction. Arch Surg 128: 765 771.

2. Evers BM : Small intestine. In : Townsend CM, Beauchamp R.D. Evers BM, Mattox. K. L (eds) Sabiston Text book of surgery : The biological basis of Modern surgical Practice 17th edn (vol 2). Saunders, Elsevier; 2004 ; 1323-1380.

3. Bastug D F, Tammell S W, Boland J P et al 1991 Laparoscopic adhesiolysis for small bowel obstruction. Surg Laparosc Endosc 1:259-262.

4. Kukor J S, Dent T L. Small intestinal obstruction. In : Nelson R L, Nyhus L M (eds) 1987 Surgery of the small intestine. 1st edn. Norwalk : Appleton & Lange, p 267-282.

5. Perry Jr JF, Smith GA, Yonehiro EG. Intestinal obstruction caused by adhesions. A review of 388 cases. Ann Surg 1955; 142; 810-816.

6. Cox M R, Gunn M c, Eastman R f et al 1993a The operative aetiology and types of adhesions causing small bowel obstruction. Aust NZJ Surg. 63; 367 - 371.

7. Ellis C N, Boggs H W, Slagel G W, Cole P A 1991 Small bowel obstruction after colon resection for benign and malignant diseases. Dis Col Rect 34:367-371.

8. Spears H, Petrelli N J, Herrera L, Mettelman A 1988 Treatment of bowel obstruction after operation for colorectal cancer. Am J Surg 155; 383 – 386.

9. Sauer M, Jarrett JC. Small bowel obstruction following diagnostic laparoscopy. Fertil Steril 1984 Oct;42(4):653-4.

10. Eltabbakh GH, Small bowel obstruction secondary to herniation through a 5mm laparoscopic trocar site following laparoscopic lymphadenectomy. Eur J Gynaecol Oncol.1999;20(4):275-6.

11. Reardon PR, Preciado A, Sarborough T, Matthews B, Marti JL, Hernia at 5mm laparoscopic port site presenting as early postoperative small bowel obstruction. J Laparoendosc Adv Surg Techn A, 1999 Dec;9(6):523-5.

12. Lajer H, Widecrantz S, heisterberg L. Hernias in trocar ports following abdominal laparoscopy. A review. Acta Obstet Gynecol Scand. 1997 May;76(5):389-93.

13. Kurtz Br, Daniell JF, Spaw AT. Incarcerated incisional hernia after laparoscopy. A case report.J Reprod Med. 1993 aug;38(8):643-4.

14. Romagnolo C, Minelli L. Small-bowel occlusion after operative laparoscopy : our experience and review of the literature, Endoscopy.2001 Jan;33(1):88-90.

15. Ogata M, Mateer J R, Condon R E. 1996, Prospective evaluation of abdominal sonography for the diagnosis of bowel obstruction. Ann Surg. 223:237-241.

16. Balthazar E J 1994 CT or small-bowel series for suspected SBO; questions and answers. Am J Radio 163:1260-1261.

17. Pain J A, Collier D St J, Hanka R 1987 Small bowel obstruction : computer-assisted prediction of strangulation at presentation. Br J Surg 74:981-983.

18. Richard WO, Garrard CL, Allos SH Non invasive diagnosis of mesenteric ischemia using a SQUID magnetometer. Ann Surg 221 : 696 – 705, 1995.

19. Stewadrsin. R.H., Bombeck, C.T., and Nyhus, L.M. : Critical operative management of small bowel obstruction. Ann. Surg., 187:189-194, 1978.

20. Sosa J, Gardner B: Management of patients diagnosed as acute intestinal obstruction secondary to adhesions. Am. Surg., 59:125-130,1993.

21. Bizer L.S., Liebling R.W., Dealny H.M., and Gliedman, M.D. : Small bowel obstruction: The role of nonoperative treatment in simple intestinal obstruction and predictive criteria for strangulation obstruction. Surgery 89: 407 – 410, 1981.

22. Keating J, Hill A, Schoeder D, Whittle D : Laparoscopy in the diagnosis and treatment of acute small bowel obstruction. J Laparoendosc Surg 1992 Oct; 2(5):239-44

23. Adams S, Wilson T, Brown AR. Laparoscopic management of acute small bowel obstruction. Aust N Z J Surg. 1993 Jan; 63(1):39-41.

24. Levard H, Mouro J, Schiffino L, Karayel M, Berthelot G, Dubois F. Celioscopic treatment of acute obstructions of the small intestine. Immediate results in 25 patients. Ann Chir. 1993; 47(6):497-501.

25. Franklin M E, Dorman J P , Pharand D 1994 Laparoscopic surgery in acute small bowel obstruction. Surg Laparosc Endosc 4:289-296.

26. Federmann G, Walenzyk J, Schneider A, Bauermeister G, Scheele C. Laparoscopic therapy of mechanical or adhesion ileus of the small intestine-preliminary results. Zentralbl Chir. 1995; 120(5):377-81.

27. Parent S, Bresler L, Marchal F, Boissel P. Celioscopic treatment of acute obstructions caused by adhesions of the small intestine. Experience of 35 cases. J Chir (Paris). 1995 Oct; 132(10):382-5.

28. I.M. Ibrahim, F. Wolodiger, B. Sussman, M. Kahn, F. Silvestri, A Sabar Laparoscopic management of acute small-bowel obstruction. Surgical Endoscopy 1996 Oct;10(10) : 1012-1015.

29. Benoist S, De Watteville JC, Gayral F. Role of celioscopy in acute obstruction of the small intestine. Gastroentrol Clin Biol. 1996;20(4):357-61.

30. Chevre F, Renggli JC, Gorebli Y, Tschantz P. Laparoscopic treatment of small bowel obstruction arising on adhesions. Ann Chir. 1997;51(10):1092-8.

31. Bailey IS, Rhodes M, O'Rourke N, Nathanson L, Fielding G. Laparoscopic management of acute small bowel obstruction. Br J Surg 1998 Jan;85(1):84-7.

32. Navez B, Arimont JM, Guiot P. Laparoscopic approach in acute small bowel obstruction. A review of 68 patients. Hepatogastroenterology. 1998 Nov-Dec; 45(24):2146-50.

33. Leon EL, Metzger A, Tsiotos GG, Schilinkert RT, Sarr MG Laparoscopic management of small bowel obstruction : indications and outcome. J Gastrointest Surg. 1998 Mar-Apr;2(2):132-40.

34. Becmeur F, Besson. R Treatment of small-bowel obstruction by laparoscopy in children multicentric study. Eur J Pediatr Surg. 1998 Dec;8(6):343-6.

35. P.Strickland, DJ Lourie, E.A. Suddleson, JB Blitz, SC stain, Is laparoscopy safe and effective for treatment of acute-small bowel obstruction? Surgical Endoscopy. 1999 July;13(7):695-698.

36. D.C. van der Zee and N.M.A. Bax Management of adhesive bowel obstruction in children is changed by laparoscopy. Surgical Endoscopy 1999 Sept; 13(9):925-927.

37. Kyzer S, Aloni Y, Charuzi I. Laparoscopic treatment of small bowel obstruction caused by adhesions. Harefuah. 1999 May 2;136(9):681-3, 755.

38. El Dahha AA, Shawkat AM, Bakr AA, Laparoscopic adhesiolysis in acute small bowel obstruction a preliminary experience JSLS 1999 Apr-Jun:3(2):131-5.

39. Chosidow D, Johanet H, Mantariol T, Kielt R, Manceau C, Benhamou G. Marmuse JP, Laparoscopy for acute small bowel obstruction secondary to adhesions. J laparoendosc Adv Surg Tech A. 2000 Jun;10(3):155-9.

40. F.Agresta, A.Piazza, I.Michelet, N.Bedin, C.A. Sartori. Small bowel obstruction laparoscopic approach Surgical Endoscopy. February 2000;14, (2):154-156.

41. A.A. Al-Mulhim. Laparoscopic management of acute small bowel obstruction. Surgical Endsocopy 2000 Feb;14(2):157-160.

42. Levard H; Boudet MJ; Msika S; Molkhou J-M; Hay J-M; Laborde Y; Gillet M; Fingerhut A. Laparoscopic treatment of acute small bowel obstruction : A multicentre retrospective study : ANZ Journal of Surgery, November 2001 Vol 71 No.11, pp 641-646.

43. Shalaby R, Desoky A. Laparoscopic approach to small intestinal obstruction in children : a preliminary experience. Surg Laparosc Endosc Percutan Tech. 2001 Oct; 11(5):301-5.

44. Bass KD, Rothenberg SS, Chang J, Laparoscopic Ladd's procedure in infants with malrotation. J Pediatr Surg 1998;33:279-281.

45. Gross E, Chen MK, Lobe TE. Laparoscopic evaluation and treatment of intestinal malrotation in infants. Surg endosc 1996;10:937-937.

46. Mazziotti MV, Strasberg SM, Langer JC. Intestinal rotation abnormalities without volvulus: the role of laparoscopy. J Am Coll Surg 1997;185:172-176.

47. Lessin MS, Luks FI. Laparoscopic appendectomy and duodenocolonic dissociation (LADD) procedure for malrotation. Pediatr Surg Int 1998; 13:184-185.

48. Wu MH, Hsu WM, Lin WH, Lai HS, Chang KJ, Chen WJ. Laparoscopic Ladd's procedure for intestinal malrotation : report of three cases. J Formos Med Assoc 2002;101:152-155.

49. Van der Zee DC, Bax NMA. Laparoscopic repair of acute volvulus in a neonate with malrotation. Surg Endosc 1995;9:1123-1124.

50. Bax NMA, Van der Zee DC. Laparoscopic treatment of intestinal malrotation in children. Surg Enodsc 1998; 12 : 1314-1316.

51. Yamashita H, Kato H, Uyama S, et al Laparoscopic repair of intestinal malrotation complicated by midgut volvulus. Surg endosc 1999;13:1160-1162.

52. Bustos B, Gomez-Ferrer F, Dalique Jb etal. Laparoscopy and septic dissemination caused by perioperative perforation of the occluded small bowel ; an experimental study. Surg Laparosc Endosc 1997 Jun; 7(3) : 228 - 31.

60

Laparoscopic Management of Intussusception

INTUSSUSCEPTION

Intussusception is the telescoping of proximal intestine (intussusceptum) into adjacent distal intestine (intussuscipien), resulting in obstruction of the lumen. Paul Barbette in the late 1600s described invaginations of one segment of bowel into another. The first successful surgical reduction was reported in 1891 by Sir Jonathan Hutchison. It is a common cause of intestinal obstruction in children under the age of two years. 80-90% of all cases occur in children between the age of 3 months to 3 years.[1] Intestinal intussusception is uncommon in adults. It constitutes only 1% of intestinal obstructions in adults and represents 5% of all cases of intussusception.[2, 3]

CLASSIFICATION - ANATOMICAL TYPES

Ileo-colic - most common type in children

Ileo-ileo-colic - second most common

Entero-enteric
  Ileo-Ileal
  Jejuno-jejunal ⎪ More common in adults
Ceco-colic
Colo-colic

AETIOLOGY

Most of the pediatric intussusceptions are idiopathic (no identifiable pathologic lead point) and involve the ileoceacal region. There is marked swelling of lymphoid tissue in the ileocecal region. In upto 30% of cases, there is a preceding viral illness (gastroenteritis, upper respiratory infection or recent administration of rota virus vaccine).[4, 5] The hypertrophied Peyer's patches may be acting as potential lead points.

A pathologic lead point is identifiable only in upto 12% of pediatric cases.[6] However, 60-67% neonates,

57% older children (>5yrs) and 97% of adults have anatomic lead points.[7] The most common anatomic lead point identified in pathological specimens is Meckel's diverticulum. Others include polyps, appendix, submucous hematomas (Henoch-Schonlein purpura), ectopic pancreatic or gastric tissue, intestinal neoplasms and intestinal duplication cysts.

Pathologic lead points for intussusception

1. Hypertrophied Peyer's patches
2. Meckel's diverticulum
3. Polyps
4. Submucous haematomas
5. Ectopic pancreatic / gastric tissue
6. Foreign body
7. Intestinal neoplasm
8. Intestinal duplication cysts

These lead points may result in areas of dysrhythmic contraction along the bowel wall during peristalsis and this non-homogenous longitudinal force along the intestinal wall results in invagination of the bowel. With each peristaltic contraction, the intussusceptum is drawn farther into the distally bowel. This leads to lymphatic obstruction, venous congestion and later on arterial compromise and necrosis of the intussusceptum. When the mucosal blood supply is compromised, mucosa sloughs off resulting in the classical "red currant jelly" stool. If untreated the process progresses to transmural gangrene and perforation of the intussusceptum.

CLINICAL PRESENTATION

Most commonly occurs in infants aged 5-10months. There is a slight male preponderance (3:2). Intussusception typically produces cyclical severe abdominal pain in an otherwise healthy infant. In between the child is comfortable. It is almost always associated with vomiting. Later on, the child develops abdominal distension and becomes toxic. Bowel ischemia results in passage of blood clots mixed with mucus ("red currant jelly" stool). A mass may be palpable in the right upper quadrant and the right lower quadrant may feel empty. Rectal examination will reveal blood staining and in late cases tip of the intussusceptum may be felt in the rectum.

Unlike children the symptoms and signs of intussusception in adults are often non specific and may be sub-acute or chronic in presentation. A palpable mass is less common and may be felt in 7-42% of cases.[2,3] Features of intestinal obstruction need not always be present.

INVESTIGATIONS

Plain X-ray abdomen will reveal small bowel obstruction

Ultrasound abdomen is the non invasive diagnostic procedure of choice. The characteristic findings include the target sign (or bulls eye) on transverse view and the "pseudokidney" sign on longitudinal view. However it is highly operator dependent.

Contrast Enema is both diagnostic as well as therapeutic

Computed Tomography is also useful in diagnosis. However, it carries the risk of radiation exposure and IV contrast administration. It is the most useful diagnostic tool in adults.[9-11] The appearance of a bowel-within-bowel configuration with or without contained fat and mesenteric vessels is pathgnomonic.

MANAGEMENT

Intussusception in infants and children less than 3 yeas of age rarely have lead point and therefore respond to non operative reduction. Older children and adults often have a surgical lead point to the intussusception and hence require operative intervention.

Idiopathic Intussusception (Infants and Young Children)

The child is resuscitated with IV fluids. Nasogastric decompression and broad spectrum antibiotics are given.

1. Non operative reduction

Hydrostatic reduction by contrast agent or pneumatic reduction by air insufflation under radiographic guidance can be attempted if there is no evidence of peritonitis/perforation and the patient is hemodynamically stable.

The hydrostatic reduction using barium or water soluble contrast has a reported success rate of 40 to 90%. It was first described by Hirschsprung.[12] Successful hydrostatic reduction depends on several factors including duration of symptoms, presence of lead points and the technique used. While using barium or water soluble contrast, the column of contrast should not exceed 100cms above the level of buttocks. An attempt is considered successful when the contrast is seen refluxing back into the terminal ileum. For pneumatic reduction, the pressure of air insufflation should not exceed 120cms of water.

When the first attempt is unsuccessful, some clinicians advocate one or two subsequent attempts.

Ultrasound guided hydrostatic reduction has the advantage of avoiding radiation exposure. Air insufflation has higher rates of reduction than saline. The results of successful reduction are immediate. The patients are kept under observation for a short period of time. The recurrence rate after non operative reduction is 5-10%.[13] Most of the recurrences occur within 72 hours of the initial event. It is treated in a similar fashion by non operative reduction. More than one recurrence suggests the presence of a lead point and in such cases, surgical exploration is indicated.

Non operative reduction is of no value in ileo-ileal intussusception, which usually is seen in older children with associated diseases like Hirschsprung's disease, hemophilia, Peutz-Jeghers syndrome or malignancies.

2. Laparotomy

Laparotomy is indicated if non operative reduction is unsuccessful or if perforation / peritonitis exists. A right transverse supra umbilical incision is preferred. Bowel is gently compressed with warm saline soaked pads to reduce edema. Apply gentle pressure at the apex - milking the intussusception proximally. Pulling out the intussusceptum carries the risk of iatrogenic perforation. Manual reduction is successful in 90% of cases. After reduction careful search for any lead points should be done and assess bowel viability. Appendicectomy is often performed if the blood supply of the appendix is compromised. A cecopexy is not necessary as the recurrence rate after surgical reduction is less than 5%. If intussusception cannot be reduced and the bowel is gangrenous, resection of the intussusception and primary anastomosis is carried out.

3. Laparoscopy

In infants with ileocolic intussusception, if non operative reduction fails, surgical reduction is indicated. There are reports of laparoscopic reduction of such cases.[14,15]

Surgical Technique

Laparoscopy is performed under general anaesthesia with the patient in supine position. The surgeon usually stands on the left side of the patient at the level of the abdomen, and the monitor is kept on the right side, opposite to the surgeon. The insufflation pressure is kept around 8mm of Hg. Umbilical trocar is used for camera and working ports are placed in left upper quadrant and left iliac fossa. Alternatively working ports may put in right iliac fossa and left iliac fossa also. The bowel should be examined thoroughly starting from the collapsed loop of bowel, moving proximally towards the dilated bowel using atraumatic instruments. The apex of the intussusceptum is stroked proximally with an intestinal clamp or atraumatic grasper while gentle traction is maintained on the distal bowel (milking out). Pneumo dissection also helps in freeing the intussusceptum from the intussuscipiens. Laparoscopic assisted hydrostatic/pneumatic reduction is preferred by some surgeons.

In one study, Schier reported that 4 of 7 intussusceptions, with failed hydrostatic reduction were successfully reduced by laparoscopy. Reduction was completed easily with squeezing and pulling with laparoscopic forceps.[14] Cuckow PM in 1996 described a laparoscopic reduction technique of infantile ileocolic intussusception. This involved grasping the ileum and stroking the neck of the intussusception back over the invaginated bowel. Reduction was achieved with persistent effort over several minutes.[15] Hay SA et al reported the use of laparoscopy in 20 patients with failed non surgical reduction.[16] Laparoscopic reduction was successful in 8 patients,

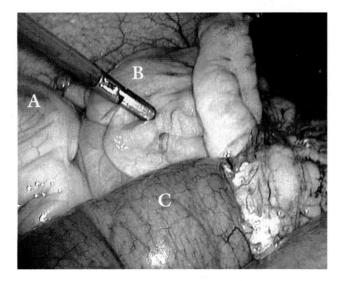

Figure 1 : Examination of the small bowel, starting from the non-dilated loop

A - Cecum
B - Normal small bowel
C - Dilated small bowel

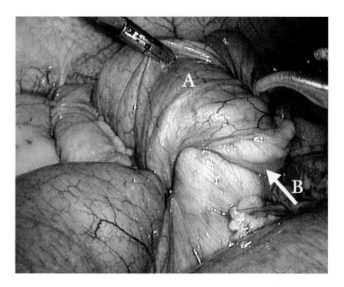

Figure 2 : Ileo ileal intussusception

A - Distal bowel
B - Mesentery of the invaginated proximal bowel

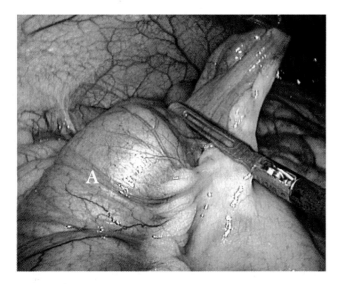

Figure 3 : Using the bowel holding forceps the intussusception of the bowel is being reduced by milking technique starting from the distal end

A - Affected segment of bowel

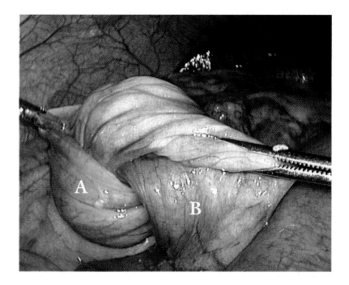

Figure 4 : Another way of reducing the intussusception of the bowel by pulling the proximal loop with the atraumatic forceps

A - Distal loop
B - Proximal loop

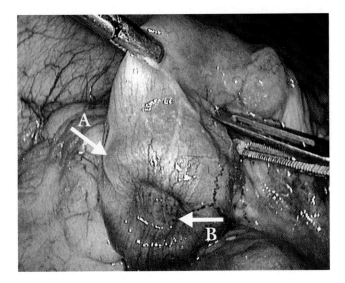

Figure 5 : After the reduction the diseased portion of the small bowel (polyp) is seen

A - Polyp in the small bowel lumen
B - Serosal involvement

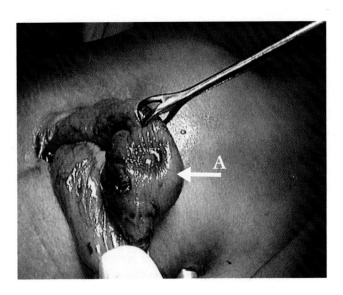

Figure 6: By extension of the umbilical port by 3cm, the affected segment small bowel is exteriorised

A - Small bowel with polyp

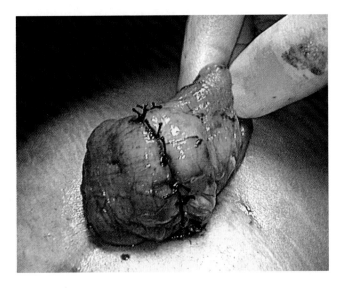

Figure 7 : Resection and hand sewn end to end anastomosis

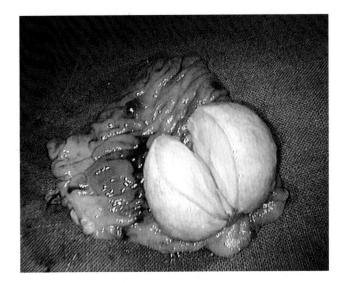

Figure 8 : Cut section of the small bowel and the polyp (biopsy showed neurofibromatous polyp in this particular case)

saline hydrostatic reduction was successful in 6 patients and in 6 patients it could not be reduced (laparotomy was done). The use of laparoscopy and hydrostatic reduction by saline during laparoscopy avoided the need for laparotomy in 70% of patients. In one study 98 infants with intussusception after a failed non operative reduction were subjected to laparoscopy. 64 (65.3%) patients had successful laparoscopic reduction and the rest required conversion to open procedure.[17]

An experimental study in dogs was done to evaluate feasibility of laparoscopy in assisting pneumatic reduction with artificially produced ileocolic intussusception. They had 94% success rate with perforation occurring in one case. Laparoscopy has a role in confirming the diagnosis and may help in reduction of difficult cases, thus avoiding laparotomy.[18]

Laan M (2001) reported that there is a role for laparoscopy in recurrent intussusception or in cases of doubtful reduction. He also stated that in patients less than 3 years of age, little is gained from laparoscopy, provided good non surgical reduction facilities are available.[19] In patients above 3 years, usually resection is needed and will not benefit from laparoscopy (if resection is not done laparoscopically). Allan M et al (2003) reported successful pneumatically assisted laparoscopic reduction of intussusception in 4 patients without any complications.[20]

These studies demonstrate that there is a role for laparoscopy in failed non surgical reduction cases. Laparoscopic reduction of intussusception is technically feasible and safe. One point which needs further clarification is if a pathological lead point is seen, can it be managed appropriately by laparoscopy. There are reports of laparoscopic resection of benign lead points.

Cunningham SD et al (1998) reported successful management of small bowel intussusception in a case of Peutz-Jeghers syndrome. They conclude that laparoscopy is a safe and effective method of managing intussusception in Peutz-Jeghers syndrome because the pathological lead point is a benign hamartoma and this could possibly eliminate the need for laparotomy and reduce the postoperative complications associated with multiple reoperations.[21]

ADULT INTUSSUSCEPTION

In contrast to infants, treatment should be operative because almost all cases have an underlying pathological process. In a review of 1024 patients from various studies, (Begos DG 1997) found the cause of colo-colic intussusception to be malignant in approximately 60% of cases[3], whereas more than 60% of small bowel intussusceptions where benign. Because of the high risk of malignancy in colo-colic intussusception some advocate enbloc resection of these lesions. Small bowel lesions are often benign, hence attempted reduction especially if the segment is long is advised.[22] In general, enbloc resection of the intussusception is done if malignancy is suspected and the bowel is necrotic.

The role of laparoscopy in adult intussusception is more controversial than in infants. Chekan EG (1998) suggests that if a benign cause is suspected preoperatively, laparoscopy should be considered.[23]

Laparoscopic assisted reduction of ileal lipoma causing ileo-ileo-colic intussusception was reported by Park KT (2001).[24] Although the role of laparoscopy is not clearly defined, it may be an alternative approach to the surgical treatment of adult intussusception in selected cases. Laparoscopic assisted resection for neoplastic lesions is feasible but should be performed only in selected cases.[25,26]

Post operative intussusception is a rare complication in the post operative period with an incidence of 0.08-0.5% of all laparotomies.[27] It is assumed to occur because of a difference in activity between segments of the intestine recovering from ileus. Rarely indwelling jejunal catheters can lead to intussusception by acting as a lead point.[28-30] Diagnosis can be made by injecting dye proximally and through the tip of the catheter. Treatment is surgical reduction.

A patient with jejuno-jejunal intussusception, induced by the feeding jejunostomy tube, following esophagectomy was treated by open reduction and closure of jejunostomy site. Laparoscopy was successful in rest of the cases. The patient with intussusception induced by worms, after successful reduction was treated with anithelminthic drugs. In other patients, resection and anastomosis were performed through a minilaparotomy with 3-4 cms

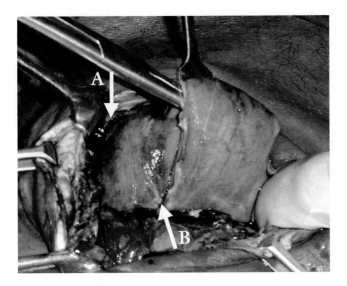

Figure 9 : Jejuno jejunal intussusception due to jejunostomy tube

A - Site of feeding jejunostomy
B - Jejuno jejunal intussusception

incision in the umbilicus. Laparoscopic assisted right hemicolectomy was performed in three patients with ileocolic and ceco-colic intussusceptions.

One of the patients had a large mass palpable in the mid abdomen. Colonoscopy and barium enema showed intussusception at the level of mid transverse colon. Laparoscopy revealed an ileo-colic intussusception and it could be reduced upto the caecum. After reduction there was a lump in the caecum. Laparoscopic assisted right hemicolectomy was performed. The specimen showed a large polyp of 5 x 5 cms with a long pedicle which was attached 10cms proximal to the ileo-caecal junction. Histopathology revealed lymphoma - an unusual clinical presentation of ileal lymphoma.

CONCLUSION

Laparoscopy is an alternative to laparotomy in children less than 3 years with intussusception not relieved by non operative reduction. Almost all forms of intussusception without bowel necrosis can be reduced using modern video laparoscopic equipment and atraumatic instruments. In adults, since the clinical features are non specific, laparoscopy has a definite role in confirming the diagnosis and if a benign cause is suspected laparoscopic assisted resection is safe and effective.

OUR EXPERIENCE

Since 1991, twelve patients with intestinal intussusception were treated here.

Type	Cause	Number of Patients	Treatment
Jejuno jejunal	Feeding tube induced	1	Open Reduction
Ileo-ileal	Round worms	1	Lap. Reduction
	Neurofibromatous polyp	2	Lap. assisted resection
	Inverted Meckel's diverticulum	4	Lap. assisted resection
	Lipoma of ileum	1	Lap. assisted resection
Ileo-colic	Mucocele of appendix - carcinoid in the base	1	Lap. assisted right hemicolectomy
	Lymphoma of ileum	1	Lap. assisted right hemicolectomy
Ceco-colic	Adenocarcinoma caecum	1	Lap. assisted right hemicolectomy

References

1. Doody DP : Intussusception. In : Oldham Kt, Colombani PM, Foglia RP, eds. Surgery of infants and Children : Scientific Principles and Practice. Lippincott-Raven; 1997 : 1241-8.

2. Azar T, Berger DL. Adult intussusception. Ann Surg. 1997;226:134-8.

3. Begos DG, Sandor A, Modlin IM. The diagnosis and management of adult intussusception. Am J Surg. 1997 Feb;173(2):88-94.

4. Chang HG, Smith PF, Ackelsberg J, et al : Intussusception, rotavirus diarrhea, and rotavirus vaccine use among children in New York State. Pediatrics 2001 Jul; 108(1) : 54-60.

5. Zanardi LR, Haber P, Mootrey GT, et al : Intussusception among recipients of rotavirus vaccine : reports to the vaccine adverse event reporting system. Pediatrics 2001 Jun;107(6):E97.

6. Young DG : Intussusception. In : O'Neill JA Jr, Rowe MI, Grosfeld EW, et al, eds. Pediatric Surgery. Vol2.Mosby-year Book;1998:1185-98.

7. Ong NT, Beasley SW : The leadpoint in intussusception. J Pediatr Surg. 25:640, 1990.

8. Barr LL : Sonography in the infant with acute abdominal symptoms. Semin Ultrasound CT MR 1994 aug; 15(4):275-89.

9. Parienty RA, Lepreux JF, Gruson B : Sonographic and CT features of ileocolic intussusception. AJR Am J Roentgeonol 1981 Mar; 136(3) : 608-10.

10. Bar-Ziv J, Solomon A. Computed tomography in adult intussusception. Gastrointest. Radiol.1991;16:264-6.

11. Gayer G, Apter S, Hofmann C et al. Intussusception in adults; CT diagnosis. Clin Radiol.1998;53:53-7.

12. Hischsprung H : Et Tilfaelde af subakut Tarminvagination. Hospitals-Tidende 1876;3:321-2.

13. Stringer MD, Pablot SM, Brereton RJ : Paediatric intussusception. Br J Surg 1992 Sep; 79(9) : 867-76.

14. Schier F. Experience with laparoscopy in the treatment of intussusception. J Pediatric Surg 1997;32:1713-4.

15. Cuckow PM, Slater RD, Najmaldin AS. Intussusception treated laparoscopically after air enema reduction. Surg Endosc 1996:10:671-2.

16. Hay SA, Kabish AA, Soliman HA. Idiopathic intussusception : the role of laparoscopy : J Pediatr Surg 1999 Apr 34(4) : 577-8.

17. Poddoubnyi IV, Dronov AF, Blinnikov OI, Smirnov AN, Darenkov IA, Dedov KA. Laparoscopy in the treatment of intussusception in children. J Pediatr Surg 1998 Aug : 33(8):1194-7.

18. Abasiyanik A, Dasci Z, Yosunkaya A, et al : Laparoscopic-assisted pneumatic reduction of intussusception. J Pediatr Surg 1997 Aug; 32(8) : 1147-8.

19. Van der Laan M, Bax NM, van der Zee DC, Ure BM. The role of laparoscopy in the management of childhood intussusception. Surg Enosc. 2001 Apr; 15(4):373-6. Epub 2001 Feb 06.

20. Allan MG, Nancy LC, Mark UM. Pneumatically assisted laparoscopic reduction of intussusception ; Pediatric endosurgery and Techniques : 2003, 7:33-37.

21. Cunningham JD, Vine AJ, Karch L : The role of laparoscopy in the management of intussusception in Peutz Jeghers syndrome : case report and review of literature.

22. Tan Ky, Tan SM, Tan AG, Chen CY, Chng HC, Hoe MN. Adult intussusception : experience in Singapore. ANZ J Surg. 2003 Dec;73(12):1044-7.

23. Chekan EG, Westcottc, Low VH. Small bowel intussusception and laparoscopy. Surg Laparosc. Endosc 1998; 8(4):324-6.

24. Park K.T., Kim SH, Song TJ: Laparoscopic-assisted resection of ileal lipoma causing ileo-ileo-colic intussusception. J Teorm Med Sc 16:119-22.

25. Alonso V, Targarona EM, Bendahan GE, Kobus C, Moya I, Cherichetti C, Balague C, Vela S, Garriga J, Trias M. Laparoscopic treatment for intussusception of the small intestine in the adult. Surg Laparosc Endosc Percutan tech 2003 Dec;13(6):394-6.

26. Hackam DJ, Saibil F, Wilson S Litwin D. Laparoscopic management of intussusception caused by colonic lipomata : a case report and review of the literature. Surg Laparosc Endosc. 1996; 6(2):155-9.

27. West KW, Stephens B, Resorla FJ, et al: Postoperative intussusception : experience with 36 cases in children. Surgery 1988 Oct;104(4): 781-7.

28. Noake T, Yoshida S, Fujita H, Ishibashi N, Shirouzu K. Intussusception during enteral nutrition: a case report. Kurume Med J. 2001;48(3):237-40.

29. Hui GC, Gerstle JT, Weinstein M, Connolly B. Small bowel intussusception around a gastrojejunostomy tube resulting in ischemic necrosis of the intestine. Pediatr Radiol. 2004 Nov;34(11):916-8. Epub 2004 July 28.

30. Ciaccia D, Quigley RL, Shami PJ, Grant JP. A case of retrograde jejuno-duodenal intussusception caused by a feeding gastrostomy tube. Nurtr Clin Pract. 1994 Feb; 9(1):18-21.

61

Laparoscopic Excision of Meckel's Diverticulum

INTRODUCTION

Meckel's diverticulum is the most common congenital abnormality of the gastrointestinal tract and is found in approximately 2% of the general population.[1] The incidence of asymptomatic diverticula is similar in both sexes. The male to female ratio of patients with symptomatic diverticula is 3:1.

Johann Friedrich Meckel, Professor of Anatomy at Halle, in 1809 described in detail its anatomy and embryonic origin, and hence it is now known by his name.[2] However, it was first reported by Hildanus in 1598.

ANATOMY

Meckel's diverticulum is a true diverticulum, containing all layer of the bowel wall and results from incomplete closure of omphalomesenteric duct or vitelline duct. It is located on the antimesenteric border of the ileum 45 to 60 cm proximal to the ileoceacal valve. Normally the vitelline duct undergoes obliteration during the fifth to ninth week of gestation.[3] Persistence of this duct may result in different forms of anomalies.

1. Fibrous cord between the umbilicus and the ileum

2. Umbilical sinus - when the umbilical side of the duct does not fully obliterate

3. Meckel's diverticulum - the intestinal end failing to obliterate

4. Umbilico-ileal fistula - when the entire duct remains patent

5. Vitelline cyst

6. Any combinations of the above[4]

It derives its blood supply from persistent vitelline vessels that are present within a distinct mesentery. The length and diameter vary. Cells lining the vitelline duct are pluripotent and heterotopic tissue can be present within the diverticulum. Most common is gastric mucosa (50%).[5] Pancreatic tissue is encountered in 5%, less commonly colonic mucosa, lipoma and other benign and malignant tumors have been reported. Incidence of heterotopic mucosa was higher in symptomatic patients (75% of bleeding Meckel's diverticulum contain ectopic gastric mucosa).

CLINICAL MANIFESTATIONS

Majority of Meckel's diverticula are asymptomatic and are discovered incidentally during laparoscopy, laparotomy or barium studies. The most common clinical presentation of a Meckel's diverticulum is gastrointestinal bleeding.

Williams in a review of 1806 collected cases found the following incidence of complications.[6]

Hemorrhage	31%
Diverticulitis	25%
Bowel obstruction	16%
Intussusception	11%
Hernial involvement	11%
Umbilical fistula or sinus	4%
Tumor	2%

Hemorrhage is the most common presentation in children aged 2 years and below. It may vary from minimal recurrent bleeding to massive hemorrhage. Another common complication is intestinal obstruction, which may occur as a result of a volvulus of the small bowel around a diverticulum associated with a fibrotic band attached to the abdominal wall, intussusception or rarely incarceration in an inguinal hernia (Littre's hernia).

Diverticulitis accounts for 10% to 20% of symptomatic presentations. This is more common in adults and clinically indistinguishable from appendicitis. Neoplasms arising from Meckel's diverticulum are rare. The most frequent one is Gastro Intestinal Stromal Tumor. Carcinoid and adenocarcinoma have also been reported.

DIAGNOSTIC STUDIES

1. Technetium pertechnate radioisotope scan is the single most accurate diagnostic test for Meckel's diverticulum in children. It is taken up preferentially by gastric mucosa and ectopic gastric tissue. Its sensitivity is 85% and specificity 95% in children. In adults it is less accurate because of reduced prevalence of ectopic gastric mucosa within the diverticulum. H_2 receptor blockers, pentagastrin and glucagon improve the accuracy of the test.

2. Superior Mesenteric Angiography may be helpful in patients presenting with acute gastrointestinal bleeding and is effective when blood loss exceeds 0.5 ml/min.

3. Laparoscopy is both diagnostic as well as therapeutic. It should be considered as an alternative diagnostic modality in patients with suspected Meckel's diverticulum, especially in paediatric age group.[7]

TREATMENT

Treatment of symptomatic Meckel's diverticulum is resection of the diverticulum or resection of ileum bearing the diverticulum. Segmental intestinal resection is required in patients with bleeding because the bleeding site usually is in the ileum adjacent to the diverticulum. Resection of non bleeding diverticulum (diverticulectomy) can be performed using either a hand-sewn technique or stapling across the base in a diagonal or transverse line so as to minimize the risk of subsequent stenosis.

Because Meckel's diverticlitis often mimics appendicitis, examine the distal ileum for Meckel's diverticulum when the appendix is discovered to be normal during exploration for suspected appendicitis.[4]

Controversy still exists regarding the ideal management of asymptamatic Meckel's diverticulum noted as an incidental finding. The resection of asymptomatic diverticula in children at laparotomy/laparoscopy is generally recommended. Most surgeons generally do not resect a Meckel's diverticulum with a wide mouth in adults. There is general agreement that diverticula that appear to have heterotopic mucosa on physical examination should be resected. Long diverticula, a narrow mouth and fibrous bands to the umbilicus or mesentery are risk factors for complications and are relative indications for resection. There are numerous reports have demonstrated the feasibility and safety of laparoscopic diverticulectomy.[7-25]

LAPAROSCOPY

Indications for resection of Meckel's diverticulum
Symptomatic Meckel's diverticulum
1. Bleeding
2. Diverticulitis
3. Bowel obstruction
4. Intussusception
5. Involvement in hernia
6. Umbilical fistula / sinus
Asymptomatic Meckel's diverticulum
1. In children
2. Thick and nodular
3. Long diverticulum
4. Narrow mouth
5. With fibrous bands/adhesions

Diagnostic laparoscopy is indicated if there is adequate clinical suspicion of Meckel's diverticulum. It should be considered in any case of lower gastrointestinal bleeding in young children. Diagnostic radiology is rarely successful and is time consuming and therefore should be avoided in patients with significant intestinal bleeding. Radioisotope scan is more reliable and can be carried out more rapidly. In case of recurrent bleeding, upper gastrointestinal endoscopy and colonoscopy should be performed prior to laparoscopy. A high index of clinical suspicion is important, particularly in children with a negative isotope scan and laparoscopy is advised in such cases with lower gastrointestinal bleed.[12,22] Immediate laparoscopic evaluation is indicated for intestinal obstruction or for mesenteric ischaemia.

Laparoscopy is both diagnostic and therapeutic. The whole small bowel can be systematically inspected and the diverticulum easily identified. Once identified, it can be resected laparoscopically or by laparoscopic assisted extracorporeal resection. Thus a formal laparotomy can be avoided.

OPERATIVE TECHNIQUE

Position of the surgeon, team and port placement are as in appendectomy. In small children umbilicus is better avoided because of the accompanying umbilical abnormalities. The Veress needle and the first trocar are placed in suprapubic area lateral to rectus muscle on the left side.

1. A Vitelline cyst if present should be removed. If the ileum is connected to the cyst, it may have to be resected

2. Embryonic bands should be divided after coagulation or using harmonic scalpel

3. Most of the diverticula are resected using a stapler or brought out and resection anastomosis performed extracorporeally. After mobilisation of the diverticulum the antemesenteric border is grasped and stretched into a tent shape and resection performed with an Endo GIA stapler, applying it diagonally or transversely to avoid bowel stenosis. Otherwise the umbilical port is widened and the bowel exteriorized and resection anastomosis performed out side.

OUR EXPERIENCE

Total No. of cases - 49

Types	No.
Incidental	26
Diverticulitis	7
Perforation	3
Small bowel obstruction	
Band	2
Volvulus around band	3
Intussusception	4
Inflammatory adhesion/kinking	4

Treatment	No.
Laparoscopic diverticulectomy using	
Endo GIA Stapler	21
Endo loop ligation	3
Laparoscopic assisted diverticulectomy	11
Laparoscopic assisted resection anastomosis	14

We had treated 49 cases of Meckel's diverticulum since 1991.

1. Incidental

Initially, when the Endo GIA stapler was not available in India, laparoscopic assisted diverticulectomy was being performed, by delivering the diverticulum through the umbilical port and resecting it extracorporeally. Now most of the incidental diverticulectomies are performed using Endo GIA stapler. Incidental Meckel's diverticulectomy was performed for the following reasons like large size, narrow neck and nodular and thickened diverticula.

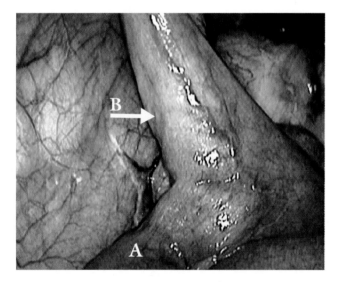

Figure 1 : Meckel's diverticula found during appendicectomy

A - Ileum

B - Meckel's diverticulum

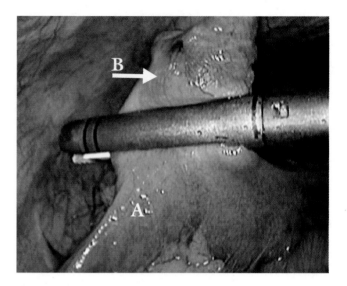

Figure 2 : Excision of Meckel's diverticulum using Endo GIA stapler

A - Ileum

B - Meckel's diverticulum

2. Diverticulitis

All these cases were picked up during diagnostic laparoscopy. A 32 year old male had recurrent attacks of intestinal colic and significant weight loss (56 -34 kg). He was on prolonged drug therapy including a course of antituberculous drugs without a definite diagnosis. Diagnostic laparoscopy showed a mass like lesion in the terminal ileum densely adherent to the right lateral pelvic wall. The whole segment was mobilized. It was a big pouch of Meckel's diverticulum with peridiverticular adhesions. Laparoscopic assisted resection anastomosis was performed. On 8 years of follow up, he is asymptomatic and put on weight substantially. In another patient, diverticular adhesion to the dome of the bladder was released and the diverticulum was resected.

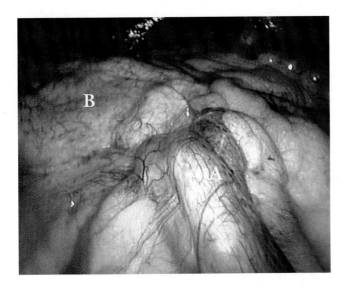

Figure 3 : Adhesion of small bowel and omentum

A - Adherent small bowel

B - Omental adhesions

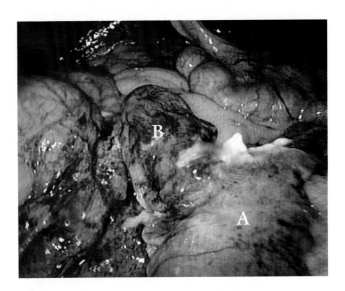

Figure 4 : Adhesions separated and Meckel's diverticulum with diverticulitis found

A - Ileum

B - Meckel's diverticulum

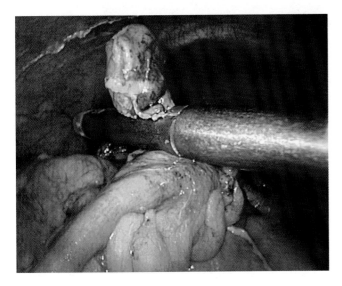

Figure 5 : Excision using Endo GIA stapler

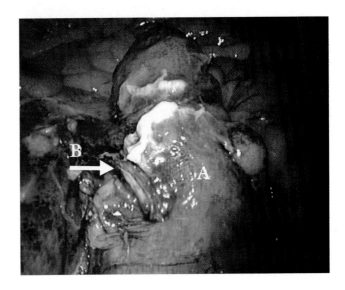

Figure 6 : Small bowel loop after diverticulectomy

A - Small bowel

B - Staple line

3. Perforation

Three patients of diverticular perforation with inter mesenteric abscesses were treated by laparoscopic approach. Diverticulectomy in one, resection and anastomosis through the extended umbilical port in the remaining two was carried out.

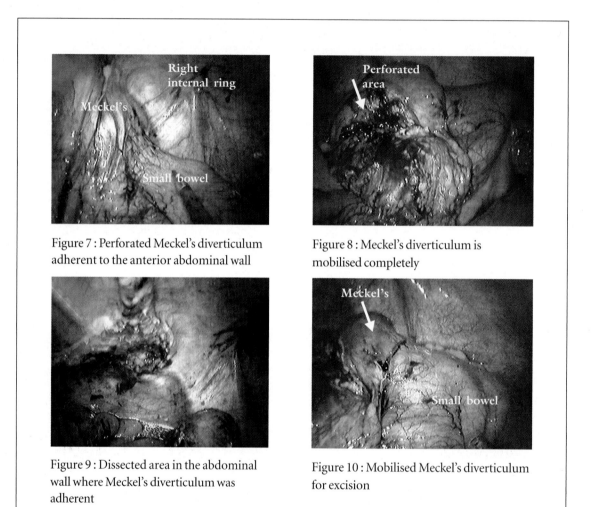

Figure 7 : Perforated Meckel's diverticulum adherent to the anterior abdominal wall

Figure 8 : Meckel's diverticulum is mobilised completely

Figure 9 : Dissected area in the abdominal wall where Meckel's diverticulum was adherent

Figure 10 : Mobilised Meckel's diverticulum for excision

4. Small Bowel Obstruction

In 3 cases of small bowel obstruction due to Meckel's diverticulum, ligamentous malfortamation of omphaloenteric duct was causing strangulation due to volvulus. All the three cases were treated successfully by laparoscopic assisted resection and anastomosis. In other cases of small bowel obstruction the obstructing band was released and Meckel's diverticulectomy was performed.

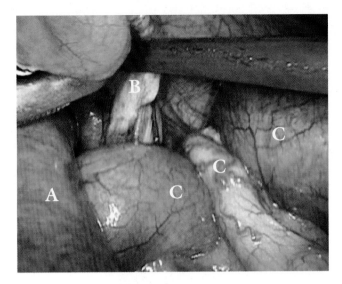

Figure 11 : Meckel's diverticulum with small bowel obstruction

A - Dilated ileum
B - Median umbilical ligament
C - Knotting of ileum

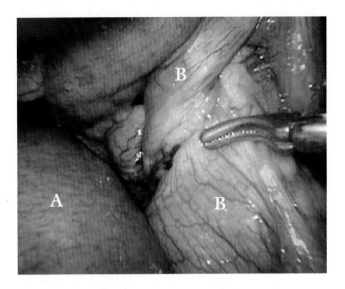

Figure 12 : Derotation of the ileal loop to find out the cause of the obstruction

A - Congested small bowel loop
B - Knotting of ileum

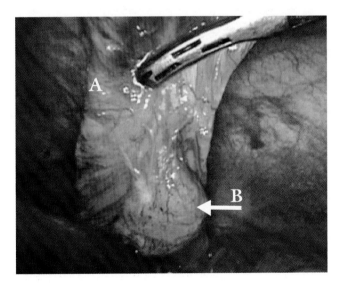

Figure 13 : Mobilisation of Meckel's diverticulum from the median umbilical ligament

A - Median umbilical ligament
B - Perforated tip of the Meckel's

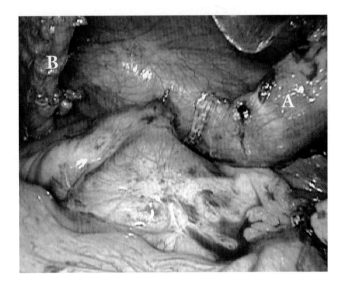

Figure 14 : Meckel's diverticulum is excised using Endo GIA stapler

A - Excised Meckel's diverticulum
B - Median umbilical ligament

5. Intussusception

In 4 cases, the Meckel's diverticulum got invaginated into the ileum like a inverted finger glove producing ileo-ileal intussusception. Reduction was attempted, the final solid mass like lesion could not be reduced. Resection and anastomosis through the extended umbilical port was performed successfully in all four.

Oral fluids was started between 24-48hrs. Most of the patients were discharged on the 4th or 5th day. The average hospital stay was 4.5 days. One of the patients with perforation was discharged on 7th POD (ileus). None of the patients had leak or wound infection.

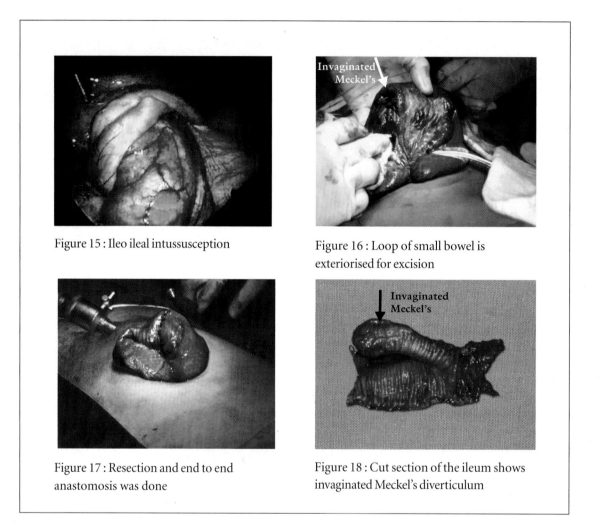

Figure 15 : Ileo ileal intussusception

Figure 16 : Loop of small bowel is exteriorised for excision

Figure 17 : Resection and end to end anastomosis was done

Figure 18 : Cut section of the ileum shows invaginated Meckel's diverticulum

DISCUSSION

Laparoscopic resection of Meckels diverticulum is safe and feasible, the published reports and studies prove it. Laparoscopy has been performed safely in cases of complicated Meckel's diverticula including bleeding, small bowel obstruction due to torsion around mesodiverticular band, intussusception and diverticulitis.

Dronov reported laparoscopic management of Meckel's diverticulum in 58 children. 33 patients had bleeding, 21 had diverticulitis and 4 had intestinal obstruction. Laparoscopic resection was possible in 56 patients. 2 patients needed conversion due to inflammation in the diverticulum and adjacent parts of the intestine. In 31 patients, Endo GIA stapler was used. Roeder's loop used in 23 patients and extracorporeal suturing used in 2 patients. One of the patient's had adhesive postoperative small bowel obstruction. There was no mortality and cosmesis was excellent is all the cases.[21]

Some of the surgeons advocate the use of pretied endoloops for ligation and resection of narrow based Meckel's diverticulum like an appendicectomy.[21] We have also done 3 cases like this with no morbidity.

Laparoscopy has a definite role in diagnosis and treatment of lower gastrointestinal bleeding of obscure origin in children. In one study, 17 children with obscure gastrointestinal bleeding had diagnostic laparoscopy. 7 patients had Meckel's diverticulum, 2 had intestinal duplication, 2 had nodular lymphoid hyperplasia of ileum and one had vascular enteritis. 4 had normal findings on laparoscopy. All patients who had positive findings had laparoscopic assisted small bowel resection except the one with extensive vascular enteritis (laparotomy). All patients made uneventful recovery without recurrence of bleeding.[22]

Mukai studied the relationship between the distribution of gastric heterotopia and the external appearance of the diverticulum for the proper selection of laparoscopic procedure. They found that long diverticula had gastric mucosa at the distal end and in short diverticula it occurred in almost any area. Hence they advocate simple transverse resection with stapler for long diverticula and for short diverticula ileal resection with end to end anastomosis.[26]

In 1976 Soltero and Bill reported that the life time risk of complications from Meckel diverticulum is 4.2% and the risk decreases with age. Their data indicated that 800 asymptomatic diverticula would have to be removed to save the life of one patient. Morbidity rates from incidental removal was reported to be as high as 12% in some studies. On that basis, they opposed surgical excision of asymptomatic diverticula.[27] This study was criticized because it was not a population based analysis.

Cullen and colleagues reported an epidemiologic, population based study on 145 patients undergoing resection of Meckel's diverticulum, in which 87% were incidentally found.[28] They calculated a 6.4%

life time risk for complications of a Meckel's diverticulum. They reported an operative morbidity rate of 2% after resection of incidentally found diverticula and found that complications does not appear to peak during childhood as originally thought. Therefore they advocate diverticulectomy for asymptomatic disease even in the older age group. This study suggests that in selected patients diverticulectomy even in the asymptomatic patient may be beneficial and safer than originally reported.

CONCLUSION

Meckel's diverticulum is an uncommon entity. A high index of suspicioun is needed for diagnosis and prompt treatment. Technetium scintigraphy is a sensitive and specific test, but in adults it is less sensitive. Diagnostic laparoscopy is indicated in clinically suspected cases especially in children with lower gastro intestinal bleeding. Laparoscopy is safe and efficient for diagnosis and definitive treatment of Meckel's diverticulum. In selected patients incidental diverticulectomy may be beneficial.

References

1. Yahchouchy EK et al : Meckel's diverticulum. J Am Coll Surg 192:658-662, 2001.

2. Meckel JF : Ueber die Divertikel am Darmkanal. Arch Physiol 9 : 421-453, 1809.

3. Di Giacomo J.C : Surgical treatment of Meckel's diverticulum, South Med J. 86:671-675, 1993.

4. Moore TC : Omphalomesentric duct malformations. Semin Pediatr Surg 5:116-123, 1996.

5. Heyman S : Meckel diverticulum : Possible detection by combining pentagastrin with hitamine H2 receptor blocker.J Nuecl Med. 35:1656-1658, 1994.

6. Williams RS : Management of Meckel's diverticulum. Br J Surg 1981; 68:477.

7. Lu CC, Huang FC, Lee SY, Huang HY. Laparoscopic diagnosis and treatment excision of bleeding Meckel's diverticulum in a child : report of one case. Acta Paediatr Taiwan 2003; 44 (1) : 41-3.

8. Sanders LE : Laparoscopic treatment of Meckel's diverticulum : Obstruction and bleeding managed with minimal morbidity. Surg Endosc. 9 : 724-727, 1995.

9. Altinli E, Pekmezci S : Laparoscopy assisted resection of complicated Meckel's diverticulum in adults. Surg Laparosc Endosc Percutan Tech 2002;12(3):190-4.

10. Rivas H, Cachione RN, Allen JW : Laparoscopic management of Meckel's diverticulum in adults. Surg Endosc.2003 April; 17(4) : 620-2.

11. Tarcoveanu E, Nicuslecu D : Meckel's diverticulum in laparoscopic era. Chirurgia 2004; 99(4):227-32.

12. Saggar RU, Krishna A : Laparoscopy in suspected Meckel's diverticulum : negative nuclear scan not withstanding. Indian Pediatrics. 2004; 41 : 747-748.

13. Negro P, Catarci M, Zaraca F, Gossetti F, Saputelli A, Scaccia M, Carboni M, Laparoscopic diverticulectomy for ileal volvulus on Meckel's diverticulum. G Chir. 1994 Mar;15(3) : 134-6.

14. Akamine M, Araki Y, Chijiiwa Y, Shimizu S, Shimura H, Nawata H. A case of Meckel's diverticulum complicated by stenosis of the colon. Am J Gastroenterol. 1997 Nov;92(11):2114-6.

15. Duca S, Al-Hajjar N, Graur F, Bala O, Indoitu G. Laparoscopic management of Meckel's diverticulum. Chirurgia (Bucur). 2004 Jul-Aug;99(4):233-6.

16. Bueno Ledo J, Serralta Serra A, Plalineeis Roig M, Dobon Gimenez F; Ibanez Palacin F, Rodero Rodero R. Intestinal obstruction caused by omphalomesentric duct remnant : usefulness of laparoscopy. Rev Esp Enferm Dig.2003 Oct;95(10):736-8, 733-5.

17. Tashjian DB, Moriarty KP. Laparoscopy for treating a small bowel obstruction due to a Meckel's diverticulum. JSLS.2003 Jul-Sep;7(3):253-5.

18. Loh DL, Munro FD. The role of laparoscopy in the management of lower gastro-itnstinal bleeding. Pediatr Surg Int. 2003 Jun; 19(4):266-7. Epub 2003 Apr 30.

19. Steffen H, Ludwig K, Scharlau U, Czarnetzki HD. Laparoscopic treatment of small bowel obstruction with intussusception, volvulus and appendicitis caused by an inflammatory Meckel's diverticulum. Zentralbl Chir. 2003 Feb;128(2):99-101.

20. Karahasanoglu T, Memisoglu K, Korman U, Tunckale A, Curgunlu A, Karter Y. Adult intussusception due to inverted Meckel's diverticulum : laparoscopic approach. Surg Laparosc Endosc Percutan Tech. 2003 Feb;13(1):39-41

21. Dronov AF, Poddubnyi IV, Kotlobovskii VI, Al'-Mashat NA, Iarustovskii PM. Video-laparoscopic surgeries in Meckel diverticulum in children. Khirurgiia (Mosk) 2002;10:39-42.

22. Lee KH, Yeung CK, Tam YH, Ng WT, Yip KF. Laparoscopy for definitive diagnosis and treatment of gastrointestinal bleeding of obscure origin in children. J Pediatr Sug. 2002 Sep;35(9) : 1291-3.

23. Schmid SW, Schafer M, Krahenbuhl L, Buchler MW. The role of laparoscopy in symptomatic Meckel's diverticulum. Surg Endosc. 1999 Oct;13(10):1047-9.

24. Valla JS, Steyaert H, Leculee R, Pebeyre B, Jordana F. Meckel's diverticulum and laparoscopy of children. What's new ? Eur J Pediatr Surg. 1998 Feb;8(1):26-8.

25. Schier F, Hoffmann K, Waldschmidt J. Laparoscopic removal of Meckel's diverticula in children. Eur J Pediatr Surg. 1996 Feb;6(1):38-9.

26. Mukai M, Takamatsu H, Noguchi H, Fukushige T, Tahara H, Kaji T. Does the external appearance of a Meckel's diverticulum assist in choice of the laparoscopic procedure? Pediatr Surg Int. 2002 May;18(4):231-3.

27. Soltero MJ, Bill AH : The natural history of Meckel's diverticulum and its relation to incidental removal : A study of 202 cases of diseased Meckel's diverticulum found in King county, Washington, over a fifteen year period Am J Surg 132:168-173, 1976.

28. Cullen JJ, Kelly KA : Surgical management of Meckel's diverticulum : An epidemiologic, population based study. Am Surg 220:564-569, 1994.

SECTION ⑩

Colon and Rectum

62

Laparoscopic Colorectal Surgery

INTRODUCTION

Laparoscopic surgery has witnessed an explosive development in the last two decades, after the acceptance of laparoscopic cholecystectomy as the gold standard by the surgical fraternity. Every organ in the abdomen was invaded by the laparoscopic surgeons and numerous reports on techniques various laparoscopic procedures were reported. This was also reflected in colorectal surgery with description of various laparoscopic procedures for benign and malignant diseases. But the pace of the development in laparoscopic colorectal surgery did not match with that of other laparoscopic surgeries like laparoscopic cholecystectomy and fundoplication.

There were numerous reasons for decreased enthusiasm like technical challenges associated with operating in several quadrants of abdomen; the fact that the colon is not a fixed organ; the need to divide major vessels; the diversity of operations performed; the longer learning curves and the presence of critical structures in close relationship that are likely to be injured during the surgery like the ureter etc.

Laparoscopic assisted left hemicolectomy was the first laparoscopic colorectal procdure that was published in 1991[1,2] which was followed by the first laparoscopic procedure for a colonic malignancy by Jacobs and colleagues.[3] The possible benefits such as shorter hospital stay, lesser pain, shorter post operative ileus and improved cosmesis were demonstrated clearly. Eventhough the authors had suggested a beneficial effect of laparoscopy for colonic resections, they had also raised certain issues like higher conversion rate, longer operative times, and higher chances of iatrogenic lesions and unclear cost effectiveness advising the future laparoscopic surgeons to adopt a selective approach.[4] The problems encountered by these surgeons were attributed to the learning curve and was expected to diminish with increasing experience.

Subsequently in a report of 74 laparoscopic assisted colonic procedures, Wexner et al had addressed these problems and had suggested tips for reducing them. This article was one of the first articles that discussed objective assessment criteria for these procedures like complications, morbidity and mortality, compliance with oncological principles.[5]

The first report of port site metastasis was reported in 1978 in a patient who had underwent diagnostic laparoscopy for ovarian cancer.[6] Port site metastasis following laparoscopic colectomy for cancer was reported in 1993 in patients in Dukes B & C cancer who had undergone colectomy with a curative intent [7]. This was further blown up by a report of 21% incidence of port site metastasis in patients who underwent laparoscopic colectomy for cancers.[8] Subsequently in an analysis of 30 reports of port site metastasis the rate was found to be around 4%.[9] The authors had issued a warning pointing to the first line of Hippocratic Oath "primum non nocere" (FIRST DO NO HARM) and had indicated that laparoscopic colorectal surgeries for malignancies should be done only in randomized trails.

In a series of subsequent reports the complications and problems encountered seemed to reducing owing to the experience gained. The recent analysis of 27 studies (each with a minimum of 50 cases) from 1993 to 2001, found an overall incidence of only 0.71 percent which is similar to the conventional surgery.[10] These reports have laid down the concerns regarding port site metastasis. The port site metastasis is not an inherent problem of laparoscopic colorectal resection, but rather unfortunate sequelae of the learning curve.

After these concerns were settled, a series of reports have appeared on various laparoscopic procedures from laparoscopic stoma creation to complex procedures like single stage Soave's pull through for Hirschpung disease, total abdominal colectomy, with ileo anal pouch anastomosis, and others.[11-18] Many of these studies have shown the beneficial effect of laparoscopic procedures both in short term and long term. Recently, long term reports of many properly conducted multi institutional randomized controlled trials have clearly demonstrated that the laparoscopic colorectal procedures are oncologically safe and the survival rates are similar to that of conventional surgeries.

INDICATIONS FOR LAPAROSCOPIC COLORECTAL PROCEDURES

1. Benign
   i. Diverticular disease
   ii. Crohns disease
   iii. Ulcerative colitis
   iv. Rectal prolapse
   v. Uncommon conditions like
      a. Colonic inertia
      b. Volvulus
      c. Fecal diversion
      d. Perforation - trauma, colonsocopic

2. Malignant
   i. Polyps
   ii. Colorectal carcinoma

BENIGN DISEASES

1. Diverticular Diseases

The laparoscopic approach for various stages of diverticular diseases such as diagnosis, assessment of disease, resection of affected segment and diversion have been shown to have favorable outcomes.[19-22] A comparative study on open and laparoscopic procedures on diverticular disease, have clearly demonstrated that patients undergoing laparoscopic surgeries have decreased hospital stay and morbidity.[20]

2. Crohns Disease

Laparoscopic resection from Crohn's disease was fist reported in 1995.[23] The subsequent reports have shown beneficial results in these patients, in spite of problems such as immuno compromised and malnourished status, dense adhesions, interloop abscess and entero cutaneous fistulas. Though the conversion rate was 16% in a multicentre trial, it can be reduced to as low as 4% if conditions like fistula, abscess and phlegmon is diagnosed preoperatively. Laparoscopy is the preferred method of resection for isolated ileocolic Crohn's disease.

They have an added advantage of reduction in post operative adhesions (which often makes future surgery difficult) and improved cosmesis and body image (which are very relevant in the younger age group patients). This is important as Crohn's disease more commonly affects patients in younger age group and the acceptance of surgery will be more when compared to laparotomies.

3. Ulcerative Colitis

Even though reports of laparoscopic approach has been described more commonly with Crohn's disease, reports on ulcerative colitis has also been published which includes subtotal, total and restorative proctocolectomies. But definitely laparoscopy in ulcerative colitis requires more advanced laparoscopic skills and expertise and is considered investigational at the current moment.[24]

4. Rectal Prolapse

The first report on laparoscopic rectopexy was published in 1992.[25, 26] Though more than hundred procedures have been described in both transabdominal and perineal approach, the transabdominal approach is preferred unless the patient is in high risk for surgery. Various reports on rectopexy, suture rectopexy, resection rectopexy, laparoscopic assisted perineal proctosigmoidectomy and others have been reported.[27-29] Compared with open surgery the laparoscopic approach resulted in shorter length of hospital stay and lower morbidity[30, 31] and even improvement in post operative anal pressures as demonstrated by anal manometric studies.[32]

5. Laparoscopic Hartman's Reversal

Reversal of Hartman's procedure is a major surgery and is often associated with increased wound infection as the mucosa is exposed and certain degree of contamination is always inevitable. The wound infection rate can be considerably reduced down in laparoscopy.[33-35]

6. Laparoscopic Stoma Creation

Temporary or permanent fecal diversion for conditions such as malignancy, trauma, perineal sepsis and for protection of distal anastomosis following surgery can be done by laparoscopy. This is the simplest surgery to start with in laparoscopic colorectal procedure. Laparoscopy is superior to laparotomy and conventional method of creation of stoma. The same procedure can be done through 10 mm incisions along with a complete and thorough intra abodminal inspection, lysis of adhesions (if needed) and mobilization. The patients recover faster with shorter ileus, conversion is rare and subsequent closure is also easy.[11, 36-41]

MALIGNANCY

Surgery for cancers of the colon has been performed by laparotomy using techniques described before the time of Halsted. It has been often judged by the dictum that 'bigger is better' along with the notion that the conventional surgery offers more chances of long term cure. This has been based on the assumption that laparotomy offers a better chance for radical resection and lymph nodal clearance. But now the concepts are slowly changing and laparoscopic resections are being more accepted.

Over the past several years, the technique of laparoscopic colectomy has been developed and refined. Laparoscopic surgery has resulted in faster recovery of bowel function, less morbidity and shorter length of hospital stay. However all these advantages would become secondary if the oncological clearance of the tumor is proven inferior. But, the important aspect that has to be understood is that the same procedure performed by laparotomy is duplicated through smaller incisions facilitated by the advanced technology. The consistent results of the recent multi-institutional randomized trials on the feasibility, oncological safety effectiveness, long term recurrence and survivals and functional outcomes has had a definitive and welcome change in the attitude of the surgeons.

The recently published multi-institutional trial involving 48 institutions and randomly assigned to 872 patients with adenocarcinoma rectum to undergo either open or laparoscopic resection by credentialed surgeons has clearly shown that the recurrence rates and the overall survival rates were similar mean follow-up of 4.4 years. This well organized trial result will definitely help in decreasing the resistance to use laparoscopic technology by some general and colorectal surgeons, surgical and medical oncologists.

> "Progress is slow, but our leaders in surgical oncology must be bold in improving minimal access surgery for cancer as their predecessors were developing bigger operations. Their patients expect nothing less".
>
> Editorial, JAMA, May 2004

BENEFITS OF LAPAROSCOPIC SURGERY

Laparoscopic colorectal surgery offers benefits like decreased postoperative pain, speedy recovery, shorter hospitalization, earlier return of bowel function, better preserved pulmonary function, decreased abdominal wound infection, reduced incidence of post operative adhesions and decreased morbidity. These benefits are more relevant in elderly population in whom colorectal disease like diverticulosis and malignancy are more common.[42] The prolonged hospital stay and other problems after open surgery might increase the morbidity in these already fragile geriatric patients.

Impact of laparoscopic approach in faster return of bowel movements is an important factor that permits early discharge. The patients can be allowed to have clear liquids on the second post operative day and regular diet the next morning. Subsequent abdominal operations will be lot more easier after laparoscopy when compared to the extensive adhesions that are found after laparotomy in some patients.

The acute phase response following laparoscopic colectomies is altered demonstrating that the systemic inflammatory response is lower in laparoscopic surgeries. Several authors have demonstrate a significant decrease in IL6[5, 43, 44] CRP[45] and granulocyte[46] and other factors. The cancer patients may already have a suppressed immune system and any further decrease in the immunity might be harmful. Laparoscopy helps in minimizing this stress response.

DISADVANTAGES OF LAPAROSCOPIC SURGERY

The advent of laparoscopic surgery has created a specific set of complications like Veress needle injury, trocar injury and electrosurgical injuries.

These were considered important during the early phase of the laparoscopy when most of the surgeons were in the learning curve. These are largely preventable with experience. The learning curve, i.e. the number of cases that a surgeon requires to perform a safe surgery has been accepted to be around 20-50 cases.[47, 48]

An important aspect that has to be understood in this context is the difference between "learning curve" and "developmental curve". The developmental curve is the period of development and refinement of a surgery by a surgeon who has no prior experience in that particular surgery. Most of the descriptions and recommendations of learning curve that were published initially were in fact describing this developmental curve.[49] Definitely a simplified approach taught by an experienced surgeon who has mastered the technique (by refinements based on his personal experience and from literature) will allow for a more rapid acquisition of skills by trainees and a definite reduction in the learning curve. In other words, the present day chief residents and laparoscopic surgery fellows can learn the refined techniques in a faster manner compared to the pioneers (for example the skills for a right hemicolectomy can be acquired in about 5 cases).[49]

Reduction in Learning Curve

1. Understanding pathophysiology of disease
2. Knowledge of anatomy
3. Adequate experience in conventional surgeries
4. Adequate laparoscopic surgery principles: dissection techniques, suturing and knotting
5. Learning from previous surgery by reviewing tapes and positive feedback.

The other supposed disadvantage of the laparoscopic surgery has been termed as the high amount of costs involved. Most studies report an increase in cost with laparoscopy[50-54] though some have shown decrease costs.[55] The main reasons for this discrepancy are the flaws in the methodology of these study designs and the impact of learning curve. It is obvious that a surgeon's operative time and the cost of the consumables are higher in the early part of learning curve and costs will naturally reduce with experience.

Use of reusable instruments, techniques like endosuturing (instead of staplers) and others will definitely reduce the cost of the procedure.

Regarding the study design, most studies discuss the charges to the patients rather the true costs, such as the immediate and quantifiable parameters such as staff cost and hospital costs. The costs saved in reduced incidence of respiratory complications, wound infections and increased productivity due to earlier recovery, quicker return to normal activity and work are difficult to quantify and yet may be substantial. A patient who recovers faster may be able to return to work faster and support his family, when compared to a patient who is still recovering from surgery. This gains more importance in developing countries like India, where the male is the sole earner of the family. His quicker return to activity may help him support his family faster.

APPROACH TO LAPAROSCOPIC COLORECTAL SURGERY

The surgeon who wishes to opt for laparoscopic surgery should understand the basic concepts of laparoscopic surgery and be experienced in basic laparoscopic surgery and 2 handed dissection techniques and suturing skills. The surgeon must be well versed with open surgeries and should have worked before in a department that is routinely performing these kinds of surgeries. He should assist the experienced surgeon initially as second assistant and then as camera assistant and later operate under the directions of the experienced surgeon. He should record the surgeries continuously and reevaluate his performance from the feedback obtained from his video tapes and comments from his fellow surgeons. Initially the procedures should be restricted to benign diseases and once the surgeon has reached the plateau of his learning curve, he can then progress to malignancies. More over, there should be adequate case load to allow for the surgeon to ascend the learning curve within a reasonable period of time i.e. 20-30 colectomeis annually.[56]

With regard to the technique of surgery in malignancy, the same extent of resection should be duplicated as performed in open surgery. The patients are being referred to tertiary centers after so called laparoscopic resections, which are mere procedures of mobilization of colon to allow it reach the abdominal wall and struggle to extract it through a minilaparotomy (which is less than adequate) and manage to resect the tumor and anastomose. This is highly unacceptable and reflects the basic lack of training and defying the oncological principles. This should be avoided at any cost, otherwise these incidences might bring disrepute to laparoscopic colorectal surgery.

It will be helpful for the surgeons if they can attempt colorectal surgeries in increasing level of difficulty staring from basic surgeries like segmental resection for benign conditions and slowly ascend to the more difficult procedures as given in the following order.

1. Segmental resection
2. Stoma formation
3. Sigmoidectomy / anterior resection
4. Right hemicolectomy
5. Left hemicolectomy
6. Transverse colectomy
7. Abdominoperinal resection
8. Repair of Hartmann's pouch
9. Low anterior resection
10. Total proctocolectomy

Difficulties in dissection of the colon & mesentery, visualization through a limited visual field, lack of 3 dimensional view and tactile feedback, handling of advanced equipments for dissection (Babcock, bowel holding, harmonic scalpel) hemostasis (staplers, ligasure) bowel division and anastomosis will be faced by all the surgeons, but can be mastered with experience. The division of rectum in the deep part of pelvis, (particularly in a male patient in case of low anterior resection) is extremely difficult because of the anatomical position.

Laparoscopic colorectal surgery has evolved to a highly specialized field in this past decade due to the developments in both technology (advanced imaging system, staplers, dissection instruments and hemostatic equipments) and more importantly due to the refinements of the technique based on previous experience, and is rapidly becoming an essential tool in the gastrointestinal surgeons armamentarium. Various benign conditions can be very effectively operated by laparoscopic approach (e.g. polyp, diverticulitis, Crohn's, tuberculosis). In regard to malignancy, the recently published well conducted multi-institutional trials have shown the fears such as trocar site recurrence, radiating of resection and complications are not true and laparoscopic surgery are as safe as open surgery in terms of oncological resection.

ANATOMY OF COLON AND RECTUM

Large intestine or colon is about 150 cm long, extending from the terminal ileum to the rectum. The divisions of colon are the cecum, colon proper, rectum and anal canal.

Cecum

The cecum, ascending colon and the hepatic flexure forms a surgical unit called the right colon. The cecum lies in the right iliac fossa and is approximately 7cm in length and width. In about 60 percent of living erect individuals it lies partly in the true pelvis. The cecum may be entirely retroperitoneal (25%) or completely free (20%).The mobile cecum is a predisposing factor to cecal volvulus or buscule. The caecum lies on the iliac and psoas muscles and overlying the genitofemoral, femoral and lateral cutaneous nerves. It also lies anterior to the testicular or ovarian vessels and the ureter. As caecum, ileoceacal junction is also extremely variable in position. In most circumstances the ileum enters obliquely into the large bowel through a horizontal slit and is partly invaginated into the caecum to form the ileo cecal valve (**Gerlach valve**).

Ascending Colon

The ascending colon is normally fused to the posterior abdominal wall and covered by peritoneum on all aspects except posterior aspect where it is attached to retroperitoeneum. In about 25% of cases, a mesentery can be identified. The ascending colon

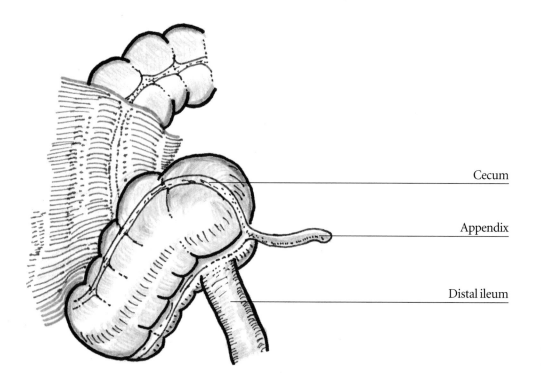

Cecum

Appendix

Distal ileum

Figure 1 : Mobile cecum, diatal ileum and proximal
right colon. This configuration is subject to volvulus

passes in front of the quadratus lumborum and transversus abdominis muscle. It extends from caecum to the hepatic flexure and averages 12-20 cm in length. The ascending colon lies anterior to the lower pole of right kidney, from which it is separated by perirenal fat and Toldt's fascia. It also relates posteriorly to the right ureter and gonadal vessels, which lie on the surface of the psoas muscle. The hepatic flexure lies immediately above the second part of the duodenum, to which it is sometimes attached by a peritoneal fold referred to as duodenocolic ligament. A tenuous adhesion from the right abdominal wall to the anterior tenia of the ascending colon has been often observed, which is referred to as **Jackson's membrane.**

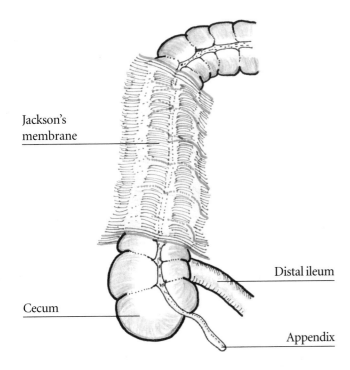

Figure 2 : Jackson's membrane or veil. May contain many small blood vessels from the second lumbar or renal arteries

Transverse Colon

The transverse colon connects the ascending and descending colon and courses horizontally across the abdominal cavity. The transverse colon has a mesentery that is attached to the anterior aspect of the pancreas. At the splenic flexure, the colon is supported by the renocolic ligament, a part of the left side of the transverse mesocolon. The root of the transverse mesocolon lies anterior to the lower pole of right kidney, head, body and tail of pancreas and hilum of left kidney. The mesocolon attachment divides the peritoneal cavity into supracolic and infracolic compartments. The duodenojejunal flexure and the ligament of Treitz lie just posterior to the root of the transverse mesocolon, caudal to the inferior border of the pancreas. The greater omentum covers the transverse colon along its entire length and is connected to it by gastro colic ligament. This ligament is divided to enter the lesser sac and to perform transverse colectomy.

The distal transverse colon is connected to the diaphragm by phrenocolic ligament. The splenic flexure lies in the left upper quadrant of the abdominal cavity. It lies in front of left kidney and forms an acute angle. It also closely related to the tail of pancreas, spleen and left adrenal gland. It lies at higher level than the hepatic flexure and is connected by flimsy adhesions to the lower pole of the spleen. This has to be released early during colonic resections. The surgical aspect regarding this part of the colon is the need to mobilize the splenic flexure during the anterior resection to achieve a tension free anastomosis at the pelvis. The phrenocolic, splenocolic ligaments should be divided completely to free the splenic flexure.

Descending Colon

The descending colon extends from the left upper quadrant to the pelvic brim and measures around 30cm. Normally it is devoid of mesentery. It descends down in the groove between the psoas and the quadratus lumborum. The surgical unit of the left colon consists of the splenic flexure and the descending and sigmoid colon. The descending colon is fixed on the posterior peritoneum through the Toldt's fascia, an important plane for bloodless dissection.

Sigmoid Colon

The sigmoid colon starts at the pelvic brim at the point where the descending colon turns medially and acquires a mesentery. Its length is variable (50-80cm). It has a long mesentery (the sigmoid mesocolon) which has short base starting at the end of

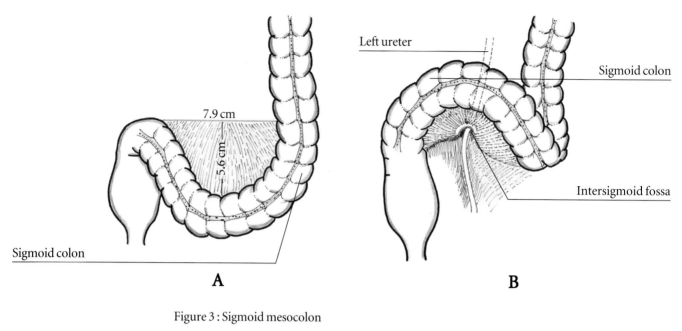

Figure 3 : Sigmoid mesocolon

A - Average measurement of sigmoid mesocolon
B - Relation of the base of sigmoid mesocolon to the left ureter

descending colon and ascending on the external iliac to the midpoint of the common iliac artery. At this point it turns downwards and to the right to enter the brim of the true pelvis (inverted V shape). The sigmoid colon terminates at the level of sacral promontory where the taenia coalesces into a diffuse longitudinal muscular layer devoid of any epiploicae. The sigmoid colon is often adherent to the lateral pelvic wall. These adhesions have to be released during anterior resection. The mesosigmoid contains a recess, referred to as the intersigmoid fossa, which can be used as a landmark for identifications of the ureter. The ureter can usually be identified deep to the intersigmoid fossa, where it courses along the surface of the psoas muscle and parallel to the gonadal vessels, medially into the pelvis above the common iliac artery bifurcation. Internal hernias can occur through the intersigmoid fossa.

Rectum and Anal Canal

The junction between the sigmoid colon and the rectum has been variously described as (a) the level at which the sigmoid mesentery disappears, (b) the diameter of colon narrows (c) teniae coli diverge a from a continuous muscle coat on the rectum (d) sacculations and epiploic appendages disappear (e) the level at which the superior rectal artery divides into right and left branches and (f) endoscopically an acute angle with variations in the mucosal pattern (rectal mucosa is smooth and flat, sigmoid forms prominent rugal folds). The length of the rectum varies depending on the build of the individual but it is around 15cm long.

It follows the curve of the sacrum and the coccyx and then runs anteriorly and inferiorly to the central lying on the anococcygeal ligament and the levator ani muscles. It then ends by turning posterior and inferior as the anal canal, immediately posterior to the central tendon of perineum and apex of the prostate in male. The lowest part of the rectum is more capacious and is known as the ampulla. The rectum is not straight; it follows the curvature of the sacrum and coccyx in the saggital plane. It is "S" shaped in the coronal plane. This gives rise to prominent folds within the lumen of the rectum at the valves of Houston. The upper 3rd of the rectum is covered by peritoneum. The middle 3rd rectum is covered anteriorly and on both sides by peritoneal layer. The lower 1/3rd is totally extra peritoneal. The lower third rectum lies behind the base of the bladder, the seminal vesicles and the prostate in the male and behind

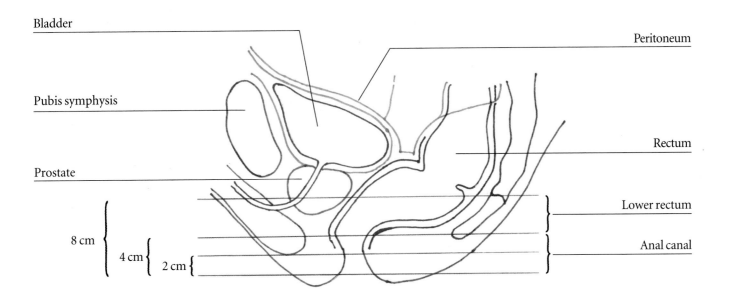

Bladder

Pubis symphysis

Prostate

8 cm

4 cm

2 cm

Peritoneum

Rectum

Lower rectum

Anal canal

Figure 4 : The lateral view of the line of peritoneal reflection on the rectum in a male.
The measurements of the anal canal and lower rectum from the anal verge are approximate

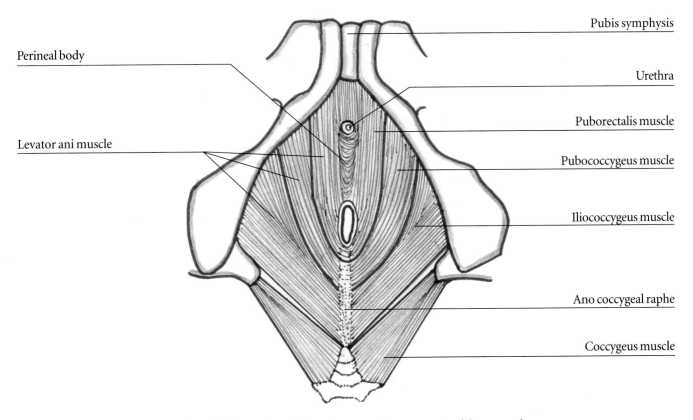

Perineal body

Levator ani muscle

Pubis symphysis

Urethra

Puborectalis muscle

Pubococcygeus muscle

Iliococcygeus muscle

Ano coccygeal raphe

Coccygeus muscle

Figure 5 : Pelvic diaphragm from below. Levator ani is composed of three muscles;
puborectalis, puboccoygeus and iliococcygeus

the vagina in the female. The surgeon considers the anal canal to be the region lying distal to the insertion of the levator ani muscle. The surgical anal canal has length of 4cm; 2cm above the pectinate line and 2cm below.

Pelvic Diaphragm and Continence

The floor of the pelvis is formed by 2 paired muscles levator ani and coccygeus. The levator ani is formed by the ileococcygeus, pubococcygeus and the puborectalis. The puborectalis muscle is very essential for maintaining rectal continence. The puborectalis with the superficial and deep parts of the external sphincter and the proximal part of the internal sphincter forms the anorectal ring. This structure must be prevented from injury during surgical procedures to avoid fecal incontinence.

VASCULATURE OF COLON AND RECTUM

Superior Mesenteric Artery (SMA)

This artery arises from aorta a few centimeters caudal to the origin of the celiac artery at body of 1st lumbar vertebra. It courses in the mesentery of small bowel. The cecum and the ascending colon receive blood supply from the branches of the SMA, the ileo colic and right colic and middle colic atrteries. The ileocolic artery is the terminal branch of the SMA. Its branches are cecal arteries, appendicular artery, ascending colic arteries and ileal branches. The right colic artery supplies the ascending colon and might be absent in some individuals. The middle colic artery supplies the transverse colon. A large a vascular window is seen to the left of the middle colic artery in that transverse mesocolon. This window is

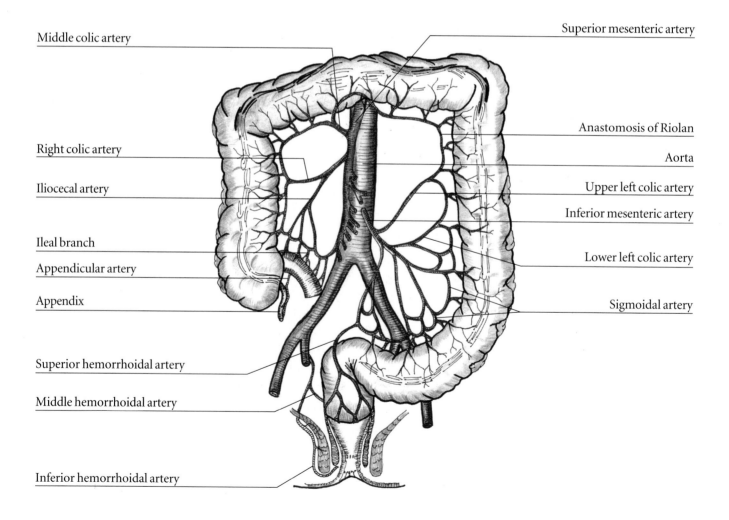

Figure 6 : Arterior supply of colon and rectum

often used for accessing the lesser sac and the posterior wall of stomach from the infracolic compartment. Any injury during this procedure will result in devascularization of the transverse colon.

The Inferior Mesenteric Artery (IMA)

The IMA arises from the aorta above its bifurcation opposite to the lower portion of the 3rd lumbar vertebra and supplies that portion of the GI tract derived from the primitive hindgut. Its branches are left colic artery, sigmoidal arteries and superior rectal artery. The left colic artery which supplies the descending colon divides into ascending and descending branches. The ascending branch anastomosis with the left branch of middle colic artery, while the descending branch anastomosis with the sigmoid arteries. The sigmoid arteries supply the sigmoid colon. The superior rectal artery, the terminal branch of IMA anastomosis with the branches of middle rectal arteries below, that arise from the internal iliac arteries.

Marginal Artery of Drummond

The marginal artery is a single arterial trunk made up of the anastomosis around the medial aspect of the colon from caecum to recto sigmoid. Vessels from this run perpendicular to the wall of colon and pierce the large intestine. The short vessels supply the mesenteric 2/3 of the bowel and large vessels the antimesenteric 1/3 of the bowel. It is formed by the anastomosis between branches of the SMA and IMA. It provides extensive collateral circulation between the vessels of midgut and hindgut.

There are several critical points where the marginal artery may not provide adequate blood supply. These are ileo-colic region, left colic flexure and the recto sigmoid junction. The **Arc of Riolan** occasionally provides a strong anastomosis between the IMA and the left branch of the middle colic artery. At the rectosigmoid region, the anastomosis between the sigmoidal and rectal arteries is weak and this junction is often called as **Sudeck's critical point**. Marginal artery is less consistent at the level of splenic flexure, the vascular anastomosis between MCA/ LCA are often absent. This area of critical blood supply is known as **Griffith critical point**

Arteries of the Rectum and Anal Canal

The superior rectal artery, middle rectal artery, inferior rectal artery and the median sacral artery supply the rectum. The superior rectal artery arises from IMA and descends to the posterior wall of the upper rectum. It divides into right and left branches to the lateral walls of the middle portion of the rectum down to the pectinate line. The middle rectal artery arises from the internal iliac artery, runs through the Denonvilliers fascia and enters the anterolateral aspect of the rectal wall at the level of anorectal ring. The inferior rectal artery is a branch of the internal pudendal arteries, which traverse Alcock's canal to enter the posterolateral aspect of ischiorectal fossa. They supply the anal canal distal to the pectinate line.

VENOUS DRAINAGE

The veins of the colon follow the arteries except for the inferior mesenteric vein which lies adjacent to the ascending branch of the left colic artery. The superior rectal vein, which drains the rectum and sigmoid colon passes upward to form the superior mesenteric vein. The inferior mesenteric vein runs in a retroperitoneal location to the left of the ligament of Treitz, continues behind the body of the pancreas, and enters the splenic vein. The superior mesenteric vein drains the caecum, ascending colon and transverse colon and joins the splenic vein to from the portal vein.

LYMPHATIC DRAINAGE

The lymph nodes of the large intestine have been divided into four groups, epicolic, (under the serosa of the intestine); paracolic (along the marginal arteries); intermediate, (along the branches of the SMA and IMA) and principal (along the root of the SMA and IMA). Wide resection of the colon should include the entire segment supplied by a major artery. This also will remove the lymphatic drainage of the segment.

The rectal lymphatics follow the same distribution as the arterial blood supply. Lymph from the upper and middle rectum drains into the inferior

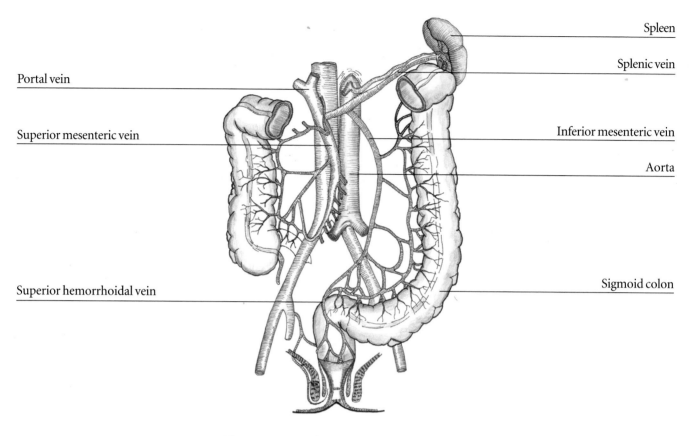

Spleen

Splenic vein

Portal vein

Superior mesenteric vein

Inferior mesenteric vein

Aorta

Superior hemorrhoidal vein

Sigmoid colon

Figure 7 : Venous drainage of colon and rectum

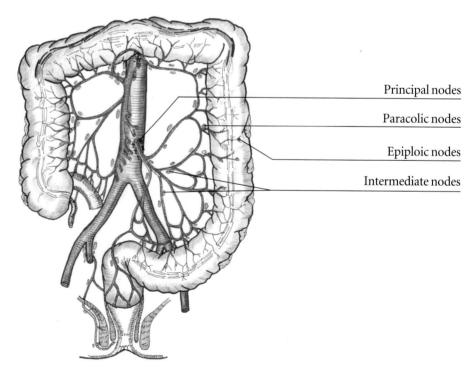

Principal nodes

Paracolic nodes

Epiploic nodes

Intermediate nodes

Figure 8 : Lymphatic drainage of colon and rectum. Four tiers of nodes are recognised;
Epiploic, paracolic, intermediate and principal lymph nodes

mesenteric nodes. The lower rectum is primarily drained by lymphatics that follow the superior rectal artery and enter the inferior mesenteric nodes. Lymph from the lower rectum can also flow laterally along the middle end inferior rectal arteries. These channels drain to the iliac nodes and subsequently to periaortic lymph nodes.

Lymphatics from the anal canal above the dentate line drain via the superior rectal lymphatics to the inferior mesenteric nodes or laterally to the internal iliac lymph nodes. Below the dentate line, the lymphatics drain primarily to the inguinal nodes, but can drain to the inferior or superior rectal lymph nodes as well.

NERVE SUPPLY

Sympathetic fibers of the right colon originate in the lower six thoracic segments of the spinal cord. They travel in the thoracic sphlanchnic nerves to the celiac plexus and then to the superior mesenteric plexus. The parasympathetic nerve supply to the right colon is by the vagus nerve. Sympathetic nerves inhibit and parasympathetic nerves stimulate peristalsis.

Sympathetic innervations of the left colon and rectum originate in the first three lumbar segments. These nerves join the preaortic plexus and become the inferior mesenteric plexus below the aortic bifurcation. The parasympathetic nerves to the left colon arise from the sacral nerves the from nervi erigentes on either side of the rectum. Extensions of the sacral parasympathetic ascend through the hypogastric plexus to the area of the splenic flexure.

Motor innervation of the internal anal sphincter is supplied by the sympathetic fibers that cause contraction and by parasympathetic fibers that inhibit contraction. Parasympathetic sacral afferent nerves mediate sensation of rectal distention. The external anal sphincter and levator ani muscles are supplied by pudendal nerve and by the 4th sacral nerve. Below the dentate line cutaneous sensations are conveyed by afferent fibers of the inferior rectal and perineal branches of the pudendal nerve. Above the dentate line the sensation is mediated probably by parasympathetic fibers.

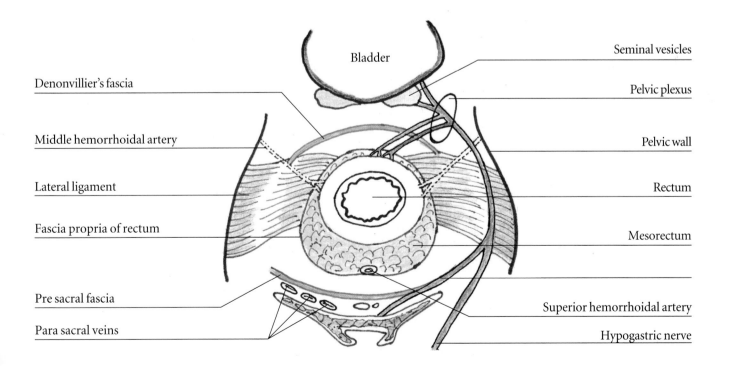

Figure 9 : Cross section of rectum showing the pelvic nerves innervation

ANATOMY OF THE MESORECTUM

The rectum is embedded in a layer of fatty tissue that contains draining lymph nodes and vessels. An adequate knowledge of anatomy is required for precise dissection outside the visceral fascia that envelopes the mesorectum. The mesorectum lies between the sacrum and the prostate and seminal vesicles in males and the vagina in females. The mesorectum at its upper level is of the shape of a half moon on transverse axis, which becomes a circle at the level of the prostate (with the rectum anteriorly placed) and becomes thinner distally after passing through the levator ani and disappears at the anus. The fascia propria is the fascial layer delineates the limits of mesorectum.

Posterior Aspect of Mesorectum

The sacrum, coccyx and the muscles of the posterior wall of the pelvis are covered by the parietal fascia, which is the continuation of transversalis fascia of the abdomen. On the bony interface this is termed as presacral fascia which at times is adherent to the periosteum of the bone. The space behind the presacral fascia is the **"Retrofascial space"** which contains the nerve bundles and vessels. This space was initially used by the surgeons for mobilization of rectum, which resulted in high incidence of nerve damage and bleeding.

The fascia propria is present just anterior to the presacral fascia (parietal layer) and this represents the visceral layer of the pelvic fascia. The space between the fascia propria and presacral fascia **"Interfascial space / Retro rectal space"** can be early dissected as this space contains only areolar tissue and is devoid of any neurovascular structures, except few branches of superior hypogastric plexus. Dissection in this space is very easy in laparoscopy due to high magnification and pneumodissection. At the caudal end of the retrorectal space, few fibres condense to connect the two of pelvic fascia, known as **retrosacral fascia**. This must be divided sharply to allow complete clearance beyond the anorectal ring.

Anterior Aspect of Mesorectum

Denonvilliers' fascia as a trapezoidal 'apron' of thickened anterior surface of the mesorectal tissue in the same plane as pouch of Douglas passing behind the prostatic capsule to reach the perineal body. The neurovascular bundles are very close to the left and right edges of the Denonvilliers' fascia. In live tissues, the Denonvilliers' fascia is intimately adherent to the anterior part of the mesorectum. In contrast the plane between the Denonvilliers' fascia and the seminal vesicles can be easily developed due to the presence of loose areolar tissue.

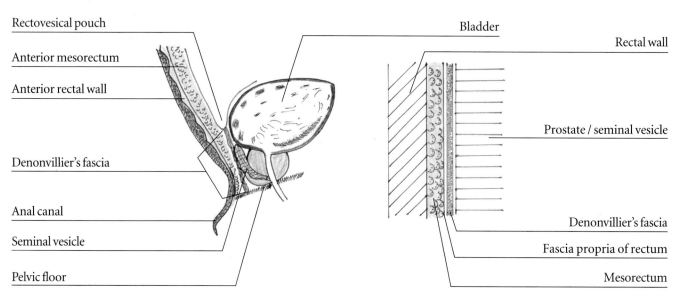

Figure 10 : Mesorectum anatomy

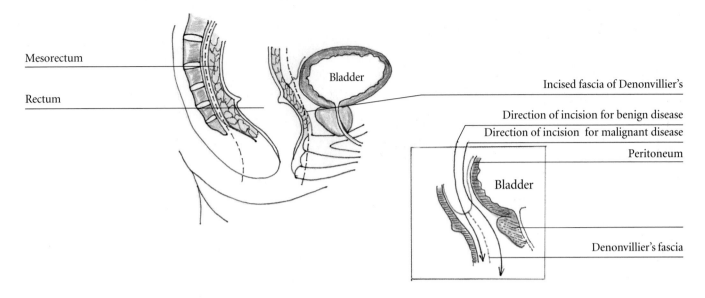

Mesorectum

Rectum

Bladder

Incised fascia of Denonvillier's

Direction of incision for benign disease

Direction of incision for malignant disease

Peritoneum

Bladder

Denonvillier's fascia

Figure 11 : The line of incision for total mesorectal excision

One can enter the plane anterior to Denonvilliers' fascia very easily by dissecting on the inner most recognizable areolar tissue during initial dissection on the anterior aspect of rectum (during total mesorectal excision). Extra care should be taken to avoid damage to the hypogastric plexus and the medially tapering neurovascular bundles at the lateral edges of the Denonvilliers' fascia.

Heald et al have compared the relevance of these anatomical points to surgical technique on two large published series that differed in the dissection of the anterior mesorectum only by the plane of excision - in front of or behind Denonvilliers' fascia.[57] Although there were no major differences in outcome for most patients, those with Dukes' stage C disease had a local recurrence rate of 21 per cent in one series (dissection behind Denonvilliers' fascia)[58], compared with 6·5 per cent when the plane of dissection was in front.[59]

Autonomic nerve damage

Risk of sympathetic nerve damage[60]

1. During ligation of the inferior mesenteric artery pedicle

2. During initial posterior rectal dissection adjacent (high in the pelvis)

Risk of parasympathetic nerve damage:[60]

1. During dissection near the pelvic plexus on the lateral aspect down in the pelvis

2. During deep dissection of the anterior aspect of the rectum away from the seminal vesicles near the cavernous nerves.

In a study of impotence rates following a trial of laparoscopic assisted versus open surgery for rectal cancer, the lap group showed ten times higher rate when compared to open group. But ejaculatory and bladder dysfunction were equivalent in the two groups. This indicates that nerve injury takes place distal to the origin of nerves supplying motor function to the bladder, distal to the pelvic plexus, i.e. injury affects the cavernous nerves during anterior dissection (which is generally the most difficult areas to obtain a good field of vision and retraction laparoscopic dissection deep in the pelvis.[61] Nocturnal penile tumescence monitoring, has been studied as an objective method of assessment for parasympathetic injury and patients with impotence after proctectomy for rectal cancer or inflammatory bowel disease have a significantly reduced number of tumescent events. Interestingly sildenafil (phosphodiesterase type 5 inhibitor) helps the patients by

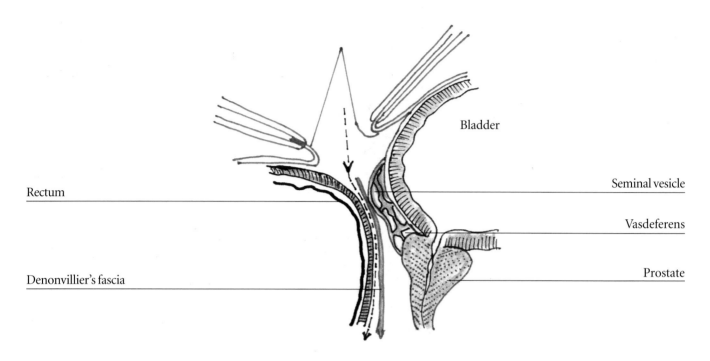

Figure 12 : Showing the line of incision for benign case of rectum

augmenting the vasodilator effect of the parasympathetic neural tone, but requires at least few intact fibres for its action. The drug is generally ineffective when there is profound nerve injury.

Appropriate plane of Anterior rectal dissection

In benign disease the choice is relatively simple. All surgeons will agree to stay posterior to Denonvilliers' fascia, some will favor close rectal dissection, but this may be technically more difficult. There is evidence now that close rectal dissection does not protect the pelvic nerves any more than mesorectal dissection. In malignancy the plane of dissection is usually anterior to Denonvilliers fascia in order to avoid recurrences.

Anatomy of the Autonomic Nerves of Pelvis

The sympathetic nerves from sphlanchnic branches from T2 to L2 form the superior hypogastric plexus just at the level of aortic bifurcation. Fibres from this plexus branches into hypogastric nerves (L & R) and course distally in the pelvis to form the inferior hypogastric plexus. These nerves bifurcate at the level of pelvic brim and pass in a plane between the fascia propria and presacral fascia (where it is closely adherent to the fascia propria). These nerves are at risk at the beginning of rectal mobilization in cancer surgeries. These nerves enter the deeper aspects of perineum in the posterolateral part.

The pelvic parasympathetic nerves (from S2, S3, S4) pierce the presacral fascia to enter the plane of pelvis and at side wall of pelvis the sphlanchnic nerves join the hypogastric nerves to form the inferior hypogastric plexus. From here fibres extend to the genital viscera. As the structures contain fibres from both sympathetic and parasympathetic fibres, these are better considered as pelvic autonomic plexus. The branches from these nerves, the **cavernous nerves** are responsible for various sexual functions. Sexual dysfunction after pelvic surgery is characterized by impotence and ejaculatory dysfunction. Impotence may be partial or complete, temporary or permanent. Ejaculatory dysfunction consists of absent ejaculation, retrograde ejaculation and painful ejaculation.

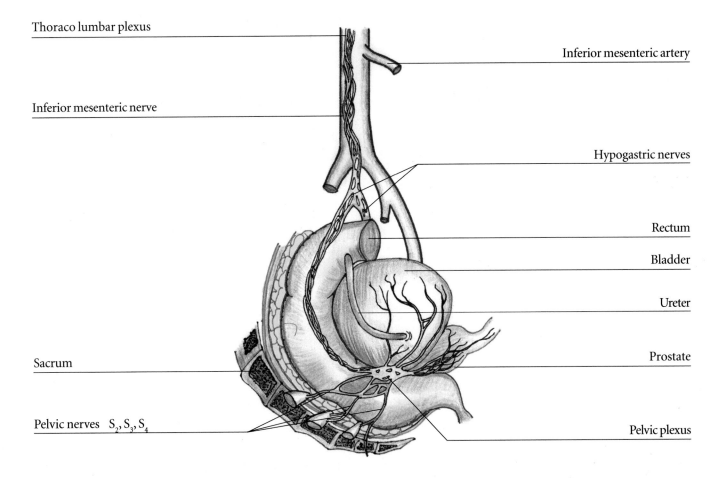

Thoraco lumbar plexus

Inferior mesenteric artery

Inferior mesenteric nerve

Hypogastric nerves

Rectum

Bladder

Ureter

Sacrum

Prostate

Pelvic nerves S_2, S_3, S_4

Pelvic plexus

Figure 13 : Parasagital section of pelvic autonomic neuroanatomy

CONCLUSION

The initial concern of complications and problems have all settled following series of reports that have appeared on various laparoscopic procedure from stoma creation to complex procedures like total proctocolectomy with ileo anal pouch anastamosis. These have shown that laparoscopic procedures are beneficial both in short term and long term. The laparoscopic colorectal procedures are oncologically safe and the survival rates are similar to that of conventional surgeries.

References

1.   Redwine DB, Sharpe DR. Laparoscopic segmental resection of the sigmoid colon for endometriosis. J Laparoendosc Surg 1991; 1(4):217-20.

2.   Schlinkert RT. Laparoscopic-assisted right hemicolectomy. Dis Colon Rectum 1991; 34(11):1030-1.

3.   Jacobs M, Verdeja JC, Goldstein HS. Minimally invasive colon resection (laparoscopic colectomy). Surg Laparosc Endosc 1991; 1(3):144-50.

4.   Guillou PJ, Darzi A, Monson JR. Experience with laparoscopic colorectal surgery for malignant disease. Surg Oncol 1993; 2 Suppl 1:43-9.

5.   Wexner SD, Cohen SM, Johansen OB, et al. Laparoscopic colorectal surgery: a prospective assessment and current perspective. Br J Surg 1993; 80(12):1602-5.

6.   Dobronte Z, Wittmann T, Karacsony G. Rapid development of malignant metastases in the abdominal wall after laparoscopy. Endoscopy 1978; 10(2):127-30.

7.   Alexander RJ, Jaques BC, Mitchell KG. Laparoscopically assisted colectomy and wound recurrence. Lancet 1993; 341(8839):249-50.

8. Berends FJ, Kazemier G, Bonjer HJ, Lange JF. Subcutaneous metastases after laparoscopic colectomy. Lancet 1994; 344(8914):58.

9. Wexner SD, Cohen SM. Port site metastases after laparoscopic colorectal surgery for cure of malignancy. Br J Surg 1995; 82(3):295-8.

10. Ziprin P, Ridgway PF, Peck DH, Darzi AW. The theories and realities of port-site metastases: a critical appraisal. J Am Coll Surg 2002; 195(3):395-408.

11. Lyerly HK, Mault JR. Laparoscopic ileostomy and colostomy. Ann Surg 1994; 219(3):317-22.

12. Milsom JW, Ludwig KA, Church JM, Garcia-Ruiz A. Laparoscopic total abdominal colectomy with ileorectal anastomosis for familial adenomatous polyposis. Dis Colon Rectum 1997; 40(6):675-8.

13. Georgeson KE, Cohen RD, Hebra A, et al. Primary laparoscopic-assisted endorectal colon pull-through for Hirschsprung's disease: a new gold standard. Ann Surg 1999; 229(5):678-82; discussion 682-3.

14. Monson JR, Hill AD, Darzi A. Laparoscopic colonic surgery. Br J Surg 1995; 82(2):150-7.

15. Decanini C, Milsom JW, Bohm B, Fazio VW. Laparoscopic oncologic abdominoperineal resection. Dis Colon Rectum 1994; 37(6):552-8.

16. Kozol RA, Kosir MA. Laparoscopic/endoscopic repair of rectal stricture. J Gastrointest Surg 1998; 2(5):426-9.

17. Prohm P, Weber J, Bonner C. Laparoscopic-assisted coloscopic polypectomy. Dis Colon Rectum 2001; 44(5):746-8.

18. Possover M, Drahonowski J, Plaul K, Schneider A. Laparoscopic-assisted formation of a colon neovagina. Surg Endosc 2001; 15(6):623.

19. Bruce CJ, Coller JA, Murray JJ, et al. Laparoscopic resection for diverticular disease. Dis Colon Rectum 1996; 39(10 Suppl):S1-6.

20. Liberman MA, Phillips EH, Carroll BJ, et al. Laparoscopic colectomy vs traditional colectomy for diverticulitis. Outcome and costs. Surg Endosc 1996; 10(1):15-8.

21. Franklin ME, Jr., Dorman JP, Jacobs M, Plasencia G. Is laparoscopic surgery applicable to complicated colonic diverticular disease? Surg Endosc 1997; 11(10):1021-5.

22. Trebuchet G, Lechaux D, Lecalve JL. Laparoscopic left colon resection for diverticular disease. Surg Endosc 2002; 16(1):18-21.

23. Bauer JJ, Harris MT, Grumbach NM, Gorfine SR. Laparoscopic-assisted intestinal resection for Crohn's disease. Dis Colon Rectum 1995; 38(7):712-5.

24. Chung CC, Tsang WW, Kwok SY, Li MK. Laparoscopy and its current role in the management of colorectal disease. Colorectal Dis 2003; 5(6):528-43.

25. Berman IR. Sutureless laparoscopic rectopexy for procidentia. Technique and implications. Dis Colon Rectum 1992; 35(7):689-93.

26. Kusminsky RE, Tiley EH, Boland JP. Laparoscopic Ripstein procedure. Surg Laparosc Endosc 1992; 2(4):346-7.

27. Allam M, Piskun G, Fogler R. Laparoscopic-assisted abdominoperineal proctosigmoidectomy for rectal prolapse. A new technique. Surg Endosc 1997; 11(2):150-1.

28. Gorey TF, O'Riordain M G, Tierney S, et al. Laparoscopic-assisted rectopexy using a novel hand-access port. J Laparoendosc Surg 1996; 6(5):325-8.

29. Reissman P, Weiss E, Teoh TA, et al. Laparoscopic-assisted perineal rectosigmoidectomy for rectal prolapse. Surg Laparosc Endosc 1995; 5(3):217-8.

30. Darzi A, Henry MM, Guillou PJ, et al. Stapled laparoscopic rectopexy for rectal prolapse. Surg Endosc 1995; 9(3):301-3.

31. Heah SM, Hartley JE, Hurley J, et al. Laparoscopic suture rectopexy without resection is effective treatment for full-thickness rectal prolapse. Dis Colon Rectum 2000; 43(5):638-43.

32. Xynos E, Chrysos E, Tsiaoussis J, et al. Resection rectopexy for rectal prolapse. The laparoscopic approach. Surg Endosc 1999; 13(9):862-4.

33. Gorey TF, O'Connell PR, Waldron D, et al. Laparoscopically assisted reversal of Hartmann's procedure. Br J Surg 1993; 80(1):109.

34. Sosa JL, Sleeman D, Puente I, et al. Laparoscopic-assisted colostomy closure after Hartmann's procedure. Dis Colon Rectum 1994; 37(2):149-52.

35. Vernava AM, 3rd, Liebscher G, Longo WE. Laparoscopic restoration of intestinal continuity after Hartmann procedure. Surg Laparosc Endosc 1995; 5(2):129-32.

36. Swain BT, Ellis CN, Jr. Laparoscopy-assisted loop ileostomy: an acceptable option for temporary fecal diversion after anorectal surgery. Dis Colon Rectum 2002; 45(5):705-7.

37. Koea JB, Guillem JG, Conlon KC, et al. Role of laparoscopy in the initial multimodality management of patients with near-obstructing rectal cancer. J Gastrointest Surg 2000; 4(1):105-8.

38. Lange V, Meyer G, Schardey HM, Schildberg FW. Laparoscopic creation of a loop colostomy. J Laparoendosc Surg 1991; 1(5):307-12.

39. Romero CA, James KM, Cooperstone LM, et al. Laparoscopic sigmoid colostomy for perianal Crohn's disease. Surg Laparosc Endosc 1992; 2(2):148-51.

40. Fuhrman GM, Ota DM. Laparoscopic intestinal stomas. Dis Colon Rectum 1994; 37(5):444-9.

41. Ludwig KA, Milsom JW, Garcia-Ruiz A, Fazio VW. Laparoscopic techniques for fecal diversion. Dis Colon Rectum 1996; 39(3):285-8.

42. Stocchi L, Nelson H, Young-Fadok TM, et al. Safety and advantages of laparoscopic vs. open colectomy in the elderly: matched-control study. Dis Colon Rectum 2000; 43(3):326-32.

43. Monson JR, Darzi A, Carey PD, Guillou PJ. Prospective evaluation of laparoscopic-assisted colectomy in an unselected group of patients. Lancet 1992; 340(8823):831-3.

44. Phillips EH, Franklin M, Carroll BJ, et al. Laparoscopic colectomy. Ann Surg 1992; 216(6):703-7.

45. Franklin ME, Jr., Rosenthal D, Abrego-Medina D, et al. Prospective comparison of open vs. laparoscopic colon surgery for carcinoma. Five-year results. Dis Colon Rectum 1996; 39(10 Suppl):S35-46.

46. Ortega AE, Beart RW, Jr., Steele GD, Jr., et al. Laparoscopic Bowel Surgery Registry. Preliminary results. Dis Colon Rectum 1995; 38(7):681-5; discussion 685-6.

47. Simons AJ, Anthone GJ, Ortega AE, et al. Laparoscopic-assisted colectomy learning curve. Dis Colon Rectum 1995; 38(6):600-3.

48. Bennett CL, Stryker SJ, Ferreira R. The learning curve for laparoscopic colorectal surgery: Preliminary results from a prospective analysis of 1194 laparoscopic-assisted colectomies. Archives of Surgery 1997; 132:41-4.

49. Hartley JE, Monson JR. The role of laparoscopy in the multimodality treatment of colorectal cancer. Surg Clin North Am 2002; 82(5):1019-33.

50. Philipson BM, Bokey EL, Moore JW, et al. Cost of open versus laparoscopically assisted right hemicolectomy for cancer. World J Surg 1997; 21(2):214-7.

51. Musser DJ, Boorse RC, Madera F, Reed JF, 3rd. Laparoscopic colectomy: at what cost? Surg Laparosc Endosc 1994; 4(1):1-5.

52. Falk PM, Beart RW, Jr., Wexner SD, et al. Laparoscopic colectomy: a critical appraisal. Dis Colon Rectum 1993; 36(1):28-34.

53. Hoffman GC, Baker JW, Fitchett CW, Vansant JH. Laparoscopic-assisted colectomy. Initial experience. Ann Surg 1994; 219(6):732-40; discussion 740-3.

54. Senagore AJ, Luchtefeld MA, Mackeigan JM, Mazier WP. Open colectomy versus laparoscopic colectomy: are there differences? Am Surg 1993; 59(8):549-53; discussion 553-4.

55. Pfeifer J, Wexner SD, Reissman P, et al. Laparoscopic vs open colon surgery. Costs and outcome. Surg Endosc 1995; 9(12):1322-6.

56. Young-Fadok TM, Pemberton JH. Discussion of: Bennett CL, Stryker SJ, Ferreira MR, Adams J, Beart RW Jr. The learning curve for laparoscopic colorectal surgery. Preliminary results from a prospective analysis of 1194 laparoscopic-assisted colectomies. Archives of Surgery 1997; 132(1):41-4 [discussion 45].

57. Heald R.J. Optimal total mesorectal excision for rectal cancer is by dissection in front of Denonvilliers' fascia. Br J Surg 2004; 91(1):121-123.

58. Killingback M, P. B, Dent O.F. Local recurrence after curative resection of cancer of the rectum without total mesorectal excision. Dis Colon Rectum, 2001; 44(4):p. 473-83; discussion 483-6.

59. MacFarlane JK, Ryall, Heald R.J. Mesorectal excision for rectal cancer. Lancet 1993; 341(8843):457-460.

60. Lindsey I, Mortensen N.J. . Iatrogenic impotence and rectal dissection. Br J Surg 2002; 89(12):1493-4.

61. Quah HM. Bladder and sexual dysfunction following laparoscopically assisted and conventional open mesorectal resection for cancer. Br J Surg 2002; 89(12):1551-6.

63

Laparoscopic Colectomy

INTRODUCTION

Laparoscopic colorectal resection has gone through a major evolution since 1991, when the first reports of laparoscopic colorectal resections had been published.[1-3] There has been an explosion of techniques in colorectal surgeries at a rapid pace ranging from benign to malignant diseases. This enthusiasm was somewhat dampened by reports of port site metastasis following laparoscopic resections for malignancies. Based on these reports, concerns about oncological safety of the laparoscopic resections arose among the surgeons. However with the recently published reports of large studies with long term follow-up, these concerns have gradually come down.[4, 5] Though laparoscopic approach for benign diseases has been well accepted, its acceptance in malignancy is slowly coming to practice due to standardization of techniques, availability of modern equipments and the results of long term randomized trials.

This chapter will focus on the various procedures of laparoscopic resection of colon (namely right, left and subtotal colectomy) laying emphasis on the concept of laparoscopic colorectal surgery in general. Difficulties in dissection, the availability of newer instruments for dissection and, mobilisation techniques will be discussed followed by complete techniques of right hemicolectomy, left hemicolectomy and subtotal colectomy. The experience gained in basic laparoscopy like technique of creation of pneumoperitoneum, trocar insertion and dissection techniques forms the foundation for advanced laparoscopic colorectal surgery.[6, 7] But there are a few unique problems specific to laparoscopic colorectal surgery that make these procedures difficult for surgeons who attempt these procedures.

UNIQUE PROBLEMS IN LAPAROSCOPIC COLORECTAL SURGERY

The colon is situated in more than 2-3 quadrants when compared to the single quadrant dissection such as cholecystectomy and appendicectomy.[8] Hence dissection and mobilization must be accomplished in more than one quadrant. The mesenteric blood vessels are numerous, large and run in a layer of opaque fat. Then are difficult to isolate, ligate and divided laparoscopically and also the procedure is time consuming.[9] Endo vascular staplers, though providing rapid and safe vascular control, are expensive (particularly in developing countries like India). Pretied vessel loops are inexpensive, but require more time to control all the vessels. Advanced hemostatic equipments like ultrasonic dissection help in avascular dissection of the colon and its vasculature.[10, 11] Visualization of colon at unfamiliar angles, handling of bulky tissue with unfamiliar tools and attempt to retract the large bowel at varied angles within the confined space are some of the other difficulties associated with laparoscopic colorectal surgery.

Due to lack of tactile sensation, the site of the lesion is not easily identified and intra operative colonoscopy is often needed to ensure removal of the correct segment of bowel. Most of the colonic malignancies are identified by palpation during conventional surgeries. This is not possible in laparoscopy due to lack of tactile feedback.[12] The introduction of hand assisted techniques helps to a certain degree to overcome this difficulty.[13-15] The mechanical manipulation during laparoscopy might lead to cellular disbursement of the malignant cells, which might jeopardise outcome. Retrieval of the resected colon requires large ports with subsequent stretching or minilaparotomy, thereby limiting the cosmetic effect. Negotiating the specimen through an inadequate opening may cause skin infection or tumor implantation. On the other hand, attempting to remove the specimen through the anus may result in either peritoneal contamination or sphincter injury. Tension free, well vascularised and circumferentially intact anastomosis is mandatory. Fashioning of the anastomosis is another challenge. Significant morbidity and mortality occurs with anastomotic leakage.

The operating time for the surgeries will be definitely longer during the initial learning curve period and this in turn increases the cost of the surgery.[16, 17] Though the concern about the cost may not be of major importance, increased duration of surgery has been the main stumbling block that prevents development of laparoscopic surgery. Though many of the surgeons in India have adequate knowledge in basic laparoscopic surgery, they are not able to move beyond basic surgeries both in private setup and government institutions. The government institutions are over loaded with patients. The operating list is so large, that they are unable to devote considerable time to laparoscopic surgery. If an advanced procedure is attempted, the remaining surgeries have to be cancelled thereby causing inconvenience. Even with the availability of equipment, patients and adequate experience, surgeons are not able to perform advanced surgeries. This situation prevails in most of the leading institutions and hospitals. Other concerns about laparoscopic surgery are the detrimental effects of conversion, incidence of port site recurrences and the safety of laparoscopic surgeries for malignancies.

Though there are various problems associated with laparoscopy, the basic technique remains the same whether it is open, lap assisted or totally laparoscopic surgery. The basic principles of conventional surgery should be replicated in laparoscopic method, the only difference being the access. The technique of traction, countertraction, dissection in correct anatomical plane, hemostasis and reconstruction are similar in both types of surgeries except that a few additional techniques have to be learnt. Avoidance of tumor spill, obtaining adequate resection margins and lymph nodal clearance form the basic of any oncological procedure.

LAPAROSCOPIC DISSECTION TECHNIQUES

The two hand manipulation; use of gravity as the second assistant to retract the bowel; technique of dissection with various electrosurgical and ultrasonic devices are some of newer surgical aspects that have to be learnt. The loss of 3 dimensional vision in laparoscopy is a major handicap for the beginners. Frequent overshooting of instruments, inability to control the bleeders, and other similar situations are experienced by all surgeons. However with practice, the surgeons usually gain the ability to judge the depth of the field. Though the introduction of three dimensional monitors and goggles has been a value added addition it is not being used routinely.[18] The technique of intracorporeal knotting and suturing will help the surgeon perform the surgery in a cost effective way. The excellent view provided by the advanced imaging technology and its magnification will help in reducing these problems to a certain extent.

TROCAR PLACEMENT

Trocar placement is a crucial but often neglected part of surgery. Basic surgeries like laparoscopic cholecystectomy and appendicectomy require a camera port (which remains the same throughout the surgery) and 2 working ports on either side of the camera. The triangular orientation is maintained throughout the surgery. However in surgeries of the colon, a single camera position will be inadequate as the colon extends over multiple quadrants. This requires the camera to be moved to various ports for complete mobilisation of the colon. The design of port placement should be such that the ports are interchangeable but still capable of maintaining the triangulation as per the ergonomics of laparoscopy. This will be a tedious task at the beginning but with experience the art of port placement can be learnt.[19] The placement of ports should be individualized to patients based on the body habitus, previous scar and the segment of bowel to be removed.

Trocar position and size of trocars should allow for change of instruments, staplers, clip appliers and retractors without any hindrance to the operating field. The retracting trocars should be always away from the working trocars and should not intrude between working trocars and camera. The trocar used for dissection and vascular control should be at least 10mm. A 10mm Babcock grasper is an ideal instrument for bowel grasping and retraction. The position of the monitor should be in front of the operating surgeon at the level of his eye to reduce strain to the neck muscles. Otherwise constant turning on one side might strain the neck muscles and produce pain.

INTRAOPERATIVE LOCALISATION

Once the trocars have been placed the abdomen should be inspected thoroughly and the lesion has to be identified. At times, there is difficulty in localizing the lesion in the large bowel.[20] This is mainly due to the loss of tactile sensation. Prior localization of the anatomical portion and the quadrant with barium enema and colonoscopy helps in locating the lesion easily. Lesions can be marked with India ink during colonoscopy so that the tattooing can be seen during laparoscopy. Tattooing may not be visible at times when the injected dye has escaped into the peritoneal cavity or when it has been applied to the colonic wall on the retroperitoneal side (that is hidden from the view). Circumferential injection of the dye (preferably on three sites) is necessary to localize the lesion. Placement of radio opaque markers and its identification with intraoperative image intensifiers has also been reported. If there is still doubt about localization of the tumors, intra operative colonoscopy can be done to confirm the position of the lesion. During intraoperative colonoscopy, an atraumatic clamp should be applied to occlude the small bowel at ileocecal junction, to prevent ballooning of the small bowel. During withdrawal, the air in the colon should be completely sucked out in order to have a complete vision of the peritoneal cavity. Semilithotomy position will be helpful if such an occasion should arise. Otherwise the patient has to be repositioned and draped in between the procedure.

LAPAROSCOPIC COLORECTAL RESECTION - BASIC COMMON STEPS

All laparoscopically assisted colon procedures have several steps that are common. These steps include

1. Localization of lesion

2. Mobilization of lesion

3. Devascularization of the specimen

4. Preventive measures for local recurrence

5. Protection of the wound during specimen retrieval

6. Restoring bowel continuity

Once the colon is identified and other lesions are ruled out, the mobilization of proposed segment of bowel is started. Only atraumatic graspers should be used to manipulate the bowel. Direct grasping of serosa of bowel should be avoided and the Babcocks should be used to grasp the adjacent pericolic fat, mesentery or at times full thickness of the bowel. This minimises the trauma to the bowel wall.

Once the colon is mobilized completely, vascular control is achieved either intracorporeally or extracorporeally. It is important that sufficient bowel is mobilized before specimen removal so that a tension free anastomosis is achieved at the end of the surgery. After vascular control, the specimen is resected by application of staplers and the anastomosis performed by endostaplers. Although technically possible, many do not prefer intracorporeal anastomosis. Transection of bowel with endo GIA staplers and extracorporeal anastomosis is often the preferred approach. Other options for resection and restoration of continuity are exteriorisation of bowel followed by resection, extracorporeal anastomosis by hand sewn technique or double stapling technique with conventional staplers.

The incidence of port site recurrence was initially considered very high (as high as 21%) but now it has been proved that there is no difference between open and laparoscopic procedures.[8, 21, 22] Exfoliated tumor cells that are viable might be present in the intraperitoneal fluid, trocars within the peritoneal cavity, serosal surfaces, instruments and the intraperitoneal gas. The desufflation of gas and the movement of trocars in the abdomen may transport the cells into the abdominal wall. Trocars must be fixed firmly to the abdominal wall to prevent the to and fro motion of the trocars.[23]

TUMORICIDAL IRRIGATION

The laparoscopic HAS era reiterated the awareness regarding liberated viable cells in the abdominal cavity because of reports about port site recurrence. Tumoricidal agents have been used either for intracolonic irrigation or for irrigations of abdominal cavity. Intraluminal colonic irrigation of tumoricidal agents has been used in an attempt to reduce recurrence rate. Similarly povidone iodine,

tauolidine, chlorhexidine, methotrexate and fluorourocil have been used for intra abdominal irrigation as a tumoricidal agent.[24] An other maneuver for prevention of wound recurrence is by preventing the displacement of trocars by methods like appropriate sized incision, screw type trocars and an anchoring stitch.

TYPES OF LAPAROSCOPIC COLORECTAL RESECTION

1. Complete laparoscopic colectomy

The dissection, resection, specimen removal and anastomosis are performed entirely within the abdomen. To accomplish the above principles by this approach is difficult, tedious, so not adopted widely.

2. Near complete laparoscopic colectomy

The dissection, resection and anastomosis are performed laparoscopically, but a small incision is made to remove the specimen and to insert the anvil of the circular stapler. This technique is well suited for anterior resection of rectum and sigmoid colon in which the anastomosis is within the reach of a circular stapler via the anus.

3. Resection-facilitated laparoscopic colectomy

The dissection and resection of the colon, sigmoid are performed laparoscopically, but retrieval of specimen and the anastomosis is performed extracorporeally.

4. Dissection-facilitated laparoscopic colectomy

The colonic mobilization is performed under laparoscopic guidance, but resection and anastomosis are performed extracorporeally. This technique allows precise inspection of the abdominal cavity and mobilization of the colon including the flexures with a limited incision. This technique is suitable to right and left colon resection.

INDICATIONS AND CONTRAINDICATIONS

The common indications for partial colectomies are Crohn's disease, diverticular disease, tuberculosis of ileocecal junction and colonic cancer. The other indicationsare benign polyps, polyposis of colon, volvulus, trauma, prolapsed rectum, endometriosis of colon etc.

Tuberculosis of Ileocecal junction

This is a common indication seen in India, which requires hemicolectomy. The disease presents as subacute obstruction due to hyperplastic tuberculosis. Hyperplastic tuberculosis needs a limited resection of caecum and terminal ileum for which the lateral to medial approach of colonic mobilisation is adequate.

Crohns disease

The ileocolic involvement of Crohns disease is one of the common indications for laparoscopic partial colectomy.[25-27] When Crohns disease involves greater omentum, this needs to be removed along with colon, which makes laparoscopic surgery difficult. Advanced stage of the disease is usually associated with inflammatory sequlae like abscess, fistula and other factors like distortion of anatomy and presence of friable tissues. These factors often make laparoscopic colorectal resection difficult and are associated with higher conversion rates. Acute inflammation, abscess, multiple fistulae are considered as contraindications for laparoscopic resection. Laparoscopic assisted colonic resection for colonic lesions, though initially uncommon are now more frequently performed.[28]

Diverticulitis

Laparoscopic resection of colon for diverticular disease forms the second common indication in the Western population,[29-32] but not among the Indian population. Here the active inflammatory process might be hindrance for laparoscopic dissection. Abscess formation, peritonitis, diverticular phlegmon are generally considered as contraindications for laparoscopy, but reports of successful laparoscopic surgery have been published.[30] It is advisable to avoid the stoma sites during port placements, as these patients might need a stoma at a later date.

Polyps

Large polyps that cannot be removed by colonoscopy can be removed by laparoscopic resection.[33] Incompletely removed malignant polyps through colonoscopy can be treated successfully by laparoscopic resection along with lymph nodal clearance.

Colon cancer

Colon cancer is the most common indication for colonic resections in Untied States. Early colon cancers can be successfully treated by laparoscopy. Colorectal resection for cancer is no longer considered as an experimental procedure. Locally advanced tumors infiltrating the adjacent organs are considered as contraindications for laparoscopic resection.

Septic shock, advanced faecal peritonitis and severe cardio vascular and pulmonary disease are considered as absolute contraindications for laparoscopic colorectal resection in any disease.[34] Morbid obesity, cirrhosis of liver, severe acute inflammatory bowel disease, large abdominal aneurysm, pregnancy, previous laparotomy, coagulopathy, blood dyscrasiasis are considered as relative contraindication.

RIGHT HEMICOLECTOMY

Laparoscopic right hemicolectomy can be performed in two ways the "medial to lateral approach" and the "lateral to medial approach". The lateral to medial approach is easier to perform especially for the beginners. This method can be adopted during the early phase of laparoscopic career of a surgeon (for benign diseases such as tuberculosis of ileocolic junction). The vascular control is obtained after exteriorization of the specimen. The medial to lateral approach is oncologically sound approach as the vessels are ligated during the initial part of dissection

Preoperative Preparation

The patient goes through the routine preoperative evaluation for diagnosis, staging and fitness for surgery. Patients are prepared with mechanical bowel cleansing solutions like polyethylene glycol and intravenous antibiotics. Adequate anticoagulation prophylaxis is given to prevent deep venous thrombosis and embolism.

Patient position

The patient is placed in supine position with arms stretched outwards. There is no need for a lithotomy position in right hemicolectomy. However, in case of detection of polyps in the distal ascending and transverse colon, it might be useful for intra operative colonoscopy (if needed). The position of the patient, team and the monitors are similar to that of appendicectomy. The operating table should be able to be controlled remotely to help in various extreme positions that is needed for colonic resection. More often gravity is used as an aid to retraction in laparoscopic colorectal resections.

The surgeon stands on the left side of the patient with the camera assistant to the left of the surgeon. The second assistant stands near the right hypochondrium of the patient and the staff nurse along with the trolley to right of the second assistant. The position of monitors is vital to reduce the stress on the neck muscles during the surgery. Two monitors are ideal for this surgery both near the head end of the patient. This reduces the unnecessary movement of the monitors during the surgery. A sand bag under the right loin increases the visibility of the ascending colon.

Position of trocars

With the patient in supine position, pneumoperitoneum is created by Veress needle technique through umbilicus. The initial camera port is made in the umbilicus and subsequent ports are made. The suprapubic port is placed in the midline and the epigastric port is placed midway between the xiphoid and umbilicus slightly to the left of the midline. This position is ideal for hepatic flexure mobilisation and control of vessels. The 10mm ports help in shifting the camera and working instruments like grasper to either suprapubic or umbilical port depending on the quadrant of dissection.

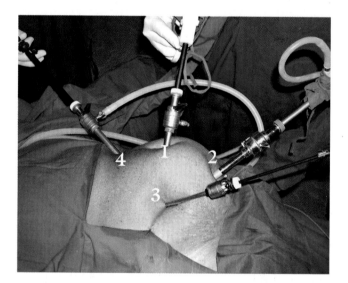

Figure 2 : Ports position for right hemicolectomy

1   -   Umbilical port 10mm (This is a right hand working port till the mobilization of cecum and ascending colon , after that it becomes camera port)
2   -   Suprapubic port 10mm (camera port, after the mobilization of cecum becomes retraction port)
3   -   Right iliac fossa port 5mm (left hand working port)
4   -   Epigastric port 10mm (Initially, a retracting port, during hepatic flexure mobilization, becomes right hand working port

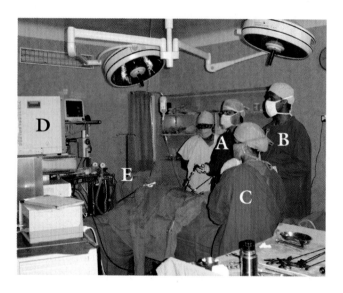

Figure 1 : Team setup for right colon resection

A   -   Surgeon
B   -   Camera surgeon
C   -   Staff nurse
D   -   Monitor
E   -   Head end of the patient

Different approaches for Mobilisation of Colon

Lateral to medial approach
  For benign lesions
  Extracorporeal vascular control, resection, anastamosis
 	
Medial to lateral approach
  For malignant lesions
  Intracorporeal vascular control

Mobilisation of Colon: Lateral to medial approach

This approach is usually performed for benign conditions such as ileocecal tuberculosis, Crohn's disease etc.

Extracorporeal vascular control, resection, anastomosis

A sand bag is placed under the patient on the right side and the table tilted to the left to keep the right colon more prominent. In this position the small bowel slides away to the left. A Babcock clamp is used to retract the colon medially and it is applied on the normal looking bowel either proximal or distal to the lesion. At no time the colonic lesion is handled directly by any instruments. The epigastric, umbilical and supra pubic ports (10mm) are all placed in midline for this approach. It is preferable to align the port incisions vertically so that the minilaparotomy at the end of surgery can be performed by joining these incisions.

Cecum and ascending colon mobilization

The cecum is gently retracted medially and slightly towards cranial side to give adequate traction to the lateral peritoneum. The suprapubic port is the camera port and the umbilical port is used as working port. The lateral peritoneum is divided by using harmonic scalpel or monopolar scissor extending towards the hepatic flexure along the white line of Toldt. During mobilisation, the right ureter, spermatic vessels and the duodenum are always identified. Meticulous hemostasis makes identification of these structures easier.

Hepatic flexure and transverse colon mobilization

The hepatic flexure is mobilized next. The camera is shifted to the umbilicus, the Babcock retractor to the suprapubic port and the epigastric port becomes the working port. The table is tilted to the reverse Trendelenburg's position and the hepatic flexure is retracted down and medially to get adequate exposure of the hepatocolic and gastrocolic ligament. This is the most difficult phase of surgery because of the risk of duodenal injury. The gastro colic ligament is divided beyond the point of resection of the transverse colon. Harmonic scalpel makes the dissection easier with control of blood vessels as well. During this maneuver the duodenum is identified and protected carefully. The greater omentum is divided from the transverse colon beyond the proposed line of resection.

Exteriorisation and vascular control

Umbilical port is extended by 5cm in the midline. The fully mobilized right colon is brought out through minilaparotomy in the sub umbilical position. Some surgeons prefer the incision in the right upper abdomen. The vessels of the ascending colon like ileo colic, right colic and right branch of middle colic are ligated extracorporeally with non-absorbable sutures and divided. If the mesentery is too short for extraction, vascular ligation and resection can be done intracorporeally. The veins are usually ligated separately.

Resection and anastomosis

Once the colonic segment has been brought outside the abdomen resection and anastomosis can be done quickly and safely in a cost effective manner. I prefer clamps for resection and end to end hand sewn anastomosis in order to reduce the cost. The incision is sutured and pneumoperitoneum is reestablished. The peritoneal cavity is reinspected for hemostasis.

The laparoscopic assisted colectomy with extracorporeal anastomosis is relatively a safe procedure, obviously faster and more cost effective than the complete laparoscopic procedure with intracorporeal anastomosis.

Medial to Lateral approach

This approach is usually performed for malignancies of the colon.

The patient position, theatre setup and the position of the trocars are similar in both the approaches. This approach helps in early identification of major blood supply for the involved segment and places the ureters at less risk of injury. Control of vessels can be done at an early phase of dissection. In case of potentially malignant neoplasms the major vessels must be ligated at their origin. The suprapubic, umbilical and epigastric ports are placed to the left of midline.

Retroperitoneal tunneling

The initial dissection begins with an incision on the peritoneum on the inferior border of the root of small bowel mesentery and is continued inferior to the caecum. Anterior and cranial traction on the mesentery opens the avascular plane over the iliac vessels and the right ureter is identified coursing over the right iliac vessels. This avascular plane between the ureter and gonadal vessels (posterior mesentery of ascending colon) is developed and the dissection is continued in a tunneling fashion cranially until

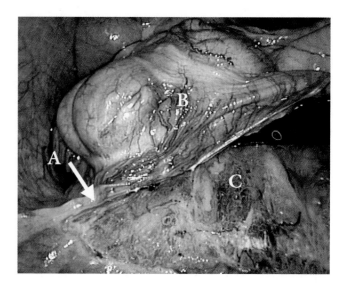

Figure 4 : Peritoneum is incised and dissection carried out behind the cecum (retroperitoneal tunneling)

A - Peritoneal incision

B - Cecum

C - Dissection behind the mesentery

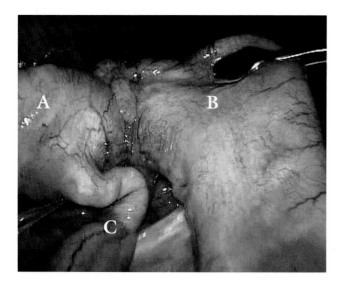

Figure 3 : Terminal ileum is retracted above and medially by using 10 mm babcock from the epigastric port

A - Cecum

B - Terminal ileum

C - Appendix

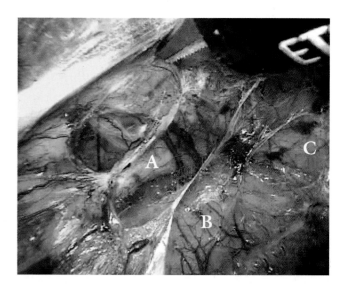

Figure 5 : Retroperitoneal dissection carried out behind the mesentery in the cranial direction

A - Right ureter

B - Inferior vena cava

C - Duodenum

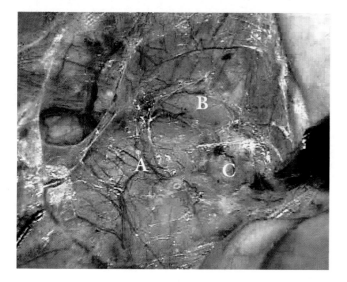

Figure 6 : Dissection carried out medially. Duodenum is seen

A - Inferior vena cava
B - Duodenum
C - Aorta

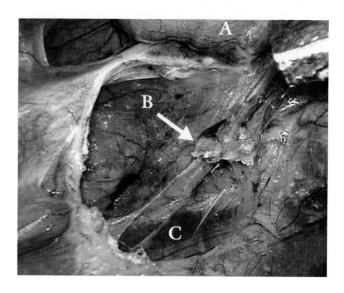

Figure 7 : Dissection behind the cecum, Right gonadal vessel is divided

A - Cecum
B - Divided end of right gonal vessels
C - Psoas muscle

the second part of duodenum is seen. The plane of dissection is kept in the areolar tissue anterior to the gonadal vessels and ureters. The Gerotas fascia is not breached unless it is infiltrated. At this phase the colon is attached to the parietal wall on lateral aspect and the mesentery with vessels on the lateral aspect. A left hand grasper from the right iliac fossa port lifts the roof of the tunnel while dissection is performed with harmonic scalpel from the umbilical port, with the camera in the suprapubic port. The lateral peritoneal attachment of the colon serves as a natural retractor to maintain the position of colon. This obviates the need for frequent manipulation of the colon which might lead to handling of the tumor, bowel injury and dissemination of tumor cells.

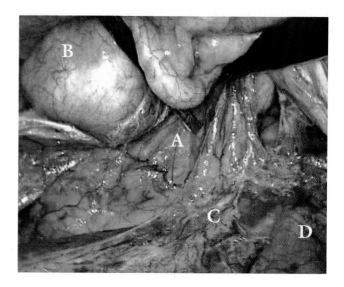

Figure 8 : Dissection carried out behind the ascending colon. Dissection continued up to the hepatic flexure

A - Posterior surface of ascending colon
B - Cecum
C - Right ureter
D - Inferior vena cava

Vascular Control

When the duodenum and the head of pancreas are seen during tunneling the ileocolic and right colic vessels can be seen on the mesentery of the ascending colon. Initial retroperitoneal dissection facilitates easy control of the vascular pedicle and clearance of lymph nodes and vessels. In obese patients, identification of these vessels is difficult. The mesentery is stretched and vessels are identified by its bow string effect. The peritoneum of the mesentery is incised over the superior mesenteric vessels at the right lateral border of the mesentery close to the origin of its branches. The ileo colic artery usually takes origin at the level of the root of superior mesenteric pedicle. The artery and veins are individually skeletonised at the origin clearing the lymphonodular and fatty tissue towards the lateral side. After skeletonisation, clipping is often adequate to control the vessels. If there is any doubt about slippage of clips, an endoloop may be applied for additional security. The incision over the mesentery is continued over the transverse mesocolon till the proposed line of division of transverse colon and the right branches of middle colic vessels are divided.

Hepatic flexure mobilisation

The table is tilted to reverse Trendelenburg position and the hepatic flexure is retracted medially and downwards. The camera from the supra pubic port is shifted to umbilicus and the right hand working port from umbilicus is shifted to epigastric port. The gastrocolic ligament between the transverse colon and stomach is divided to enter the lesser sac. The peritoneum over the head of pancreas and second part of duodenum is divided next and further division is continued towards right lateral side. The hepato colic ligament is incised till the hepatic flexure. The division of hepato colic ligament (the fibres strands on the lateral side of hepatic flexure) release the transverse colon medially. Now the colon is attached to the retroperitoneum only by the transparent mesocolon. The right branch of the middle colic artery is divided close towards origin after clipping. At the end of this phase of dissection, the entire ascending colon, hepatic flexure and proximal transverse colon are mobilized and devascularised. The small bowel mesentery is also divided upto the proposed line of transection of ileum. Finally the lateral attachment of the colon is

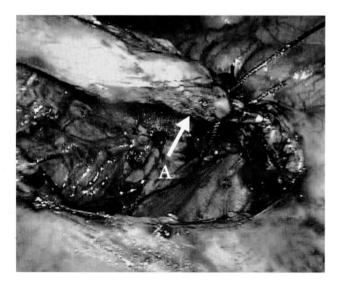

Figure 9 : Ligation of iliocolic artery with silk

A - Ilio colic artery

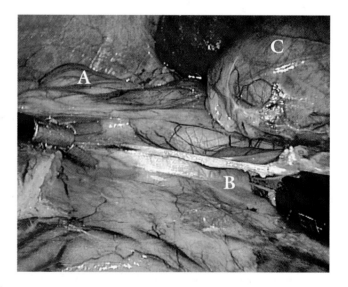

Figure 10 : Mobilization of transverse colon and hepatic flexure

A - Hepatic flexure
B - Duodenum
C - Gall bladder

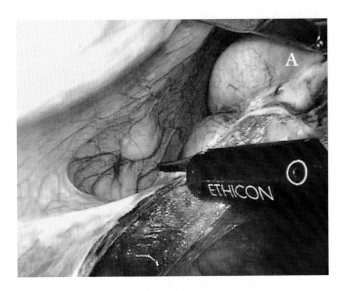

Figure 11 : Division of lateral attachment of the cecum and ascending colon

A - Cecum

divided by sharp dissection from the caecum upto the hepatic flexure.

Resection

The resection of specimen can be done either intracorporeally or extracorporeally. In extracorporeal resection, a small subumbilical incision is made, the mobilized bowel brought out through a protective sheath, and resection and anastomosis is performed as described previously.

Intracorporeal resection can be accomplished by application of linear endostaplers over the transverse mesocolon and ileum. The specimen is placed in an endobag and extracted outside through subumbilical incision. The divided edges of the bowel are exteriorized and continuity is restored by either hand sewn or stapled anastomosis.

A total intracorporeal stapled anastomosis is possible with the currently available instrumentation, but it is tedious and does not offer any additional benefit. The extraction of specimen mandates a subumbilical incision, which can be used for exteriorization of the bowel and extracorporeal anastomosis. The

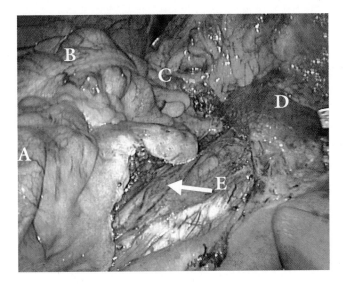

Figure 12 : Completion of right colon mobilization

A - Terminal ileum
B - Ascending colon
C - Hepatic flexure
D - Right kidney
E - Right ureter

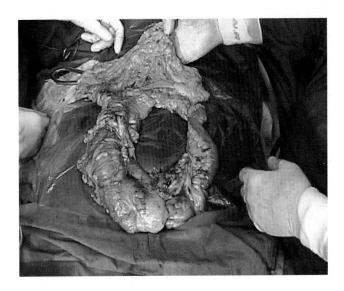

Figure 13 : Mobilized colon and terminal ileum is exteriorised by minilaparotomy

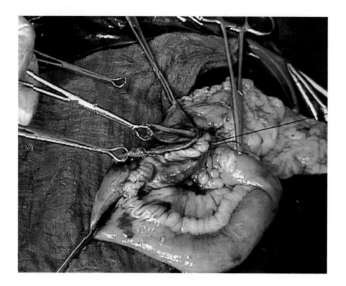

Figure 14 : Resection and end to end anastomosis is done

mesenteric defect is closed and bowels are replaced into the peritoneal cavity. The incision is closed with prolene and pneumoperitoneum recreated. A thorough wash is given and drainage tube is kept. The ports are closed with a port closure needle.

LIMITED RESECTION OF ILEOCEACAL JUNCTION

Limited resection of ileoceacal junction by laparoscopy is an ideal treatment for benign diseases like hyperplastic tuberculosis of ileoceacal junction. There is no need for complete mobilisation of the ascending colon, hepatic flexure and transverse colon in these types of resection. Limited mobilisation of the proximal ascending colon and the terminal ileum as described in lateral to medial approach is sufficient for the specimen to be brought out through a subumbilical incision. Vascular control, resection and anastomosis can be performed extracorporeally. The patient position, theatre setup and position of ports are identical to that of laparoscopic right hemicolectomy. This surgery can be done as the first procedure by surgeons interested in performing laparoscopic colonic resection.

Our Experience

Between 1992 and June 2005, a total of 190 patients underwent laparoscopic right hemicolectomy at our institution. The indications include ileoceacal tuberculosis with obstruction (89), right side colonic growth (adenocarcinoma - 82, lymphoma – 15) and carcinoid in 3, diveritcular bleed in cecum in 1 and ilecolic intussusception due to ileal polyp in 2). All patients with malignant tumors were stage III disease or below according to AJC staging system. We excluded those cases with extensive involvement of parties, fixed growth and very bulky lesion (>15cm) for laparoscopic approach.

There were 124 men and 66 women with a mean age of 57.4 years (range 18 to 83). 36 patients had prior abdominal surgeries for some reason. More than 60% of our study patients were above 55 years of age group.

Classical right hemicolectomy was performed in all malignant patients and limited ileo-colon resection for non-malignant patients.

Patient Characteristics	
Total	190
Male (%)	124 (65.26 %)
Female (%)	66 (34.73 %)
Mean Age (yr)	57.6
Age Range (yr)	18-83
>55 yr	54
ASA Status	
ASA I (%)	89 (46.84 %)
ASA II (%)	71 (37.36 %)
ASA III (%)	20 (10.52 %)
Indications	
Ileocecal TB	89 (46.84%)
Adenocarcinoma	82 (43.15 %)
Lymphoma	15 (7.89 %)
Carcinoid	3 (2.38%)
Diverticular bleed in cecum	1 (1.57 %)
Ileocolic intussusception	2 (1.05 %)

Results	
Conversion	2 (1.05 %)
Mean Operative time	82 mts
Mean operative time (Range)	183 - 66 mts
Mean blood loss	55ml
Range	125 - 35 ml
Flatus (Mean POD)	1.9 days
Stool (Mean POD)	3.1 days
Postoperative hosptial stay	
Mean	5 days
Uncomplicated	4 days
Complicated	9.2 days
Return to normal work	14.2 days

Complications	
Mortality	Nil
Morbidity	
Leakage	3
Post op. bleeding	1
Ileus	3
SI. obstruction	2
Wound infection	3
Respiratory infection	1
Urinary retention	3

Two patients required conversion to open due to bulky lesions. Mean operative time was 82 minutes (range 183-66). Mean blood loss was 55ml (Range 125-35ml). All patients were mobilized from day one. Liquids started after 48 hours. The mean day for passing flatus was 1.9 and for feces were 3.1. The mean post op hospital stay was 5 (Range 9-4) the mean day of return to normal work was 14. All tuberculosis patients were given a full course of ATT post operatively (4 drugs - 2 months and 2 drugs - 4 months). Two of them presented with recurrent intestinal obstruction during their course of ATT therapy and required stricturoplasty. Mean follow up was 4.2 years (range 4 months - 7.3 years).

All malignant patients were seen by medical oncologist and post op chemotherapy were given to 36 (40%) of patients. There is no mortality in our series.

Regarding morbidity, we had one patient with leak which was managed conservatively. Three patients had ileus due to which their hospital stays prolonged. Three patients developed wound infection (all were DM), and required daily dressing for 10 days. 3 patients developed respiratory infection which settled with higher version of antibiotics. Three patients had urinary retention and require recatheterization. Two patients developed local recurrence, for whom laparotomy and resection done. Both of them had poorly differential adenocarcinoma.

LEFT HEMICOLECTOMY

Patient position, theatre set up

The patient is placed in a semilithotomy position Trendelenburg position as for laparoscopic anterior resection. The thighs are minimally flexed (15°) so that they do not impede the movement of the instruments. The position of ports and theatre set up are similar to that of anterior resection.

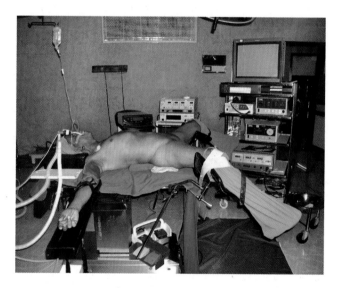

Figure 15 : Position of the patient. Lithotomy with trendelenberg position and sandbag below the hip. (Surgeon stands initially on the right side of the patient, for transverse colon mobilization he moves between the legs)

Peritoneal incision and vascular control

The left side of the patient is raised while maintaining Trendelenburg position to allow the small bowel to fall out of the pelvis. After initial assessment of

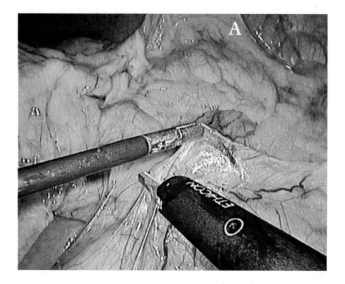

Figure 16 : Peritoneal incision over the mesentery

A - Splenic flexure of colon

the lesion liver and the peritoneal cavity, an incision is made over the medial aspect of the mesosigmoid at the level of sacral promontory. A 10mm grasper from the left midclavicular port retracts the sigmoid laterally to facilitate this dissection. The incision is deepened with a combination of blunt and sharp dissection in a plane anterior to the ureter, gonadal vessels and inferior mesenteric pedicle. Ureter should be carefully protected from injury during this dissection. The inferior mesenteric pedicle is isolated and dissected. The vessels are divided close to their origin after intracorporeal ligation with silk.

Mobilisation of sigmoid and descending colon

The dissection in the avascular plane proceeds from medial to lateral aspect. During this dissection the ureters and gonadal vessels are carefully protected. The dissection is continued laterally till the level of the splenic flexure in a similar manner. The retroperitoneal dissection facilitates easy mobilisation of mesentery of the left colon. The dissection extends cranially upto inferior border of the pancreas, laterally upto the lateral abdominal wall. The dissection

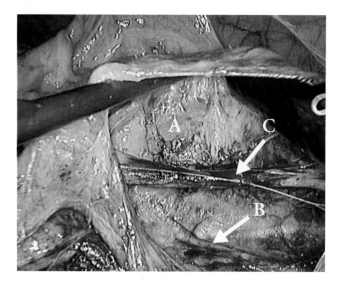

Figure 17 : Dissection carried out behind the mesentery (medial to lateral dissection)

A - Left kidney
B - Left ureter
C - Left gonadal vessels

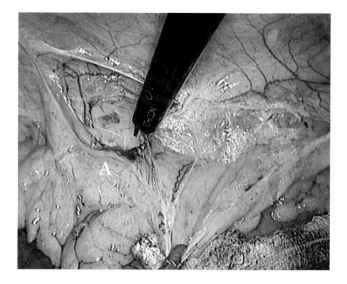

Figure 18 : Division of lateral peritoneal attachment of the desending colon

A - Descending colon

is maintained in the fascial plane anterior to the ureter and gonadal vessels. Creation of a plane of dissection deeper to Gerota's fascia will lead to bloody dissection. With gentle medial traction of the sigmoid colon from the right side port, the lateral peritoneal attachment along the white line of Toldt is divided from the level of sigmoid to proximal part of the descending colon.

Mobilisation of splenic flexure

This phase of dissection is performed by standing in between the legs of the patient. The splenic flexure is retracted medially and downwards by a 10mm grasper. Care should be taken to avoid injury to the splenic hilum. The greater omentum is divided from the attachment to the colon for adequate mobilisation of the splenic flexure. The lateral peritoneal incision is extended cranially till the splenic flexure is reached. The splenocolic and renocolic ligaments are divided to free the splenic flexure. The attachment of the transverse mesocolon over the ventral aspect of the pancreas is divided till the proposed line of division.

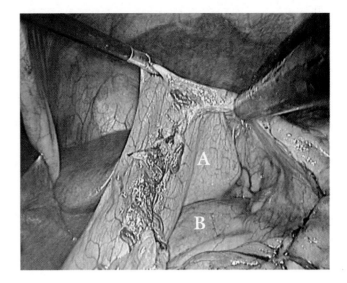

Figure 20 : Division of gastrocolic omentum

A - Posterior surface of the stomach

B - Pancreas

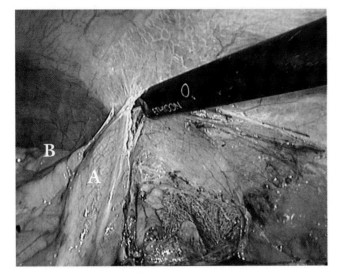

Figure 19 : Mobilization of splenic flexure of colon

A - Spleen

B - Descending colon

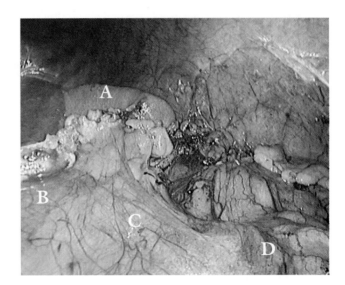

Figure 21 : Completion of splenic flexure mobilization

A - Spleen

B - Pancreas

C - Transverse mesocolon

D - Transverse colon

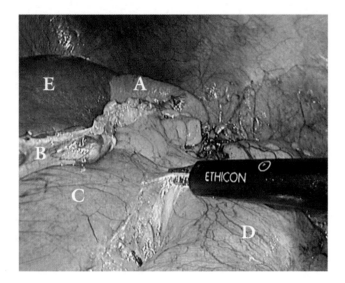

Figure 22 : Division of transverse mesocolon

A - Spleen
B - Stomach
C - Pancreas
D - Transverse colon
E - Left lobe of liver

Rectal mobilisation

After mobilisation of the splenic flexure, the surgeon returns to the right side of the patient for rectal dissection. The avascular plane between the visceral and parietal layer of pelvic fascia is entered and dissected upto the proposed level of transection. The mesorectum is divided at this level upto the rectum with harmonic scalpel. A clamp is applied on the rectum and a washout is given with povidone iodine to reduce the risk of implantation of exfoliated tumor cells. The rectum is divided with a linear endo GIA stapler from the right iliac port.

Minilaparotomy, Resection, Anastomosis

The divided end of the sigmoid is exteriorized through a pfannensteil incision after protecting the wound with a plastic sheath. The proximal transection is completed and the specimen removed. The restoration of continuity can be performed either intracorporeally or extracorporeally. If the length of the rectal stump is adequate, anastomosis can be performed by conventional hand sewn technique.

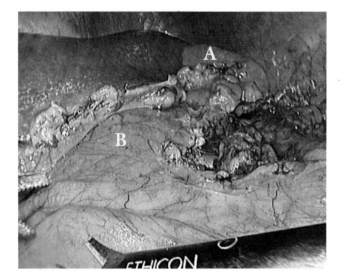

Figure 23 : Completion of transverse colon mobilization

A - Spleen
C - Pancreas

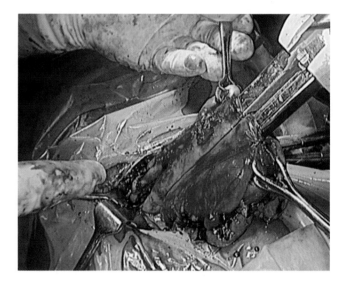

Figure 24 : Mobilized colon is exteriorised by minilaparotomy and resected. Side to side anastomosis is done by using stapler

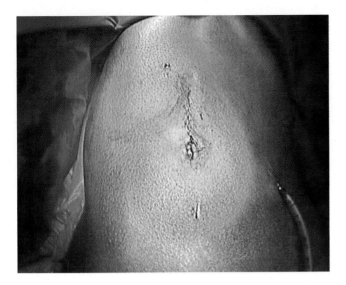

Figure 25 : Ports and minilaparotomy after completion of laparoscopic left colon resection

The bowel is replaced inside and the abdomen closed after insertion of drain. Otherwise, if the distal stump is short, the anastomosis can be performed by circular stapler technique as described in laparoscopic anterior resection. The anastomosis is checked by filling the pelvic cavity with saline and insufflating air through the rectum. It can also be done by injection of methylene blue through the rectum under laparoscopic visualization.

POST OPERATIVE MANAGEMENT

The nasogastric tube is removed on the same day or on the next day morning. Urinary catheter is removed on the first post operative day. Clear liquids are started after passage of flatus (usually second day) and semisolids a day after. The patient is usually discharged between 4-6 days.

Our Experience

Between 1992 and June 2005, a total of 75 patients underwent laparoscopic left hemicolectomy. There were 58 (77.33 %) men and 17 (22.66 %) women with a mean age of 52.6 years (range 40 to 72). Adenocarcinoma was the indication in all patients except in 1 patient who had carcinoid tumor of left colon. As in right hemicolectomy we excluded those

cases with infiltration to parietal wall and those which were very bulky. The mean operative time was 95 minutes and the mean blood loss was 70 ml. There was no conversion in our series as we had excluded bulky lesions and lesions that were infiltrating the parietes. There was no operative or perioperative mortality in our series. The mean hospital stay was 6 days and the patients returned to normal work in 15 days. Four patients had postoperative leak which was successfully managed by conservative measures alone. Wound infection in five, urinary retention in four, respiratory infection in three, portsite herniation in one and deep venous thrombosis in one were the complications in our series.

CONCLUSION

Laparoscopic segmental resections are feasible and safe in the hands of experienced laparoscopic surgeons. The patients gain short term benefits such as faster return of bowel function and work, faster recovery, decreased wound and pulmonary complications. The operative time and the costs involved are more in the early phase; they are expected to reach the same as conventional surgery in the future. Laparoscopic colorectal surgery for benign conditions such as tuberculosis, Crohn's and diverticulitis has been well accepted. The controversy regarding laparoscopy for colorectal cancer is slowly decreasing with the published reports of various long term multi institutional trials which confirm that laparoscopic surgeries are as safe as conventional surgery in terms of radicality of resection, recurrence and survival.

References

1. Redwine DB, Sharpe DR. Laparoscopic segmental resection of the sigmoid colon for endometriosis. J Laparoendosc Surg 1991; 1(4):217-20.

2. Schlinkert RT. Laparoscopic-assisted right hemicolectomy. Dis Colon Rectum 1991; 34(11):1030-1.

3. Jacobs M, Verdeja JC, Goldstein HS. Minimally invasive colon resection (laparoscopic colectomy). Surg Laparosc Endosc 1991; 1(3):144-50.

4. The Clinical Outcomes of Surgical Therapy Study Group. A comparison of laparoscopically assisted and open colectomy for colon cancer. N Engl J Med 2004; 350(20):2050-9.

5. Theodore N. Pappas, Danny O. Jacobs. Laparoscopic Resection for Colon Cancer - The End of the Beginning? N Engl J Med 2004; 350(20):2091-2.

6. Palanivelu C. Basic Instrumentation. *In* Palanivelu C, ed. Text Book of Surgical Laparoscopy. Coimbatore: Gem Digestive Diseases Foundation, 2002. pp. 7 - 14.

7. Palanivelu C. Laparoscopic Space Access and Physiological Significance. *In* Palanivelu C, ed. Text Book of Surgical Laparoscopy. Coimbatore: Gem Digestive Diseases Foundation, 2002. pp. 31-39.

8. Kieran JA, Curet MJ. Laparoscopic colon resection for colon cancer. J Surg Res 2004; 117(1):79-91.

9. Steven Wexner, Eric G Weiss. Laparosocpic COlectomy: The concerns and the benefits. *In* J.G Geraghty, J M Sackier, H L Young, eds. Minimal Access Surgical Oncology. London: Grenwhich Medical Media, 1998. pp. 69-82.

10. Msika S, Deroide G, Kianmanesh R, et al. Harmonic Scalpel ™ in laparoscopic colorectal surgery. Dis Colon Rectum 2001; 44:432-436.

11. Araki Y, Noake T, Kanazawa M, et al. Clipless hand-assisted laparoscopic total colectomy using Ligasure Atlas. Kurume Med J 2004; 51(2):105-8.

12. Hartley JE, Monson JR. The role of laparoscopy in the multimodality treatment of colorectal cancer. Surg Clin North Am 2002; 82(5):1019-33.

13. Nakajima K, Lee SW, Cocilovo C, et al. Hand-assisted laparoscopic colorectal surgery using GelPort. Surg Endosc 2004; 18(1):102-5.

14. Maartense S, Dunker MS, Slors JF, et al. Hand-assisted laparoscopic versus open restorative proctocolectomy with ileal pouch anal anastomosis: a randomized trial. Ann Surg 2004; 240(6):984-91; discussion 991-2.

15. Nakajima K, Lee SW, Cocilovo C, et al. Laparoscopic total colectomy: hand-assisted vs standard technique. Surg Endosc 2004; 18(4):582-6.

16. Bouvet M, Mansfield PF, Skibber JM, et al. Clinical, pathologic, and economic parameters of laparoscopic colon resection for cancer. Am. J. Surg. 1998; 176:554.

17. Khalili TM, Fleshner PR, Hiatt JR, et al. Colorectal cancer:Comparison of laparoscopic with open approaches. Dis. Colon Rectum 1998; 41:832.

18. Kourambas J, Preminger GM. Advances in camera, video, and imaging technologies in laparoscopy. Urol Clin North Am 2001; 28(1):5-14.

19. Palanivelu C. Laparoscopic Colorectal surgery. *In* Palanivelu C, ed. Text Book of Surgical Laparoscopy. Coimbatore: Gem Digestive Diseases Foundation, 2002. pp. 437-452.

20. Hill ADK, Banwell PB, Darzi A. Laparoscopic colonic surgery: the unseen lesion. Minimally Invasive Therapy 1993; 1:13-5.

21. Wexner SD, Cohen SM. Port site metastases after laparoscopic colorectal surgery for cure of malignancy. Br J Surg 1995; 82(3):295-8.

22. Lin KM, Ota DM. Laparoscopic colectomy for cancer: an oncologic feasible option. Surg Oncol 2000; 9(3):127-34.

23. Ziprin P, Ridgway PF, Peck DH, Darzi AW. The theories and realities of port-site metastases: a critical appraisal. J Am Coll Surg 2002; 195(3):395-408.

24. Stocchi L, Heidi Nelson. Basic Instrumentation for Laparoscopic Surgery. *In* Greene FL, Heniford BT, eds. Minimally Invasive Cancer Management. New York: Springer-Verlag, 2001. pp. 200-214.

25. Bauer JJ, Harris MT, Grumbach NM, Gorfine SR. Laparoscopic-assisted intestinal resection for Crohn's disease. Dis Colon Rectum 1995; 38(7):712-5.

26. Hamel CT, Pikarsky AJ, Wexner SD. Laparoscopically assisted hemicolectomy for Crohn's disease: are we still getting better? Am Surg 2002; 68(1):83-6.

27. Wexner SD, Moscovitz ID. Laparoscopic colectomy in diverticular and Crohn's disease. Surg Clin North Am 2000; 80(4):1299-319.

28. Wexner SD, Cera SM. Laparoscopic surgery for ulcerative colitis. Surg Clin North Am 2005; 85(1):35-47.

29. Bruce CJ, Coller JA, Murray JJ, et al. Laparoscopic resection for diverticular disease. Dis Colon Rectum 1996; 39(10 Suppl):S1-6.

30. Franklin ME, Jr., Dorman JP, Jacobs M, Plasencia G. Is laparoscopic surgery applicable to complicated colonic diverticular disease? Surg Endosc 1997; 11(10):1021-5.

31. Liberman MA, Phillips EH, Carroll BJ, et al. Laparoscopic colectomy vs traditional colectomy for diverticulitis. Outcome and costs. Surg Endosc 1996; 10(1):15-8.

32. Trebuchet G, Lechaux D, Lecalve JL. Laparoscopic left colon resection for diverticular disease. Surg Endosc 2002; 16(1):18-21.

33. Prohm P, Weber J, Bonner C. Laparoscopic-assisted coloscopic polypectomy. Dis Colon Rectum 2001; 44(5):746-8.

34. Chung CC, Tsang WW, Kwok SY, Li MK. Laparoscopy and its current role in the management of colorectal disease. Colorectal Dis 2003; 5(6):528-43.

64

Laparoscopic Total and Subtotal Colectomy

INTRODUCTION

Laparoscopic total colectomy is the most complex and demanding procedure in laparoscopic colorectal surgery, requiring significant experience in advanced laparoscopic surgery. It has been shown that these procedures are technically possible and safe. The demanding technical nature of the procedure has been reported to result in greatly prolonged operating time compared with open procedures.[1, 2] However, with increasing experience, this difference may be minimal.[3]

Various procedures such as subtotal colectomy, total colectomy and total proctocolectomy are performed for indications such as ulcerative colitis, crohn's disease or familial polyposis coli.[4, 5] Few years ago, these procedures had to be performed through a long midline incision from xiphisternum to pubic symphysis due to the anatomical position of the colon.[6] Hence these procedures were invariablely associated with increased postoperative pain and delayed recovery. Currently the same procedures can be performed through laparoscopy. This is mainly due to experience gained in partial and segmental colonic resections.[7] These have had a significant impact in the early postoperative recovery and cosmetic outcome. The better cosmesis gains importance as these procedures are commonly performed in younger age group because it helps them to maintain their body image.[8] These procedures are performed in cases of inflamatory bowel disease (IBD) that no longer respond to conservative treatment or in patients with familial colonic polyposis.[9] Peters performed the first successful laparoscopic total proctocolectomy with an ileostomy in two patients with severe ulcerative colitis.[5]

While perioperative morbidity rates remain high when compared with simpler segmental resections, quality-of-life studies uniformly support the performance of these major procedures.[8-11] Patients report excellent long-term overall satisfaction and improved scores for physical, emotional, and social well-being.

LAPAROSCOPIC SUBTOTAL COLECTOMY

Preoperative preparation

The preoperative preparation for total colectomy is the same as the open procedure. Bowels are prepared with polythelene glycol solution and intravenous antibiotics. The consent for stoma and the psychological preparation for accepting the stoma should be taken before surgery. The patient should be assessed for fitness for surgery with regard to cardiac and pulmonary status and started on antithrombotic prophylaxis as these surgeries are involved with sufficiently longer operative times. A nasogastric tube and a urinary catheter are inserted before the starting the procedure.

Principles

The basics of total colectomy are the combination of various phases of mobilisation and ligation of vessels (left, right and transverse colectomy). The procedure starts with the mobilisation of sigmoid and the rectosigmoid, which is continued cranially towards the descending colon. This phase is done with the surgeon on the right side of the patient. The surgeon moves to in between the legs of the patient for mobilisation of splenic flexure and transverse colon. The ascending colon and hepatic flexure are mobilized from the left side of the patient. The surgeon returns back to the right side for rectal mobilisation and resection. Resection and anastomosis can be performed either by intracorporeal or extra corporeal method.

Patient position and placement of ports

The patient is placed in a semilithotomy position with arms outstretched. The thighs are flexed minimally so as to not to impede the movement of laparoscopic instruments. The importance of a remote controlled operating table that can be tilted on any axis cannot be over emphasized. It is gravity that is most often used as a retractor to keep the bowels away from the operating area. More importantly this relieves the

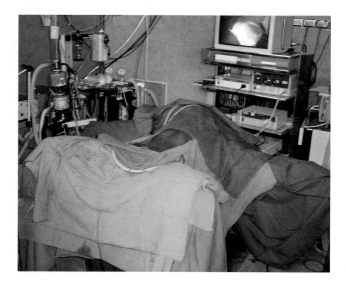

Figure 1 : Position of the patient. Lithotomy with trendelenberg position. Surgeon stands between the leg, for right colon mobilization he moves to right side of the patient

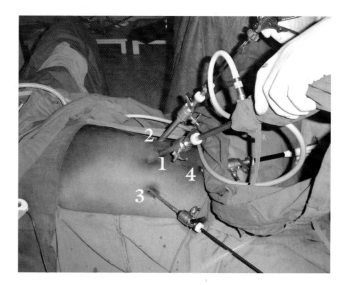

Figure 2 : Ports position

1 - Camera port 10mm
2 - Right hand working port 10mm
3 - Left hand working port 5mm
4 - Retracting port 10mm

ports for retractor can be used for other working instruments.

Phase 1: Recto sigmoid mobilisation

The patient is placed in a steep Trendelenburg position with left side up. This allows the small bowels to fall out of the pelvis and stay in the peritoneal cavity without any retraction. A 10mm Babcock grasper from the left hypochondrial port retracts the sigmoid colon laterally by holding the apex of the sigmoid. This maneuver exposes the medial aspect of the sigmoid colon. An incision is made on the medial aspect of the mesosigmoid, on the peritoneum near the origin of the inferior mesenteric vessels at the level of sacral promontory. This incision is deepened and avascular plane is entered between the mesosigmoid and the Toldt's fascia. This dissection is performed with the harmonic scalpel, which helps in maintaining absolute hemostasis. The origin of the inferior mesenteric vessels is identified and the peritoneum over the vessels is incised to expose the vessels. The artery and vein are identified and dissected out, the artery is ligated with 2-0 silk and divided between ligatures at the level of aortic

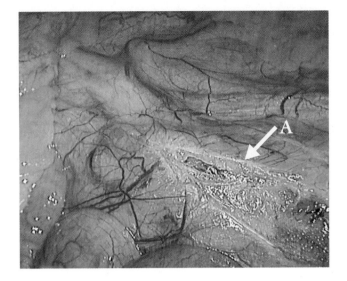

Figure 4 : Peritoneal incision for medial to lateral dissection

A - Peritoneal incision

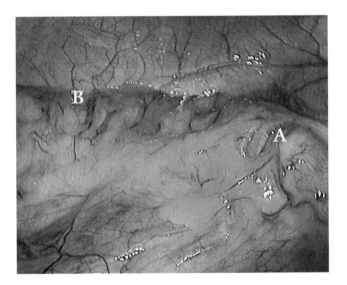

Figure 3 : Exposure of mesosigmoid. Small bowels were retracted to the right

A - Sigmoid colon
B - Descending colon

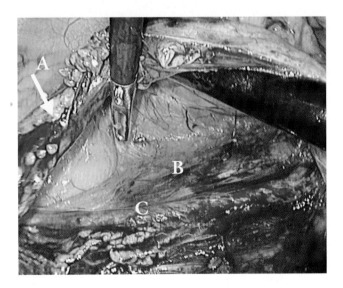

Figure 5 : Dissection carried out behind the mesentery towards lateral side

A - Inferior mesenteric pedicle
B - Psoas muscle
C - Left ureter

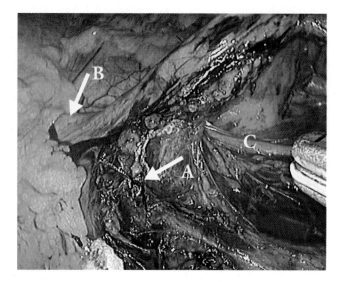

Figure 6 : Inferior mesenteric artery is ligated and divided

A - Divided end of inferior mesenteric artery
B - Inferior mesenteric artery
C - Left ureter

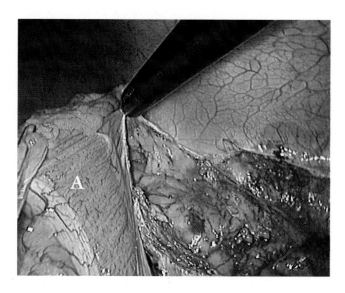

Figure 8 : Division of lateral peritoneal attachment of colon (White line of Toldt)

A - Descending colon

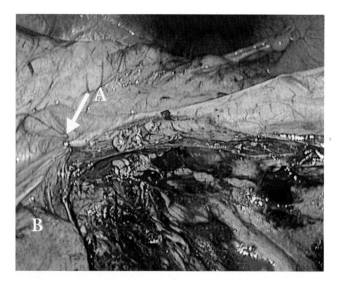

Figure 7 : Inferior mesenteric vein is clipped at the level of duodenojejunal flexure

A - Clipped inferior mesenteric artery
B - Duodenojejunal flexure

origin. The left ureter and gonadal vessels are identified in the plane and are carefully dissected off posteriorly. The dissection continues in a medial to lateral aspect towards the splenic flexure. The lateral peritoneal attachment is divided at the end of this phase along the white line of Toldt.

Phase 2: Splenic flexure and transverse colon mobilisation

The splenic flexure is attached to the spleen and the diaphragm through the peritoneal attachments namely splenocolic and phrenocolic ligaments. Due to its various attachments, the mobilisation of splenic flexure is considered as the most difficult part of the surgery.

This is best performed by standing in-between the legs of the procedure. The transverse colon and the descending colon are retracted medially and downward to expose the peritoneal attachments of the splenic flexure. The change of position of patient to reverse Trendelenburg position with right lateral tilt, exposes the flexure and allows the small bowel and omentum to fall away from the field of vision.

The phrenocolic and splenocolic ligaments are divided with harmonic scalpel to free the splenic flexure. Now the splenic flexure is connected only by mesentery of the colon. The mesocolon of the splenic flexure is divided in an avascular space. The incision on the mesentery of left colon is continued over the splenic flexure and the transverse colon. The course of left ureter is identified coursing over Gerota's fascia.

The mobilisation of transverse colon begins with division of gastrocolic ligament from the colon. This division is started from the splenic flexure and continued until the hepatic flexure. The lesser sac is entered at this juncture. The mobilized gastrocolic omentum (greater omentum) is placed over the stomach so that it does not obscure the operating field. Now the colon is attached only by transverse mesocolon (attached to the ventral surface of the pancreas extending towards the hilum of spleen). The mesocolon is divided with harmonic scalpel after ligating the middle colic artery at its origin. Inadvertent ligation of superior mesenteric artery for

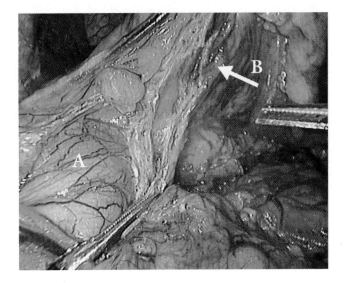

Figure 10 : Division of gastrocolic omentum

A - Transverse colon
B - Posterior surface of antrum of stomach

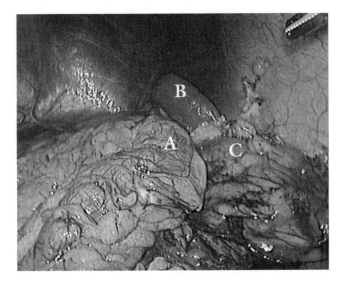

Figure 9 : Completion of mobilization of splenic flexure of colon

A - Splenic flexure
B - Spleen
C - Left kidney

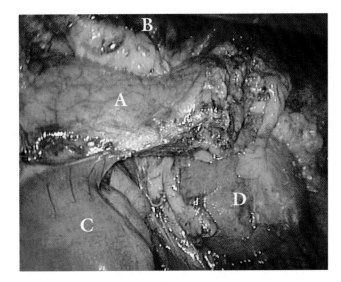

Figure 11 : Completion of transverse colon mobilization on the left side

A - Pancreas
B - Stomach
C - Duodenojejunal flexure
D - Left kidney

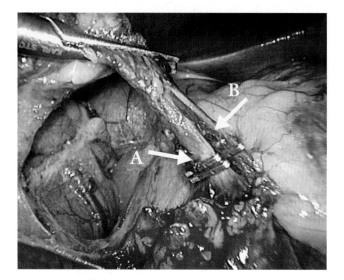

Figure 12 : Division of middle colic vessels

A - Clipped middle colic artery

B - Clipped middle colic vein

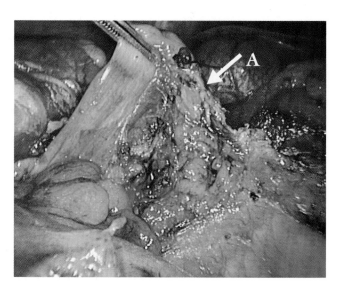

Figure 13 : Dissection of Ileocolic vessel

A - Ileocolic vessel

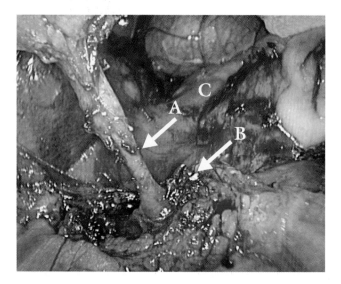

Figure 14 : Completion of Dissection of ileocolic artery

A - Illeocolic artery

B - Divided end of vein

C - Duodenum

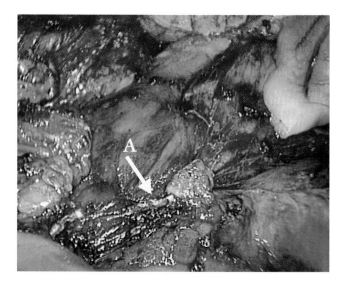

Figure 15 : Ileocolic artery is clipped and divided

A - Divided end of ileocolic artery

middle colic artery should be avoided at any cost as this might lead to disastrous complications. The ligament of Trietz must be identified and the proximal jejunum protected from being injured.

Phase 3 : Ascending colon and hepatic flexure mobilisation: Retroperitoneal tunnel technique

This procedure is similar to 'medial to lateral mobilisation' of right hemicolectomy. The surgeon stands on the left side of the patient and starts the dissection with the patient tilted to left side (Right side up). A peritoneal incision is made below the distal ileum and caecum. An avascular plane is entered and the plane is continued upwards between the mesentery of ascending colon and Toldt's fascia. The right ureter is seen over coursing the iliac vessels, which is protected by sweeping it posteriorly. The dissection continues in the avascular plane in a tunneling fashion up to the second part of duodenum. (Retroperitoneal tunnel). The mesentery of the ascending colon is divided with harmonic scalpel,

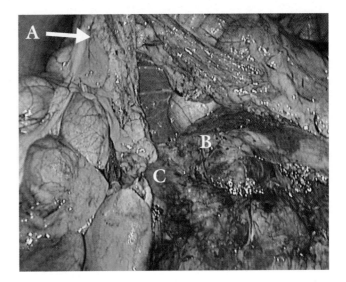

Figure 17 : Completion of hepatic flexure mobilization

A - Hepatic flexure
B - Duodenum
C - Right kidney

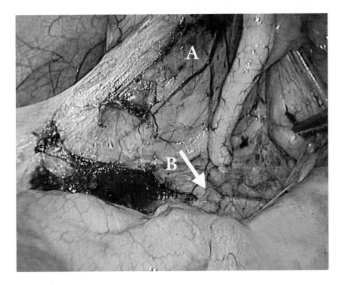

Figure 16 : Cecum and terminal colon is lifetd up, dissection carried out behind the mesentery (retroperitoneal tunneling)

A - Inferior surface of cecum
B - Right ureter

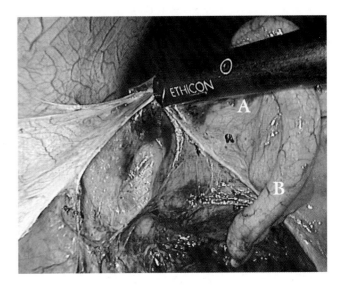

Figure 18 : Division of lateral peritoneal attachment of the ascending colon

A - Cecum
B - Appendix

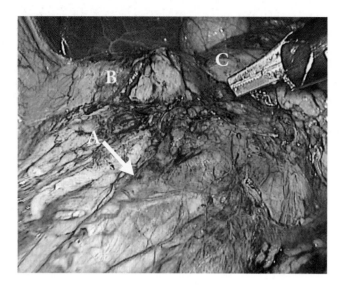

Figure 19 : Completion of right colon mobilization

A - Right ureter
B - Right kidney
C - Duodenum

carefully clipping and dividing the ileocolic and right colic vessels. The peritoneal attachment on the lateral aspect along the white line of Toldt is divided at the end of mobilisation. Now the peritoneal attachments on superior aspect of the hepatic flexure are divided. Medial and downward traction of the hepatic flexure aids in division of these ligaments. The transverse colon is slowly mobilized from the gall bladder and the duodenum during this part of the dissection. This completes the mobilisation of entire colon from caecum to recto sigmoid junction.

Phase 4 : Mobilisation of Rectum

This procedure is similar to anterior resection. The patient is repositioned back in steep Trendelenburg position with left side tilt up to expose the rectum completely. A 10mm Babcock from the left lumbar port retracts the rectum superiorly and to the left to expose the posterior aspect of the mesorectum. An avascular plane between the visceral and parietal layers of the pelvic peritoneum is entered and this plane of dissection is continued distally in the hollow of sacrum.

If the plane of dissection enters deep to the presacral fascia (parietal layer of pelvic fascia), then the incidence of injury to the autonomic nerve plexus is very high. This is an important cause for sexual dysfunction following mobilisation of rectum. The bleeding due to injury to sacral plexus is again difficult to control as these branches retract into the sacral foramina. Coagulation of these veins is almost impossible.

Phase 5 : Completion of colectomy

The level of the division of recto sigmoid area is identified and divided with the application of linear endo GIA staplers from the right iliac fossa port. Usually 2-3 firings of 45mm endo GIA staplers are needed for complete division of the sigmoid. Once the sigmoid is divided, a minilaparotomy (Pfannensteil incision) is made and the specimen is exteriorized through the wound with the help of wound protector. A wound protector is a plastic sheath opened on either end. An appropriate sized plastic sheath is taken and inserted into the wound. The entire depth of wound is covered with wound protector and is best held by 2 retractors on the sides of the wound. The edge of the specimen is held by a 10mm Babcock retractor before minilaparotomy is made. The Babcock is introduced through the Pfannenstiel incision and the distal bowel is slowly eased out through the plastic sheath. This facilitates the extraction of specimen that is still attached to the bowel at one end and wound protector is used. The entire colon is pulled out of the wound to expose the distal ileum and is divided.

Phase 6 : Reconstruction

The restoration of continuity can either be done with circular stapler or by hand sewn anastomosis. If the rectum can be mobilized into the external wound, the ileorectal anastomosis can be performed extracorporeally. The same anastomosis can be performed by intracorproeal suturing.

The terminal ileum is closed over the anvil of the circular stapler and replaced inside the abdominal cavity, wound is closed and pneumoperitoneum is recreated. The shaft of the circular stapler is introduced through the anus and once the shaft touches the stapled portion, the center spike is pierced through it. The shaft and the anvil are docked with each other and fired. The anastomosis is checked for leak by filling the pelvic cavity with saline and

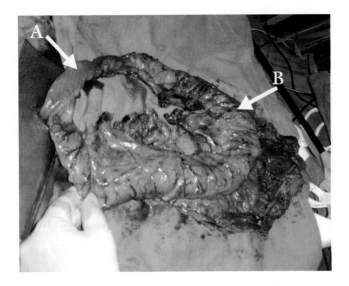

Figure 20 : Specimen is exteriorised by minilaparotomy

A - Ileum

B - Colon

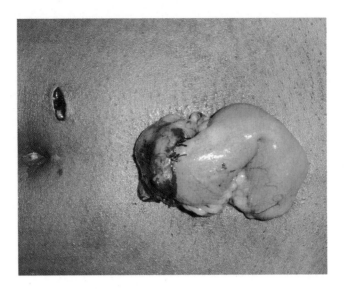

Figure 21 : Resection and end to end ileocolic anastomosis is done

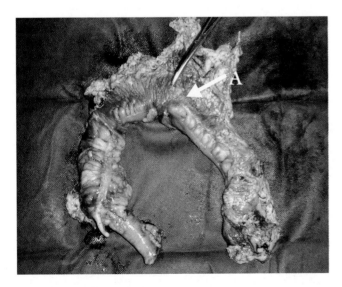

Figure 22 : Excised colon

A - Growth

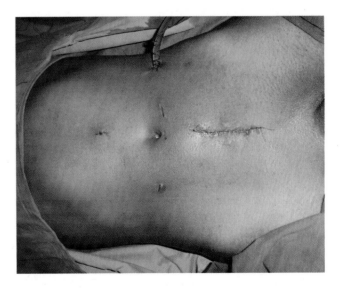

Figure 23 : Position of ports and minilaparotomy after laparoscopic subtotal colectomy

insufflating air through rectum. The mesenteric defect is closed and a drainage tube kept. Ports are closed.

LAPAROSCOPIC TOTAL PROCTOCOLECTOMY

This procedure combines subtotal colectomy with resection of the rectum, creation of jejunal pouch and pouch anal anastomosis. The entire procedure is the same as subtotal colectomy till the complete mobilisation of the colon. This is followed by rectal mobilisation and division.

Rectal mobilisation

The dissection is continued in the avascular plane between the visceral and parietal layer till the rectum is circumferentially mobilized. Laparoscopy offers a clear advantage compared to open surgery in the pelvic dissection. The excellent magnification by laparoscopy helps in easy identification and preservation of neurovascular structures. The rectal mobilisation starts in the posterior aspect and proceeds distally up to the coccyx. Division with harmonic scalpel aids bloodless dissection in this plane. After the posterior mobilisation, the rectum is retracted to the left and upwards, exposing the lateral ligament on the right, which is divided. The lateral ligaments, which are the condensation of the endopelvic fascia often contain the middle rectal artery. Injury at this level to the nerves erigentes might lead to sexual dysfunction. The anterior mobilisation between the seminal vesicles and rectum in males and vagina and rectum in females may be in a plane posterior to the Denonvilliers fascia in benign conditions. The dissection is continued till the levator ani. Resection of the lower end of the rectum is difficult due to the narrow angle f the pelvis. It is often impossible obtain a straight line of division in distal rectum. The use of roticulating staplers has reduced this difficulty.

Surgeons have described a new method to divide the rectum by conventional linear staplers through a Pfannensteil incision. The specimen retrieval and division of the ileum is performed in a similar manner as subtotal colectomy. The perineal dissection is no different from the conventional dissection. The specimen can be extracted through the perineum and pelvic wound closed in layers.

Creation of J pouch

The intestinal continuity can be performed by creation of the various types of pouches; the J pouch is the most commonly used pouch for reconstruction. The ileocolic artery is divided at the level of the origin so that the small bowel reaches up to the bottom of the pelvis. There are few other methods of lengthening of short small bowel like mobilisation of the small bowel mesentery up to the level of the pancreas and others. If there is difficulty for the small bowel to reach the pelvis, either an ileostomy or J pouch anastomosis over a large rectal cuff is the only alternative.

The distal ileum is exteriorized and is folded on itself to create a J shaped pouch. An enterotomy is made at the apex of the pouch and a linear stapler is introduced into the small bowel and is fired. Two or three more applications of stapler on the same loop of the bowel creates an adequate pouch of 15 cms.

Reconstruction

A purse string is applied on the apex after introduction of the anvil and a circular anastomosis is

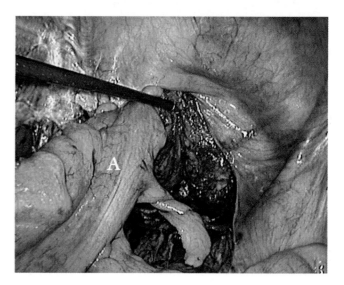

Figure 24 : Dissection of rectum on the right side

A - Rectum

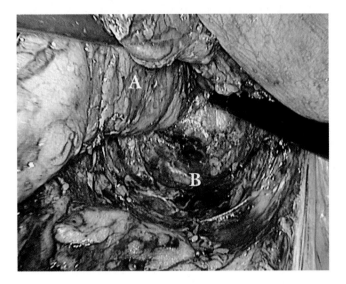

Figure 25 : Posterior dissection of rectum in the holy plane (plane between the mesorectum and presacral fascia)

A - Mesorectum
B - Presaral fascia

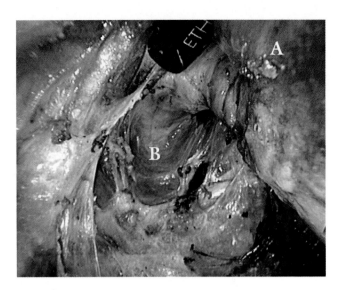

Figure 26 : Dissection of the rectum on left side

A - Rectum
B - Levator ani muscle

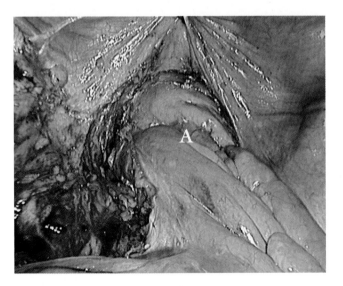

Figure 27 : Dissection of the retum anteriorly

A - Rectum

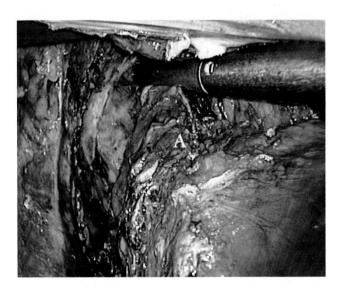

Figure 28 : Division of the rectum using Endo GIA stapler

A - Rectum

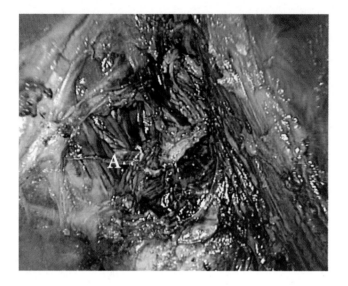

Figure 29 : Completion of rectal transection

A   -   Levator ani

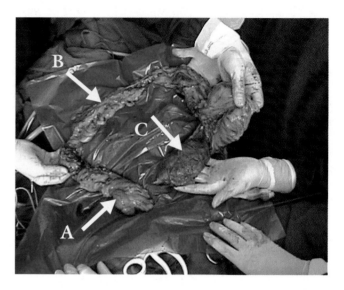

Figure 30 : Mobilized coln and divided rectum is brought out by minilaparotomy

A   -   Cecum
B   -   Transverse colon
C   -   Rectum

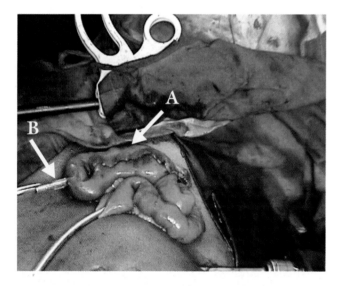

Figure 31 : Colon and rectum is excised, ileal pouch is formed by stapler and anvil of the circular stapler is placed

A   -   Ileal pouch
B   -   Anvil of the circular stapler

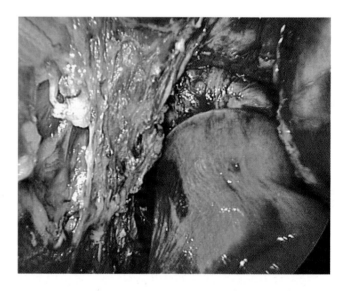

Figure 32 : Ileal pouch is placed in the peritoneal cavity and anastomosed to anal canal

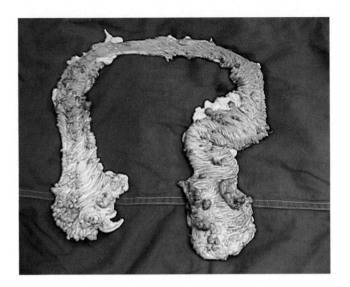

Figure 33 : Cut section of excised colon and rectum

created in a similar fashion. The adequacy of anastomosis is tested. A diverting ileostomy is usually performed to protect the stoma.

OUR EXPERIENCE

Eight cases of Familial Adenomatous Polyposis (FAP) with malignant transformation (Rectal malignancy in four, rectal and cecal malignancy in the other four) underwent laparoscopic total proctocolectomy followed by reconstruction using ileal "J" pouch. Fourteen patients underwent subtotal colectomy with ileorectal anastamsosis for ulcerative colitis. Ten patients were males and four were female and the mean age was 34 years (16 - 56). The mean duration of surgery was 150 minutes (100 - 230). Oral fluids were started on 3 rd day (1-3 days) and the first solid diet was started on 4 th postoperative day. The mean length of hospital stay was 8 days. There were no intra-operative surgical complications or deaths. There was no postoperative mortality. One patient developed wound infection and one patient had postoperative urinary retention. One patient had subacute obstruction after 6 months which was treated conservatively. None of the patients had problems with potency, orgasm sensation, ejaculation, micturition. All the patients are highly satisfied with functional outcome and cosmesis.

DISCUSSION

Subtotal or segmental colectomy with an end ileostomy or colostomy with oversewing of the rectal stump may be indicated because a primary anastomosis for patients with diffuse intra-abdominal sepsis, acute diverticulitis, toxic colitis, or mechanical obstruction of the large bowel is associated with a high risk for dehiscence.

Laparoscopic colectomy involves the entire mobilization of the colon in all the quadrants before resection. This mobilization alone can be performed by laparoscopy and resection anastomosis by conventional method (limited Pfannenstiel incision) as described by various laparoscopic assisted procedures.[9, 12] These laparoscopic assisted procedures greatly help in reducing the operating time of these procedures, as some of the initial reports of laparoscopic total proctocolectomy claimed that these were associated with significantly longer operating times. Those advocating a purely laparoscopic approach, on the other hand, argue that the use of a laparoscopically assisted technique reduces the potential benefits of the minimally invasive approach, especially with regard to the most obvious advantage, improved cosmesis.

Even if operation time and hospital stay might be longer in some series, the protection of the abdominal wall integrity and subsequent cosmetic outcome are very important in this patient group, as there usually is a reluctance to accept this major surgical intervention. The possibility to perform it with maximal cosmetic outcome will help them to overcome their psychological barrier.

Schmitt et al, compared the duration of the postoperative ileus and hospitalization between conventional and laparoscopic assisted proctocolectomy and ileal pouch anastomosis in a prospective randomized study. Neither the length of time for ileus resolution nor the hospital stays were reduced after the laparoscopic procedure. They concluded that laparoscopic assisted approach did not offer any theoretical advantages associated with other laparoscopic procedures.[13] Although these results were expected to improve as more cases are performed, dramatic differences in rates of postoperative recovery had not been realized.

But in subsequent studies it was found that the though operating time was comparable with the conventional approach, the nasogastric tube removal and the passage of stools were earlier than in the conventional group[14]. Various studies that compared the laparoscopic with the open technique in a group of patients with slow transit constipation found that the cosmetic advantage was remarkable, even if the operating time was longer in the laparoscopic group.[15, 16]

Prophylactic laparoscopic total colectomies are performed for carriers of FAP gene for prevention of cancer. The concept of prophylactic surgery for HNPCC gene mutation carrier was first proposed by Henry Lynch. [17] Marc Pocard et al have reported the use of laparoscopic prophylactic surgery for HNPCC gene mutation carrier. Recommending extensive surgery for HNPCC mutation carriers who do not yet have disease, cannot be recommended universally as these individuals have a high risk of developing several types of tumour (not only colonic lesions), and not all mutation carriers will develop tumours. Prophylactic surgeries for HNPCC should be performed routinely after development of international expert consensus guidelines.

CONCLUSION

Laparoscopic total and subtotal colectomy are safe and feasible in the hands of experienced laparoscopic surgeons. The use of laparoscopic assited approaches help in reducing the operative time when compared to totally laparoscopic approaches. The cosmetic outcome of these surgeries greatly helps the young patients in accepting these treatment options to prevent the occurence of cancer in patients with FAP gene.

References

1. Santoro E, Carlini M, Carboni F, Feroce A. Laparoscopic total proctocolectomy with ileal J pouch-anal anastomosis. Hepatogastroenterology 1999; 46(26):894-9.

2. Bernstein MA, Dawson JW, Reissman P, et al. Is complete laparoscopic colectomy superior to laparoscopic assisted colectomy? Am Surg 1996; 62(6):507-11.

3. Seow-Choen F, Eu KW, Leong AF, Ho YH. A consecutive series of open compared to laparoscopic restorative proctocolectomy with ileo-pouch anal anastomosis for familial adenomatous polyposis. Tech Coloproctol 1999; 3:83-6.

4. Wexner SD, Johansen OB, Nogueras JJ, Jagelman DG. Laparoscopic total abdominal colectomy. A prospective trial. Dis Colon Rectum 1992; 35(7):651-5.

5. Peters WR. Laparoscopic total proctocolectomy with creation of ileostomy for ulcerative colitis: report of two cases. J Laparoendosc Surg 1992; 2(3):175-8.

6. Corman ML. Carcinoma of the colon. Philadelphia: J.B. Lippincott Company, 1933.

7. Jacobs M, Verdeja JC, Goldstein HS. Minimally invasive colon resection (laparoscopic colectomy). Surg Laparosc Endosc 1991; 1(3):144-50.

8. Dunker MS, Bemelman WA, Slors JF, et al. Functional outcome, quality of life, body image, and cosmesis in patients after laparoscopic-assisted and conventional restorative proctocolectomy: a comparative study. Dis Colon Rectum 2001; 44(12):1800-7.

9. Milsom JW, Ludwig KA, Church JM, Garcia-Ruiz A. Laparoscopic total abdominal colectomy with ileorectal anastomosis for familial adenomatous polyposis. Dis Colon Rectum 1997; 40(6):675-8.

10. Maartense S, Dunker MS, Slors JF, et al. Hand-assisted laparoscopic versus open restorative proctocolectomy with ileal pouch anal anastomosis: a randomized trial. Ann Surg 2004; 240(6):984-91; discussion 991-2.

11. Pace DE, Seshadri PA, Chiasson PM, et al. Early experience with laparoscopic ileal pouch-anal anastomosis for ulcerative colitis. Surg Laparosc Endosc Percutan Tech 2002; 12(5):337-41.

12. Reissman P, Salky BA, Pfeifer J, et al. Laparoscopic surgery in the management of inflammatory bowel disease. Am J Surg 1996; 175:47-51.

13. Schmitt SL, Cohen SM, Wexner SD, et al. Does laparoscopic-assisted ileal pouch anal anastomosis reduce the length of hospitalization? Int J Colorectal Dis 1994; 9(3):134-7.

14. Araki Y, Isomoto H, Tsuzi Y, et al. Clinical aspects of total colectomy-laparoscopic versus open technique for familial adenomatous polyposis and ulcerative colitis. Kurume Med J 1998; 45(2):203-7.

15. Ho YH, Tan M, Eu KW, et al. Laparoscopic-assisted compared with open total colectomy in treating slow transit constipation. Aust N Z J Surg 1997; 67(8):562-5.

16. Thibault C, Poulin EC. Total laparoscopic proctocolectomy and laparoscopy-assisted proctocolectomy for inflammatory bowel disease: operative technique and preliminary report. Surg Laparosc Endosc 1995; 5(6):472-6.

17. Lynch HT. Is there a role for prophylactic subtotal colectomy among hereditary nonpolyposis colorectal cancer germline mutation carriers? Dis Colon Rectum 1996; 39:109-10.

65

Laparoscopic Anterior Resection

INTRODUCTION

To address the problem of high recurrence rates following rectal surgeries, Miles combined radical and perineal approach[1] to remove the pelvic mesocolon and the "zone of upward spread". But even this was associated with poor quality of life due to permanent colostomy and damage to autonomic plexus resulting in sexual[2,3] and bladder dysfunction[4] affecting the quality of life after surgery. Introduction of mechanical stapling devices[5] have lead to resection at lower levels with reconstruction providing the patient with functional anal sphincter, avoiding permanent colostomy.

The introduction of concept of total mesorectal excision (Heald)[6-8] markedly improved local control and survival. In this technique, the entire mesorectum enveloping the rectum is removed carefully preserving the pelvic autonomic nerves, by entering a relatively bloodless plane by sharp dissection under direct vision in the true pelvis. This reduces the incidents of sexual and urinary dysfunction. In fact now TME has become the standard of care for rectal cancers, replacing conventional techniques. With this technique the local recurrence rates after 5 yrs is < 5% and the 5 yr survival rate is 80%.[9]

Sexual dysfunction following abdominoperineal in the early stages (1942), were about 95%. Nerve preservation significantly increases the quality of life of patients undergoing surgery for rectal carcinoma. Jones identified "destruction of sympathetic nerve fibers, including the nervi erigentes" as the cause for impotence, but concluded: "I know of no way to prevent it if one is to do a radical operation for cancer".[10] Deliberate tracking and preservation of the autonomic nerves in conjunction with TME was introduced by Enker in 1991.[11] Japanese surgeons have extended to complete, partial, or unilateral nerve-sparing techniques with iliac or obturator lymphadenectomy and total mesorectal excision. Now the male sexual functions like erection and ejaculation is maintained with nerve preservation techniques.[12, 13]

LeRoy performed the first laparoscopic total mesorectal excision in 1991[14] which was followed by many such reports. Adequate experience in open mesorectal excision and laparoscopic suturing skills and familiarity of working with laparoscopy in deep structures of pelvis is an important factor for the success of the surgery. With an adequate experience in laparoscopic surgeries for both benign and malignant colorectal conditions, we have opted to offer laparoscopic mesorectal excision for patients with low rectal cancers. Since 1993, we have been performing laparoscopic colorectal resections (low anterior resection, ultra low anterior resection, coloanal anastomosis and laparoscopic assisted abdomino perineal resection) and we have standardized most of the techniques in laparoscopic colorectal surgeries.[25]

ROLE OF LAPAROSCOPY

The advantages of laparoscopy like early return of bowel function, reduction in pain, decreased disability; shorter hospitalization and better cosmesis have been proved in the management of benign colorectal surgeries. The reservations about its use in malignancies of the colon are slowly reducing with the publication of long term results which conclude that laparoscopic surgeries are as effective open surgeries.[15] Although several multi institutional randomized trails are being done for laparoscopic management of colorectal cancer, most of the trials have excluded rectal cancer, because of the complexity of the techniques required both in laparoscopy and open techniques. However several authors have shown that laparoscopic anterior resection is feasible and safe through laparoscopy, with sphincter preservation.

PREOPERATIVE PREPARATION

A thorough preoperative assessment includes physical examination, liver function, and radiograph of the chest, CEA, colonoscopy and CT examination of the abdomen to rule out distant metastasis. We follow TNM AJCC staging system. Patients with advanced stages and infiltration into the prostate, bladder, sacrum and other tissues were referred for preoperative chemo-radiotherapy. Only patients whose tumors were situated beyond 5cm of anal verge were offered laparoscopic anterior resection. This was assesed by digital examination and sigmoidsocopic evaluation.

Total mesorectal Excision (AR) should aim at the following goals.

1. Radical resection
2. Sphincter preservation
3. Autonomic nerve preservation

All patients with middle and lower rectal cancers are candidates for sphincter saving mesorectal excision. There are certain risk factors, where sphincter saving might not be possible and abdominoperineal resection may the better choice.

Indications

1. Rectosigmoid and rectal cancers without infiltration to adjacent organs (T2 lesions)
2. Endoscopically untreatable benign rectal polyps.

Absolute Contraindications

1. Contraindication to laparoscopy
2. Perforated and obstructed rectal cancers
3. Low lying anaplastic cancers of the rectum
4. Prior prostatectomy or radiotherapy for cancer prostate

Relative Contraindications

1. Bulky tumor just above the anorectal ring due to difficult dissection
2. Cancers located 2-3cm from the Anorectal ring
3. Anteriorly located tumors in obese males
4. Extensive diverticular disease or prior left colectomy
5. Poor preoperative sphincter function

Word of caution

An important difference between the open surgery and laparoscopy lies in decision making in low rectal cancers. In conventional surgeries if the level of the distal transection is difficult to anticipate preoperatively, the surgeon can always attempt for a trial pelvic dissection and decide about sphincter preservation during the course of the surgery. But during laparoscopic surgery the assessment of the level of distal transection is impossible due to the lack of tactile sensation. So it is imperative that the type of surgery (either sphincter sparing or removing) should be decided preoperatively if laparoscopic management is considered. During the section if there is any doubt about the distal extent of the tumor, it can be assessed by peroperative sigmoidoscopy and endorectal ultrasound, if facilities are available.

LAPAROSCOPIC TOTAL MESORECTAL EXCISION:

Patient position

The patient is placed in semi lithotomy position with hip flexed for adequate exposure for perineal approach as described in abdominoperineal resection. The stirrups should be positioned such that the thighs are maintained semi flexed, (rather than flexion to 90 degrees) because flexed thighs obstruct the movement of laparoscope and instruments. The presence of a hydraulic operating table that can be remotely operated is ideal for frequent change of position that is ideal.

Theatre set up

The theatre set up is as shown in the figure. The position of the surgeon, camera assistant, second assistant and the staff nurse are similar to that of the abdominoperineal resection described previously. The initial dissection is completed and the perineal

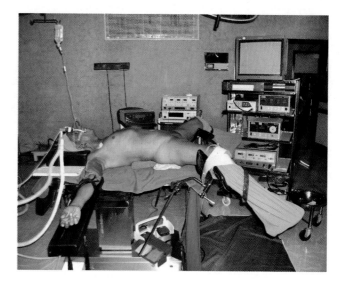

Figure 1 : Position of the patient. Lithotomy with trendelenberg position and sandbag below the hip. Surgeon and camera surgeon stand on the right side of the patient

surgeon joins the procedure for the creation of circular anastomosis by transanal approach.

Position of trocars

The patient is draped completely and the bladder is catheterized. During draping, care should be taken to drape the abdomen widely for placement of lateral trocars. The patient is placed in a Trendelenburg position and carbon dioxide pneumoperitoneum is established with a Veress needle technique. After insufflation of pneumoperitoneum to a pressure of 14mm Hg, the Veress needle is replaced with a 10mm trocar for the camera just above and to the right of the umbilicus. Some surgeons choose the umbilical

Types of Laparoscopic Sphincter saving procedures

Lap High Anterior Resection	Anastomosis above the peritoneal reflection
Lap Low Anterior Resection	Anastomosis below the peritoneal reflux
Lap Ultra Low Anterior Resection	Anastomosis within 2cm of dentate line
Lap Coloanal anastomosis	Anastomosis at or below the level of dentate line

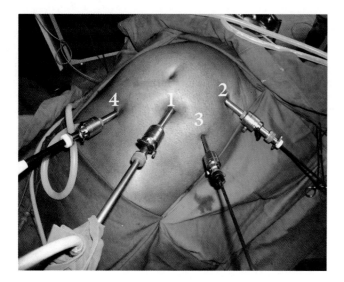

Figure 2 : Port position

No.	Instruments	Place	
1	Camera	Supraumbilicus, right of midline	10mm
2	Right hand working port	Right iliac fossa	10 mm
3	Left hand working port	Right lumbar	5mm
4	Colon retracting port	Left lumbar	10mm

or infraumbilical position for placement of camera. But we feel that right laterally placed camera port greatly facilitates medial to lateral dissection and gives an unobstructed view during the mobilization of mesorectum. The camera at infraumbilical or umbilical position might be obstructed by a bulky tumor that fills the narrow pelvis.

The remaining trocars two 10mm, two 5mm are placed under visual guidance, taking care to avoid injury to the inferior epigastric vessels. The right hand working trocar is placed to allow easy transection of rectum with linear endostapler.

Technique

Exploration of Peritoneal cavity

The peritoneal cavity is thoroughly assessed for distant metastasis on the liver, peritoneal surface and small bowel. Assessment of the pelvis follows upper abdomen and adhesions if any due to previous surgeries are lysed.

Division of Inferior mesenteric pedicle

The left side of the patient is raised up to allow the small bowel to fall out of the pelvis. The critical angle of Trendelenburgh beyond which the small bowel falls out of pelvis varies from person to person. The apex of the sigmoid is held up and to left by the

second assistant positioned near the left shoulder of the patient. The sacral promontory is identified and the peritoneum over it is incised on the medial aspect of the mesosigmoid. A window is made between the mesocolon over the inferior mesenteric artery and the Toldt's fascia. The left ureter and gonadal vessels are identified and carefully preserved during this part of the dissection.

Once the origin of inferior mesenteric pedicle is identified, the peritoneum over its anterior aspect is incised and the pedicle skeletonized. The incision is further extended over the pedicle and extended upto the level of duodenojejunal flexure. The inferior mesenteric artery and vein are dissected, preserving the sympathetic roots of dorsolumbar origin at the level of the sacral promontory. The dissection at this phase is usually done with the harmonic scalpel. The vessels are individually ligated and divided either by endostapling, intracorporeal suturing or bipolar coagulation. The inferior mesenteric artery is ligated after it gives off the left colic branch. Further cranial dissection is performed to identify the vein at the lower border of pancreas and is doubly clipped and divided. The IMV lies close to the ascending branch of the left colic artery. In 15-20% of the cases an accessory left colic artery is found at this region, care should be taken to prevent injury to the artery.

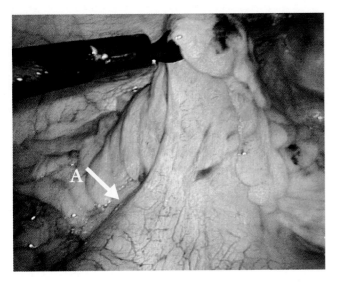

Figure 3 : Colon is lifted up by 10 mm babcock and inferior mesenteric pedicle is exposed

A - Inferior mesenteric pedicle

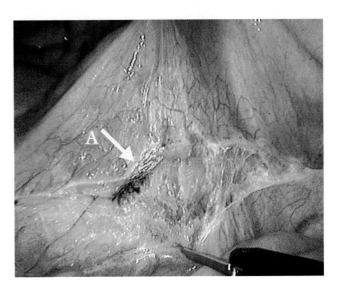

Figure 4 : Peritoneum is opened just right of the midline using harmonic scalpel

A - Peritoneal incision

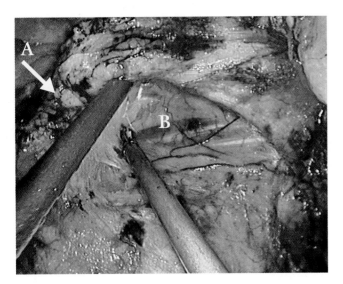

Figure 5 : Dissection carriedout behind the mesocolon and Toldt fascia (medial to lateral dissection)

A - Inferior mesenteric pedicle
B - Psoas muscle

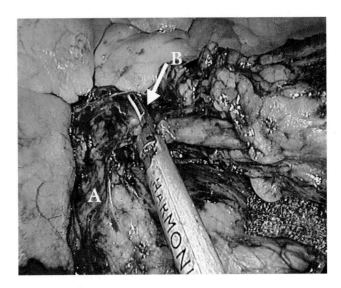

Figure 6 : Division of inferior mesenteric artery using Harmonic Ace

A - Aorta
B - Inferior mesenteric artery

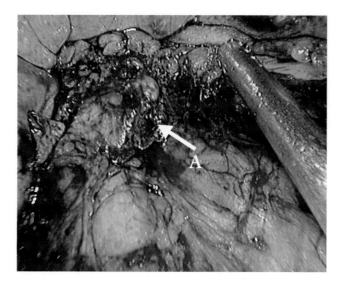

Figure 7 : Completion of inferior mesenteric artery division

A - Divided end of Inferior mesenteric artery

Mobilization of descending colon, splenic flexure and transverse colon

After ligation, the plane of dissection is continued from medial to lateral aspect, proceeding towards the lateral parietal wall between the mesocolon and Toldts fascia. This is aided by adequate traction of the mesentery from left lumbar port. Once exact plane is entered, the dissection is done in a tunneling fashion both cranially and caudally maintaining the lateral attachment of the colon to the parietal wall. The course of the gonadal vessels and the ureter is completely traced and preserved during this phase of dissection.

Extreme care must be taken in detaching the mesenteric attachment of the splenic flexure, because of the risk if injury to marginal vessels of left colon. Identification of the lower border of pancreas is the limit of the cranial dissection. Subsequently the lateral peritoneal attachment is incised from the sigmoid to the level of splenic flexure.

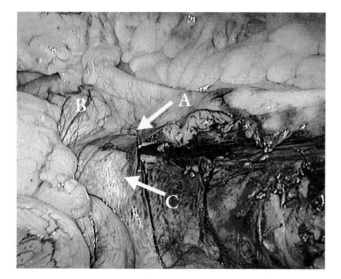

Figure 8 : Inferior mesenteric vein is dissected and clipped at the level of inferior border of pancreas

A - Clipped inferior mesenteric vein
B - Pancreas
C - Duodenojejunal flexure

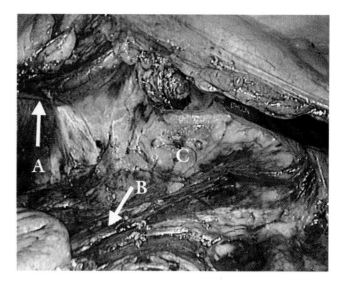

Figure 9 : Completion of medial to lateral dissection

A - Mesocolon is lifted by the hand instrument
B - Left ureter
C - Toldt fascia

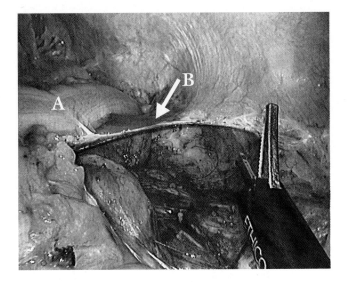

Figure 10 : Division of lateral attachment of desending colon

A - Descending colon
B - White line of Toldt

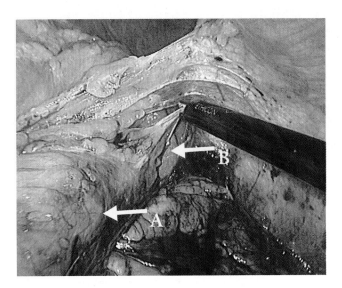

Figure 11 : Mobilization of splenic flexure of colon

A - Colon is pulled medially
B - Spleen

Splenic flexure and transverse colon Mobilization

The splenic flexure and the left colon should be mobilized in all cases of sphincter saving mesorectal excision, for tension free anastomosis. Division of the splenocolic and retro colic ligaments releases the splenic flexure. The gastrocolic portion of the greater omentum on its left end and the attachment of transverse mesocolon to the inferior border of pancreas are released separately. The marginal vessels of the colon are protected by keeping the level of division at inferior border of the pancreas. It is easy to perform the procedure by standing between the two legs using the left lower ports.

The descending colon, splenic flexure and the distal transverse colon are completely mobilized at the end of this phase. This helps to obtain a adequate length of proximal colonic segment for tension free anastomosis at the level of the pelvic floor.

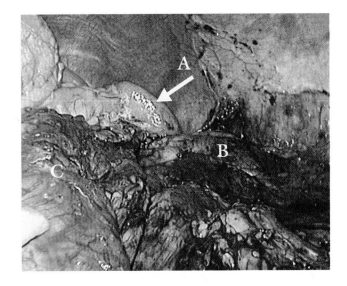

Figure 12 : Splenic flexure of colon is mobilized

A - Spleen
B - Left kidney
C - Splenic flexure of colon

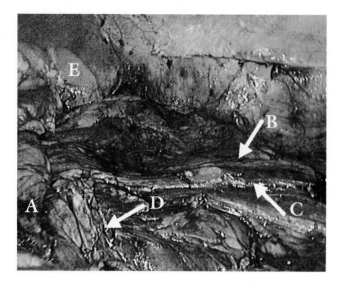

Figure 13 : Completion of colon mobilization

A - Desending colon
B - Left ureter
C - Left gonadal vessels
D - Divided end of inferior mesenteric artery
E - Spleen

Pelvic Dissection

It is during this phase the camera position at a point above and to the right of the umbilicus is highly appreciated. If the camera post is in umbilicus or subumbilical position, the mobilized rectum when lifted out of the pelvis completely obscures the field of vision. The role of the camera assistant during the pelvic dissection is very important. The 30 degree scope should be used to its maximum potential by adjusting the angle of the scope. This is very important when there is a bulky tumor with a large mesentery in a male patient as the mobilized rectum of the fills the whole of pelvis. The camera trocar at the right side of umbilicus helps in solving this problem.

Pelvic dissection starts with the identifications of the avascular plane of Heald. This is a potential space that lies between the parietal (presacral fascia) and visceral (fascia propria) layer of pelvic fascia which is of utmost importance in total mesorectal excision.

The peritoneum overlying the sacral promontory is incised and is continued distally along the right side of the rectum into the pelvis. The mesosigmoid is retracted to the left and the plane is entered by sharp dissection with harmonic scalpel. With the advanced imaging systems and magnification it is virtually impossible to miss this plane of dissection. At this point of dissection, the pelvic autonomic plexus (or superior hypogastric plexus), and the left and right hypogastric nerves emerge sagitally below the level of bifurcation of aorta. They divide below the prom-ontory as 'wishbone' and course distally to the semi-nal vesicles. Anterior traction on the rectum can tent the pelvic autonomic nerve plexus and help in its identification and preservation. The peritoneal inci-sion is made on the left side of the rectum and is continued distally into the pelvis. Both the incisions are joined down to the anterior reflections in a U shaped manner (retrovesical fold in males and retrovaginal fold in females).

Posterior mobilization

The posterior dissection is the continued down into the pelvis just above the fascia propria as low as pos-sible as this helps in subsequent lateral and anterior dissection. Multiple slips of thin fascia extend from the parietal fascia posteriorly into the visceral mesorectal fascia. These are the rectosacral fibres. These are divided at the level S4 to enter the pelvic floor which straightens the rectum from the sacrum curvature. The levators are now cleared on both sides. The division of midline rhape completes the poste-rior dissection. By this approach rectum is length-ened to 4-5cms.

Lateral mobilization

Laparoscopically, the most difficult of the dissection is the lateral and anterior mobilization (medial seg-ment of pelvic autonomic nerve plexus and its branches enter through the lateral ligament). This is composed of thickened pelvic fascia and these con-tain the middle rectal artery in between its layers. These ligaments are divided with harmonic scalpel not at is origin, but at its medial portion to preserve pelvic nerves.

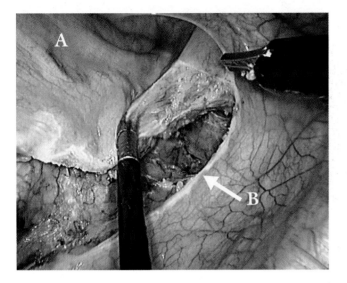

Figure 14 : Dissection of the rectum. Division of the peritoneum on the right side

A - Rectum
B - Peritoneal incision

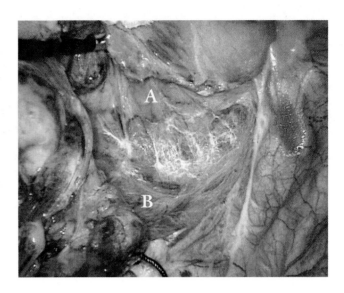

Figure 15 : Dissection carriedout posterior to the rectum in
the plane between the mesorectum and the presacral fascia
(Holy plane)

A - Mesorectum
B - Presacral fascia

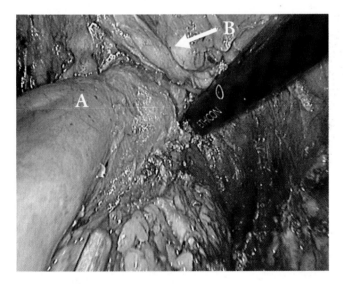

Figure 16 : Dissection of the rectum laterally on right side

A - Rectum
B - Seminal vesicle

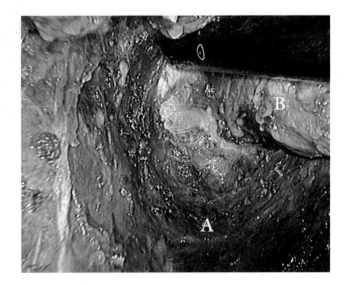

Figure 17 : Completion of posterior dissection

A - Presacral fascia
B - Mesorectum

Anterior mobilization

The dissection is started in the midline. The dissection is continued in front of the Denovillers fascia including it along with the mesorectum. The dissection is continued distally in this plane posterior to the prostatic capsule upto the pelvic floor.

The lower rectal dissection is made easier by the retraction of the rectum. The dissection is pursed by alternating lateral, anterior and posterior dissection down to the pelvic floor until circumferential mobilization of the bowel is accomplished. The longitudinal muscle of the rectum and the levator ani should be clearly visualized at the end of the dissection **(Denudation, Muscularisation)**. Denudation of the rectal tube result is removal of fat and fascia propria till the muscle of the rectum is seen.

After complete mobilization, distal limit of tumor and clearance below can be assessed by digital examination or proctoscopy. At the end of dissection, the entire mesorectum is excised upto the level of levator ani. The stapler has to be applied only after complete denudation. The entire dissection is performed under vision using sharp dissection technique and minimal application of low levels of electrocoagulation.

Distal Occlusion and Rectal Washout

The distal resection line, 2-5cm distal to the tumor is precisely identified using sigmoidoscopy. Once the distal resection line has been freed from the mesorectum, a right angle bowel clamp or stapler line is applied to occlude the lumen distal to the growth. A distal rectal washout is then given transanally with 4% povidone-iodine, to reduce the risk of implantation of exfoliated tumor cells.

Rectal Transection

The rectum is transected at a level just below the occluding stapler line with two or three applications of the 30 mm linear endostapler that has been passed through the right-lower-quadrant trocar as perpendicular to the bowel as possible. It is also important to keep the transection line as straight as possible when the multiple cartridges are applied. Endoflex endo GIA (roticulating staplers) is found to be highly beneficial in transecting the bowel in a straight line. At times the right iliac port may not help in a

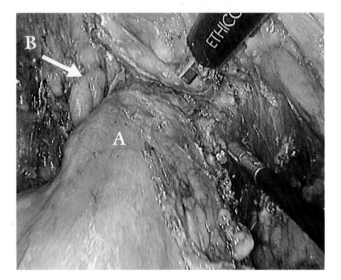

Figure 18 : Dissection of the rectum anteriorly

A - Rectum

B - Seminal vesicle

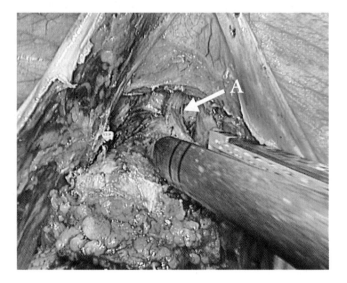

Figure19 : Division of the rectum using Endo GIA stapler. One stapler is fired and partially divided rectum is seen

A - Partially divided rectum

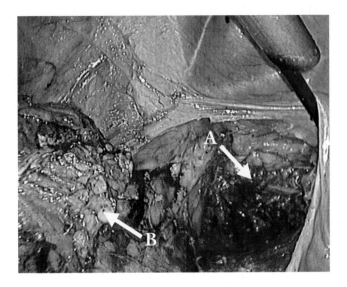

Figure 20 : Completion of rectal transection

A - Distal end
B - Proximal end of the rectum

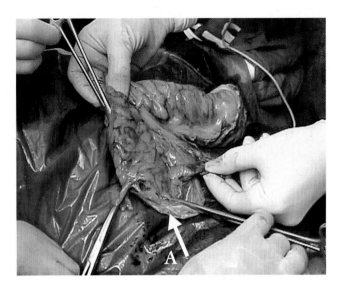

Figure 21 : Rectum and desending colon is brought out through the minilaparotomy

A - Wound protection sheet

perpendicular division of the rectum. An additional port at the suprapubic region for the stapler may solve this problem. In ultra low anterior resection assistant keeps his first on the perineum, to push the anal sphincter and levator ani into the pelvis to facilitate transaction at the level of anorectal ring

Some surgeons prefer a Pfannensteil incision and division of the rectum by a conventional linear stapler. More over the distal line of the tumor can be felt and the adequacy of distal margin can be verified also be verified at this juncture. The specimen is resected extracorporeally, abdomen closed and pneumoperitoneum recreated to complete the anastomosis.

Specimen Removal

The suprapubic port site is extended transversely (5 cm or more) depending on the size of the growth. The distal end of the bowel is brought outside the abdomen through a protective sheath, till the proposed level of transection of the bowel. The mesentery is divided and bowel transected keeping 5-6 cms of the bowel extending beyond the pubic symphysis, in order to avoid tension in the bowel after anastomosis, particularly in low rectal anastomosis.

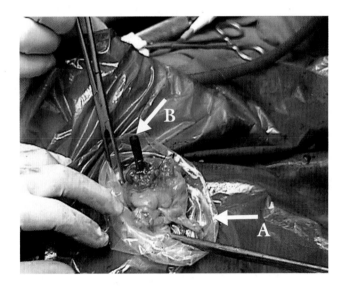

Figure 22 : After the resection, anvil of the circular stapler is inserted and purse string stitch is applied

A - Wound protection sheet
B - Anvil of the circular stapler

Site of Growth	Type of Anastomosis
> 2 cm proximal to dentate line	Low anterior resection
< 2 cm proximal to dentate line	Ultra low anterior resection
At or below dentate line	Colo anal anastomosis

Anastomosis

Reconstruction following mesorectal excision of cancers of the rectum is usually of 3 types, namely low anterior resection, ultra low anterior resection and coloanal anastomosis depending of the distal limit of the tumor. Tumors located more than 2 cm proximal to the dentate line is suited for low anterior resection, within 2 cm of dentate line for ultra low anterior resection and colo-anal anastomosis for growths located at or below the level of dentate line.

Low anterior resection

The anvil of a 31 or 33 mm circular stapler is placed in the proximal end of the divided colon, and purse string suture is applied with 2-0 prolene. The bowel along with the anvil is carefully replaced inside the abdomen without twisting its mesentery. The abdominal wound is closed 1-0 ethilon and the pneumoperitoneum is reestablished.

The shaft of the circular stapler is inserted transanally under laparoscopic guidance. A braided silk suture is threaded through the cap of the puncture cone of the shaft. The knob of the stapler is rotated in a clockwise direction, till the cap of the puncture cone protrudes through the divided rectal stump. A small enterotomy is made with scissors, hook or harmonic scalpel and the puncture cone along with the cap is pushed into the peritoneal cavity. The entry of the cone is adjusted so that it lies either on the anterior or posterior aspect of the rectal stump. The thread is pulled to safely dislodge the plastic cap form the puncture cone and is removed out. The point at which the puncture enters should be at centre of the occluding line, as too lateral displacement results in ischemia and leakage of anastomosis. For lower bulky tumors it is advisable to perform the dissection under intra anal finger guidance, to avoid accidental damage to other structures.

The full length of the shaft is pushed inside the peritoneal cavity by counter clock wise movement of the knob. 10mm or 5mm Allies forceps is used to manipulate the shaft to dock into the circular anvil. The anvil and the shaft are approximated and the stapler is fired to create a circular anastomosis. The knob is rotated clockwise to release the stapler and is carefully removed through the anus by gentle rotatory movements.

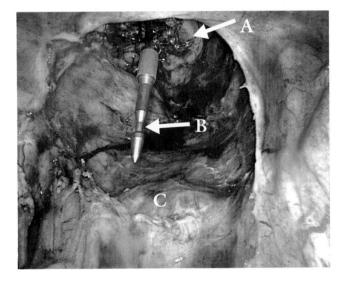

Figure 23 : Shaft of the circular stapler is inserted transanally and the cone is protrudes through the divided rectal stump

A - Rectal stump
B - Cone of the circular stapler
C - Sacral promontary

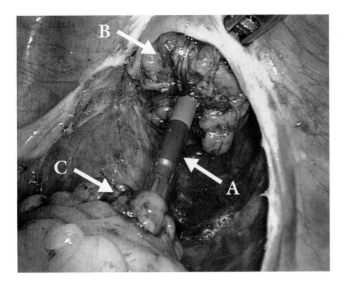

Figure 24 : Docking the anvil and shaft

A - Cone of the shaft is locked into the anvil

B - Distal rectal stump

C - Proximal end of colon

Ultra Low anterior resection

The dissection should reach the levator ani to achieve an adequate distal margin. Firm pressure on the perineum by the assistant on the perineal side pushes the anal sphincter and levator ani into the pelvis to facilitate transection at the level of anorectal ring. The anastomosis is performed in the same type as low anterior resection.

Coloanal anastomosis

By this technique the anastomosis is created on the anal verge with out disturbing the integrity of the sphincter. When the pelvis is very narrow and stapled resection near levator ani is not possible, rectal mucosectomy can be done and a true colo-anal anastomosis can be done through perineum. The specimen is removed through the anal verge.

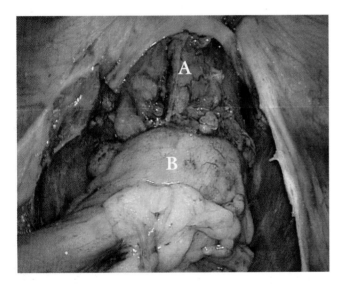

Figure 25 : Approximation of colon and rectum before firing

A - Rectal stump

B - Proximal colon

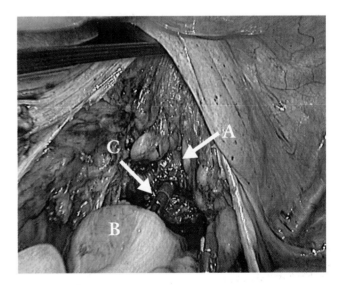

Figure 26 : Ultra low anterior resection. Approximation of distal rectal stump to the proximal colon

A - Rectal stump

B - Proximal colon

C - Anvil is locked with the cone of the shaft

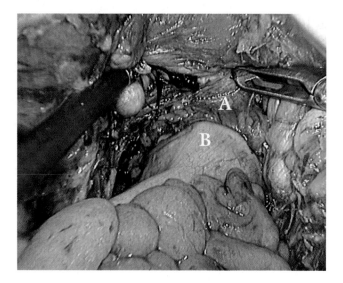

Figure 27 : Approximation and firing of the circular stapler

A - Rectal stump

B - Proximal colon

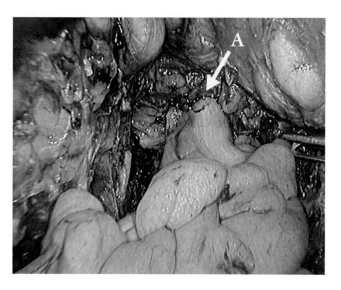

Figure 28 : Ultra low anastomosis of rectum and colon

A - Anastomotic line

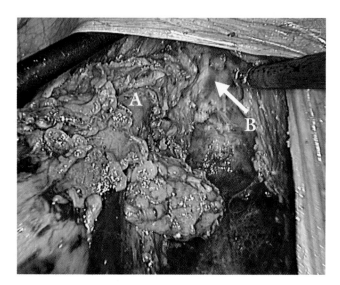

Figure 29 : Dissection of the rectum below the levator ani muscle for coloanal anastomosis

A - Rectum

B - Levator ani

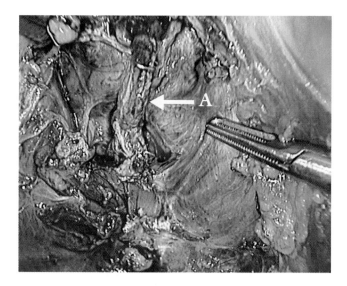

Figure 30 : Transection of the rectum using Endo GIA stapler(anus is pushed by the perineal surgeon and simultaneously rectum is pulled laparoscopically to get the ultra low level of the rectum before firing)

A - Rectal stump

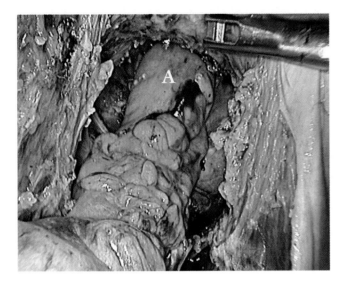

Figure 31 : Approximation and firing of the circular stapler. Completion of colo anal anastomosis

A   -   Colon

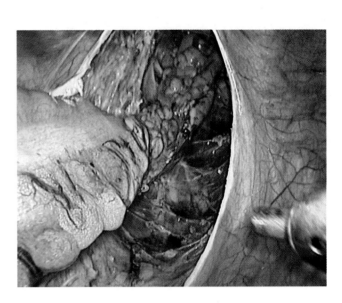

Figure 32 : Position of the colon after colo anal anastomosis

Assessment of anastomosis

Pelvis is filled with saline to submerge the anastomotic line and air insufflation of the rectum is performed with a proctoscope to test for leakage. During this maneuver the proximal colon is occluded with a clamp to prevent escape of air into proximal part of colon. The tissue donuts are checked for completeness and sent for hisotpathological analysis.

A 24 size drainage tube is placed through the right lateral port for drainage. At the completion of the procedure irrigation and a final examination of the peritoneal cavity is carried out to ensure hemostasis. The greater omentum is released from the transverse colon on its attachment to the right half of the transverse colon taking adequate care in protecting the blood vessels intact on its left and is used to fill the pelvic cavity. Apart from preventing adhesion of small bowel to the pelvic cavity, it also prevents urinary bladder getting folded especially in male patients. A diverting transverse colostomy is done if the anastomosis is in doubt. The presence of stoma does not obviate the development of leaks, but it does offer protection from their adverse consequences. Some surgeons routinely do contrast enema contrast in the post operative period to detect leaks, but we do not routinely do contrast studies.

MANAGEMENT OF RECTAL MALIGNANCIES WITH OBSTRUCTION

Obstructed rectal or rectosigmoid cancer with grossly dilated proximal loops may be treated by conventional resection techniques. Locally advanced rectal cancers with obstruction should undergo a preliminary diversion. Rectal resection should be considered at a lateral stage after chemo radiation. A stoma can be created by laparoscopic approach. Low sigmoid loop colostomy is preferred as it is away from the radiation field and is also amenable to be resected as part of low anterior resection. Distal loop ileostomy will not decompress the obstructed colon and transverse loop colostomy should not be performed as it may interfere with mobilization of the transverse colon and splenic flexure.

OUR EXPERIENCE

We have operated on 170 patients of rectal malignancy by laparoscopic anterior resection. 90 (52.94%) underwent high anterior resection, 52 (30.58 %) low anterior resection, 20 (11.76%) ultra low anterior resection and 8 (4.7 %) coloanal anastamsosis. There were no intraoperative complications or mortality. The mean operating time was 130 minutes (range 110-240 minutes), and the mean operative blood loss was 40 mL (range 5-60 mL). The mean hospital stay was 7 days (range 6-12 days). Two patients had developed a small anastamotic leak (demonstrated by gastrograffin study) which was managed by conservative measures. One patient developed blow out of the anastamosis and we had to do laparoscopic peritoneal toileting and decompression transverse colostomy. The anastamosis was repaired and colostomy closed in a staged manner at a later date. After this we changed our policy to perform a routine transverse colostomy in all our patients. After surgery, 2 patients had urinary retention and one had wound infection.

DISCUSSION

Surgical management of rectal cancer has undergone a significant change during the past two decades and a new concept of total mesorectal excision (TME), is now considered the golden standard for management of rectal cancer. Developed and popularized by Heald, 1 this technique has been reported with local recurrence rate at 5 and 10 years of 4% in curative cases and a 5-year tumor-free survival rate of 78%. Even though TME is a difficult and time-consuming procedure associated with a clinical leak rate in the range of 10% to 16% and a postoperative complication rate up to 50%, its optimal oncologic results make TME an acceptable risk for surgery of rectal cancer.

Like other diseases, various surgeries for malignancies of colon are being routinely performed. But laparoscopic surgeries for rectal carcinomas have not been commonly done. Factors like inadequate operative vision and limitation of the narrow pelvis, associated steep learning curve deter the routine use of laparoscopy in rectal cancer.[16] The area below the peritoneal reflection and 8 cm from anal verge is considered as a **blind zone** and the area within 5 cm as **forbidden zone**, because of the greater difficulty of dissection and leak rates following anastamosis. Due to these problems there are a very few published series about laparoscopic total mesorectal excision.[14,17-23]

Laparoscopic total mesorectal excision appears to be feasible in safe and has also been shown to achieve a level of cancer control comparable to open surgery with good quality of life. The various series have demonstrated that the laparoscopic mesorectal excision can be performed safely without defying the oncological principles. In a review of 100 laparoscopic TMEs for low and mid-rectal tumors, with distal limit on average 6.1 (range 3–12) cm from the anal verge. The conversion rate was 12% and the overall postoperative morbidity was 36%, including 17 anastomotic leaks with 100 % preservation of the sphincters. Studies like these confirm the safety of the procedure in the hands of experienced surgeons. In a study with long-term outcomes of laparoscopic total mesorectal excision, Leroy et al has shown 91.8 % curative resection with a 3% conversion rate. The overall morbidity, mortality and leak rates were 27%, 2% and 17 % respectively. The local recurrence rates (6%), cancer-specific survival of all curatively resected patients (75% at 5 years), overall survival rate (65% at 5 years) and a mean survival time was 6.23 years. The authors had concluded that laparoscopic TME is feasible and safe and did not jeopardize the safety in terms of long-term recurrence and survival.

A large number of multicentre prospective randomized trails on colorectal cancers have paved a way to allay the fears about the oncological safety of laparoscopic surgeries.[15] But most of these studies have excluded rectal cancers from their studies due to the higher level of technical skill that is required to perform these skills. As these procedures are still in the process of standardization, these are better done in highly specialized centers. In multicentre trials of outcomes are more dependants on the variable degrees of expertise of the operating surgeons rather than reflecting the efficacy of the technical approach itself. The optimum time for the multi institutional randomized trails would be after the standardization of the procedure.

	Leroy, J., 2004 [14]	Morino, M., 2003 [16]	Zhou , 2003 [17]	Bretagnol, F. [24]	Hartley, J. E. [22]	Tsang [18]	GEM
Patients	102	100	82	50	42	44	170
Conversion	3	12		6 pts	33	0	0
Morbidity	27	36		28			10
Mortality	2	2		2		0	0
Leak rate	17	17	1 pt				0
Trocar mets	0	1.4		0			0
Operative time (mts)		250 (110-540)	120 (110-120)		180 (168-218)	180*	130 (110-240)
Hospital Stay (days)		12.05(5-53)					7 (6-12)
Blood loss (ml)			20 (5-120)			80	40 (5-60)

* median

The anastomotic leak rate following laparoscopic mesorectal excision is around 16 -20%.[16,22] though the general morbidity is low. The risk factors associated with leakage are identified are male sex, obesity, anastomosis < 5cm from anal verge, surgery performed in emergency basis and undue tension in the staple lines. Stapling from right iliac fossa or suprapubic port results in an unduly long stapler line and this puts a longer segment of bowel at risk. The roticulating staplers can help to apply the stapler at right angle to the bowel, resulting a shorter stapler line and a potential reduction in the ischemic zone and thus reducing the leak rate. Other alternative is to perform colo anal hand sewn anastamosis through a suprapubic incision, which can also be used for specimen extraction.

The conversion rates vary from 3 - 33 % among the reported series. The morbidity of the procedure is around 25 - 30 % and has minimal mortality of around 2% in many of the series. The conversion rates, morbidity and leak rates are expected to fall with the combination of experience and optimization of the technique, technological advancements.

The histological assessments of laparoscopic TME resection specimens are encouraging and suggest that initial cancer clearance may be comparable to that which can be achieved using conventional methods with regards to oncologic safety.[22] The dissected retroperitoneal area that contacts directly with carbon dioxide is extensive in laparoscopic total mesorectal excision with anal sphincter preservation surgery. It is important to clarify whether the immune response in these patients is suppressed more severely than that of open surgery. In the study by Hu et al, there were no significant differences in the following factors (IL 6,IL 2, CD3+ and CD56+ T19).

Advantages of laparoscopic approach

1. Greater patient comfort and early return to work

2. Improved visualisation: Magnification and clarity offered by the recent imaging equipments enables surgical precision and dissection in an other wise difficult in the narrow pelvis where the surgeon has to struggle and most often proceed with the feel of tissues. It behave like a third eye of a surgeon

i. Identification and preservation of nerves plexus and branches

ii. Identification and entry of the holy plane of Heald

iii. Increased hemostasis due to minimally invasive sharp dissection.

3. Enhanced teaching ability: During conventional surgeries only the surgeon will be able to see the structures when compared to the ability to demonstrate the complete pelvic dissection to the entire team. The videos can be recorded and reviewed by the surgeon or in case of the resident it can allow the consultant to offer practical advice and help in standardization of the surgery and improve the outcomes.

Disadvantages:

1. Longer operative time

2. Lack of tactile feedback and 3 D resolution

3. Technical constraints in working in narrow pelvis

4. Long learning curve

5. Difficult assessment of distal limit of transection

CONCLUSION

Laparoscopic total mesorectal excision for tumors of middle and distal one third of rectum have proven to be feasible and safe in the hands of experienced laparoscopic colorectal surgeons and the long term results are comparable with the conventional TME (The current gold standard for rectal Ca). With the advancement in the technological front like better mechanical staplers (roticulating), robots and increased experience, both the short term (conversion & anastomotic leak) and long term results (survival and local recurrence) are likely to improve further.

Reference

1. MILES, E., A method of performing abdominoperineal excision for carcinoma of the rectum and the terminal portion of the pelvic colon. Lancet, 1908. 2: p. 1812-13.

2. Havenga, K., et al., Male and female sexual and urinary function after total mesorectal excision with autonomic nerve preservation for carcinoma of the rectum. J Am Coll Surg, 1996. 182(6): p. 495-502.

3. van Driel, M.F., et al., Female sexual functioning after radical surgical treatment of rectal and bladder cancer. Eur J Surg Oncol, 1993. 19(2): p. 183-7.

4. Petrelli, N.J., et al., Morbidity and mortality following abdominoperineal resection for rectal adenocarcinoma. Am Surg, 1993. 59(7): p. 400-4.

5. Kyzer S and G. PH., Experience with the use of the circular stapler in rectal surgery. Dis Colon Rectum, 1992. 35: p. 696 - 706.

6. Enker, W.E., Potency, cure, and local control in the operative treatment of rectal cancer. Arch Surg, 1992. 127(12): p. 1396-401; discussion 1402.

7. Aitken, R.J., Mesorectal excision for rectal cancer. Br J Surg, 1996. 83(2): p. 214-6.

8. Heald, R.J. and N.D. Karanjia, Results of radical surgery for rectal cancer. World J Surg, 1992. 16(5): p. 848-57.

9. Murty, M., W.E. Enker, and J. Martz, Current status of total mesorectal excision and autonomic nerve preservation in rectal cancer. Semin Surg Oncol, 2000. 19(4): p. 321-8.

10. Jones, T., .Complications of onestage abdominoperineal resection of the rectum. JAMA, 1942. 120: p. 104-7.

11. Enker, W.E., et al., Total mesorectal excision in the operative treatment of carcinoma of the rectum. J Am Coll Surg, 1995. 181(4): p. 335-46.

12. Masui, H., et al., Male sexual function after autonomic nerve-preserving operation for rectal cancer. Dis Colon Rectum, 1996. 39(10): p. 1140-5.

13. Sugihara, K., et al., Pelvic autonomic nerve preservation for patients with rectal carcinoma. Oncologic and functional outcome. Cancer, 1996. 78(9): p. 1871-80.

14. Leroy, J., et al., Laparoscopic total mesorectal excision (TME) for rectal cancer surgery: long-term outcomes. Surg Endosc, 2004. 18(2): p. 281-9.

15. A comparison of laparoscopically assisted and open colectomy for colon cancer. N Engl J Med, 2004. 350(20): p. 2050-9.

16. Morino, M., et al., Laparoscopic total mesorectal excision: a consecutive series of 100 patients. Ann Surg, 2003. 237(3): p. 335-42.

17. Zhou, Z.G., et al., Laparoscopic total mesorectal excision of low rectal cancer with preservation of anal sphincter: a report of 82 cases. World J Gastroenterol, 2003. 9(7): p. 1477-81.

18. Tsang, W.W., C.C. Chung, and M.K. Li, Prospective evaluation of laparoscopic total mesorectal excision with colonic J-pouch reconstruction for mid and low rectal cancers. Br J Surg, 2003. 90(7): p. 867-71.

19. Hu, J.K., et al., Comparative evaluation of immune response after laparoscopical and open total mesorectal excisions with anal sphincter preservation in patients with rectal cancer. World J Gastroenterol, 2003. 9(12): p. 2690-4.

20. Chung, C.C. and M.K. Li, Laparoscopic total mesorectal excision. Surg Endosc, 2003. 17(2): p. 356.

21. Pikarsky, A.J., et al., Laparoscopic total mesorectal excision. Surg Endosc, 2002. 16(4): p. 558-62.

22. Hartley, J.E., et al., Total mesorectal excision: assessment of the laparoscopic approach. Dis Colon Rectum, 2001. 44(3): p. 315-21.

23. Weiser, M.R. and J.W. Milsom, Laparoscopic total mesorectal excision with autonomic nerve preservation. Semin Surg Oncol, 2000. 19(4): p. 396-403.

24. Bretagnol, F., et al., Technical and oncological feasibility of laparoscopic total mesorectal excision with pouch coloanal anastomosis for rectal cancer. Colorectal Dis, 2003. 5(5): p. 451-3

25. Palanivelu C. Laparoscopic colorectal surgery In: Palanivelu C, ed. Text Book of Surgical Laparoscopy. Coimbatore: Gem Digestive Diseases Foundation, 2002:437-460

66

Laparoscopic Abdominoperineal Resection

INTRODUCTION

A new concept in the carcinogenesis of rectal cancer has developed recently, indicats that lymphatic spread of rectal carcinoma occur in three directions namely upward, lateral and downward. It was necessary to remove the entire rectum, anus, sphincters, most of the sigmoid colon, and the lymphatics. Until now many techniques have been described for the resection of rectal tumors which had high incidence of recurrence. The first Abdominoperineal resection was performed on these principles by West Ernest Miles in 1908. Even though the mortality of the procedure was initially high, improved long term survival of patients justified its use.

Since then, three major improvements in the operative technique has considerably reduced the morbidity and mortality and increased survival after surgical treatment. Stapling for low rectal anastomosis, the concept of Total Mesorectal Excision (TME) and the introduction of Minimal access approach.

The incidence of rectal cancers that are being treated with abdominoperineal resection is slowly coming down due to technical advancements and the availability of newer therapeutic options. The introduction of staplers have completely revolutionized colorectal surgery as it is now possible to attempt low and even ultra low anastomosis, even upto the levator ani. Rectal preservation has also been made possible with the advent of transanal microsurgery procedures. The routine abdominoperineal resection surgeries are now restricted to patients with invasive advanced tumor involving the anal sphincter and low rectal cancers.

The concept of total mesorectal excision for rectal tumors has shown improved 5 year survival rates from 45% to 70% and reduced local recurrences rates of 50-70% to 11-13%. The technique of resecting the rectum and mesorectum en-bloc using sharp dissection between the well defined planes of pelvic fascia permits identification and preservation of the pelvic autonomic nerve plexus that controls sexual and urinary function.

The third development is the minimal access approach in colorectal surgery. Because of concerns about the efficacy of laparoscopic resection of cancers, there has been less enthusiasm for laparoscopic approaches initially due to concerns about recurrence, port site metastasis and oncological safety. Now, laparoscopic abdominoperineal resection appears to be an ideal operation that maximizes the advantages of laparoscopic surgery without compromising the oncological principles. Laparoscopy offers excellent magnified view of the finer structures in the pelvis which is otherwise not visible during conventional surgery. This would greatly facilitate sharp dissection of the mesorectum and preservation of pelvic nerves during the dissection. Laparoscopic abdominoperineal resection(APR) is unique in the sense that it is totally laparoscopic as there is no need for a minilaparotomy incision to remove the specimen, as this is usually performed through the perineal route. The first laparoscopic APR was performed by Sackier et al in 1991.

Laparoscopic Abdominoperineal Resection: Who should do ?

Laparoscopic Abdominoperineal resection is a safe and effective procedure in the hands of surgeons experienced in laparoscopic colorectal surgery. The surgeon attempting this procedure should be adequately qualified and should have enough experience by assisting various lap. colorectal procedures.

LAPAROSCOPIC ABDOMINOPERINEAL RESECTION

The indications and patient selection are identical to that of open abdominal perineal resection. In majority of cases, the abdominoperineal resection is offered as a treatment for invasive lower rectal carcinomas where sphincter saving surgery is not an oncologically safe treatment. Although in a few selected cases this procedure is indicated for treatment of inflammatory bowel disease and diseases like severe radiation proctitis, anorectal malignancies, sarcomas of pelvic floor muscles. Tumor necrosis, perforation and obstruction are considered as absolute contraindications for laparoscopic approach.

Indications

1. Rectal cancers within 1 cm from the sphincter complex
2. Cancers limited to the rectum without infiltration into adjacent organs.

Contraindications

1. Cardio respiratory compromised patients.
2. Previous lower abdominal incision.
3. Locally advanced tumors.
4. Disseminated malignancies.
5. Grossly obese patients.

Selection of patients for laparoscopic APR is based on patient-related issues as well as tumor characteristics.

Patient-related issues

The patients with significant cardio respiratory compromise may not be able to withstand the effects of prolonged duration of pneumoperitoneum and its antecedent complications. The absorbed CO_2 in normal patients is washed off by the respiratory reserve function, which when defective might lead to respiratory acidosis and cardiac arrhythmias. The patients, who are obese, especially tend to have their fat around the viscera, which makes dissection cumbersome. Previous pelvic surgery evokes dense adhesions in the pelvis which preclude dissection in that area. Operating in males with bulky tumors is also difficult due to the narrow pelvis, and the more frequent infiltration around the seminal vesicles and prostate. It is advisable that the surgeons, who are attempting APR in their early laparoscopic career, refrain from selecting these types of cases.

Tumor characteristics

Tumors that invade pelvic sidewall, bladder, or uterus warrant open APR in most cases. However, invasion into the posterior vagina can be managed during the abdominal portion of the procedure and is not a contraindication for laparoscopic APR in our experience. Large bulky tumors that occlude the pelvic brim prevent adequate exposure of the posterior surface of the rectum.

Preoperative Preparation

All patients should be evaluated thoroughly before deciding to perform a laparoscopic abdomino-perineal resection to exclude synchronous tumors and metastatic disease. This always helps the surgeon to plan the procedure and minimize intra operative surprises, and maximizes the chance of a good outcome. Patients with doubtful local extension on preoperative imaging investigations might benefit from neo adjuvant therapy.

All patients should be evaluated by an enterostomal therapist if available or properly counseled about the permanent colostomy and its implications. The planned site of the stoma should be marked preoperatively and the patients should be educated well about the care of the stoma. Bowel preparation by mechanical bowel cleansers, deep vein thrombosis (DVT) prophylaxis and periopertive intravenous antibiotics are mandatory. We do not use oral antimicrobial prophylaxis in our department. The patients are catheterized and also a nasogastric tube is inserted before starting the procedure.

Operative technique

Patient Position

The patient is placed in semi lithotomy position with hip flexed for adequate exposure for perineal approach. The stirrups should be positioned such that the thighs are maintained semi flexed, (rather than flexion to 90 degrees) because flexed thighs obstruct the movement of laparoscope and instruments. The gravity should be fully utilized to retract the viscera out of the operating field by tilting the table accordingly. The presence of a hydraulic operating table that can be remotely operated is an added advantage. Alternatively, some surgeons use a bean bag to position the patient. The critical angle of Trendelenberg is usually 30-40 degree steep down

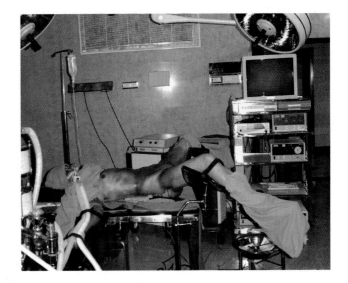

Figure 1 : Position of the patient. Lithotomy with trendelenberg position and sandbag below the hip. Laparoscopic trolley kept in the left foot end of the patient

and left side up (ie. the angle beyond which the small bowel fall out of the pelvis), but it might vary from patient to patient.

Theatre Set up

The surgeon stands on the right side of the patient and the camera assistant to the left of the operating surgeon, near the right shoulder of the patient. The second assistant usually stands near the left shoulder of the patient to retract the small bowel and rectum during various phases of dissection. The staff nurse stands on the right side of the patient, to the right of the operating surgeon. The entire laparoscopic dissection is performed in this setting and the surgeon moves to the left of the patient for fashioning of colostomy. The perineal resection may be performed by the same surgeon who moves to stand in between the legs of the patient after the division of colon. The monitor is placed near the left side of the foot end of the patient as shown in the figure. An optional second monitor at the head of the patient can also be used for added comfort.

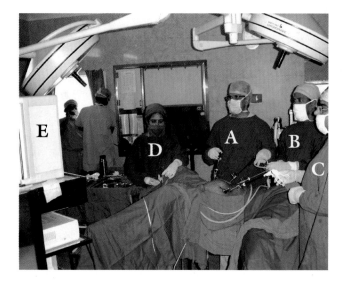

Figure 2 : Surgeon and camera surgeon stand on the right side of the patient.

A - Surgeon
B - Camera surgeon
C - Assistant surgeon
D - Staff nurse
E - Monitor

Position of Trocars

During draping care should be taken to drape the abdomen widely for placement of lateral trocars. The anus is closed with a double purse string suture to prevent the rectal fluid contaminating the perineum. The patient is placed in a Trendelenberg position and carbon dioxide pneumoperitoneum is established with a Veress needle placed through an incision that is to the right and above of the umbilicus. After insufflation of CO_2 to a pressure of 14-15mm Hg, the Veress needle is replaced with a 10mm trocar for the camera. We have gradually shifted the camera trocar from the umbilicus to the right lateral position to facilitate the medial to lateral approach, as the view from this position helps in complete visualization of the sigmoid colon, mesosigmoid, descending colon and the rectum without any hindrance. The other trocars are placed under vision to avoid any visceral injuries.

The right lower abdominal trocar should be placed as low as possible on the right iliac fossa (preferably 12mm for Endo GIA stapling). A 5 mm left hand working trocar is placed in the left lumbar region. The trocar on the left lumbar area can be positioned at the proposed site of colostomy. Fifth port (10mm) for colon retraction with Babcock is made as per the convenience of the surgeon, preferable in the left lumbar region.

After creation of the above mentioned ports a complete and thorough staging laparoscopy is done with attention to the extent of the tumor and its spread. The liver is examined for metastasis and if necessary laparoscopic USG can be done to exclude deeper lesions in the liver. A thorough assessment of the omentum, small bowel and large bowel is also made. Any suspicious nodule should be biopsied for confirmation.

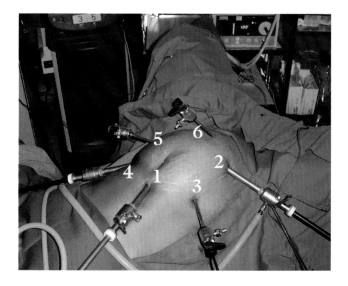

Figure 3 : Ports position

1 - Camera port 10mm
2 - Right hand working port 10mm
3 - Left hand working port 5mm
4 - Colon retracting port 10mm
5 - Left hand working port during rectal mobilisation 5 mm (placed at the level of colostomy site)
6 - Optional port for retraction of bladder 5mm

Steps of abdominoperineal resection

Phase I: Mobilisation of Sigmoid Colon

   i.   Control of inferior mesenteric pedicle.

      a) Endo Ligature Method
      b) Endo Stapling technique
      c) Clipping the vessels

   ii. Retroperitoneal dissection of sigmoid (medial to lateral dissection)

   iii. Division of lateral attachement of colon

Phase II: Mobilization of Rectum

   i.   Posterior mobilization of rectum

   ii. Division of lateral ligament.

   iii. Anterior Mobilization of the rectum.

Phase III : Division of Sigmoid Colon

Phase IV : Lateral mobilization of Omentum

Phase V : Perineal dissection and extirpation of specimen

Phase VI : Omentoplasty of pelvic cavity and formation of Terminal Colostomy

Phase I : Mobilisation of Sigmoid Colon

Any adhesions between the bowels and the pelvis should be carefully divided at this stage and the small bowel is retracted out of the pelvis. Apart from the position, retractors from the left lumbar port held by an assistant standing near the left shoulder of the patient also helps in retraction. In females, the uterus and adnexa should be elevated and fixed to the anterior abdominal wall. This is facilitated by a silk thread with needle inserted percutaneously that sutures the fundus of the uterus and is tied outside the body.

i. Control of inferior mesenteric pedicle.

The left side of the patient is raised while maintaining the Trendelenberg position. The apex of the sigmoid colon is retracted towards the abdominal wall by the assistant. Peritoneum is incised on the right of the aorta by harmonic scalpel, monopolar hook or scissor and extended caudally upto the sacral promontory. The dissection is continued cephalad towards the trunk of the inferior mesenteric artery, and its origin from the aorta. At the origin of the artery, the

pedicle is skeletonized by stripping the lympho fatty tissue. The dissection is continued beyond the origin of the left colic artery. The inferior mesenteric vein is dissected upto the inferior border of pancreas. The division of the inferior mesenteric artery and vein can be done by any of the three methods.

a) Endo Ligature Method

The more economical way of ligation of pedicle would be intracorporeal knotting with conventional non absorbable sutures. Though extracorporeal knotting has been described, intracorporeal ligation with a single thread is ideal, since many ligatures can be performed without increasing the operative time significantly. Extracorporeal knots are useful for surgeons who are not well experienced in intracorporeal suturing and knotting.

b) Endo Stapling / Clipping Technique

This can be also done by using Endo vascular stapler (25mm) through the right hand working lower port. Inferior mesenteric artery and later vein are divided close to its origin. This might not be a cost effective way of performing the operation in centers where the staplers are not freely available. Alternatively some surgeon prefers division of the artery with PDS Clips.

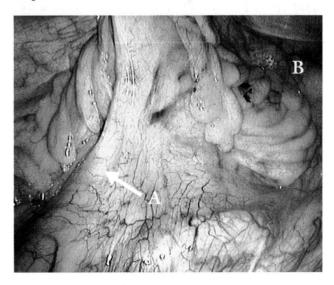

Figure 4 : Sigmoid colon is lifted up, inferior mesenteric pedicle is streched

A - Inferior mesenteric pedicle
B - Rectum

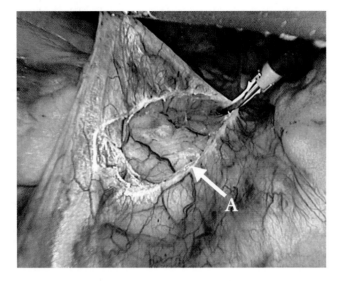

Figure 5 : Division of the peritoneum on the rigt side using 5mm harmonic scalpel

A - Peritoneal incision

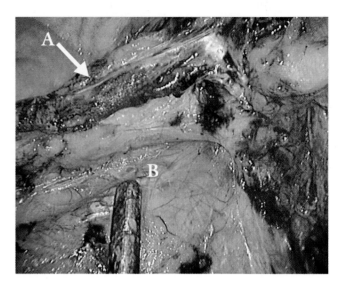

Figure 6 : Dissection behind the mesocolon from medial to lateral direction

A - Inferior mesenteric pedicle
B - iliac artery

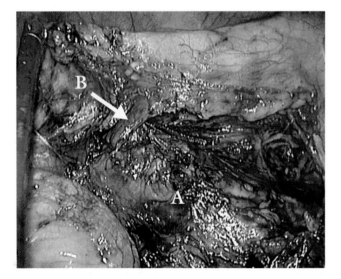

Figure 7 : Dissection of inferior mesenteric artery

A - Aorta
B - Inferior mesenteric artery(IMA)

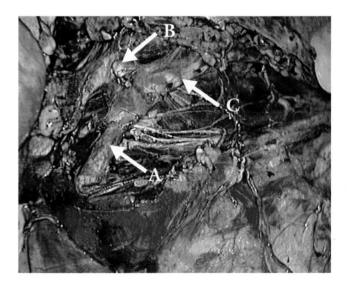

Figure 8 : Dissection of left colic artery

A - Inferior mesenteric artery
B - Left colic artery
C - Sigmoid branch of IMA

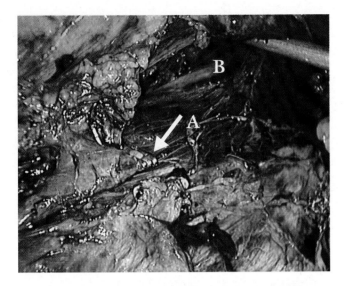

Figure 9 : Division of sigmoid branch of IMA after clipping

A - Divided end of sigmoid artery

B - Left ureter

approach). The left ureter, gonadal vessels and sympathetic branches of the pelvic autonomic nervous system are identified and swept posteriorly. Undue bleeding hampers the surgery as the light is absorbed by the red blood corpuscles resulting in a dark image. Dissecting too anteriorly can lead to creation of a plane within the mesentery of sigmoid and descending colon and this can result in troublesome bleed. Conversely, careless dissection posteriorly can lead to creation of a plane behind the ureter and some times even behind the kidney. Splenic flexure mobilization is not necessary. The mesocolon is divided up to the colonic edge of sigmoid colon at the proposed level of transection.

c) Vessel Sealant and Division

The recently available modified versions of bipolar; the bipolar vessel sealing system (Ligasure) can also be used for coagulation and division of inferior mesenteric artery and vein. These instruments can be safely used to coagulate vessels up to 7 mm in diameter and it has been estimated that the burst pressure that is required to open the seal formed by these instruments is more than 3 times the systolic blood pressure. Harmonic ACE, a new versatile 5mm instrument is highly effective in dissecting as well as dividing the inferior mesenteric artery and vein.

ii. Medial to Lateral Dissection

After division of the vascular pedicle the dissection proceeds in a medial to lateral fashion towards the lateral parietal wall. The tunnel that is created under the peritoneum is extended cranially and caudally. Identification of correct plane is the key to blood less dissection in this phase. The plane of dissection is developed posterior to the recto sigmoid in the retroperitoneum towards the left (medial to lateral

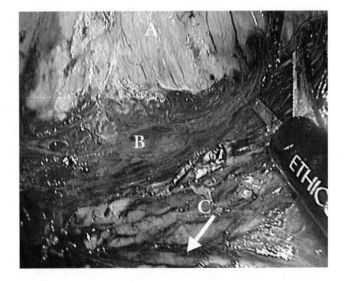

Figure 10 : Medial to lateral dissection in the plane between the mesocolon and Toldt fascia

A - Mesocolon

B - Toldt fascia

C - Left ureter

iii. Division of Lateral Attachement of Colon

After mobilization of the colon in a tunnelling fashion in a medial to lateral approach, the lateral peritoneal attachment of the colon is divided along the white line of Toldt upto the level of the splenic flexure.

Phase II: Mobilisation of Rectum

After mobilization of the sigmoid and the descending colon the next step is the dissection of the presacral space. The Babcock retractor is replaced at the upper part of rectum and is retracted cranially and anteriorly to expose the presacral space. The right iliac vessels and the right ureter are seen during this phase of dissection.

i. Dorsal mobilization of rectum

The peritoneum overlying the sacral promontory is incised and is continued distally along the right side of the rectum into the pelvis. With continuous traction from above, the areolar plane between the fascia propria of the mesorectum and the Waldeyer's fascia is identified and dissected with sharp dissection. Entry into this plane can be easily identified by the presence of areolar tissue. Further dissection is done with harmonic scalpel between the rectum and the sacrum, thereby lifting the rectum anteriorly. The dorsal fascial gap is opened up, down to the floor of the pelvis. The mesorectum is enveloped by the endopelvic fascia which prevents the invasion of rectal cancer. Adequate care should be taken to avoid breaches in this fascial covering. The rectosacral fascia is sharply divided to identify the levator ani. Finally the division of median raphe completes the posterior dissection. At this time the rectum appears attached to only to the levator ani. While transecting the Waldeyer's fascia care is taken not to injure the presacral vascular plexues.

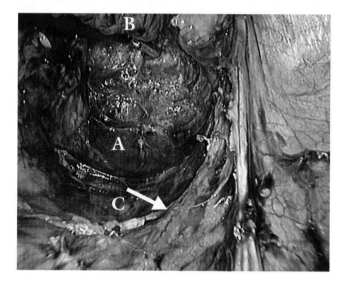

Figure 12 : Completion of posterior dissection

A - Presacral fascia
B - Mesorectum
C - Right hypogastric nerve

During completion of dissection the rectum is attached to the lateral wall of pelvis only by the peritoneum on the left side of the pelvis. The peritoneal incision is extended on the left side of the rectum and is continued distally into the pelvis and joined with the opposite side incision in a U shaped manner.

ii. Division of lateral ligaments

This stage marks the end of the rectal mobilization. The rectum and the meso rectum are retracted to

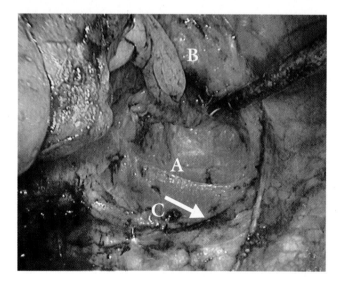

Figure 11 : Mobilisation of rectum posteriorly

A - Presacral fascia
B - Mesorectum
C - Right hypogastric nerve

the left for division of right lateral ligaments, and vise versa for division of the left lateral ligament. The rectum is completely mobilized circumferentially. Dissection with harmonic scalpel aids in blood less dissection in this phase. Nerves or vessels that directly enter the mesorectum are divided under direct vision. Great care must be exercised to avoid injury to either the mesorectum or the autonomic nerves.

dissection easier. At times the retraction of the bladder can be accomplished by a 5 mm port at the supra pubic region. The plane of the dissection should start in the recess of Denonviller's fascia in male and in the female through obliterated fascial gap dorsal to the vagina. The plane of dissection should proceed anterior to the Denovillers fascia. Dissection should be done up to the pelvic floor.

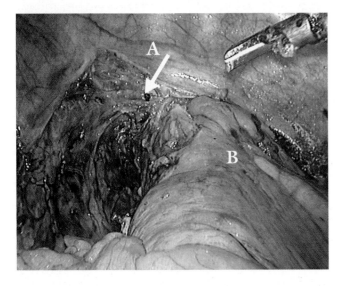

Figure 13 : Lateral mobilisation of rectum

A - Completion of lateral dissection on left side
B - Rectum

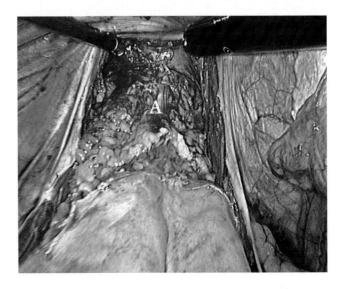

Figure 14 : Anterior dissection of rectum

A - Rectum

The aim of the dissection should be to remove intact rectum and mesorectum with a complete visceral fascial envelop (the fascia propria of the rectum). The autonomic nerves should be preserved at the end of the dissection.

iii. Anterior Mobilization of the rectum

The anterior mobilization of the rectum is more difficult than the posterior mobilization, especially in the males due to the presence of prostate and seminal vesicles. The rectum is pushed posteriorly to facilitate dissection in this area. In female patients intrauterine probe manipulation makes the anterior

Phase III: Division of Sigmoid Colon

Following mobilization of the rectum, the proximal colon is transected in preparation for the perineal dissection and ultimate delivery of the specimen. The remaining mesosigmoid is divided up to the proposed site of colostomy, which lies usually at the junction of descending and sigmoid colon. The site of the colostomy is identified laparoscopically by indenting the preoperatively marked stoma site from outside. The stapled end of the colon is grasped with a grasper and elevated to the stoma site to verify the mobility of the colon. If the colon is under tension, the ligamentous attachments that tether the colon

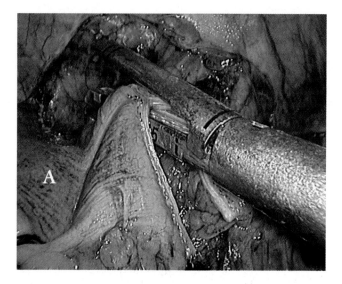

Figure 15 : Sigmoid colon is divided using Endo GIA stapler
A - Proximal end of sigmoid colon

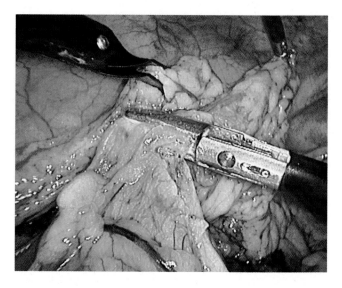

Figure 16 : Greater omentum is mobilized from the transverse colon to fill up the pelvic cavity

should be divided. If necessary, some of the sigmoid mesenteric vessels can also be divided to ensure a tension-free colostomy.

Phase IV: Lateral Mobilization of Omentum

The greater omentum is mobilized from the transverse colon starting from the right towards midline, taking adequate care in preserving its blood supply. This is used to fill the pelvic cavity at the end of surgery. If the blood supply to the omentum is accidentally divided then it is better to remove the omentum rather than risking postoperative necrosis of the devitalized omentum.

Phase V: Perineal Dissection and Extirpation of the Rectum

Pneumoperitoneum is deflated, keeping the ports in place to check for bleeding in the pelvis and to fill the pelvic cavity with the mobilized greater omentum after the completion of perineal procedure. The peritoneal portion of the operation is the same as in conventional procedure. A circumferential perineal skin incision is made. The dissection is advanced through the subcutaneous tissues and ischiorectal

fossa to the levators. The coccyx is identified and the anococcygeal ligament is divided. With entry into the presacral space, a finger is inserted deep to the levator muscles and divided circumferentially over the finger with electrocautery. The anterior pelvic floor structures are then divided beginning with the superficial transverse perineal muscle. The plane anterior to the rectum is bluntly dissected, and the anterior dissection is completed after division of the rectourethralis and puborectalis muscles. The surgeon can then slide the hand around to the anterior rectal plane from the left and right sides, bluntly dissecting any remaining attachments and completing the circumferential dissection. The specimen is then removed via the perineal wound. With increasing clinical experience, laparoscopic mobilization of the rectum can be carried out as far as the pelvic floor, so that only the levator ani on either side of the rectum needs to be divided stepwise before removal of specimen. Perineal wound is closed in layers using thick chromic catgut after approximating the levator ani on both sides, anterior to coccyx. The ischiorectal fat is also closed with interrupted stitches. No drainage is necessary at the perineum.

Phase VI: Omentoplasty of Pelvic cavity and formation of Terminal Colostomy

The pneumoperitoneum is recreated and the pelvic cavity is thoroughly rinsed with saline and checked for hemostasis. The mobilized greater omentum is brought down to the pelvic cavity medial to the descending colon and the colostomy and placed in the pelvic cavity. Filling up the pelvic cavity has three important advantages. It prevents fluid collection and minimizes the chance of infection. Following APR the residual urine tends to be accumulate more particularly in the aged people. Omentum reduces the chance of residual urine. Small bowel adhesion to the pelvic diaphragm is known occur following repair of the levator ani. Omental filling prevents small bowel adhesion to the pelvis. A final examination of the colon is made to ensure that there is no tension and the colon is not twisted at the site of colostomy. A closed tube drain is placed to the pelvic cavity through the right lower part and trocars are removed.

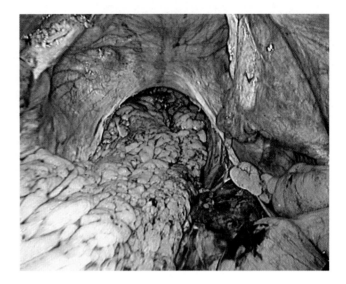

Figure 18 : Pelvic cavity is filled with omentum

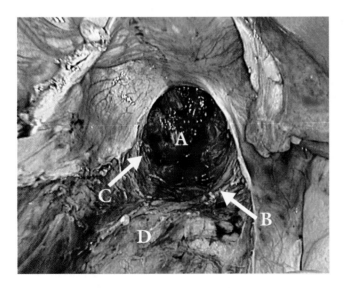

Figure 17 : Rectum and anal canal is excised, pelvic cavity is inspected for hemostasis

A - Pelvic cavity
B - Right hypogastric nerve
C - Left hypogastric nerve
D - Sacral promontary

The terminal colostomy can be performed either by staplers or extracorporeal division. In the first method, the colon is divided with 45mm Endo GIA Staplers (blue cartridege) through the 12 mm right lower quadrent working port. Subsequently the left lumbar port is enlarged to 20mm and the proximal colon is brought out through the incision with Babcock forceps and the terminal colostomy is fashioned in the usual way. Endo GIA stapler is highly useful for preventing intra peritoneal contamination. The same can be performed in a cost effective way without the use of staplers. The colon is brought out as a loop through the enlarged incision on the left lumbar port and divided extracorporeally. The distal colon is closed and replaced inside the abdomen. After the completion of perineal procedure, the terminal colostomy is fashioned with proximal colon.

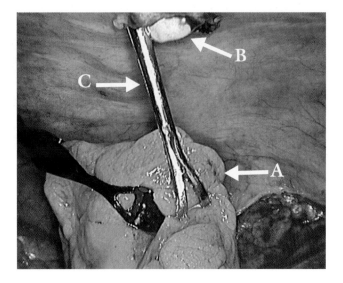

Figure 19 : Proximal end of colon is held by the babcock after the resection which is brought out for end colostomy

A - Proximal end of colon
B - Colostomy site (tip of finger is seen)
C - Conventional babcock is used to take the colon out

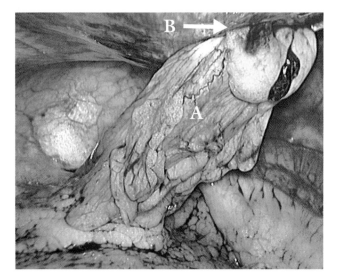

Figure 20 : Laparocopic view of the colon after end colostomy

A - Descending colon
B - Colostomy site

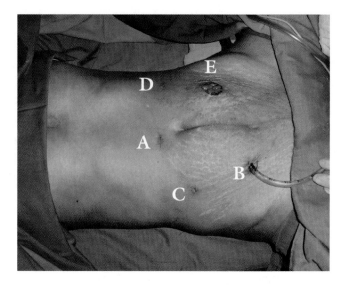

Figure 21 : Position ports and colostomy site after the completion of laparoscopic abdominoperineal resection

A - Camera port
B - Right hand working port
C - Left hand working port
D - Colon retracting port
E - Left hand working port is converted to colostomy site

OUR EXPERIENCE

Between 1992 and June 2005, a total of 145 patients underwent laparoscopic AP resection for adenocarcinoma of the rectum (except 1 who had melanoma of rectum). There were 108 men and 37 women with a mean age of 60.3 years (range 40 to 69). There was conversion in 4 patients due to infiltration near the prostate and seminal vesicle. Mean operative time was 70 minutes (range 60-110) and the mean blood loss was 40 ml. The mean post operative hospital stay was 5 (Range 4-10) and the mean day of return to normal work was 10 days. The movement of the bowels was noticed in a mean duration of 2 days and the oral intake was started in second postoperative day. There was no intra operative or peri operative mortality in any of our patients.

DISCUSSION

The number of patients undergoing abdominoperineal resection has considerably come down due to factors such as the improvement of surgical techniques resulting from development of mechanical suture devices, better knowledge about dissemination of rectal cancers and more recently, due to neoadjuvant treatment through chemo and radiotherapy. These advancements have lead to substantial increase in sphincter preserving surgeries and lesser number of abdominoperineal resections. However, abdominoperineal resection (APR), is still the choice operation for cancers which are very distally located in the rectum, especially when infiltrating anorectal ring and sphincteric system.

Laparoscopic surgery is more frequently applied in the field of colorectal surgery both in benign and malignant diseases. Increasing evidence concerning benefits originated from laparoscopic colorectal surgery such as less morbidity and pain, earlier recovery of bowel function, shorter hospital stay, and early return to work have virtually consolidated this approach. Doubts such as the cost-effectiveness and other factors like port site recurrences, steep learning curve, and our inability to find adequate animal models to practice; larger occurrence of complications during initial experience, concern about oncological safety and the adequacy of resection were present in the early days of laparoscopic colorectal surgery. These were considered as the main barrier to the application of laparoscopic approach for radical surgical treatment of colorectal cancer.

In spite for all these concerns, APR represents the ideal surgery to be performed by laparoscopic approach. The following factors are in favor of laparoscopic approach to rectal cancers. The concerns about port site recurrence are not a problem here as the location of the tumor is well below the peritoneal reflection and the tumor manipulation occurs only during the perineal phase. Moreover there is no need for abdominal incision to remove the surgical specimen as this also minimizes the chances of wound recurrence and also easy to handle the colostomy bags. The complexity of the surgery is also less, as there is no anastomosis to be performed. Due to these factors, several authors have suggested that the laparoscopic abdominoperineal resection for rectal cancer can be considered as a safe and effective treatment option.

Decanini et al in a study performed in fresh corpses, demonstrated laparoscopic abdominoperineal resec-

tion can be performed according to oncological principles with proximal vascular ligation of inferior mesenteric artery, wide clearance of pelvic side walls, and complete removal of mesorectum.[1] It has been consistently demonstrated that Laparoscopic APR represents feasible and safe operation with benefits already observed by several authors.[2-9]

Since the status of resected lymph nodes is related to prognosis after curative colorectal cancer surgery, it is not a surprise that this aspect constitutes an endpoint of critical evaluation. With respect to APR, several clinical trials involving a larger number of patients demonstrated similarity in the extent of lymphadenectomy provided by the lap APR and conventional APR [7, 10-15].

In the only available randomized study to evaluate the safety and efficacy of lap APR compared to open APR for rectal cancer after chemoradiation by Araujo et al in 28 patients (13 lap, 15 conventional surgery) there was no significant difference in complications, need for blood transfusion, hospital stay, length of resected segment and pathological staging. Mean operation time was 228 minutes for lap APR versus 284 minutes for conventional approach. After a mean follow-up of 47.2 months, local recurrence was observed in two patients in the conventional group and in none in the lap group. They concluded that lap APR was feasible, similar to conventional approach concerning surgery duration, intra operative morbidity, blood requirements and post operative morbidity.[2]

Laparoscopic abdominoperineal resection for cancers does not compromise cancer-specific survival outcomes in the long term. In a retrospective review of 89 patients who underwent APR (28 lap, 61 open) there was no difference in mean length of overall survival (open = 30.3 months; laparoscopic = 40.8 months), recurrence rates or in the disease-free survival. There was no difference in the number of lymph nodes harvested from the resected specimens, and the distance to lateral margins or involvement of tumor in the lateral margins between the two groups.[4]

A multi institutional study of the laparoscopic Colorectal Surgery Study Group (2000), involving a total of 18 institutions in Germany and Austria concluded that laparoscopic APR was oncologically safe and offered considerable benefits to the patients in early post operative period.[6] The subsequent results from the same group in 2002, showed an overall survival rate of 86.6%, with 62.4% disease-free survival for APR (mean follow-up of 24.8 months).[3]

CONCLUSION

Laparoscopic abdominoperineal resection is technically possible and safe surgery for anorectal malignancies.[16] The excellent view of the pelvic structures provided by advanced imaging systems, the advanced electrosurgical dissection devices like harmonic scalpel and ligasure help the surgeon to achieve an oncologically adequate resection. With the growing evidence, laparoscopic abdominoperineal resection will be more commonly embraced by the surgeon's world over when compared to conventional methods.

Reference

1. Decanini, C., et al., Laparoscopic oncologic abdominoperineal resection. Dis Colon Rectum, 1994. 37(6): p. 552-8.

2. Araujo, S.E., et al., Conventional approach x laparoscopic abdominoperineal resection for rectal cancer treatment after neoadjuvant chemoradiation: results of a prospective randomized trial. Rev Hosp Clin Fac Med Sao Paulo, 2003. 58(3): p. 133-40.

3. Scheidbach, H., et al., Laparoscopic abdominoperineal resection and anterior resection with curative intent for carcinoma of the rectum. Surg Endosc, 2002. 16(1): p. 7-13.

4. Baker, R.P., et al., Does laparoscopic abdominoperineal resection of the rectum compromise long-term survival? Dis Colon Rectum, 2002. 45(11): p. 1481-5.

5. Leung, K.L., et al., Laparoscopic-assisted abdominoperineal resection for low rectal adenocarcinoma. Surg Endosc, 2000. 14(1): p. 67-70.

6. Kockerling, F., et al., Laparoscopic abdominoperineal resection: early postoperative results of a prospective study involving 116 patients. The Laparoscopic Colorectal Surgery Study Group. Dis Colon Rectum, 2000. 43(11): p. 1503-11.

7. Fleshman, J.W., et al., Laparoscopic vs. open abdominoperineal resection for cancer. Dis Colon Rectum, 1999. 42(7): p. 930-9.

8. Sousa Junior, A.H., et al., [Laparoscopic abdominoperineal resection of rectum. Analysis of 18 cases]. Rev Hosp Clin Fac Med Sao Paulo, 1998. 53(5): p. 242-8.

9. Mehigan, B.J. and J.R. Monson, Laparoscopic rectal-abdominoperineal resection. Surg Oncol Clin N Am, 2001. 10(3): p. 611-23.

10. Darzi, A., et al., Laparoscopic abdominoperineal excision of the rectum. Surg Endosc, 1995. 9(4): p. 414-7.

11. Chindasub, S., et al., Laparoscopic abdominoperineal resection. J Laparoendosc Surg, 1994. 4(1): p. 17-21.

12. Ramos, J.R., et al., Abdominoperineal resection: laparoscopic versus conventional. Surg Laparosc Endosc, 1997. 7(2): p. 148-52.

13. Seow-Choen, F., et al., A preliminary comparison of a consecutive series of open versus laparoscopic abdominoperineal resection for rectal adenocarcinoma. Int J Colorectal Dis, 1997. 12(2): p. 88-90.

14. Larach, S.W., et al., Laparoscopic assisted abdominoperineal resection. Surg Laparosc Endosc, 1993. 3(2): p. 115-8.

15. Wu, J.S., E.H. Birnbaum, and J.W. Fleshman, Early experience with laparoscopic abdominoperineal resection. Surg Endosc, 1997. 11(5): p. 449-55

16. Palanivelu C. Laparoscopic colorectal surgery In: Palanivelu C, ed. Text Book of Surgical Laparoscopy. Coimbatore: Gem Digestive Diseases Foundation, 2002:437-460

67

Laparoscopic Management of Rectal Prolapse

INTRODUCTION

The complete rectal prolapse or procidentia indicates a full thickness eversion of the rectal wall through the anal canal. It is a distressing condition that has long fascinated surgeons as evidenced by the multitude of proposed operative approaches for its correction.

HISTORY

The earliest clinical case of rectal prolapse was identified in a male mummy from Antinoe, Egypt (400 to 500 BC). Hippocrates recognized rectal prolapse as a clinical disorder and described several treatments. Vesalius (1514 to 1564) Dehumani Corpus, published in 1543, meticulously describes colorectal and anal anatomy, including the levator ani and anal sphincter. Renaissance surgeons well able to construct etiologic theories of rectal prolapse based on these noval anatomic concepts. Morgagni (1682 to

1771) attributed rectal prolapse to a laxity of rectal suspensory ligaments and was the first to suggest rectal intussusception. Von Haller demonstrated the first experimental model of rectal prolapse. John Hunter (1728 to 1793) was the first to differentiate between the intussusception and procidentia. In the early twentieth century, Moschwitz observed deep rectovaginal or rectovesical cul de sac in prolapse patients and advocated a sliding hernia theory.

As surgeons understanding of pelvic floor colorectal and anal anatomy improved, so did the operative procedures devised to treat rectal prolapse. Twentieth century surgeons have described an array of surgical procedures aimed at correcting the anatomic defects associated with rectal prolapse. More than 100 operations have been described to correct these pathologic anatomies. The approaches for these procedures are usually transabdominal or transperineal. Perineal procedures which are usually preserved for elderly high risk patients, produce higher recurrence rate than transabdominal procedures as well as inferior functional results.

Several abdominal procedures have been readily adapted to a laparoscopic approach. This approach leads to decreased morbidity, fewer pulmonary complications, earlier return to a normal diet and earlier discharge. Patients who must undergo transabdominal operations for the treatment of rectal prolapse are ideal candidates for the application of laparoscopic surgery. Conventional transabdominal rectopexy and rectopexy with sigmoid resection are currently the most common surgical procedures for rectal prolapse. Since its introduction in 1992, laparoscopic rectopexy with posterior mesh fixation has gained popularity because it is simple and easily accomplished. The feasibility of laparoscopic rectopexy with posterior mesh fixation and laparoscopic assisted resection rectopexy is well established. Only a few large series have included data on the functional results and changes in symptoms after surgery.

TYPES OF RECTAL PROLAPSE

The complete rectal prolapse must be distinguished from other types of prolapse prior to the consideration of surgical intervention.

1. Mucosal Prolapse

Mucosal prolapse is an abnormal descent of the rectal mucosa. This results in partial thickness prolapse in which only the mucosa and submucosal protrudes through the anal canal. Prolapsing internal haemorrhoids also is included in this category. It is characterized by radial or linear folds of mucosa and absence of perineal sulcus.

2. Internal Prolapse (Intussusception)

Also known as occult rectal prolapse, is an incomplete rectal prolapse, that does not prodtrude through the anal canal.

3. Complete Rectal Prolapse (procidentia)

Complete rectal prolapse is characterized by concentric rings of mucosa, and a sulcus is palpable between the protruding mucosa and perianal skin.

ETIOLOGY AND PATHOGENESIS

Complete rectal prolapse is more frequent in children before the development of the normal toddler's lordosis and the acquisition of a normal anorectal angle. Spontaneous resolution is the rule when these children become ambulant. In the elderly population excessive straining at stool appears to be the most common cause. The Male : Female incidence ratio was 1:6 in Western literature, which does not correlate to the Indian scenario of 1:1. In our study group there were more male than females. The age group varies, though it is rare in men older than 45 years and in women younger than 20 years. A high percentage of younger patients have neurologic or mental disorders. The other conditions associated with procidentia includes pelvic neuropathies such as tabes dorsalis, multiple sclerosis and pelvic trauma.

Differntial diagnosis of Rectal Mucosal Prolapse and Procidentia

Type	Rectal Mucosal Prolapse	Procidentia
Size	< 5 cm	> 5 cm
Bowel lumen	Central	Posterior
Folds	Radial	Circular
Haemorroids	Readily visible	Not visible
Thickness	Only mucosa	All layers
Sphincter tone	Maintained	Diminished

Various Types of Rectal Prolapse

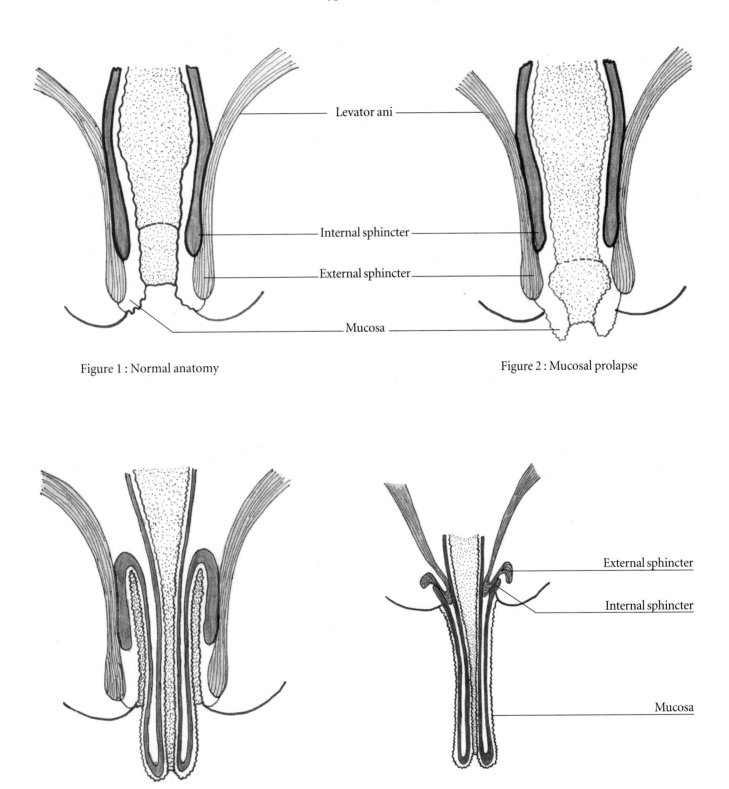

Figure 1 : Normal anatomy

Figure 2 : Mucosal prolapse

Levator ani

Internal sphincter

External sphincter

Mucosa

External sphincter

Internal sphincter

Mucosa

Figure 3 : Intussusception of the rectum through the anus

Figure 4 : Eversion of the rectal wall

The anatomic features associated with rectal prolapse include abnormally low descent of the peritoneum covering the anterior rectal wall, loss of posterior fixation of the rectum to the sacral curve, lengthening and downward displacement of the sigmoid and rectum, diastasis of the levator ani and an incompetent anal sphincter mechanism.

Circumferential intussusception is the precursor for complete rectal prolapse. This was confirmed by Theurkalf and colleagues with the help of cinedefecography.

Porter demonstrated that a non relaxing puborectalis muscle may have a role in the development of rectal prolapse by causing severe constipation and excessive straining at stool.

CLINICAL FEATURES

The most common symptom is the protruding mass itself. The prolapse may occur spontaneously or during defecation, coughing or walking. If the history suggests a rectal prolapse but the prolapse can not be seen on examination, then the patient should be asked to sit on the toilet and strain, and visual or digital examination of the patient's rectum can confirm the diagnosis. Other complaints includes tenesmus and mucosal discharge and bleeding from the protruding rectal mucosa. The majority of patients have difficulty in managing their bowels and complain of constipation, incontinence or both. Occasionally some patients presents with incarceration of the prolapsed rectum.

Complications of procidentia

1. Fecal incontinence
2. Constipation
3. Ulceration
4. Bleeding
5. Strangulation
6. Gangrene
7. Rupture with evisceration

INVESTIGATIONS

A complete clinical history should include the duration of symptoms, the presence or absence of fecal incontinence, constipation and any co-morbid diseases or risk factors. Physical examination should include digital examination to verify the presence of complete rectal prolapse.

All the patients should undergo colonoscopy or double contrast barium enema to rule out concomitant malignancy.

Anorectal manometry, pudental nerve terminal motor laterncy studies, and videodefecography may be useful in patients with incontinence and may assist the surgeon in selection of the surgical procedure. Similarly, colonic transit studies should be considered in patients with constipation. In addition, anorectal manometry can exclude outlet obstruction in constipated patients.

Currently no absolute criteria exist for choosing the best procedure to use for any given patient with rectal prolapse. The results obtained from studies using these expensive assessments do not provide evidence that the outcome is superior. Actually, Boccasanta[11,12,13] found that the statistically significant improvement in anal pressures post operatively was of no clinical significance in terms of symptoms resolution.

PATIENT SELECTION

The aims of surgical treatment of prolapse are to eradicate the external prolapsing of the rectum. More than 100 abdominal and perineal operations have been described for the surgical treatment of rectal prolapse, which suggests that no operation has yielded completely satisfactory results.

Optimally the goal should be to restore anatomic configuration and improve the functional outcome. The selection of appropriate procedure must be made after evaluating several patient factors. The patient age, gender, comorbid conditions, bowel function and degree of continence which can significantly affect the operative course and post operative results. These factors must therefore be considered before planning surgical intervention.

Abdominal procedures include pelvic floor repair, sacral fixation of the rectum and resection of the sigmoid colon and rectum with or without rectosacral fixation. All of the most popular traditional abdominal operations for repair of rectal prolapse have been adapted for laparoscopy.

Abdominal procedures are generally reserved for younger and more robust patients who are better able to tolerate a major operation and general anaesthesia. The perineal procedures are adopted to those elderly patients deemed unfit for a major abdominal procedure and general anasthesia.

The potential advantage of abdominal procedures is fixation of the rectum in a more appropriate anatomic location without sacrifice of the compliant rectal reservoir. In addition, these approaches generally are considered superior because of the lower recurrence rates, improvement in symptoms, and better functional results. Perineal approaches that eradicate the rectal ampulla with a coloanal anastomosis or plicate the prolapse are felt to be superior in older, high risk patients because of less surgical trauma. It is clear, however that these procedures typically are associated with higher recurrence rate.

Laparoscopic management of rectal prolapse was first introduced by Baerman in 1992. Laparoscopic access may produce a means of paving the reduction in surgical stress associated with a perineal approach and the low recurrence rates achieved with abdominal repair of the prolapse.

Even when a laparoscopic approach is selected a choice must be made between a rectopexy with suture or artificial material and a sigmoid colectomy with or without rectopexy. Patients with normal bowel habits or constipation without symptoms of anal incontinence will be benefited with laparoscopic resection rectopexy. Patients with symptoms of incontinence or preop diarrehoea will be benefited with Laparoscopic posterior mesh rectopexy (LPMR).

PERINEAL PROCEDURES

These are preferred for treating elderly and debliated patients, who are poor candidates for general anaesthesia and with other co-morbid illness and whose life expectancy is limited.

1. Theirsche Anal Encirclement

This was described by Thiersche in 1891. Non-absorbable suture like 1-ethilon or prolene can be used. It requires only local or regional anaesthesia. Two small incision anterior and posterior to the anus are created through which the non-absorbable suture material is passed. Recurrence rates are high and with post operative complication like disruption of the suture material, fecal impaction and infections.

2. Delorme procedure

This was reported in 1899 by a French surgeon called Delorme. This procedure involves stripping the mucosa from the prolapsed bowel, plicating the denuded muscularis layer and reanastomising the

Laparoscopic Surgical Options for Procidentia

Symptoms		Surgical Option
Diarrhoea with /without Incontinence		LPMR
Constipation	Normal anal tone	LPMR
	Hypotonic anal canal	LRR
Incontinence		LPMR
Normal bowel function / No Incontinence		LPMR/LRR

LPMR - Laparoscopic Posterior Mesh Rectopexy, LRR - Laparoscopic Resection Rectopexy

mucosal ring. This can be performed in poor risk patients under LA. It is well tolerated and associated with few complications. The major disadvantage is the high recurrence rate and the tedious dissection needed in larger prolpases.

3. Altemeier Procedures - (Perineal Rectosigmoidectomy)

This procedure can be performed under SA or GA. Procedure includes excision of redundant bowel, obliterating the hernial sac, and approximation of the levator ani in front or behind the rectum. It is associated with low morbidity and is a viable option for elderly patients. Incontinence may persists partly because of the loss of the rectal vault.

ABDOMINAL PROCEDURES

In the management of complete rectal prolapse the abdominal procedures are considered superior to perineal procedures because they give better functional results and low recurrence rate. Though varieties of abdominal procedures have been described in the literature, few procedures have become standardised after various modification during the past decades. They are suture rectopexy, posterior mesh rectopexy, sigmoid resection with or without suture rectopexy, anterior resection and pelvic floor repair. All these open abdominal procedures have been adopted for laparoscopy and have shown comparable results to that of open procedures.

I. Laparoscopic Posterior Mesh Rectopexy (LPMR)

Indication

All patients with complete rectal prolapse who are fit for GA with or without any comorbid illness. Patients with excess redundant sigmoid with severe constipation features should undergo LRR.

Preoperative Preparation

All patients were advised to take soft diet 2 days prior to surgery. Exelyte or Peglec preparation was given the night before surgery. Colonoscopy is mandatory in all cases prior to surgery to rule out malignancy and any leading cause for the prolapse.

At the induction of anaesthesia a third generation cephalosporin with aminoglycoside and metronidazole were administered and continued for 3 days post operatively. Prophylactic anticoagulation and compressive elastic stockings were used in every patient.

Theatre Setup and Port Placement

Patient was placed in modified lithotomy position with Trendelenburg tilt. Monitor was kept at foot end and the surgeon and camera person stand at head end of the patient. The surgeon commences the procedure on the patient's right hand side. Pneumoperitoneum is created by closed method using Veress needle. Four ports were used, two 10mm and two 5mm. The 10mm umbilical port is the camera port. A 30° telescope is used in all cases. The 10mm right lower pararectus is the right hand working port and the 5mm left lower pararectus is the left hand working port. Another 5mm or 10mm at the left lumbar is used for the traction of sigmoid colon.

In all female patients, the uterus is fixed to the anterior abdominal wall temporarly using 1.0 ethilon/prolene stitch or the same can be done with one extra supraumbilical 5 mm port using an atraumatic instrument.

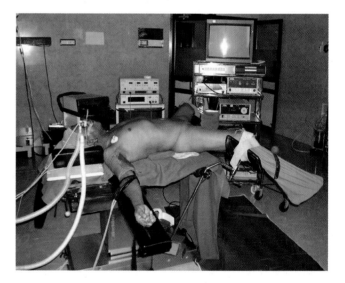

Figure 5 : Position of the patient. Lithotomy with trendelenberg position. Surgeon and camera surgeon stands on the right side of the patient

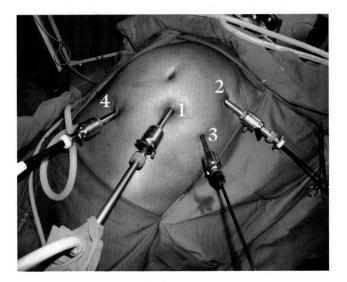

Figure 6 : Ports position

1 - Camera port 10mm
2 - Right hand working port 10mm
3 - Left hand working port 5mm
4 - Colon retracting port 10mm

Operating Technique

Identifying the Ureter and Presacral Nerves

Mobilization of the rectum is commenced on its right lateral side of the inferior mesenteric pedicle. Over the sacral promontory medial to the right ureter care should be taken, not to injure the ureter while dissecting over the sacral promontory as the mesorectum is lax here and the ureter is also mobile. The rectosigmoid is retracted anterior and cephalad with a Babcock. The surgeon applies counter traction to the peritoneum and incises the parietal peritoneum over the sacral promontory to carefully enter the plane between the visceral layer of pelvic fascia covering the mesorectum anteriorly and the presacral fascia covering presacral nerves posteriorly. This avascular presacral areolar tissue contributes the "holy plane" in mesorectal mobilization. The plane is developed in this way down into the pelvis incising the peritoneum along the right pelvic side wall and continued anteriorly to reach the rectovesical or rectovaginal pouch. The right ureter is carefully protected and the dissection continued in the retroperitoneum medial to the ureter.

The right sided plane of dissection is extended towards left from medial to lateral, keeping presacral nerves posteriorly intact. Most often the left ureter is identified by right sided dissection.

Posterior Mobilization of Rectum

Mobilization of the recto sigmoid on its left side is now performed. The apex of the sigmoid and rectosigmoid are held with Babcock to the right and the operation table tilted with left side up. While applying countertraction with an atraumatic grasper the lateral peritoneal reflection is incised. The left ureter is identified through the window in the mesocolon to avoid the risk of inadvertent damage to a "tented up" left ureter approached from the lateral side. In the medial to lateral approach the left ureter is already dissected away from peritoneum, thus unlikely to be injured. The right sided plane of dissection is connected to that on the left through the presacral space. The peritoneal incision is extended downwards keeping the left ureter lateraly. The entire mesorectum is dissected off the presacral fascia upto the levator ani. In elderly patients the lateral ligaments can be divided, in doing so we always divide close to the rectum to preserve the parasympathetic nerves. We usually try to preserve the lateral ligament.

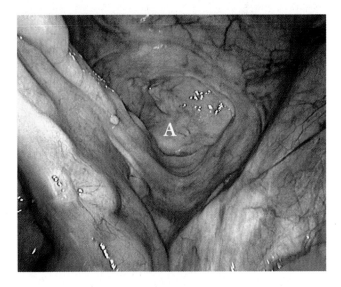

Figure 7 : Redundant rectum is pulled cranially by using 10mm babcock from the left hypochondrial port

A - Rectum

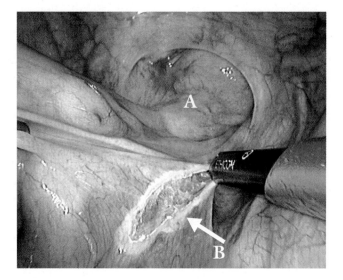

Figure 8 : Peritoneal incision on the right side starting at the level of sacral promontary

A - Rectum
B - Peritoneal incision

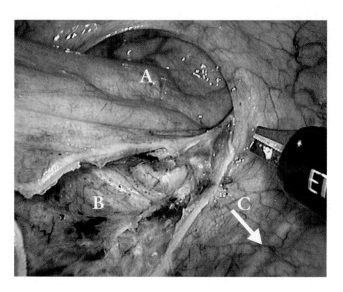

Figure 9 : Rectum is dissected laterally and posteriorly

A - Rectum
B - Presacral fascia
C - Right ureter

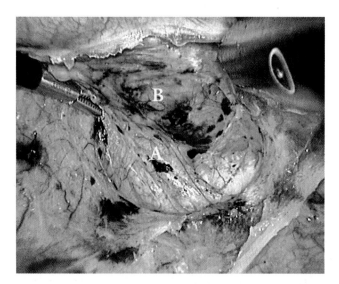

Figure 10 : Continuation of posterior dissection in the plane between the mesorectum and presacral fascia

A - Mesorectum
B - Presacral fascia

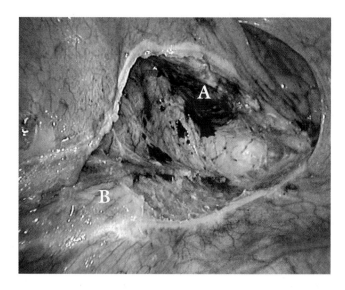

Figure 11: Posterior dissection is continued and left lateral side of the rectum is also mobilized

A - Mesorectum
B - Sacral promontary

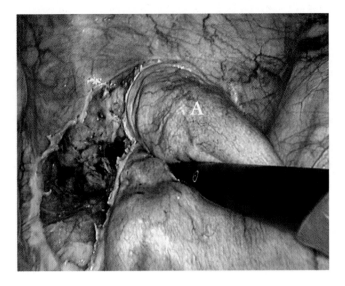

Figure 12 : Peritoneal attachment on the left side of the rectum is divided

A - Rectum

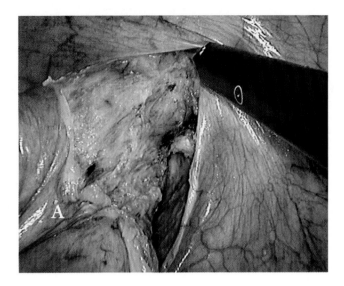

Figure 13 : Anterior dissection of the rectum

A - Rectum

Anterior Mobilization of Rectum

Having connected the pelvic incision anteriorly the surgeon retracts the rectum toward the sacrum commences the anterior dissection following the plane of Denonvillier's fascia, utilizing an atraumatic retractor to provide anterior countertraction on the bladder or vagina. Anterior dissection is carried out about 5 cm beyond peritoneal reflection. After completion of anterior and poster dissection, rectum can be retracted cranially. The presacral median veins if present should be coagulated using bipolar cautery in order to avoid bleeding during mesh fixation.

Presacral mesh fixation

15 x 10 cm size polypropylene mesh narrowed at its caudal end is introduced into the pelvis using the metal sleeve or through the trocar after removal of the head. The prolene mesh is carefully aligned over the sacrum reaching caudally upto the levator ani. Three or four prolene stitches are used to fix the prolene mesh to the presacral fascia, the most proximal one at the sacral promontory.

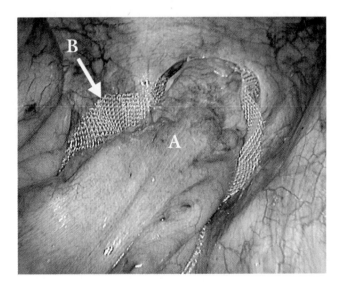

Figure 14: Polypropylene mesh kept behind the rectum and size of the mesh is assessed

A - Rectum
2 - Polypropylene mesh

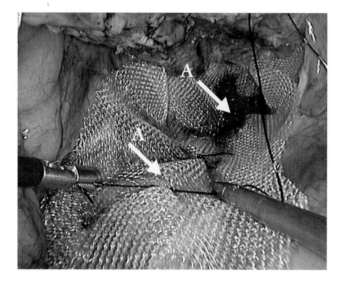

Figure 15 : Rectum is retracted up and the prolene mesh is sutured to the presacral fascia in the midline using prolene stitches

A - Stitch to the presacral fascia

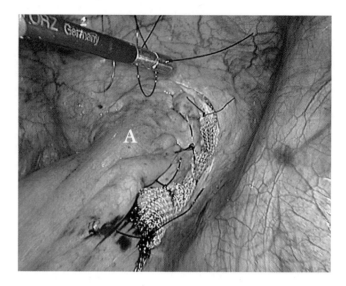

Figure 16 : Completion of the fixation of the mesh on the right side. Mesh is sutured to the lateral side of the rectum on the right side using prolene stitches

A - Rectum

The course of the presacral nerves should be identified before placing the sutures. Proper fixation of the mesh can be assessed by moving the mesh over the sacrum keeping cranial traction on the rectum. The mesh is wrapped over the mesorectum at the junction of the peritoneal reflection of the mesorectum over the rectal wall, where the peritoneum is usually thicker. The excess of the mesh is cut and the proximal corners are trimmed according to individual requirement.

The rectum is fixed to the prolene mesh by anchoring the lateral ligaments and the mesorectum using two or three 2-0 nonabsorbable prolene stitches. The mesh is wrapped to the side wall of the rectum and fixed with 2 or 3 prolene stitches on either side of the rectum. We use to wrap the rectum partially (½) unlike in conventional method where 2/3rd or ¾th of the rectal wall is wrapped. The higher incidence of constipation following conventional 2/3rd wrap made us to modify this approach. In this combined mesh and suture fixation, we have found complete correction of prolapse without incontinence and with

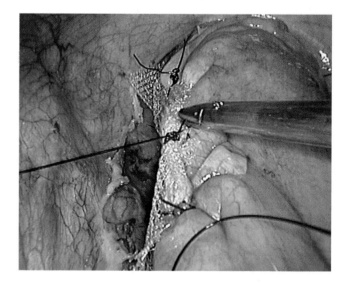

Figure 17 : Fixation of the mesh to the rectum on the left side using interrupted prolene stitches

decreased incidence of postoperative constipation. Laxicity of the mesorectum over the presacral fascia is the cause for prolapse. After adequate fixity of the mesorectum only partial wrapping of the rectum is required. In this method of partial wrapping, the rectal wall is so pliable that the normal peristalsis is unaffected and the so called functional block is prevented. In addition, the prolene mesh induces fibrosis between the mesorectum and the presacral fascia thus helping further in the prevention of prolapse.

Peritoneal Closure

The mesh is extraperitonealised by resuturing back the divided peritoneal folds. Tube drain is kept in the pelvis in selected cases where we think the dissection is extensive.

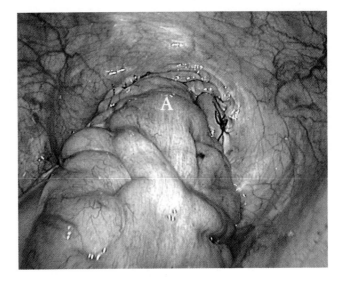

Figure 19 : Position of the rectum after the completion of the posterior mesh rectopexy

A - Rectum

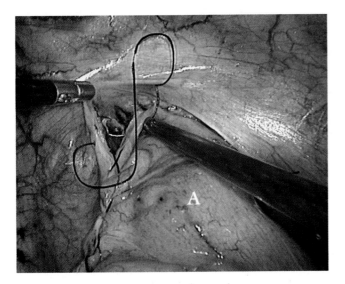

Figure 18 : Peritoneal closure using 2 0 vicryl (continuous suture)

A - Rectum

II. Laparoscopic Sigmoid Resection with Rectopexy or Laparoscopic Resection Rectopexy (LRR)

This procedure is often used for young, healthy patients with constipation and excess redundant sigmoid colon causing kinking. The theatre setup, position and port placement are similar to that of anterior resection. The mobilization was carried out upto the splenic flexure. The sigmoidal vessels were clipped or stapled or divided using harmonic scalpel. The bowel was divided with an endoscopic stapler and exteriorized for the final resection through a mini-laparotomy at the level of the left lower trocar site. After closure of the wound and re-creation of the pneumoperitoneum a double stapled anastomosis was performed with a circular stapling instrument. Sutured rectopexy was performed by anchoring the mesorectum to the presacral fascia below the promontory or from the lateral ligaments to the sacral promontory using 2 or 3 non-absorbable (prolene) stitches intracorporeally. The anastomosis is checked with a rigid sigmoidoscope and air insufflation for hemostasis and integrity.

III. Laparoscopic Anterior Resection

Procedure and team setup are similar as described for LAR. Here the rectum was mobilized all the way to levator ani that is necessary to take up the slackness of the rectum. The upper rectum along with the redundant sigmoid colon is resected and primary anastomosis is positioned above the anterior peritoneal reflection because the lower risk of anastomatic dehiscence at this level when compared to the standard AR. A tube drain is inserted through a trocar and positioned near the anastomosis.

OUR RESULTS

Till today we have treated 88 patients of complete rectal prolapse with laparoscopic LPMR. 52 were male and 36 were female. In contrast to the Western studies, we have more male patients than female patients. Age ranges between 24 to 78 years. 24 patients were above 50 years of age. The mean operating time was 89 minutes. The procedure initially took a longer time but with experience it could be completed within an hour. Oral liquids were started 24-48 hours in all patients. Drainage tube removed on 3rd or 4th postoperative day. The mean length of hospital stay was 5 days (4 to 9 days). There was no mortality in our study group and there was no recurrence of prolapse as well.

Laxatives were given routinely to all patients for a period of four weeks postoperative and they were advised not to strain more during each defecation. Two patients underwent laparoscopy resection rectopexy, since both had significantly more redundant sigmoid.

Pre and postoperative courses of patients were determined with particular interest in terms of constipation, continence, sexual function and recurrence. Follow up was obtained in terms of physical examinations and symptoms in OPD basis for a mean period of 5½ years (3 weeks - 10 years).

Three out of 8 patients who had constipation preoperatively continue to have the same, which was managed by using laxatives. All those patients with persistent post operative constipation had 2/3rd wrap of the rectum. One patient had prolonged drainage

LPMR - Our Results	
Mean operation time	89 mts
Range	160-58 mts
Mean blood loss	45 ml
Range	25-110 ml
LOS 5 days	
Range	4-9 days
Return to normal work	12 days
Follow-up	
Mean	5½ years
Range	3 wks-10 yrs

Complication	
Mortality	Nil
Morbidity	
Port site Hernia	Nil
Mesh infection	1
Wound infection	1
UTI	2
Recurrence	Nil

and has to stay in the hospital for eleven days. There were no port site wound infection. One patient developed mesh infection with sigmoid perforation 6 month after surgery and required sigmoid resection and mesh removal.

All the patients who had preoperative incontinence showed excellent improvement post operatively except three due to wide anal opening for whom we did Theirsche anal encirclement using 1.0 loop ethilon and they become normal. Mucus soiling were noticed in 10 patients lasted for 2-3 months, improved by regular sphincter stimulation exercises.

Sexual function was preserved in all. There was no incidence of premature or retrograde ejaculation. 10 female patients in reproductive age group conceived within 5 years of the operation.

Functional outcome at 24 months after LPMR

Pre operative status and post operative outcome	No.(%)
Incontinence before operation	
Total	22
Unchanged	3 (13.6%)
Worse	0
Continence restored	19 (86.3%)
Constipation before operation	
Total	8
Unchanged	3 (13.6%)
Worse	0
Constipation improved	5 (62.5%)

LPMR - Demographic Profile

Age (median) yr	44.6
Age (Range) yr	24-78
Duration of prolapse (yr)	3½
Previous abdominal surgeries	12
ASA I (%)	30 (34)
ASA II (%)	52 (59)
ASA III (%)	6 (7)
No. of patients with constipation	8 (9%)
No. of patients with incontinence	22 (25%)

DISCUSSION

Laparoscopy has been proposed as a feasible and effective procedure for complete rectal prolapse. Studies comparing the laparoscopic and open surgical approach for rectal prolapse have demonstrated that laparoscopy confers benefits related to postoperative pain, length of hospital stay and return of bowel function. Currently, no absolute criteria exist for choosing the best procedure to use with any given patient who has rectal prolapse. The goal is to achieve the best possible functional outcome with the least morbidity and risk of recurrence.

Current laparoscopic surgical technique include posterior suture or stapled rectopexy, posterior mesh rectopexy and resection of sigmoid and upper rectum with or without suture rectopexy. The use of foreign material for fixation adds the potential benefit of a greater degree of rectal fixation. However, it poses a potential risk if used with resection should an anastomotic complication occur. Therefore mesh rectopexy generally is not performed with bowel resection.

Suture rectopexy is technically less demanding and avoids the risk of foreign material, but there is a higher recurrence late and a similar risk of post operation constipation. Resection rectopexy gives good results in terms of recurrence and avoidance of post operative constipation. However it adds the risk of anastomotic complications and longer hospital stays with added problem of post operative incontinence.

Darzi et al[1] reported only a 20% rate of incontinence improvement after LRR. Xynos et al[2] despite the use of extensive physiologic testing, still found that 40% of cases needed post operative anal sphincteroplasty for incontinence after LRR. It therefore appears that clinical identification of significant incontinence symptoms may be predictive of poor functional results after LRR.

Our patients achieved restoration of anal continence within 3-6 months after anatomical correction of prolapse. According to other investigators the restoration of anal continence after prolapse repair is related to the resolution of the patient's chronic recto anal inhibition and recovery of internal sphincter electromyographic activity together with an increase in anal resting pressure. Other contributing factors include an increases in maximal voluntary contraction pressure, reflex ting recovery of the external anal sphincter as well as improved anorectal sensation.

LPMR has gained popularity because it gives the best results in terms of recurrence and avoidance of complication including incontinence. The only

Tabel 1 : Results from laparoscopic Management of Rectal prolapse

Investigator(ref)	Year	Lap. Procedure	Mean Operative Time (in minutes)	Mean Blood Loss (ml)	Conversion (%)	LOS (Days)
Madbouley et al[3]	2003	LRR,	128	81	9	3.6
		LPMR	80	69-91	-	2.3
Kellokumpu et al[4]	2000	LPR	225	NA	NA	LRR - 5
		LSR	150			LSR - 3.6
Darzi et al[1]	1995	LPMR	113.5	-	-	2.7
Xynos et al[2]	1999	LRR	225	-	-	5
Bruch et al[5]	1999	LSR	130	-	1.4	15
		LRR	227			
Soloman et al[6]	1998	LPMR	198	-	14	6.3
Stevenson et al[7]	1998	LRR	185	-	0	5
Palanivelu et al[8]	2004	LPMR	88	45	0	5

LOS – Length of hospital stay, LRR – Laparoscopic Resection Rectopexy, LPMR – Laparoscopic Posterior Mesh Rectopexy, LSR – Lap suture rectopexy

disadvantage which surgeon is worried is the post operative constipation, which has also reduced to a great extend in our study, since we preserve the parasympathetic innervation by avoiding the division of lateral ligaments.

Many studies in the literature have shown that preoperative constipation is unchanged or worsen after LPMR. The definition of constipation and the operating techniques (e.g. division of lateral ligaments) have varied in different studies, making comparison of the results difficult. Impaired rectal motility caused by division of the lateral mesorectal tissue with parasympathic denervation, functional obstruction caused by kinking of the redundant sigmoid colon above the fixed rectum and fibrosis related to the use of mesh are all regarded as etiological factors for postoperative constipation after rectopexy alone. Madbouly et al[3] have reported that constipation has improved in 100% of the patients after LPR and was unchanged after LPMR. Kessler et al[9] had 6% incontinence and 15% obstructed defecation after suture rectopexy. Zittle et al[10] identified similar incidence of evacuation problems after suture rectopexy although there was no post operative incontinence cases. We strongly believe that the

Table 2 : Functional outcome after Laparoscopic Management of Rectal Prolapse

Investigator (ref)	Lap. Procedure	Improvement of Pre op Constipation (%)	Improvement of Pre op Incontinence (%)	Development of Post Op constipation (%)	Recurrence (%)
Madbouly et al[3]	LRR LPMR	95	80	0	0
Kellokumpu et al[4]	LRR LSR	68	100	12	7
Darzi et al[1]	LPMR LRR LSR	0 100 0	100 75 80	32 0 25	0
Xynos et al[2]	LRR	100	70	0	0
Bruch et al[5]	LSR LRR	76	64	0	0
Solomon et al[6]	LPMR	-	-	-	0
Stevenson et al[7]	LRR	64	70	0	0
Palanivelu et al[8]	LPMR	62.5	86.3	3.4	0

division of the lateral rectal ligaments results in parasympathetic denervation and leads directly to evacuation problems. This contension is supported by the persistence of constipation in 18% of patients after LRR with division of lateral stalks in the publications by Darzi[1] et al. Bruch et al[5] also found that preservation of lateral ligaments leads to significant improvement of constipation after both LRR and suture rectopexy as compared with lateral ligament dissection. It is generally agreed that after nonresectional repairs, constipation-related symptoms remain unchanged or even increases if the lateral ligaments are divided during the rectal mobilization. Symptoms attributed to difficult rectal evacuation however, were significantly ameliorated in our mesh rectopexy group, as was also reported in a previous study comparing various form of rectopexy. The tables 1 & 2 show the operative and functional outcome of various laparoscopic procedures for rectal prolapse.

Our results show that LPMR effectively cure the prolapse and can be performed safely in majority of patients who are fit for GA. The primary disadvantage is the long operative time during the learning curve and need for surgeon with experience in intracorporeal suturing techniques. However, a reduction in operating time can be expected with increasing experience. The median post operative hospital stay of 5 days in our study and other laparoscopic series compares with the 7-11 days reported with conventional abdominal surgery. Complications are not infrequent with abdominal procedure to repair rectal prolapse. In recent review they occurred in 21% of patients. This findings is also in line with our results.

Conventional resection rectopexy is associated with a recurrence rate of 0-9%, whereas the recurrence rate for abdominal rectopexies is 0-12%. But in our series there is no recurrence till date.

CONCLUSION

Currently, no absolute criteria exist for choosing the best procedure to use with any given patient who has rectal prolapse. Our experience has shown that LPMR for rectal prolapse is safe and effective technique which can be performed with no mortality and less morbidity rates compared to those of conventional techniques. Since our Indian patients present with less severe constipation and bowel symptoms when compared to western population due to their dietary habits, this procedure can be safely performed in majority of all complete rectal prolapse. The use of clinical criteria for selection of operative approach appears to result in good functional outcome in terms of both constipation and incontinence symptoms. Preservation of lateral rectal ligaments and avoidance of injury to the hypogastric nerves also may play a role in the good functional results. Apart from less recurrence rates when compared to other studies who have reported recurrence of 3-8%, it gives all the advantages of laparoscopic surgery to the patients like shorter hospital stay, early return to work, etc. We strongly recommend this technique for all the patients with complete rectal prolapse in the Indian subcontinent, provided the surgeon has good experience in intracorporeal suturing technique.

Reference

1. Darzi A, Henry MM, Guillou PJ, et al. Stapled laparoscopic rectopexy for rectal prolapse. Surg Endosc 1995; 9(3):301-3.

2. Xynos E, Chrysos E, Tsiaoussis J, et al. Resection rectopexy for rectal prolapse. The laparoscopic approach. Surg Endosc 1999; 13(9):862-4.

3. Madbouly KM, Senagore AJ, Delaney CP, et al. Clinically based management of rectal prolapse. Surg Endosc 2003; 17(1):99-103.

4. Kellokumpu IH, Vironen J, Scheinin T. Laparoscopic repair of rectal prolapse: a prospective study evaluating surgical outcome and changes in symptoms and bowel function. Surg Endosc 2000; 14(7):634-40.

5. Bruch HP, Herold A, Schiedeck T, Schwandner O. Laparoscopic surgery for rectal prolapse and outlet obstruction. Dis Colon Rectum 1999; 42(9):1189-94; discussion 1194-5.

6. Solomon MJ, Young CJ, Eyers AA, Roberts RA. Randomized clinical trial of laparoscopic versus open abdominal rectopexy for rectal prolapse. Br J Surg 2002; 89(1):35-9.

7. Stevenson AR, Stitz RW, Lumley JW. Laparoscopic-assisted resection-rectopexy for rectal prolapse: early and medium follow-up. Dis Colon Rectum 1998; 41(1):46-54.

8. Palanivelu. Laparoscopic Management of Rectal Prolapase In Textbook of Laparoscopic Surgery Eds C Palanivelu, Gem Digestive Diseases Foundation, Coimbatore 2002.461-466

9. Kessler H, Jerby BL, Milsom JW. Successful treatment of rectal prolapse by laparoscopic suture rectopexy. Surg Endosc 1999; 13(9):858-61.

10. Zittel TT, Manncke K, Haug S, et al. Functional results after laparoscopic rectopexy for rectal prolapse. J Gastrointest Surg 2000; 4(6):632-41.

11. Boccasanta P, Rosati R, Venturi M, et al. Comparison of laparoscopic rectopexy with open technique in the treatment of complete rectal prolapse: clinical and functional results. Surg Laparosc Endosc 1998; 8(6):460-5.

12. Boccasanta P, Rosati R, Venturi M, et al. Surgical treatment of complete rectal prolapse: results of abdominal and perineal approaches. J Laparoendosc Adv Surg Tech A 1999; 9(3):235-8.

13. Boccasanta P, Venturi M, Reitano MC, et al. Laparotomic vs. laparoscopic rectopexy in complete rectal prolapse. Dig Surg 1999; 16(5):415-9.

14. Brown AJ, Horgan AF, Anderson JH, et al. Colonic motility is abnormal before surgery for rectal prolapse. Br J Surg 1999; 86(2):263-6.

15. Cuschieri A, Shimi SM, Vander Velpen G, et al. Laparoscopic prosthesis fixation rectopexy for complete rectal prolapse. Br J Surg 1994; 81(1):138-9.

16. Huber FT, Stein H, Siewert JR. Functional results after treatment of rectal prolapse with rectopexy and sigmoid resection. World J Surg 1995; 19(1):138-43; discussion 143.

17. Solomon MJ, Eyers AA. Laparoscopic rectopexy using mesh fixation with a spiked chromium staple. Dis Colon Rectum 1996; 39(3):279-84.

18. Berman IR (1992) Sutureless laparoscopic rectopexy for procidentia. Dis Colon Rectum 32:689-693.

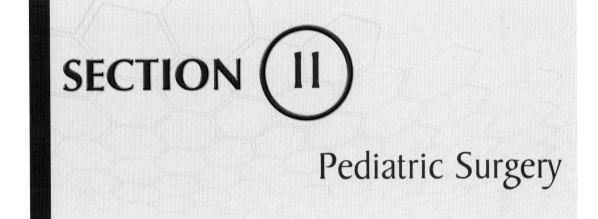

SECTION II

Pediatric Surgery

68

Laparoscopy in Pediatric Surgery

INTRODUCTION

Pediatric laparoscopic surgery is a highly developing field of minimal access surgery that is being embraced by the pediatric surgeons at present. The main reason for the growth is the development of better instrumentation and imaging systems. There has been an explosion in the development of instrumentation for laparoscopic surgery. The Hopkins Rod lens telescope has revolutionized the field of laparoscopy.

The abdominal wall of the children is thin and elastic which poses two problems the placement of needle or trocar in the subcutaneous plane and parietal wall insufflation by Veress needle technique. Postoperatively, the trocar sites should be sutured as there is greater likelihood of a hernia in a trocar site.

The imagination and creativity of surgeons world over armed with the experience in adults has led to a broad array of surgeries that can now be performed in pediatric populations which includes herniotomy, appendicectomy, fundoplication and even fetal surgeries. Through laparoscopy, it is easy to gain access to the abdomen and perform the same procedure from inside the abdominal cavity without the external incision. We have been accustomed to see children who get operated in the morning (eg lap cholecystectomy, herniotomy) regaining their potential and springing back to normalcy and playing in the wards within 3-4 hours of surgery. Now with the improvement of laparoscopic techniques and the development of miniscope (2 mm), shorter instruments specially designed for pediatric use and greater understanding of the physiological impact of pneumoperitoneum in infants and children, increasing number of surgeons prefer laparoscopic repair of hernias in children.

INGUINAL HERNIA

The incidence of inguinal hernia in childhood is approximately 0.8% to 4.4% of term infants and is greatest in the first year of life.[1] If a clinical hernia develops on one side, the risk of developing a contralateral hernia during the child's lifetime increases to 15% to 20%. The risk increases to 40% if the herniorrhaphy is performed before 1 year of age.[2] For this reason, many advocate routine contralateral exploration of groin in all infants and small children.[3,4,5,6] Failure to examine the contralateral inguinal ring can result in the subsequent development of a clinically apparent contralateral hernia in 10% or more of children undergoing unilateral repair.[7] Contralateral surgical exploration is not an absolutely safe procedure, but includes risks such as injury to the vas deferens and testicular blood supply for eg 1.6% risk of vasal injury.[8] In addition, animal studies by Shandling [9] have revealed a 10% incidence of vasal luminal narrowing even with gentle manipulation of the cord during dissection. Other potential complications include testicular atrophy (1-2%) and decreased testicular size (2.7-13%) in patients after herniorrhaphy.[10] These potential complications have raised serious concerns regarding the need for such an exploration in the absence of a clinically detectable hernia. Diagnostic laparoscopy now appears to end this debate by providing a safe and foolproof method to avoid the occurrence of contralateral hernias in these children.

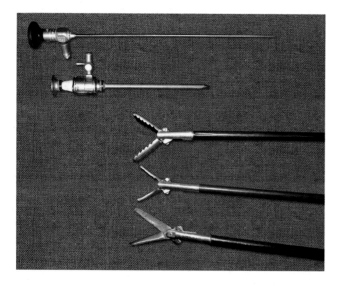

Figure 1 : Miniscope, trocar, instruments

Indications for Laparoscopy

1. **Inguinal Hernia**
   i. Laparoscopic herniotomy
   ii. Laparoscopic exploration of the contra lateral groin in unilateral hernias
   iii. Laparoscopic inguinal herniorrhaphy

2. **Hiatus Hernia**
   Laparoscopic fundoplication in sliding hiatus hernia

3. **Diaphragmatic Hernia**
   Laparoscopic/thoracoscopic repair of diaphragmatic hernia

1. Laparoscopic Herniotomy

This technique adheres to the essential principles of hernia surgery. We identify and ligate the hernial sac at the level of the internal ring. After creation of the pneumoperitoneum the 3 mm trocar is introduced in the umbilicus. Miniscopes are extremely useful in pediatric population as they reduce the incision size further. These miniscopes necessitate the use of advanced cameras systems that provide maximum clarity. Three chip digital cameras are excellent solutions for this, but the cost of the equipment is a deterrent factor. The 2 working ports are created in the right and left para rectus and 3 mm working instruments are used. The inguinal area is visualized and the presence of hernia confirmed. In young children with small defects, ligation of the sac is the ideal procedure. We use non absorbable sutures like 4 0 absorbable suture for this purpose. The 3 mm trocars might not allow these needles to pass through the trocar. We follow any one of the following methods for introducing the needles into the peritoneal cavity.

i. After removing the trocar, 3 mm instrument is used to hold the thread close to the needle and then introduced into the abdomen along with the trocar

ii. The needles are inserted through the abdominal wall by direct puncture and pulled from inside the peritoneal cavity.

The internal ring is approximated by intracorporeal purse string sutures with 4-0 vicryl or prolene. The peritoneal layer easily glides over the cord structures during suturing. The spermatic vessels and vas deferens are well visualized and protected during the circumferential passage of the suture, ensuring that they are excluded from the suture ligation. Injection of saline at the sub peritoneal plane, separates the vas deferens and vessels away from the peritoneum during this maneuver. Cord structures, particularly the vas deferens should not be handled with the grasper during manipulation as ischemic stenosis of vas deferens is known to occur. The port are closed with 4-0 vicryl taking care to include the muscle in the suture to prevent development of port site hernias.[11] The child is allowed to take liquids as soon the effect of anesthesia wear off; solids after 8 hrs and discharged on the first post operative day. No restriction is placed on the physical activities of the child and is allowed to play normally as they recover.[25,26]

Polypropylene can be used for suturing, unfortunately; it takes time for complete occlusion of the internal ring. A small gap in the suture site might

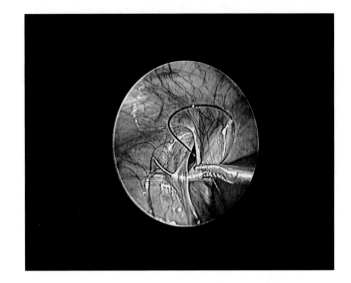

Figure 3 : Occlusion of Internal ring

Continuation of purse string suture on the inferior aspect of the internal ring

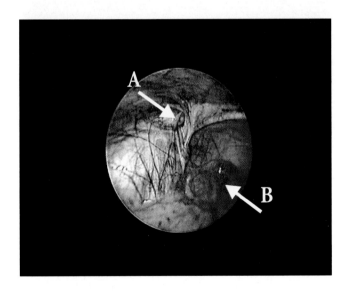

Figure 2 : Left congenital hernia viewed by 3 mm telescope

A - Defect

B - Uterus

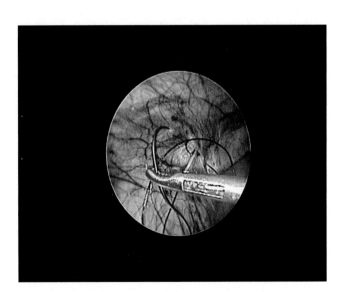

Figure 4 : Occlusion of Internal ring. Final suture on the superior aspect of internal ring

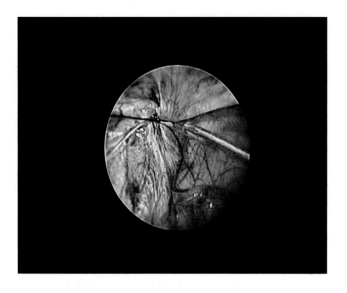

Figure 5 : Completion of the purse string suture

not allow the bowel or the omentum to herniate, but will readily permit seepage of the peritoneal fluid resulting in congenital hydrocele. We had this complication in one of our cases, which was repaired through relaparoscopy. Now we use 4 0 absorbable suture.

2. Laparoscopic Exploration of the Contra Lateral Groin

Studies have shown about 29 percent incidence development of hernias on the contralateral unexplored side in open hernia repairs. Laparoscopy is the ideal method of exploring the contralateral sides in cases of unilateral hernias in children. We have found a patent contralateral processus vaginalis in 20% of children.

3. Laparoscopic Inguinal Herniorrhaphy - Iliopubic Tract Repair

Ligature of the hernial sac at the internal ring alone is not adequate in cases associated with dilated internal ring. Iliopubic tract repair is performed by approximating the transversus arch to the iliopubic tract with non absorbable sutures. This repairs the inguinal floor and the dilated internal ring.

After creation of ports, saline is injected in the sub peritoneal plane over the cord structures at the level

of internal ring. The peritoneum is incised anterior to the defect in a similar fashion to TAPP repair in adults. The hernial sac is divided circumferentially. The iliopubic tract and the transversus arch bordering the internal ring are defined clearly. In presence of large hernial sac, the sac is divided longitudinally on the lateral aspect of the cord structures. Usually dissection is kept to minimum to avoid trauma to the cord structures. The iliopubic tract is approximated with the transversus arch using interrupted sutures with 2-0 non absorbable suture. The approximation of the internal ring should not be very tight. The number of sutures required to approximate the internal ring depends on its size. Care is taken to avoid suturing on too lateral aspect (nerve injury) or below the iliopubic tract (iliac and femoral vessels). The peritoneum is sutured over the repair with absorbable continuous sutures (3-0 vicryl). Accidental trauma to the testicular artery may produce testicular atrophy later. Extensive dissection may cause scrotal and testicular swelling. Similar procedure is performed in association with laparoscopic orchidopexy.

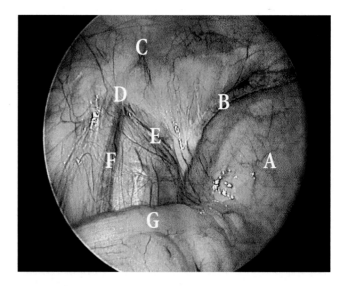

Figure 6 : Normal left inguinal anatomy

A - Bladder
B - Medial umbilical ligament
C - Inferior epigastric vessels
D - Internal ring
E - Vas deferens
F - Testicular vessels
G - Sigmoid colon

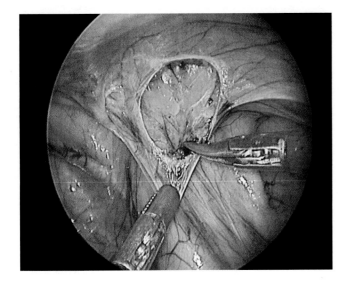

Figure 7 : Peritoneal incision

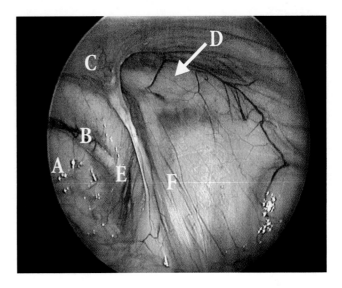

Figure 8 : Right indirect hernia

A - Bladder

B - Medial umbilical ligament

C - Inferior epigastric vessels (displaced medially)

D - Dilated internal ring

E - Vas deferens

F - Testicular vessels

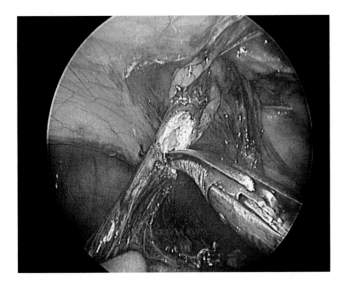

Figure 9 : Division of the sac

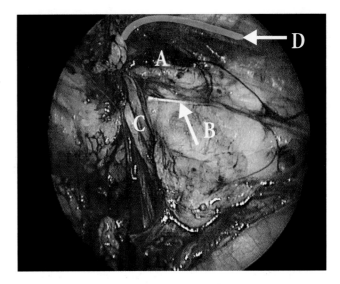

Figure 10 : Completion of dissection

A - Dilated internal ring

B - Iliopubic tract

C - Cord structures

D - Transverse fascial arch

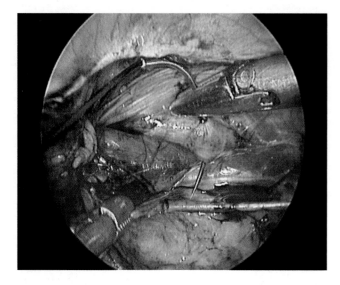

Figure 11 : Approximation of transverse fascial arch and iliopubic tract

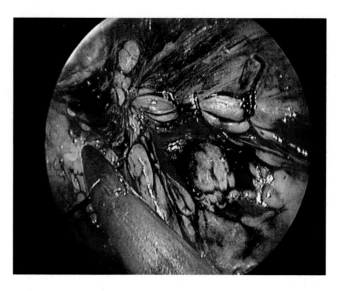

Figure 12 : Completion of iliopubic tract repair.

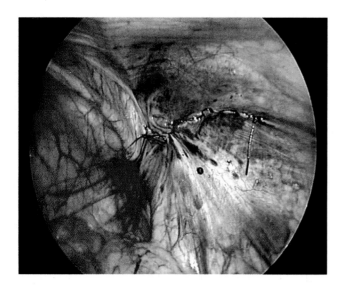

Figure 13 : After peritoneal flap closure

Our Results

We have treated 64 children with inguinal hernias. All our patients have had minimal postoperative discomfort and all resumed normal activities immediately after surgery. As there is no longitudinal skin incision in the abdominal wall, cosmetic results were excellent and the risk of infection is almost nil. In our experience we had one recurrence of congenital hydrocele, treated by re laparoscopy. One child had scrotal swelling which subsided with analgesic and antibiotics.

56 male, 8 female - 29 were bilateral. Over this period 22 iliopubic tract repair has been done successfully. On seven years of follow up there were 2 recurrences. Both were treated with laparoscopic iliopubic tract repair. Early data in the literature suggest a lower recurrence rate with extra peritoneal high ligation technique.

DISCUSSION

Once the technique of intracorporeal suturing in a limited space is mastered, laparoscopic herniorrhaphy is safe, reproducible, and technically easy for experienced laparoscopic surgeons.[25,26] The laparoscopic procedure is gaining increasing as a acceptable technique in the management of inguinal hernias in children as it combines diagnosis and the potential for immediate treatment.

Some surgeons use laparoscopy to diagnose the contralateral hernia while performing the repair by conventional method. This novel technique known as "Transinguinal Laparoscopic Examination of the Contralateral Groin" is performed in the following way. The surgery starts as a routine conventional hernia repair. After dissection of the hernial sac, it is opened and a 5 mm or a smaller trocar is placed intraperitoneally through the opening in the hernial sac. The abdomen is insufflated with CO_2 and the opposite side internal ring and inguinal canal inspected with a 70-degree laparoscope. This permits excellent exposure of the internal ring and determination of a patent processus vaginalis (PPV) or unsuspected hernia. The abdomen is deflated of CO_2, and the laparoscope and trocar are removed. The symptomatic hernia is repaired in the usual fashion, and contralateral repair was undertaken only if indicated by positive findings on laparoscopy.[12,13,14,15]

In a meta analysis of laparoscopic evaluation of the pediatric inguinal hernia it was found that laparoscopy was the ideal tool to diagnose a contralateral patent processus vaginalis intraoperatively. It is sensitive, specific, fast, and safe. All available studies of children with a unilateral hernia who had exploration of the contralateral groin by laparoscopy were analyzed and compared with open exploration or development of a metachronous hernia as the gold standard. Out of 946 patients contralateral hernia was diagnosed on laparoscopy in 376 patients. This was confirmed by open exploration in 373 patients (sensitivity of laparoscopy was 99.4%). Out of the remaining 588 patients, 62 underwent open exploration as there was a clinical suspicion and only one child had a true hernial sac. The remaining 526 patients were followed for 1 month to 3 years and only one hernia developed (specificity of laparoscopy was 99.5%). Laparoscopy added an average of 6 minutes to the surgical time and was accurate regardless of the technique.[16]

The essential step in the conventional method for inguinal hernia repair in children is simple ligation of the hernial sac without narrowing the open ring. From our point of view, one needs to identify two things. First and the most obvious one is the confirmation of the hernia and look for the contralateral side. The second aspect is the size of the internal ring. Internal ring closure is essentially a high ligation of the indirect hernia sac, which is the preferred technique in pediatric patients. Many surgeons have reported similar laparoscopic repair.

Also, ligature of the hernial sac at the internal ring alone is inadequate in cases with dilated internal ring (24% children), as it does not take care of the component of the dilated ring. We perform an Iliopubic tract repair without placing a mesh. We first started with Laparoscopic Iliopubic tract repair (LIPTR) in 1994. We believe that in children with a dilated internal ring, a routine laparoscopic ring closure would be inadequate. This is also observed in our two recurrences with one of them occurring within 5 months of LRC. Following LIPTR, there have been no recurrences. Recurrence following LRC can be dealt with LIPTR. The long-term follow-up of LIPTR is awaited.[27]

In patients with recurrences after laparoscopic herniorrhaphy, the surgeon has an undisturbed anatomy for groin incision; the risk of an injury to the vas deferens, subsequent testicular atrophy, and the risk of superior displacement of the testicle seem less likely.[16] On the contrary, the chances of injury to these organs are more in the conventional repair as the surgeon has to dissect through the scarred tissue to perform a durable repair.

HIATUS HERNIA

Laparoscopic Management of Sliding Hiatus Hernia

Gastroesophageal reflux disease (GERD) is a common problem in the pediatric population. Most children can be managed successfully with feeding regimens and medication, but children whose reflux fails to respond become surgical candidates. During the past 2 decades, GERD has been recognized more frequently because of increased awareness of the condition and because of the more sophisticated diagnostic techniques that have been developed for both identifying and quantifying the disorder.

Laparoscopic Nissen fundoplication as described by Nissen[18] is the procedure most commonly performed for GERD. The principles of the operation include increasing the length of intrabdominal esophagus, creating a valve-like mechanism at the gastroesophageal junction by wrapping a portion of the gastric fundus around the esophagus at that location, and creating a wrap sufficiently loose to allow the patient to relieve gastric distention by belching.

In our series of pediatric patients with GERD, five children (below the age group of 12 years) had significant reflux. These patients had associated sliding hiatus hernia and did not respond to medical therapy. They were operated successfully by laparoscopic method. We routinely use 5 mm laparoscopes with 5 and 3 mm instruments for this procedure. The placement of trocar sites is similar to fundoplication in adults.   The technique of laparoscopic Nissen

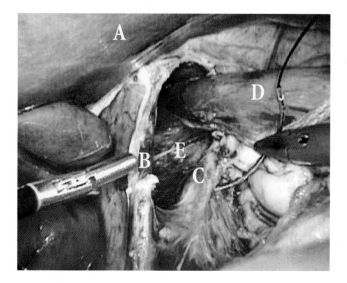

Figure 15 : Completion of dissection

A   -   Left lobe of liver
B   -   Right crus
C   -   Left crus
D   -   Esophagus
E   -   Hiatal defect

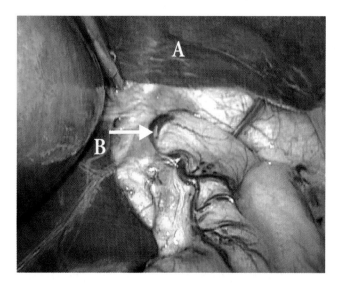

Figure 14 : Laparoscopic view of sliding hiatus hernia

A   -   Left lobe of liver
B   -   OG junction inside the hiatus

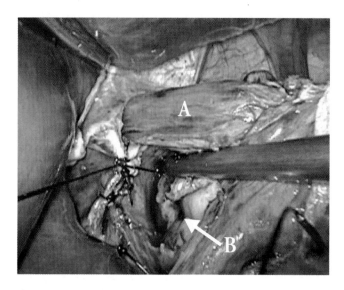

Figure 16 : Hiatal repair with interrupted prolene suture

A   -   Esophagus
B   -   Window for gastric fundus

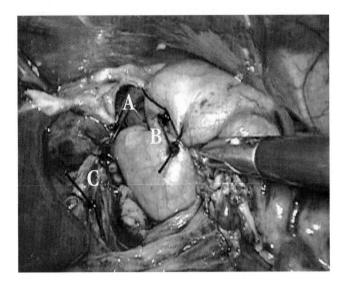

Figure 17 : Completion of Nissen fundoplication

A - Esophagus
B - Fundal wrap
C - Repaired crura

fundoplication is similar to the procedure described in chapter 19. We found 5 mm harmonic scalpel an excellent tool for dissection.

Mattioli et al report a comparison of laparoscopic and open approaches to fundoplication. Mostly children were between 1 and 14 years of age. 17 patients were treated with open fundoplication while 49 underwent laparoscopic Nissen. The latter group averaged 22 minutes less intraoperatively and 5 days less in the hospital.[19]

Esposito recorded 25 complications in 289 patients who underwent antireflux surgery. Fifteen had intraoperative events including pleural perforation, vagus nerve injury, esophageal perforation, gastric perforation, and pericardial perforation. They described 10 postoperative complications: 1 undetected esophageal perforation, 5 cases of fat herniated into port sites, 3 cases of dysphagia (all of which resolved), and 1 case of delayed gastric emptying that required surgery.[20]

Indications of laparoscopic procedures in children

Incidence of various laparoscopic procedures in children- GEM experience			
Appendectomy	1150	Mesenteric cyst	3
Cholecystectomy	35	Foreigh body magnet	1
Undescended testis	12	Splenectomy	7
Small bowel obstruction	14	Meckel's diverticulectomy	8
Malrotation of gut	3	Vagotomy and GJ	5
Peritonitis	3	Rectal prolapse	1
Inguinal Hernia	64	Rec abdominal pain	50
Nissen fundoplication	5	Pseudocyst pancreas	6
Liver Biopsy	7	Adhesiolysis	11
Achalasia cardia	24	Ovarian cyst	5
Nephrectomy	2	Re laparoscopy	22
Choledochal cyst	8	Intersex	3
Adnexal Tumor	6		

LAPAROSCOPIC REPAIR DIAPHRAGMATIC HERNIA

In 1995 Van der Zee and Bax did the first laparoscopic repair of a posterolateral diaphragmatic hernia in a six month old infant. The minimally invasive approach to diaphragmatic hernia should be considered only for children who are hemodynamically stable.[20] Older children with minimal symptoms are the suitable candidates for laparoscopic approach. The technique of laparoscopic repair of diaphragmatic hernia is similar to adults. Paraesophageal hernia[22], Morgagni hernias[23] and posttraumatic diaphragmatic hernias[24] have also been operated by laparoscopic approach. The reader is advised to go through chapter 18 for a detailed review of diaphragmatic hernia repair.

References

1. Rowe MI, Clatworthy HW Jr. The other side of the pediatric inguinal hernia. Surg Clin North Am 1971; 51:1371-6

2. Sparkman RS. Bilateral exploration in inguinal hernia in juvenile patients. Surgery 1962;51:393.

3. Rowe MI, Marchildon MB. Inguinal hernia and hydrocele in infants and children. Surg Clin North Am 1981;61:1137-45.

4. Clausen EG, Jake RJ, Binkley FM. Contralateral inguinal exploration of unilateral hernias in infants and children. Surgery 1958;44:735-49.

5. Shun A, Puri P. Inguinal hernia in the newborn: a 15 year review. Pediatr Surg Int 1988;3:156-7.

6. Tepas JJ III, Stafford PW. Timing of automatic contralateral groin exploration in male infants with unilateral hernias. Ann Surg 1966;52:70-1.

7. Surana R, Puri P. Is contralateral exploration necessary in infants with unilateral inguinal hernia? J Pediatr Surg 1993;28:1026-7.

8. Sparkman RS. Bilateral exploration in inguinal hernia in juvenile patients. Surgery 1962;51:393

9. Shandling B, Janik JS. The vulnerability of the vas deferens. J Pediatr Surg 1981;16:461-4

10. Fischer VR, Mumenthaler A. Ist bilaterale herniotomie bei Sauglingen und Kleinkindern mit einseitiger Leistenhernie angezeigt? Helv Chir Acta 1957;24:346-50

11. Waldenhausen JHT. Incisional hernia in a 5-mm trocar site following pediatric laparoscopy. J Laparoendosc Surg 1996;6(supp 1):S89-90

12. Chu C, Chou C, Hsu T, et al. Intraoperative laparoscopy in unilateral hernia repair to detect a contralateral patent processus vaginalis. Pediatr Surg Int 1993;8:385-9

13. Zitsman JL. Transinguinal diagnostic laparoscopy in pediatric inguinal herniorrhaphy. J Laparoendosc Surg 1996;6(suppl):S15-20.

14. Delarue A, Galli G, Contralateral transinguinal laparoscopy in unilateral inguinal hernia;Arch Pediatr. 1999 Jan;6(1):22-6.

15. Yerkes EB, Brock JW ; Laparoscopic evaluation for a contralateral patent processus vaginalis, Urology. 1998 Mar;51(3):480-3.

16. Miltenburg DM, Laparoscopic evaluation of the pediatric inguinal hernia-a meta-analysis. J Pediatr Surg. 1998 Jun;33(6):874-9

17. C.M. Gorsler, F.Schier; Laparoscopic herniorrhaphy in children; Surg Endosc (2003) 17:571-573

18. Nissen R. Gastropexy as the lone procedure in the surgical repair of hiatus hernia. Am J Surg. 1956;92:389

19. Mattioli G, Repetto P, Carlini C, et al. Laparoscopic vs open approach for the treatment of gastroesophageal reflux in children. Surg Endosc. 2002;16:750-752

20. Esposito C, Montupet P, Amid G, Desruelle P. Complications of laparoscopic antireflux surgery in childhood. Surg Endosc. 2000;14:622-624

21. van der Zee DC, Bax NM. Laparoscopic repair of congenital diaphragmatic hernia in a 6-month-old child. Surg Endosc. 1995;9:1001-1003

22. Van der Zee DC, Bax NM, Kramer WL, Mokhaberi B, Ure BM. Laparoscopic management of a paraesophageal hernia with intrathoracic stomach in infants. Eur J Pediatr Surg. 2001;11:52-54

23. Lima M, Domini M, Libri M, Morabito A, Tani G, Domini R. Laparoscopic repair of Morgagni-Larrey hernia in a child. J Pediatr Surg. 2000;35:1266-1268

24. Ugazzi M, Chiriboga A. Laparoscopic treatment of incarcerated post-traumatic diaphragmatic hernia. J Laparoendosc Surg. 1996;6:S83-S88

25. Palanivelu C. Role of Laparoscopy in Paediatric Surgery. In: Palanivelu C, ed. Text Book of Surgical Laparoscopy. Coimbatore: Gem Digestive Diseases Foundation, 2002:469-480.

26. Palanivelu C. Role of Laparoscopy in Paediatric Surgery. In: Palanivelu C, ed. CIGES Atlas of Laparoscopic Surgery. Second ed. New Delhi: Jaypee Brothers Medical Publishers Pvt. 2003:271-280.

27. Vijaykumar Malladi, Palanivelu Chinnaswamy, Kalpesh V. Jani, Parthasarthi R., Roshan A. Shetty, Alfie Jose Kavalakat, Anand Prakash. Laparoscopic inguinal hernia repair in children: initial experience of 93 herniae. JSLS. 2005 (in press).

69

Laparoscopic Management of Midgut Malrotation

INTRODUCTION

Midgut malrotation has been defined as intestinal nonrotation or incomplete rotation around the superior mesenteric artery (SMA). It involves anomalies of intestinal fixation as well. Interruption of typical intestinal rotation and fixation during fetal development can occur at a wide range of locations, and this leads to a variety of both acute and chronic presentations of disease. The most common type found in pediatric patients is incomplete rotation predisposing to midgut volvulus, which can result in short-bowel syndrome or even death. Many embryonic variants exists, ranging from nonrotation to reversed rotation.[1,2] The most common anomaly is malrotation.[3]

HISTORY

Case reports of malrotation exist prior to the 1900s. During the 20th century, understanding of the embryology and anatomy of malrotation became more complete, along with changes in surgical approaches to the problems.[4] In 1936, William E. Ladd wrote the classic article on treatment of malrotation, and his surgical approach (ie, Ladd's procedure) remains the cornerstone of practice till today.[5]

FREQUENCY

Intestinal malrotation occurs at a rate of 1 in 500 live births.[6] Most infants with gastroschisis, omphalocele, or congenital diaphragmatic hernia have associated intestinal malrotation. Approximately 50% of patients with duodenal atresia and 33% of patients with jejunoileal atresia have a malrotation as well. Also, intestinal malrotation occurs in association with Hirschsprung's disease, gastroesophageal reflux, intussusception, persistent cloaca, anorectal malformations like imperforate anus and extrahepatic anomalies.

Mortality/Morbidity

Younger patients have higher rates of morbidity and mortality. In infants, the mortality rate ranges from 2-24%. The presence of necrotic bowel at surgery increases the mortality rate by 25 times for infants, and the presence of other anomalies increases the risk by 22 times.[7]

Sex

Male predominance exists in neonatal presentations at a male-to-female ratio of 2:1. No sexual predilection exists in patients older than 1 year.

Age

Up to 40% of patients with malrotation present within the first week of life, and 75% by the age of 1 year. The remaining 25% of patients who present after the of age 1 year and into late adulthood, many are recognized intraoperatively during other procedures or at autopsy.[8]

PATHOPHYSIOLOGY

The cause of intestinal malrotation is disruption in the normal embryological development of the bowel. A full understanding of normal development aids in understanding the etiology of malrotation.[1]

Normal embryology

Normal rotation takes place around the SMA as the axis. It is described by referring to 2 ends of the alimentary canal, the proximal duodenojejunal loop and the distal cecocolic loop, and usually is divided into 3 stages. Both loops make a total of 270° in rotation during normal development, starting in a vertical plane parallel to the SMA and ending in a horizontal plane.[2]

Stage I: It occurs between the 5th and 10th weeks of gestation. It is the period of physiologic herniation of the bowel into the base of the umbilical cord. The duodenojejunal loop begins superior to the SMA at a 90° position and rotates 180° in a counterclockwise direction. At 180°, the loop is to the anatomical right of the SMA, and by 270°, it is beneath the SMA. The cecocolic loop begins beneath the SMA at 270°. It rotates 90° in a counterclockwise manner

and ends at the anatomical left of the SMA at a 0° position. Both loops maintain these positions until the bowel returns to the abdominal cavity. Also during this period, the mid gut lengthens along the SMA, and, as rotation continues, a very broad pedicle is formed at the base of the mesentery. This broad base protects against midgut volvulus.

Stage II: It occurs during the 10th week of gestation, the period when the bowel returns to the abdominal cavity. As it returns, the duodenojejunal loop rotates an additional 90° to end at the anatomical left of the SMA, the 0° position. The cecocolic loop turns 180° more as it reenters the abdominal cavity. This turn places it to the anatomical right of the SMA, a 180° position.

Stage III: It lasts from 11 weeks of gestation until term. It involves the descent of the cecum to the right lower quadrant and fixation of the mesenteries.

Nonrotation

Arrest in the development during stage I results in nonrotation. Subsequently, the duodenojejunal junction does not lie inferior and to the left of the SMA, and the cecum does not lie in the right lower quadrant. The mesentery in turn forms a narrow base as the gut lengthens on the SMA without rotation, and this narrow base is prone to clockwise twisting leading to midgut volvulus. The width of the base of the mesentery is different in each patient, and not every patient develops midgut volvulus.

Incomplete rotation

Stage II arrest results in incomplete rotation and is most likely to result in duodenal obstruction. Typically, peritoneal bands running from the misplaced cecum to the mesentery compress the third portion of the duodenum. Depending on how much rotation is completed prior to arrest, the mesenteric base may be narrow and, again, midgut volvulus can occur. Internal herniations may also occur with incomplete rotation if the duodenojejunal loop does not rotate but the cecocolic loop does rotate. This may trap most of the small bowel in the mesentery of the large bowel, creating a right mesocolic (paraduodenal) hernia.

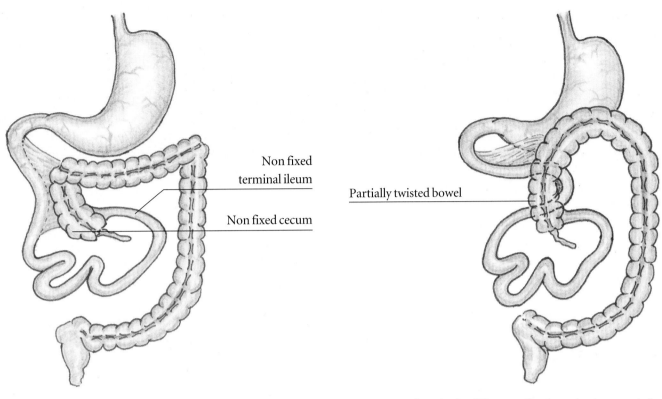

Non fixed
terminal ileum

Non fixed cecum

Partially twisted bowel

Figure 1 : Malrotation (The non-fixed terminal ileum and
cecum - 180^0-270^0 rotation)

Figure 2 : Early volvulus (The non-fixed area begins to twist)

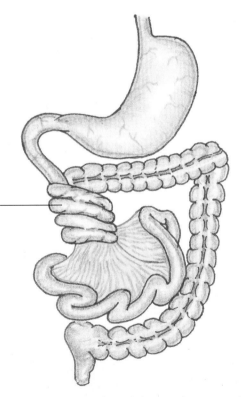

Twisted bowel

Figure 3 : Late volvulus (Here the twisting continuous, until intestines
are obstructed and the blood supply to that area is cut-off)

Incomplete fixation

Potential hernial pouches form when the mesentery of the right and left colon and the duodenum do not become fixed retroperitoneally. If the descending mesocolon between the inferior mesenteric vein and the posterior parietal attachment remains unfixed, the small intestine may push out through the unsupported area as it migrates to the left upper quadrant. This creates a left mesocolic hernia with possible entrapment and strangulation of the bowel. If the cecum remains unfixed, volvulus of the terminal ileum, cecum, and proximal ascending colon may occur. Arrested cecal descent occurs where the cecum lies in the subhepatic position but does not descend to the right iliac fossa. In the strictest use of the term this is not a malrotation but instead is a maldescent. This condition can cause neonatal obstruction due to Ladd's bands. Also it can cause partial recurrent volvulus in older children due to the narrow mesenteric attachment between the cecum and the duodenojejunal flexure. The condition is often asymptomatic and may only cause problems if the patient develops acute appendicitis.

A Ladd's band is a peritoneal band that stretches from the cecum to the subhepatic region. Ladd's bands are a cause of intestinal obstruction in cases of small intestinal malrotation and arrested cecal descent. In incomplete rotation of the gut, the rotation of the extraembryonic coelom is only about 90 degrees counter- clockwise. The colon and cecum return first to the abdomen and occupy the left side. The right side of the abdomen is filled by the small bowel. The small bowel is suspended by a very narrow 1 cm mesenteric attachment between the cecum and the duodenojejunal flexure. This condition carries a high risk of volvulus in the early days of life with resultant total small bowel infarction.[9]

SYMPTOMS AND SIGNS

They vary according to acute or chronic presentation as well as according to the type of rotational defect. About 25 to 50% of adolescents with malrotation are asymptomatic. Adolescents who become symptomatic present with acute intestinal obstruction or history of recurrent episodes of abdominal pain with less frequent vomiting and diarrhea.[10]

Acute midgut volvulus

Most patients present in the first year of life, the primary presenting sign of acute midgut volvulus is sudden onset of bilious emesis. Abdominal distention is frequently present, and the infant appears in acute pain. As vascular compromise persists, intraluminal bleeding may occur, which leads to bleeding per rectum and sometimes hematemesis. Abdominal guarding is usually present and prevents palpation of intestinal loops. As symptoms persist, the infant may develop signs of shock, including poor perfusion, decreased urine output, and hypotension. Patients may have signs of peritonitis, including abdominal tenderness and discoloration of the skin.

Chronic midgut volvulus

This is due to intermittent or partial twisting that leads to lymphatic and venous obstruction, the main presenting features are recurrent abdominal pain and malabsorption syndrome. Other clinical features include recurrent bouts of diarrhea alternating with constipation, intolerance to solid food, obstructive jaundice and gastroesophageal reflux. Physical examination may be completely normal if the patient presents during a period when the obstruction is relieved. If partial twisting is present at the time of examination, the patient may have signs and symptoms similar to those of acute midgut volvulus.

Acute duodenal obstruction

This anomaly usually is recognized in infants and is due to compression or kinking of the duodenum by peritoneal bands (Ladd's bands). Patients present with forceful vomiting, which may or may not be bile stained depending on location of the obstruction with respect to the entrance of the common bile duct (ampulla of Vater). Abdominal distention and gastric waves may be present. Passage of meconium or stool can be present. These patients usually do not have signs of peritonitis or shock unless volvulus is also present distal to the obstruction.

Chronic duodenal obstruction

The typical age at diagnosis ranges from infancy to preschool. The most common symptom is vomiting, which is usually bilious. Patients may also have failure to thrive and intermittent abdominal pain.

Physical examination may be completely normal at the time of presentation. Abdominal distention and tenderness may be present. Diagnosis is usually made by history and enough suspicion to obtain radiologic studies; physical examination findings are very unreliable.

Internal herniation

It may progress from intermittent to constant. Patients have vomiting and recurrent abdominal pain as well as constipation at times. They are often misdiagnosed to have psychosocial problems. Physical examination findings can be unremarkable and diagnosis is made by radiologic studies and high index of suspicion only. Patients with left mesentericoparietal hernias may have findings related to mesenteric venous obstruction, such as hematochezia, hemorrhoids, and dilated anterior abdominal veins. If the bowel of the patient is obstructed at the time of presentation, abdominal tenderness and guarding may be present, and a soft globular mass may be palpated at the location of the hernia.

INVESTIGATIONS

Lab Studies

Complete blood cell count: An elevated or decreased WBC count may indicate sepsis as a reason for abdominal distention and bilious emesis. A decreased platelet count may indicate a platelet consumptive process like necrotizing enterocolitis. A decreased hemoglobin/hematocrit gives evidence of blood loss, possibly through GI bleeding.

Arterial, capillary, or venous blood gas: Metabolic acidosis provides evidence for ongoing ischemia as observed with necrotizing enterocolitis or strangulated bowel (volvulus).

Blood chemistries: Correct any electrolyte imbalances if possible prior to surgery. Ongoing sodium, chloride, and bicarbonate losses occur through suctioned GI secretions. Furthermore, patients may have increased potassium levels due to metabolic acidosis and hemolysis.

Urinalysis and urine culture: Complete these tests only if abdominal distention is suspected because of another ongoing infectious process and not because of GI rotational or obstructive malformations.

Blood type and screening: Keep this test current because these infants often need emergent surgery and may need blood replacement.

Prothrombin time (PT) and activated partial thromboplastin time (aPTT): Perform clotting studies in older infants and children in whom surgery is highly likely.

Imaging Studies

Plain abdominal radiography

Plain radiography has limited use in suspected malrotation as infants may have a gasless abdomen or one that is almost normal. The classic pattern for duodenal obstruction, if present, is the double-bubble sign produced by an enlarged stomach and proximal duodenum with little gas in the remainder of the bowel. Distended bowel loops and possibly pneumatosis intestinalis may be observed if necrotising enterocolitis is present. If concern for free air in the abdomen exists, order a left lateral decubitus radiograph as well.

Upper gastrointestinal series

It is the study of choice. Normal rotation is present if the duodenal C-loop crosses the midline and places the duodenojejunal junction to the left of the spine at a level greater than or equal to the pylorus. If contrast ends abruptly or tapers in a corkscrew pattern, midgut volvulus or some other form of proximal obstruction may be present. Barium is the contrast of choice in patients who are stable or have chronic symptoms. Contrast studies may not be possible in patients who are actively vomiting or are otherwise unstable and need immediate surgical exploration. Water-soluble agents should be used if the study must be performed prior to imminent surgery.[11]

Lower gastrointestinal series (contrast enema)

Occasionally, upper GI series findings may be indeterminate for the location of the duodenojejunal junction. In these cases, lower GI series may be used to identify location of the cecum. Lower GI series can also rule out colonic obstruction and ileal atresia. However, a normally placed cecum does not unequivocally rule out a malrotation, and clinical judgment must be exercised. Conversely, maldescent of the cecum does not predict malrotation in all cases.

Ultrasonography

In the hands of experienced radiologists, ultrasonography has been shown to be very sensitive (approximately 100%) in detecting neonatal malrotation. Highest sensitivity is achieved when inversion of the SMA and the superior mesenteric vein (SMV) relationship is shown. Other diagnostic findings are fixed midline bowel loops and duodenal dilation with distal tapering. Also, volvulus is highly probable if the SMV is shown to be coiling around the SMA.[12] Detection rate is enhanced if water is instilled by nasogastric (NG) tube. The presence of ascites and thickened bowel wall were not found to be statistically significant predictors of malrotation with midgut volvulus.

Computed tomography scanning

CT scanning is not well standardised for diagnosing malrotation and midgut volvulus. Scattered case reports of its use exist, but it is not recommended as the principal diagnostic tool.[13]

MANAGEMENT

The first step is directed toward stabilizing the patient.

Nasogastric tube (NG) insertion: NG tube should be inserted in all patients with bilious emesis and suspected malrotation. Adjust the NG tube to low intermittent suction in order to decompress the bowel proximal to any obstruction that may be present.

Central venous catheter placement: Patients may require long-term intravenous access after surgery, especially if midgut volvulus is present.

Fluid and electrolyte deficits are corrected and broad-spectrum antibiotics are administered prior to surgery. If a patient has signs of shock, administer appropriate fluids, blood products, and vasopressor medications to correct hypotension. Dopamine is used as the first-line therapy because of its possible effects to increase splanchnic blood flow. If the patient is unstable, do not delay surgical intervention

for upper gastrointestinal and laboratory studies. Quick surgical intervention, not prolonged medical management, produces the best results if midgut volvulus is suspected.

Surgical Care

The Ladd's procedure remains the cornerstone of surgical treatment for malrotation today. Prior to William Ladd's publication in 1936, surgical treatment for malrotation with or without volvulus had a mortality rate higher than 90%. In fact, at Ladd's own institution, the mortality rate was 100% before the development of his new technique.[5] A classic Ladd's procedure is described as reduction of volvulus (if present), division of mesenteric bands, placement of small bowel on the right and large bowel on the left of the abdomen, and appendectomy. Published reports for laparoscopic Ladd's procedure are now appearing in the literature as well.

Midgut volvulus

If midgut volvulus is present, the entire small intestine along with the transverse colon is delivered out of the abdominal incision, where the volvulus can be reduced. Because the volvulus usually twists in a clockwise direction, reduction is accomplished by twisting in a counterclockwise direction. After the blood supply has been restored by detorsion, the surgeon must make a decision about viability of the involved bowel. The outcome is better when no gangrenous bowel is present or when a small localized gangrenous segment is present, which can be resected and a primary anastomosis performed. Enterostomy is performed when questionable viability exists at the ends of a gangrenous area that is resected. If multiple areas of questionable viability are present, many surgeons choose to leave the areas and perform a second-look operation in 24-48 hours if the patient is not showing clinical recovery.

Duodenal obstruction

After the volvulus is reduced or if no volvulus was present, identify any extrinsic obstruction to the duodenum. Peritoneal bands crossing the duodenum are divided with careful attention to protecting the superior mesenteric vessels. The bands may also obstruct the ileum or the jejunum and sometimes run to the gallbladder and liver. Extrinsic obstruction may also be due to the cecum, colon, or SMA impinging on the duodenum; relief is obtained by placing the cecum with its mesentery in the left upper quadrant and exposing the anterior duodenum through its entire length. After extrinsic obstruction has been relieved, determine that no intrinsic obstruction exists by passing an NG tube through the duodenum.

Appendectomy: It is advisable because the normal anatomical placement of the appendix is disrupted when the cecum is placed on the left side of the abdomen.

OUR EXPERIENCE

Between 2001 and 2005, we managed three children with malrotation of gut laparoscopically. All cases had presented with acute symptoms suggestive of upper gastrointestinal obstruction. Age was between 7-12 years, 2 were females and 1 was male. Laparoscopy was done and classical findings of malrotation were noted - cecum overlying the duodenum, colon was on the left side and Ladd's bands going across the duodenojejunal flexure, that was on the right side. The bands were divided and the cecum and colon were released medially from the duodenum and the pancreas. Anterior leaf of the narrow mesentery was lifted and divided to widen the base of the mesentery. Duodenum was straightened and placed along the right paracolic gutter and the cecum placed in the left hypochondrium. Small bowel loops were placed on the right side and colon on the left side. Appendectomy was also done. In essence, all the classical steps of Ladd's procedure were performed easily laparoscopically.

Postoperative care

Volume status is a major issue in the immediate postoperative period, so carefully infuse intravenous fluids. However, take care not to cause volume overload in these patients because this could be detrimental to wound healing and bowel healing if edema and ascites worsen. Broad-spectrum antibiotics are continued as per the hospital protocol. NG tube decompression is typically required postoperatively, and the clinician must replace ongoing fluid and electrolyte losses from this source. Infants tend to require more days with suctioning than older children, and patients with midgut volvulus also take longer to recover bowel function. One retrospective study found infants younger than 1 year had an average of 6.7 days on NG suctioning with a range from 1.5-16 days, and older children had 4.3 days of suctioning with a range from 2-8 days. With the presence of midgut volvulus, NG suctioning was required for an average of 8.4 days (no range reported). Patients require central venous catheter access for total parenteral nutrition until full oral feedings can be reestablished. Furthermore, most of these patients have some degree of protein calorie malnutrition prior to surgery. Achieve positive nitrogen balance as soon as possible by use of intravenous amino acid solutions. Total parenteral nutrition is maintained until the patient is able to consume at least 50% of the daily caloric requirement. Parenteral nutrition can then be weaned slowly as full enteral intake is being achieved.

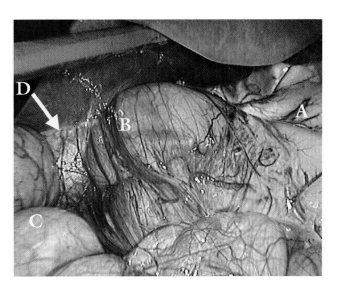

Figure 4 : Malrotation of gut

A - Stomach

B - Duodenum

C - Small bowel

D - Gall bladder

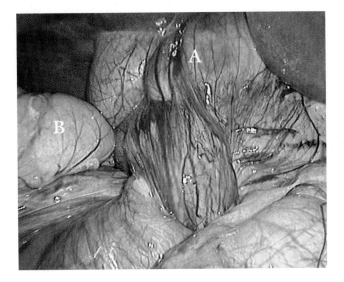

Figure 5 : Partially rotated small bowel

A - Duodenum
B - Small bowel

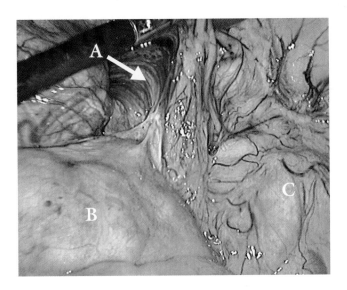

Figure 6 : Deroration is done and band (Ladd's) is seen

A - Band
B - Small bowel
C - Cecum

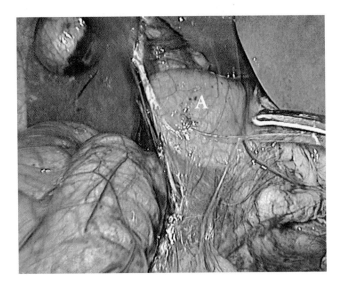

Figure 7 : Division of the band

A - Duodenum

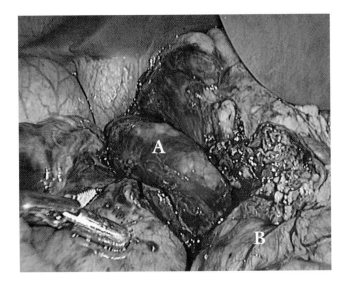

Figure 8: Completion of band division

A - Duodenum
B - Cecum

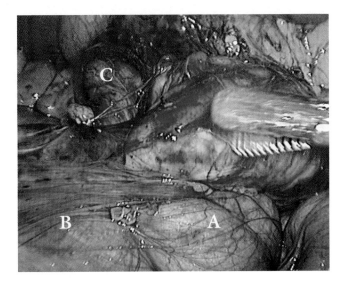

Figure 9 : Narrow mesentry

A - Cecum

B - Small bowel

C - Duodenum

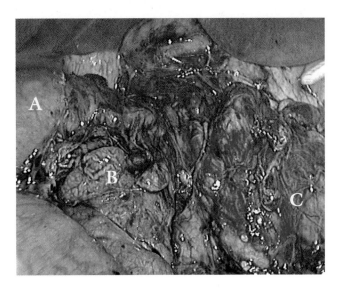

Figure 10 : Anterior leaf of mesentry is divided, base of the mesentry is widened

A - Duodenum

B - Pancreas

C - Cecum

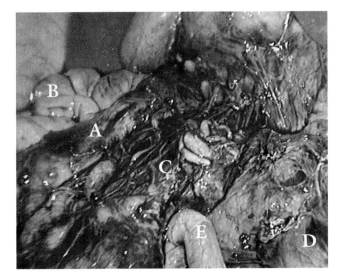

Figure 11 : Completion of dissection. Duodenum is straightened and placed on right side, Cecum is placed in the left upper abdomen

A - Duodenum

B - Small bowel

C - Pancreas

D - Cecum

E - Appendix

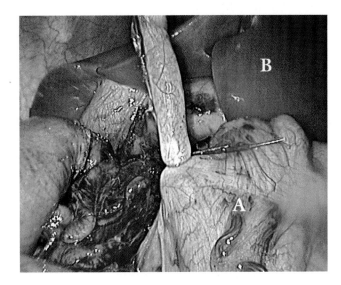

Figure 12 : Appendectomy is being performed

A - Cecum

B - Left lobe of liver

DISCUSSION

Laparoscopy has been used to repair malrotation with signs of duodenal obstruction but no midgut volvulus.[14] The Ladd's procedure, including widening of the mesenteric base and dissection of peritoneal bands, has been performed successfully and has resulted in shorter hospital stays.[15]

In 1996, Gross and Waldhausen, in separate centers first reported laparoscopic surgery for malrotation of intestine.[15,16] Since then, there have many cases reported in the literature. At the present time, laparoscopy is not adviced for midgut volvulus. Most of the published data report laparoscopic Ladd procedure in infants and very young children (5 days – 3years of age).[17,18]

Postoperative complications

Short-bowel syndrome is the most common complication of midgut volvulus with bowel necrosis. These patients have longer delays to recovery of bowel motility and function. They are at high risk for malabsorption and can require long-term parenteral nutrition. Furthermore, they have more complications from treatment and much longer hospital stays than patients with malrotation and no volvulus. Infection: Wound infections and sepsis can occur in the immediate postoperative period, requiring extended treatment with intravenous antibiotics. Patients may also have infection because of long-term placement of central venous catheters. Translocation of enteric bacteria and superimposed candidal infection further complicate the hospital course. Reoperation: In a series of 56 patients by some authors, 8 required reoperation for various complications, including volvulus of the cecum (1), recurrence of midgut volvulus (1), bowel obstruction due to adhesions (3), insertion of central venous catheter (2), abdominal wall cyst (1), and wound dehiscence (1).[19] In the same series of 56 patients, 13 had persistent (>6 months) gastrointestinal symptoms, including constipation (6), intractable diarrhea (1), abdominal pain (2), vomiting (3), and feeding difficulties (1).

In general, older children do better than infants.[20] The presence of midgut volvulus prolongs hospital-ization, and prognosis is based on how much bowel is preserved. The biggest pitfall is delay in diagnosis of midgut volvulus. The quicker a patient is taken to surgery, the better the chance for full bowel recovery. Rule out malrotation with midgut volvulus as quickly as possible in any pediatric patient with bilious emesis. Chronic duodenal obstruction is frequently misdiagnosed as colic in patients who present with intermittent abdominal pain and failure to thrive. Upper gastrointestinal series should be performed to confirm appropriate placement of the duodenojejunal junction.

CONCLUSION

Our results suggest that laparoscopic Ladd's procedure is an effective technique and can be performed safely in patients with malrotation of the gut. In addition, patients are expected to benefit from the smaller incision, earlier feeding, shorter hospital stay, and fewer complications compared with traditional Ladd's procedure. It can be performed in times equivalent to standard open techniques. Laparoscopy may also be used for the diagnosis of patients with intestinal malrotation. It may be especially helpful to verify the diagnosis in patients who do not have classic radiographic findings. Laparoscopy can he used to determine the position of ligament of Treitz and whether the cecum is fixed in the right lower quadrant. If the patient is judged to be at risk for volvulus like a shortened mesenteric pedicle, a Ladd's procedure can be accomplished laparoscopically with good long-term results.

References

1. Snyder WH Jr., Chaffin L. Embryology and pathology of the intestinal tract: presentation of 40 cases of malrotation. Ann Surg 1954;140:368-80.

2. Lister J. Malrotation and volvulus of the intestine. In: Lister J, Irving IM, eds. Neonatal surgery. 3rd ed. London: Butterworth; 1990. p. 442-5.

3. Touloukian RJ, Smith EI. Disorders of rotation and fixation. In: O'Neil JA, ed. Pediatric surgery. Vol 2. 5th ed. Baltimore:Mosby; 1998. p.1199-203.

4. Ladd WE: Congenital Obstruction of the Duodenum in Children. N Engl J Med 1932; 206: 277-80.

5. Ladd WE: Surgical Diseases of the Alimentary Tract in Infants. N Engl J Med 1936; 215: 705-8.

6. Steward DR, Colodny AL, Daggett WC.: Malrotation of the bowel in infants and children: a 15 year review. Surgery 1976;79:716-20.

7. Spigland N, Brandt ML, Yazbeck S: Malrotation presenting beyond the neonatal period . J Pediatr Surg 1990 Nov; 25(11):1139-42.

8. Brandt ML, Pokorny WJ, McGill CW, Harberg HJ.: Late presentation of midgut malrotation in children Am J Surg 1985;150:767-71.

9. Skandalakis JE, Gray SW, Ricketts R, Richardson DD. The small intestine. In: Skandalakis JE, Gray SW, eds. Embryology for surgeons. 2nd ed. Baltimore: Williams & Wilkins; 1994. p. 184-200.

10. Smith EI: Malrotation of the Intestine. In: Welch KJ, Randolph JG, Ravitch MN, et al, eds. Pediatric Surgery. 4th ed. Vol 2. St Louis, Mo: Mosby-Year Book; 1986: 882-95.

11. Simpson AJ, Leonidas JC, Krasna IH, Becker JM, Schneider KM. Roentgen diagnosis of midgut malrotation: value of upper gastrointestinal radiographic study. J Pediatr Surg 1972;7:243-52.

12. Zerin JM, DiPietro M. Superior mesenteric vascular anatomy at ultrasound in patients with surgically proved malrotation of the midgut. Radiology 1992;183:693-4.

13. Ai VH, Lam WW, Cheng W, et al: CT appearance of midgut volvulus with malrotation in a young infant. Clin Radiol 1999 Oct; 54(10): 687-9.

14. Mazziotti MV, Strasberg SM, Langer JC: Intestinal rotation abnormalities without volvulus: the role of laparoscopy. J Am Coll Surg 1997 Aug; 185(2): 172-6.

15. Gross E, Chen MK, Lobe TE.: Laparoscopic evaluation and treatment of intestinal malrotation in infants. Surg Endosc. 1996 Sep;10(9):936-7.

16. Waldhausen JH, Sawin RS.: Laparoscopic Ladd's procedure and assessment of malrotation. J Laparoendosc Surg. 1996 Mar;6 Suppl 1:S103-5.

17. Wu MH, Hsu WM, Lin WH, Lai HS, Chang KJ, Chen WJ.: Laparoscopic Ladd's procedure for intestinal malrotation: report of three cases. J Formos Med Assoc. 2002 Feb;101(2):152-5.

18. Bass KD, Rothenberg SS, Chang JH: Laparoscopic Ladd's procedure in infants with malrotation. J Pediatr Surg 1998 Feb; 33(2): 279-81.

19. Nair R, Hadley GP.: Intestinal malrotation - experience with 56 patients. S Afr J Surg 1996;34:73-5.

SECTION (12)

Hernia

70

Laparoscopic Trans Abdominal Preperitoneal Hernioplasty (TAPP)

INTRODUCTION

The era of laparoscopy which exploded with the introduction of cholecystectomy is continuing to march forward through various advanced laparoscopic surgeries. Even though hernia repairs were reported as early as 1982,[1] the widespread interest in laparoscopic herniorrhaphy did not occur till the 1990's. Disappointing early recurrence rates (even upto 25%),[2,3] excessive cost and the steep learning curve were the major stumbling blocks which prevented the routine use of laparoscopy in the management of inguinal hernias.

The preperitoneal placement of mesh that was popularized by Nyhus[3] and colleagues after the pioneering works of Cheatle (1920),[4] Henry (1936)[5] and Mc Evedy(1950)[6] has been considered as more physiological, safe and secure technique of groin hernia repair. The concept of preperitoneal mesh was applied in minimally invasive surgery with the added advantages of decreased pain, discomfort and early return to work. In 1991, Arregui reported Trans Abdominal Preperitoneal (TAPP) technique for inguinal hernias.[7] With the introduction of TAPP, the previous laparoscopic techniques such as closure of internal ring, plug and patch and intraperitoneal onlay mesh have slowly faded away due to their high complication and recurrence rates.

The TAPP procedure represents an amalgamation of the principles of conventional preperitoneal repair and minimally invasive surgery. The preperitoneal mesh uses the forces available within the abdomen to keep the mesh sandwiched between the layers of the abdomen. It is very difficult to dislodge a mesh in the preperitoneal space, as the intra abdominal pressure is exerted uniformly over the entire prosthesis thereby helping to fix it. Any increase in the intraabdominal pressure forces the prosthesis against the potentially defective area, guarding against herniation. This is in contrast to the anteriorly placed meshes (Lichtenstein) where the increase in the abdominal pressure during straining forces the mesh away from the defect. With more than a decade of laparoscopic preperitoneal repairs the experiences have consolidated, the learning curves stabilized, recurrence rates reduced and the complications diminished.[8]

INDICATIONS

The TAPP approach can be performed in almost all types of inguinofemoral hernia depending on the level of expertise of the surgeon.

1. Any type of groin hernia
   - Direct
   - Indirect
   - Bilateral
   - Recurrent
   - Femoral hernia

RELATIVE CONTRAINDICATIONS

1. Prior laparoscopic hernia repair on the same side
   - Although some experts suggest that such a recurrence can be successfully repaired by the TAPP procedure, it is considerably more difficult than a primary repair. This is certainly dependent on the experience of the surgeon and the desire of the patient.

2. Prior pelvic lymph node dissection or other pelvic surgeries like radical prostatectomy.

3. Prior groin irradiation or other inflammatory process.

4. Very large scrotal hernia:
   - Injury to the bowel or omentum is possible while attempting reduction. If laparoscopy is attempted, the TAPP approach may be safer.

5. Small congenital hernias (Nyhus-I)
   - For which mesh is not required.

6. Morbid obesity.

- However, the potential of more rapid mobilization may be advantageous to such patients. After gaining adequate experience in laparoscopic surgery, it is more preferable than open approach.

ABSOLUTE CONTRAINDICATIONS

1. Patients unsuitable for general anaesthesia:
   - Although local and epidural anaesthesia may be possible in some cases, the suitability for general anesthesia seems to be a prudent criteria. Those who are unable to tolerate this type of anaesthesia may not be able to benefit from the purported advantages of laparoscopic hernioplasty.

2. Active infection or inflammatory process:
   - eg. peritonitis. It would have a deleterious complication such as infection of the mesh.

3. An incarcerated hernia.
   - Diagnostic laparoscopy and a gentle attempt at reduction can be considered. This should allow for the assessment of the entrapped viscera. However the risk of perforation should confine this effort only to the most experienced surgeons.

4. Large irreducible long standing scrotal hernia (scrotal abdomen)

ADVANTAGES OF TAPP OVER TEP

1. Assessment of hernial defect and recognition of important landmarks during dissection is easier, particularly for beginners.

2. Adhesion between the omentum, intestine and the sac can be released without injuring the structures.

3. Even patients with irreducible hernias can be managed with ease in TAPP approach.

4. Sliding Hernia can be recognized immediately and dissection performed safely.

5. Control of bleeding is possible without injuring the adherent intestinal wall.

6. It is possible to combine this procedure with diagnostic laparoscopy and other surgeries like cholecystectomy

TRANS ABDOMINAL PRE PERITONEAL HERNIOPLASTY (TAPP)

Operative Room Setup

The patient is in supine position with arms by the side. The position of the surgeon is initially to the left side of the patient during creation of pneumoperitoneum and placement of trocars. Then the surgeon moves to the head end and stands on the right side while the camera assistant stands on the left side. The patient is given 10 degree head down position at this time to allow the bowel loops to fall away from the groin region. The position of the surgeon and the camera assistant is always on the same position regardless of the side of the hernia. In contrast to the other reports of changing position of the surgeons depending on the side of the hernia,

I find this approach very effective and comfortable. The scrub nurse usually stands on the right side of the patient along with the laparoscopic trolley. The monitor is placed at the foot end of the patient.

Instruments required

30 degree 10 mm telescope, Veress needle , one 10 mm trocar, two 5 mm trocars, holding forceps, Maryland dissector, scissors, 10 mm to 5 mm reducing sleeve, 5 mm needle holder, electrosurgical apparatus- monopolar/bipolar, 15 x12 cm prolene mesh, conventional suture materials- 1-0 prolene, 3-0 vicryl.

We find the use of 10 mm, 30 degree telescope more helpful than the 0 degree scope, as we can visualize the anterior layers such as the rectus muscle, peritoneum clearly. The important aspect that has to be kept in mind during the selection of the scope is the experience of the camera assistant. 30 degree scope demands basic familiarity in laparoscopy to assist the surgeon during advanced laparoscopic surgeries.

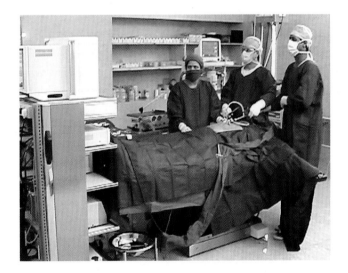

Figure 1 : Team Setup. The surgeon stands on the left side of the patient for creation of pneumoperitoneum and ports. Subsequently the surgeon moves to the head end of the patient with the camera assistant on left side. The staff nurse stands on the right side with the monitor at the foot end of the patient.

If a surgeon is operating alone with the help of trainees who stay in the department for a short time, then 0 degree scope will be a better option.

Operative Technique

Pneumoperitoneum

1. Umbilical Puncture By Veress Needle

In the absence of operative scar, periumbilical site (thinnest site) is the most preferred site for Veress needle insertion. Depending on the shape of umbilicus either transverse or vertical stab is made with a 15 size or 11 sized knife. By lifting the abdominal wall midway between the pubic symphysis and umbilicus by the non-dominant left hand as shown in the Figure 2, the Veress needle is inserted perpendicular to the abdomen with a slight degree of tilt so that tip of the needle faces the pelvis. The needle should be held by the right hand on the shaft, keeping the distal length just adequate for the tip to pierce the full thickness wall of the abdomen.

Aspiration test is used to confirm the position of the needle in the abdominal cavity.[9,10] Five ml of saline is injected through the Veress and aspirated. If aspiration does not yield the injected solution, then

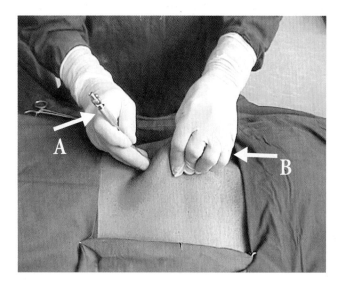

Figure 2 : Method of insertion of Veress needle

A - Needle direction towards pelvis
B - Abdominal wall lifted by left hand

the position of the needle in the peritoneal cavity is confirmed. If the saline is aspirated back into the syringe then it indicates that the needle is within the layers of the abdominal wall or the presence of adhesions.

In patients who had undergone surgeries before, we prefer insertion of the Veress needle in either Right or Left hypochondrium (Palmer's point) for creation of pneumoperitoneum. We routinely use 3 mm scope initially through the first port and under vision we create the umbilical port, subsequently changing the scope to 10 mm. The epigastric and the right iliac fossa are the other sites for needle insertion.

After creating the pneumoperitoneum with Veress needle, 1 cm transverse or vertical incision according to the shape of the umbilicus is made and the camera trocar is inserted. The 10 mm pyramidal trocar with the obturator is inserted into the abdominal cavity by rotational movements, keeping the abdominal wall under tension to avoid slipping on the fascia. By this technique, inadvertent injury to the intestines or vessels can be prevented. We found this technique useful in almost in all the cases.

2. Open Laparoscopy Technique

We rarely use the technique of open access by Hasson cannula that has been advocated to decrease the incidence of injuries associated with the blind introduction of the Veress needle and initial trocar. Hasson proposed a blunt minilaparotomy access called open Hasson's Technique. Hasson's open access device has an olive sleeve that slides up and down the shaft of the canula to allow for the variation in the abdominal wall thickness. The trocar is held in place by the stay sutures that are placed through the fascial edges and attached to the body of the cannula. These cannulas are available as both reusable and disposable ones. Injuries following the use of Hasson Cannula has also been reported.[11,12]

An infraumbilical incision (1-3 cm) is made and the subcutaneous tissue is bluntly dissected and retracted.[13,14] Two clamps are used to lift the line alba and a horizontal or vertical incision of about 1.5 cm is made. The preperitoneal fat is dissected and the peritoneum is incised after lifting it with a hemostat. Excessive dissection in the preperitoneal space should be discouraged, as the peritoneum falls away from the fascia and the surgeon feels lost in this plane. Two absorbable sutures, preferably Vicryl are placed on either side of the fascial defect. The Hasson's cannula with the blunt obturator is advanced into the peritoneal cavity until the olive abuts the fascia. The obturator is removed and the sutures are secured firmly to create a seal. The laparoscope is then introduced.

Port Placement

We place the camera port in the umbilicus in majority of the patients and the two working trocars just lateral to rectus sheath on either side of umbilicus, few cms below the camera port. 5 mm ports are sufficient for mesh fixation by suturing or by fixation devices such as tackers (USSC) or anchors (Ethicon endo surgery). If stapler fixation is planned, a 12 mm port is placed on the ipsilateral side of hernia. In the first few years many centres including our institute were using staplers for fixation. Since 1995 we have discontinued the practice of hernia stapler.

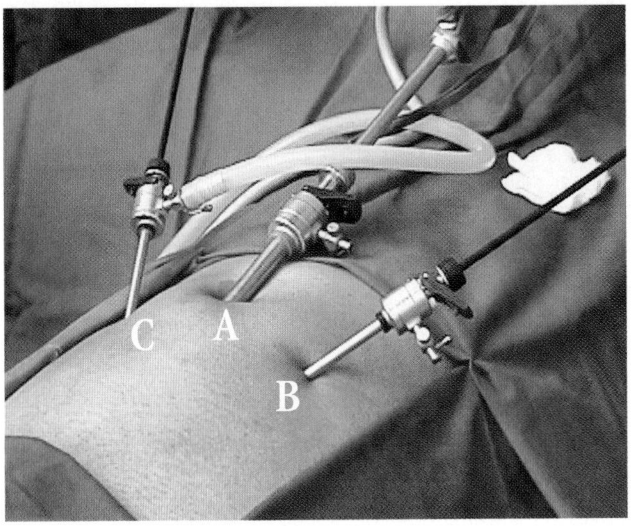

Figure 3 : Position of Ports

A - Umbilical 10 mm camera port (in case of low placed umbilicus, the camera port can be shifted to supra umbilical position)

B - Left pararectus 5 mm left hand working port

C - Right pararectus 5 mm right hand working port

We do not use tacker due to high costs involved. More over endosuturing is highly effective and has fewer side effects. In patients with low placed umbilicus, it is preferable to place the camera port in supra umbilical position. This aids in better visualization of the inguinal region without interference with the working instruments.

Reduction of contents

When the scope is directed towards the groin the hernial defect is immediately identified without any difficulty. In certain situations the small bowel, omentum or colon is seen hanging from the abdominal wall. The contents of the sac are gently pulled into the abdominal cavity. In some patients the medial ligament is well developed and obstructs the field of vision during surgery. In these situations it is advisable to retract the ligament medially by a percutaneous silk stitch on the peritoneum.

Peritoneal incision

A peritoneal flap is created by a horizontal incision 2 cm above the defect extending from the medial umbilical ligament to the level of anterior superior iliac spine. The incision is curved down like a hockey stick on the lateral aspect. The dissection is continued downwards beyond the ilio pubic tract by raising a flap of peritoneum. Peritoneal incision should not be extended medial to the medial umbilical ligament as this might result in increased incidence of bleeding from the perivesical plexus of vessels and patent umbilical vessels. Dissection of the entire Hasselbach's triangle and the retro pubic space can be performed easily even without medial extension of the peritoneal incision.

Medial Dissection

Dissection of direct hernias is relatively an easy task. The thinned out transversalis fascia termed as pseudosac, can be readily identified by its glistening appearance. The peritoneum and the preperitoneal fat can be easily separated from this pseudosac by gentle traction with the left hand, while the right hand instrument pushes the pseudosac away from the peritoneum. Sharp dissection in this area in an attempt to resect the pseudosac will produce troublesome bleeding.

The dissection should reach the pubic symphysis on the midline. This dissection is useful for identification of a supra symphytic defect in a recurrent hernia and to create a wider space for wrinkle free placement of the mesh. The dissection is restricted to the areolar tissue in order to avoid injury to the bladder, particularly in cases of large direct hernia which might be associated with a sliding component with bladder as its content. In such cases the bladder wall should be carefully retracted by the left hand.

Dissection should always be performed in the avascular, cobweb like areolar tissue. The two handed dissection with active assistance from the left hand is essential for a proper dissection of the preperitoneal space. The right hand instrument is used to dissect the preperitoneal fatty tissue away from the abdominal muscles, while the left hand grasper maintains traction on the peritoneal flap. Very few blood vessels may be encountered during this maneuver. The peritoneal and sub peritoneal blood vessels are coagulated immediately with monopolar cautery, to maintain a clear operative field.

Early identification of certain anatomical structures at this stage is considered vital for safe completion of the surgery. Epigastric vessels, symphysis pubis, pubic ramus and Cooper's ligament are the important structures that require prompt recognition. Care is taken during dissection beneath the iliopubic tract to avoid injury to nerves (Triangle of Pain) and vessels (Triangle of Doom).

The abnormal obturator artery and vein with many collaterals in this region should be protected from injury. The obturator foramen and its contents are identified. This forms the inferior limit of the dissection. The bladder should be continuously drained by an indwelling catheter (particularly in patients with previous surgery, prostatism or irradiation) to prevent accidental injury.

Lateral Dissection

The dissection in the lateral compartment is more challenging as the sac is densely adherent to the cord structures in long standing hernias. The operating table is tilted towards the surgeon, to relieve the arm working at the level of the lateral trocar. (eg. mild Right lateral tilt in right sided hernia). The hernial

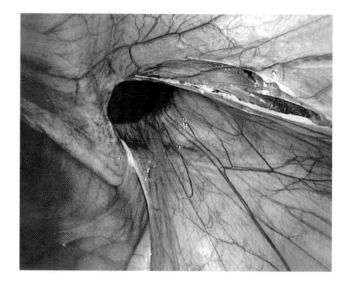

Figure 4 : Peritoneal incision above the defect. Wide internal ring with medial displacement of inferior epigastric vessels and lateral umbilical ligament.

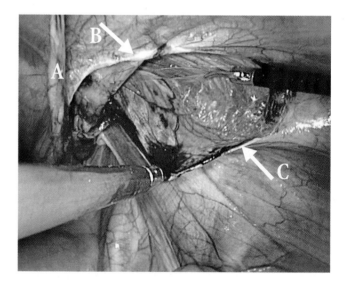

Figure 5 : Completion of peritoneal incision

A - Medial umbilical ligament
B - Superior flap
C - Inferior flap

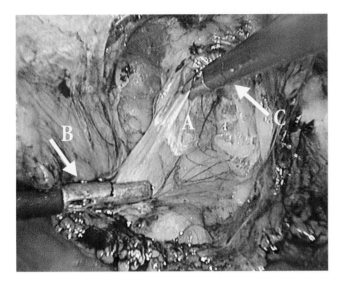

Figure 6 : Medial dissection in direct hernia - Separation of pseudo sac

A - Transversalis fascia (pseudo sac)

B - Traction on the peritoneum with the left hand grasper

C - Counter traction on pseudosac by right hand instrument

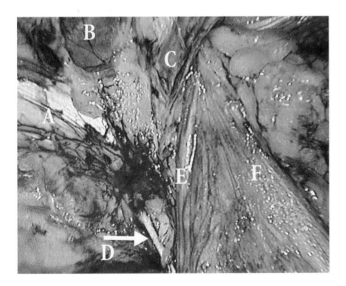

Figure 7 : After completion of medial dissection

A - Right pubic ramus

B - Direct defect

C - Inferior epigastric vessels

D - Obturator vessels

E - Vas deferens

F - Testicular vessels

sac should be dissected   close to the peritoneal flap. The relationship of the hernial sac and cord structures is usually constant. The hernial sac is usually present above and lateral to the spermatic cord. At the level of the deep ring the vas deferens curves medially over the iliac vessels after emerging out of the pelvis. The testicular vessels are located on the lateral aspect. The transversalis sling separates the sac and the inferior epigastric vessels. Injury to inferior epigastric vessels can be prevented if the dissection (during separation of the sac from the cord structures) is not continued medially beyond the level of the transversalis sling. Similarly, injury to cord structures can be prevented if the separation of the sac is performed on the upper half of the internal inguinal ring, as the cord structures are usually present on the inferior aspect. Simultaneous traction and application of short bursts of electrocautery helps in severing the dense adhesions between the sac and the cord structures.

Small indirect sacs can be easily dissected out completely into the peritoneal cavity. The sac is separated by a combination of blunt and sharp dissection along with electro coagulation. In cases of longer sac, the dissection is continued distally into the inguinal canal after creating a window between the sac and cord structures. In these cases, it might need a strong tug with the left grasper to separate the sac from its attachments in the inguinal canal. The dissection should be confined close to the hernial sac. For larger sacs extending deep into the scrotum, particularly congenital type, complete mobilization of the sac is more traumatic and chances of injury to cord structures are increased. In these situations, hernial sac is divided beyond the internal ring within the canal, leaving the distal end of the sac in situ. The proximal sac is separated from the cord structures, high ligation performed at the neck by endoloop ligation and excess sac is excised. In our experience of 275 scrotal hernias, we could dissect out the entire sac in 260 patients without injuring the testicular vessels or creating extensive hematoma.

Apart from the structures visualized during medial dissection, laterally placed structures like ilio pubic tract, Triangle of Doom and Triangle of Pain are

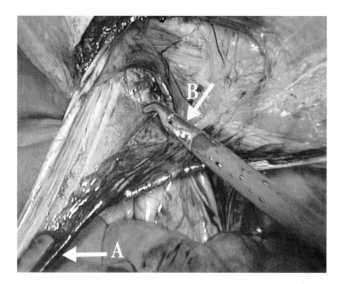

Figure 8 : Lateral dissection : Indirect hernia

A - Traction of hernial sac by left hand grasper

B - Cord structures pushed by right hand dissector

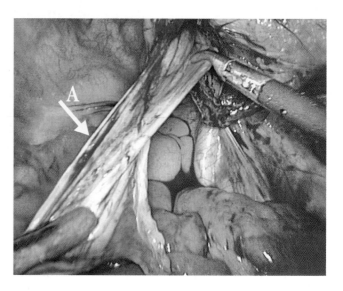

Figure 9 : Dissection of sac that extends into the inguinal canal

A - Sac

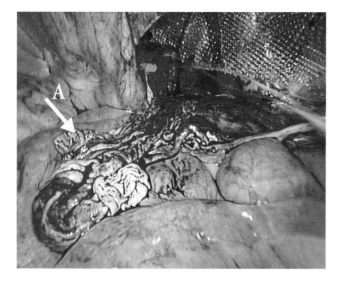

Figure 10 : Completion of dissection with entire sac lying in the peritoneal cavity

A - Separated sac

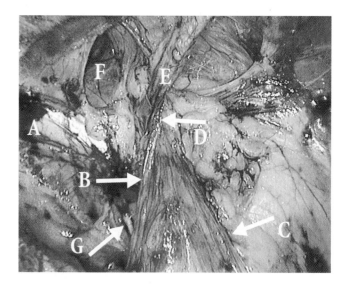

Figure 11 : After completion of medial and lateral dissection

A - Right pubic ramus

B - Vas deferens

C - Spermatic vessels

D - Internal ring

E - Inferior epigastric vessels

F - Direct defect

G - Obturator vessels

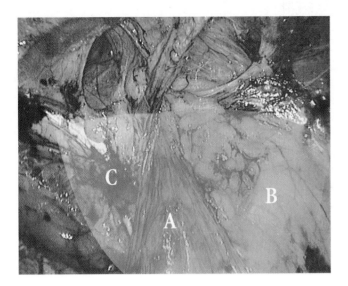

Figure 12 : Extended Square of doom - GEM

A - Triangle of doom
B - Triangle of pain
C - Circle of death

also exposed during this dissection. It is desirable to retain the preperitoneal fat along with the peritoneum and continue the dissection just underneath the fascia and visible muscle fibres. Any bleeding that obscures the vision must be immediately coagulated to the maintain the clarity of the visual field. Monopolar or bipolar cautery may be used minimally as these pose risk of injury to nerves and vas deferens.

Parietalisation

Once the hernial sac is reduced or divided, the peritoneum is separated from the vas and gonadal vessels towards the cranial aspect. This procedure is known as parietalisation. The parietalisation is carried out as far as the middle of the psoas muscle so that the peritoneum is no longer in contact with vas deferens or the vessels in the inguinal region. Extensive parietalisation is important to position the currently recommended larger sized (15 x12 cm) unslit mesh. Inadequate mobilization leads to displacement and folding of the mesh and eventually

to recurrence. The dissection should be atleast 1-2 cm beyond the edges of the mesh on all sides.

Extent of Dissection

Before placement of the mesh flap should be lifted and the extent of dissection verified. The dissected space should extend beyond the midline on the medial aspect, beyond the anterior superior iliac spine exposing the psoas muscle on the lateral aspect, inferiorly up to the symphysis pubis and the level of obturator foramen and superiorly up to the level of working trocars. The peritoneum should be free from the vas deferens and testicular vessels. This wide dissection is needed to ensure problem free placement a 15 x12 cm mesh.

Placement of Mesh

The corners of the mesh are trimmed and the lateral ends narrowed to accommodate the space beyond the internal ring. 15 X 12 cm sized prolene mesh adequately covers the entire dissected area reinforcing the myopectineal orifice. Various methods have been described to introduce the mesh into the peritoneal cavity. The usual practice is to roll the mesh and tie it with a suture to maintain it in the rolled position. This is then taken through the trocars and the stitch is removed once the mesh is inside the abdomen. In practice we found that it was very cumbersome to unroll the mesh in the dissected space. We routinely fold the mesh, which is very similar to the practice of folding plantain leaves in the villages of India. These leaves are traditionally used as disposable plates for eating.

The folded mesh is reverse loaded into 10-5 mm reducer after trimming the edges. The laparoscope is withdrawn and the mesh is taken into the abdominal cavity by blind insertion through the 10 mm trocar. Once inside the dissected space, the mesh most often unfolds by itself and spreading of the mesh becomes much easier. To avoid unnecessary manipulation of the mesh inside the preperitoneal space, it is advisable to place the narrow end of the mesh on the lateral side. The mesh is positioned to cover the entire myopectineal orifice of Fruchaud (direct, indirect and femoral defects).

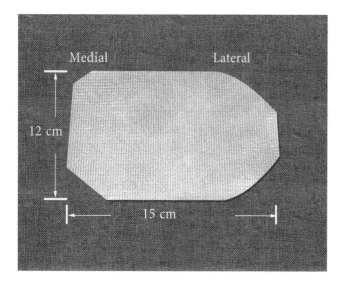

Figure 13 : Size of the mesh for right side hernia (Trimmed edges of the mesh is oriented towards the lateral inguinal hernia. Lower border of the medial side the mesh is trimmed to prevent covering over the bladder)

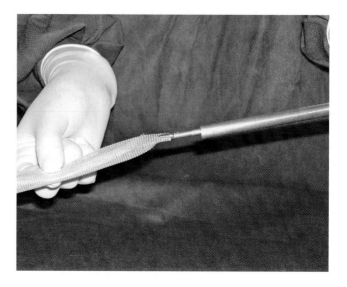

Figure 14 : Reverse loading of the mesh into a 10-5 mm reducing sleeve with a needle holder

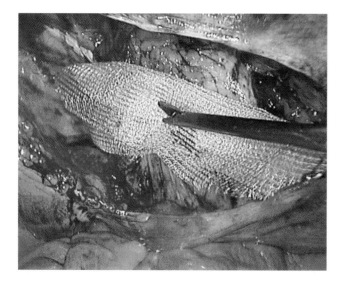

Figure 15 : Mesh kept over the dissected area (before unfolding)

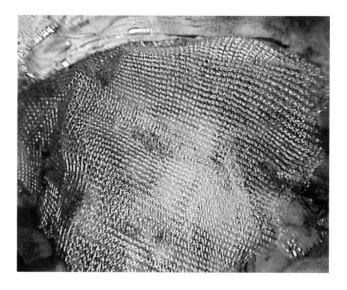

Figure 16 : Unfolded mesh covering the entire dissected area

Fixation of mesh

We prefer to fix the mesh with intracorporeal suturing with 1-0 prolene.[15] The conventional needle of 1-0 prolene is slightly straightened, reverse loaded on to a 10-5 mm reducer and introduced into the abdomen like the introduction of mesh. The mesh is fixed to the Cooper's ligament inferiorly and to the rectus muscle on the superomedial aspect of the mesh, medial to the inferior epigastric vessels. Before fixing to the Cooper's ligament, the dangerous area of Corona mortis should always be carefully inspected. Apart from these areas, we do not fix the mesh on the lateral aspect. As the area of Triangle of Doom and Triangle of Pain are totally avoided, the incidence of vascular injuries and neuralgias are negligible following this approach.

Alternatively the mesh can be fixed by the mechanical fixation devices such as hernia stapler (12 mm),[16] tacker (5 mm)[17] and anchors (5 mm). We prefer suturing as it is more effective and reduces the cost of surgery. Stapling, suturing or any other form of fixation lateral to the cord structures and below the iliopubic tract (Triangle of Pain) is contraindicated. Such procedures have shown to produce higher incidence of neuralgias.

Peritoneal closure

After the placement of the mesh the peritoneum is sutured over the mesh to prevent adhesions of bowel or omentum. The peritoneal flap can be closed either by suturing or with the help of hernia staplers or tackers. Suturing of the peritoneum completely closes the flap without any gap. We prefer to suture the flaps. More effective peritoneal closure is facilitated by reducing pneumoperitoneum to 8 mm Hg at this stage. We routinely close the peritoneum with continuous suture using 2-0 vicryl. This technique has helped me to master the art of endo suturing. Richter's types of hernia can occur if the flaps are closed improperly by leaving gaps in between during the use of staplers. A long acting local anaesthetic can be injected into the peritoneal space at this stage to reduce postoperative discomfort.

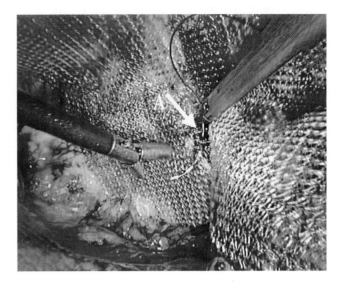

Figure 17 : Fixation of the mesh to the Cooper's ligament

A - Stitch to the Cooper's Ligament

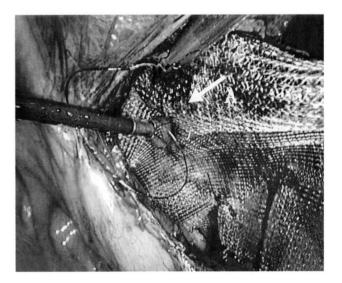

Figure 18 : Fixation of the mesh to the inferior surface of rectus muscle

A - Needle crossing the rectus muscle

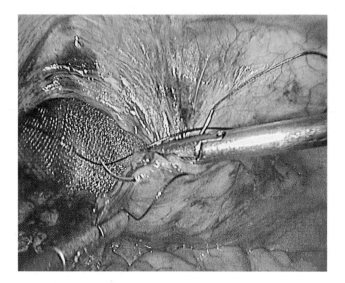

Figure 19 : Closure of peritoneal flap using continuous vicryl sutures

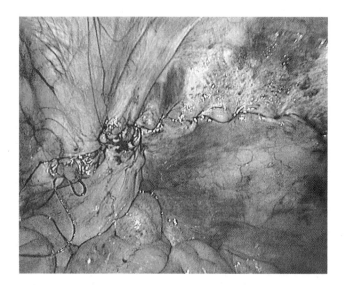

Figure 20 : Completion of peritoneal closure

The working trocars are removed under direct vision. The bleeding vessels near the ports can be controlled by cautery or by port closure technique. The 5 mm trocar sites are closed with subcuticular sutures with 3-0 vicryl. The camera port requires closure of the rectus sheath separately before closing the skin to prevent trocar site herniation.

In case of large scrotal hernias, a closed suction drain is kept through a separate stab incision at the route of the scrotum. A 5 mm trocar is introduced into the peritoneal cavity through the sac or the dissected space from the scrotum. A suction drain is introduced through the trocar and is positioned between the mesh and the abdominal wall. The drain is usually removed after 2-3 days.

DISCUSSION

The two major controversies regarding the prosthesis in laparoscopic hernia repair are the fixation of the mesh and avoidance of splitting of the mesh.

Slitting of mesh

Recurrence through the area of the slit (due to loss of integrity of the mesh), increased risk of injury to the testicular vessels and testicular atrophy are the main disadvantages of slitting of the mesh. Injury to the iliac vessels may occur during dissection posterior to the cord structures in this region. It is dangerous to dissect with electro cautery. More over, the cord structures can get incorporated into the scar tissue that forms around the internal ring.[18] We no longer recommend slitting of the mesh. In our method, we do not dissect posterior to the vas or the testicular vessels and hence these complications are not encountered in our series.

Fixation of the mesh

Fixation of the prosthesis represents a major ongoing controversy. Fixation or anchoring of the mesh to multiple areas was the recommended procedure when these repairs were introduced. There were multitudes of reports of nerve injuries, vascular injuries due to indiscriminate use of fixation devices in all areas.[20] The concept of Stoppa's repair in open preperitoneal approaches produced successful results without fixation. The large increase in the abdominal pressure helps to keep the mesh in place between the layers of abdominal wall.[19] There was no significant movement of mesh which was studied postoperatively at 1, 7, 28 days & 3 months after laparoscopic hernia repair.[20] Various trials have shown that there are no differences in the recurrence rates of stapled versus non stapled mesh repairs.[18,19,21] Other authors focus on lack of fixation as major cause for recurrence.[22,23] Application of numerous staplers/tackers rises the chances for vascular & nerve damage, whereas fixation at selective few points allows the mesh to adapt to the contours of the abdominal wall in a more satisfactory manner.

The major argument for fixation is the potential prosthetic migration or roll up or dislodgment of the mesh. In keeping a large sized mesh without fixation, patient can develop a large fibrous mass, which can be felt in the inguinal region particularly following surgery for a large direct sac. The arguments against fixation are the risk of injuries and the cost reduction without compromising on the recurrence. Though this debate is to continue till more clear results are published, at present majority agree that the fixation should be reduced to as minimum as possible.

The laparoscopic hernia repair has undergone significant changes from its initial description of closure of internal ring to the recent versions of TAPP & TEP. The advantages of the laparoscopic hernia repair have been highlighted previously. The potential disadvantages are those related to laparoscopy such as bowel perforation, breach of peritoneum, adhesive complications, need for general anesthesia

We have discussed the relevant practical aspects of the technique of laparoscopic inguinal hernia repair (TAPP and TEP) in this book. The readers are advised to refer the "Operative manual of laparoscopic hernia surgery" written by the author for a detailed description of the various types of hernias, their anatomy, types of laparoscopic repair and a more comprehensive review of the current literature on laparoscopic management of hernia.

and increased cost due to expensive equipment. Several studies comparing TAPP to mesh repairs and non mesh repairs have shown consistent benefits in several parameters studied such as decreased pain and analgesic requirements, faster return to work and improved quality of life.

CONCLUSION

TAPP is more widely used because of its relative ease to learn this technique. Invasion into the peritoneal space for treatment of defect in the abdominal wall is one of the major drawbacks of this technique. The peritoneal incision and its closure might increase the chances of postoperative adhesions and small bowel obstruction. Insufficient closure of this incision will lead to formation of internal hernias with its antecedent complications. The size of the mesh which is kept inside is comparatively smaller than in TEP procedure. As documented by various studies this smaller mesh might produce increased recurrence rates. Because of these concerns, laparoscopic surgeons are now switching to TEP repair. A surgeon who is interested in performing laparoscopic hernia repair should begin with TAPP approach, as the inguinal anatomy is less complex and easy to learn in the initial period. With adequate number of cases the surgeon will be more confident in performing extra peritoneal approach. Still TAPP will remain as an ideal approach for management of difficult inguinal hernias such as incarcerated hernias, sliding hernias and other complex hernias.

References

1. Ger R. The management of certain abdominal herniae by intra-abdominal closure of the neck of the sac. Preliminary communication. Ann R Coll Surg Engl 1982;64:342-4.

2. Fitzgibbons RJ, Jr., Camps J, Cornet DA, Nguyen NX, Litke BS, Annibali R, Salerno GM. Laparoscopic inguinal herniorrhaphy. Results of a multicenter trial. Ann Surg 1995;221:3-13.

3. Vogt DM, Curet MJ, Pitcher DE, Martin DT, Zucker KA. Preliminary results of a prospective randomized trial of laparoscopic onlay versus conventional inguinal herniorrhaphy. Am J Surg 1995;169:84-9; discussion 89-90.

4. Cheatle G. An operation for the radical cure of inguinal and femoral hernia. Br Med J 1920;2.

5. Henry A. Operation for femoral hernia by midline extraperitoneal approach: with a preliminary note of the use of

this route for reducible inguinal hernia. Lancet 1936:531-533.

6. McEvedy P. Femoral hernia. Ann R Coll Surg. 1950;7:484-496.

7. Arregui ME, Davis CJ, Yucel O, Nagan RF. Laparoscopic mesh repair of inguinal hernia using a preperitoneal approach: a preliminary report. Surg Laparosc Endosc 1992;2:53-8.

8. Felix EL, Harbertson N, Vartanian S. Laparoscopic hernioplasty: significant complications. Surg Endosc 1999;13:328-31.

9. Palanivelu C. Laparoscopic Space Access. In: Palanivelu C, ed. CIGES Atlas of Laparoscopic Surgery. Second ed. New Delhi: Jaypee Brothers Medical Publishers Pvt. Ltd, 2003:11-16.

10. Palanivelu C. Laparoscopic Space Access and Physiological Significance. In: Palanivelu C, ed. Text Book of Surgical Laparoscopy. Coimbatore: Gem Digestive Diseases Foundation, 2002:31-39.

11. Voitk A, Rizoli S. Blunt hasson trocar injury: long intra-abdominal trocar and lean patient-a dangerous combination. J Laparoendosc Adv Surg Tech A 2001;11:259-62.

12. Hanney RM, Carmalt HL, Merrett N, Tait N. Use of the Hasson cannula producing major vascular injury at laparoscopy. SurgEndosc 1999;13:1238-40.

13. Palanivelu C. Laparoscopic Trans Abdominal Pre Peritoneal Hernioplasty. In: Palanivelu C, ed. Text Book of Surgical Laparoscopy. Coimbatore: Gem Digestive Diseases Foundation, 2002:227-236.

14. Palanivelu C. Laparoscopic Transabdominal Preperitoneal Hernioplasty (TAPP). In: Palanivelu C, ed. CIGES Atlas of Laparoscopic Surgery. Second ed. New Delhi: Jaypee Brothers Medical Publishers Pvt. Ltd, 2003:91-96.

15. Palanivelu C, Rajan PS, Sendhilkumar K, Parthasarathi R. Results of Hand Sutured Laparoscopic Hernioplasty : Effective method of Repair. Surg Endosc 1998;12:596.

16. Smith AI, Royston CM, Sedman PC. Stapled and nonstapled laparoscopic transabdominal preperitoneal (TAPP) inguinal hernia repair. A prospective randomized trial. Surg Endosc 1999;13:804-6.

17. Douglas JM, Young WN, Jones DB. Lichtenstein inguinal herniorrhaphy using sutures versus tacks. Hernia 2002;6:99-101.

18. Davis CJ, Arregui ME. Laparoscopic repair for groin hernias. Surg Clin North Am 2003;83:1141-61.

19. Stoppa RE. The treatment of complicated groin and incisional hernias. World J Surg 1989;13:545-54.

20. Irving S. Does the mesh Move after TAPP hernia Repair. Minimal Invasice ther;4:54.

21. Khajanchee YS, Urbach DR, Swanstrom LL, Hansen PD. Outcomes of laparoscopic herniorrhaphy without fixation of mesh to the abdominal wall. Surg Endosc 2001;15:1102-7.

22. Tetik C, Arregui ME, Dulucq JL, Fitzgibbons RJ, Franklin ME, McKernan JB, Rosin RD, Schultz LS, Toy FK. Complications and recurrences associated with laparoscopic repair of groin hernias. A multi-institutional retrospective analysis. Surg Endosc 1994;8:1316-22; discussion 1322-3.

23. Felix EL. A unified approach to recurrent laparoscopic hernia repairs. Surg Endosc 2001;15:969-71.

71

Laparoscopic Totally Extraperitoneal Hernioplasty (TEP)

INTRODUCTION

The revolutionary success of laparoscopic cholecystectomy, has resulted in an intense effort to apply this concept of minimally invasive surgery to other operative procedures like inguinal hernia. The laparoscopic hernia surgery was initially a controversial topic with various studies publishing contradictory results. Unfortunately the initial enthusiasm in laparoscopic herniorrhaphy, was met with a disappointing early recurrence rate, which was as high as 25% in some series.[1,2] But now with a decade of experience in lap hernia surgery, the dust seems to be settling down more towards accepting the superiority of the laparoscopic repairs over conventional repairs. This is mainly due to the proper understanding of endoscopic inguinal anatomy, effacement of initial procedures like plug and patch technique, refinement of the techniques, introduction of the preperitoneal placement of mesh etc.

Laparoscopic hernioplasty has several advantages over its "open" counter parts. First and foremost aspect from the patients point of view is the reduced post operative pain and short recovery period.[3,4,5] Second, the entire myopectineal orifice can be inspected, allowing for repair of any unexpected hernias thereby reducing the chance for recurrence. Third, laparoscopic hernioplasty avoids the previous operative scar site in patients with recurrent hernias.[6-11] The disadvantages of laparoscopic repair include the need for general anesthesia, the breach of peritoneum in TAPP repairs and the cost of the procedure. The most vital factor to be kept in mind before a general surgeon opts to treat his patients through laparoscopy is the difficult and prolonged learning curve, in order to perform the procedure in a safe and efficient manner.[12,13,14,15]

Totally extraperitoneal laparoscopic hernioplasty is the minimally invasive approach equivalent to the open preperitoneal approach of groin hernia repair. It potentially offers several advantages over TAPP. It eliminates the complications related to violation of the peritoneal layer to reach the preperitoneal space and reduces the operative time especially for bilateral hernias.[12]

To start with, TAPP may be a better approach to gain adequate working knowledge and understanding of the inguinal anatomy. After adequate experience, if one proceeds to adopt TEP the learning curve can be minimized. Disappointments and failures may be reduced to a major extent.

INDICATIONS

A surgeon must be experienced in conventional anterior approaches as well as both laparoscopic approaches (TAPP and TEP) in order to make a rational decision in selecting the appropriate hernioplasty for an individual. For most patients we prefer TEP approach because it avoids entry into the peritoneal cavity, requires less operative time and is associated with less complications when compared to TAPP. We choose TAPP in selected patients where TEP cannot be done like incarcerated hernia, very large scrotal hernia etc. For patients with chronic lower abdominal pain of unknown etiology who need diagnostic laparoscopy or who have undergone pelvic surgeries like radical prostatectomy and children are the candidates for TAPP approach.

The laparoscopic approach is ideal for recurrent hernias; whether TAPP or TEP approach should be dependent upon the expertise of the surgeon. The dissection of the recurrent hernial sac can be difficult using the TEP approach and requires more experience.

EXTRAPERITONEAL APPROACH

The extraperitoneal approach is made possible by the fact that the peritoneum in the suprapubic region can be easily separated from the anterior abdominal wall. This space can be enlarged to help in dissection of the hernial sac and insertion of mesh. Several techniques have been used to create this space eg. Phillips, McKernan and Dulucq's technique. Our approach is the posterior rectus sheath approach, where the trocar enters the plane between the rectus muscle and posterior rectus sheath just above the preperitoneal space. In Dulucq approach the preperitoneal space is created initially and the trocar is inserted directly into preperitoneal space. Another method is followed by Phillips, where pneumoperitoneum is created and the laparoscope is introduced into the

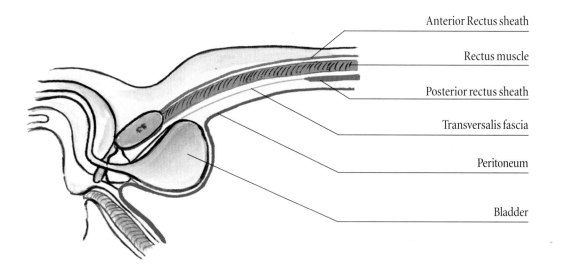

Figure 1 : Normal preperitoneal anatomy

Anterior Rectus sheath

Rectus muscle

Posterior rectus sheath

Transversalis fascia

Peritoneum

Bladder

peritoneal cavity. Under vision the 2 working ports are placed in the preperitoneal space. Subsequently the laparoscope is withdrawn and reintroduced into the preperitoneal space. After port placement the method of dissection remains the same in all approaches. In the following paragraphs we discuss these methods and the essential difference between them.

1. Phillips Technique (TEP with Peritoneoscopy)

Pneumoperitoneum is created initially and a 10 mm trocar is inserted through a subumbilical incision. The sites of the two working ports are marked lateral to the rectus muscle on either sides of the camera port. Saline or local anaesthetic solution is injected on the planned trocars sites to create a subperitoneal blister, under laparoscopic guidance. A 10 mm incision is made and a curved Kelly clamp is used to dissect through the muscle and transversalis fascia to reach the preperitoneal space. The entry of the clamp can be seen through the peritoneal layer. A 10 mm trocar is placed into this space and blunt instruments are introduced through the trocar. The preperitoneal space is widened by to and fro movements of the instrument. Insufflation of the space is done through the side channel of 10 mm port. Similar procedure is performed on the other side. Instruments in the preperitoneal space are seen through the thin layer of the peritoneum, as the laparoscope is in the abdominal cavity. The laparoscope and the cannula are withdrawn gradually till the peritoneum slips past the trocar tip and the preperitoneal fat is seen. The scope along with the cannula is slowly guided into the newly developed preperitoneal space.[16]

2. McKernan's Technique

This is a totally extraperitoneal approach without entering the peritoneal cavity. A two cm infraumbilical incision is created and the rectus sheath is exposed. The rectus sheath is lifted and incised vertically exposing the rectus muscles. Retractors are placed beneath the rectus muscle and a tunnel is developed between the rectus muscle and the underlying posterior rectus sheath. A 10 mm Hassons cannula is inserted into this tunnel and further space is created by blunt probing or by balloon dissector. The other working ports are placed in the midline

lower to the umbilical port. First 5 mm port is placed approximately one finger breadth above the pubis and second 10 mm trocar is placed half way between the pubis and the upper trocar. To cover the hernial defect, 7.5 x 12.5 cm mesh is fashioned with a slit to accommodate the cord structures.[16a]

3. Dulucq's Technique

In this approach the Veress needle is first inserted in the midline just above the pubis.[17] It penetrates the linea alba with slight resistance and enters the suprapubic space of Retzius. The CO_2 insufflation is started with the needle in this position. Free flow of CO_2 at the rate of one litre per minute indicates the correct position of the needle. After 0.5 - 1 litre gas is insufflated the needle is gently manipulated in various direction to allow the gas to increase the preperitoneal space. The insufflation is stopped after 1.5 liters of CO_2 had entered the space.

A 1 cm transverse or vertical subumbilical incision is made; 10 mm trocar is inserted in the subcutaneous plane in a horizontal direction. Then it is slowly lifted up and introduced at an angle of 60 degree towards the sacrum. The linea alba should be pierced at the level of arcuate line, a point roughly in level with the anterior superior iliac spine. The trocar pierces the linea alba to enter into the newly created preperitoneal space. The laparoscope is then introduced and the space is expanded by blunt dissection with 0° telescope. The cobweb areolar tissue is dissected by to and fro movements of telescope. The retro pubic space of Retzius and the space of Bogros are easily expanded by the telescopic approach. At this stage a 5 mm working trocar is made in the midline mid way between the camera port and symphysis pubis. Thereafter the preperitoneal space is widened by alternate sharp and blunt dissection under laparoscopic guidance. Second working trocar is placed either in the midline or in the midclavicular line on the side of hernia.

In this technique 15 x 12 cm mesh is used to reinforce the myopectineal orifice. Prof. Dulucq a gifted surgeon, who innovated this technique, has completed over 4000 hernias without any recurrence. I have witnessed his surgeries where he takes just 15-20 minutes for laparoscopic hernioplasty.

This technique is safe, easy and fast when performed by experienced laparoscopic surgeons. The difficult part of this operation is the needle placement, particularly in very thin patients with minimum preperitoneal fat.

4. Sub Fascial Approach

In this approach the linea alba below the umbilical is incised and a tunnel is made between the peritoneum and the linea alba with blunt dissection. The first trocar is placed in this space. Many surgeons do not recommend this approach due to the increased incidence of peritoneal laceration.

COMPARISON BETWEEN THE TECHNIQUES

A fundamental and important difference between our approach and Prof Dulucq is the plane of entry. The trocar in the Dulucq approach pierces the posterior lamina of the transversalis fascia (in midline) to enter the true preperitoneal space superficial to peritoneum. The entry into this space is at the level of the arcuate line. Further identification of the anatomy and dissection of the sac is much simpler with this approach. The difficulty is the insertion of the Veress needle in this correct plane which needs good experience.

In our approach the trocar is inserted into the space between the rectus muscle and posterior rectus sheath.[19,20] When compared to Dulucq's approach our trocar enters in a plane above the posterior lamina of the transversalis fascia more cranially, lateral to the linea alba. The preperitoneal space is then entered from this plane by dividing the posterior lamina of transversalis fascia.

The posterior lamina is attached to linea alba at the midline. This should be divided to enter the contra lateral side. There is no need for this maneuver in Dulucq's technique as the trocar enters deeper to the posterior lamina of transversalis fascia.

The preperitoneal space is more wider in our approach when compared to Dulucq's approach. This can be easily explained by the fact that the trocars enter more cranially in our approach (Our approach - Subumbilical, Dulucq approach - Arcuate line).

TOTALLY EXTRA PERITONEAL HERNIOPLASTY (TEP)

Instrumentation

TEP approach does not demand use of specialized instruments. Extraperitoneal space creation can be done comfortably with the blunt introduction of 10 mm laparoscope (0 degree). We use 0 degree scope for initial creation of space and then change to 30 degree scope for rest of the dissection. Some surgeons prefer a balloon dissector to create the space, but this is not mandatory. Two atraumatic graspers (one straight and one curved) are needed to perform the dissection. Endoloop sutures to ligate an indirect sac or a peritoneal tear are also needed. A suction irrigator will be needed to aspirate the blood if accidental laceration of vessels occurs. We have designed a unique retractor to facilitate the dissection and retraction of the rectus sheath and muscle. Two 5 mm trocars are used as working channels. Some use Hasson Cannula or balloon trocar to prevent gas leakage.[21] 5 mm anchors or tackers, depending on the surgeon's preference of mechanical fixation of the mesh are needed, but we prefer endo suturing using 1-0 polypropylene by Ethicon endoneedle holder. The prolene mesh is trimmed to 15x12 cm.

Operative Room Setup

With the patient in supine position, I start the procedure from the left side of the patient and introduce the subumbilical trocar. Then the 5 mm working port is created on the contralateral side of the hernia (eg. Right side hernia : first 5 mm port just to the left of mid line) and the preperitoneal space in the side of hernia dissected to create space for the placement of the next trocar. Further dissection and placement of the second trocar can be performed from the head end of the patient.

Operative Technique

Incision

We begin the procedure with a 12 mm subumbilical incision extending up to linea alba. The skin and subcutaneous tissue are retracted to the side of the hernia or to the dominant side (usually the right). The

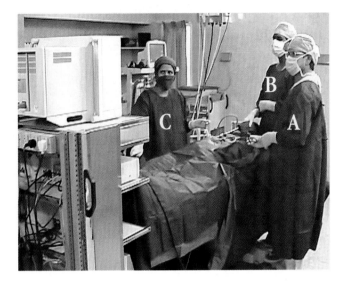

Figure 2 : Team Setup. Surgeon on the left side of the patient, assistant surgeon on the right side of the surgeon

A - Surgeon
B - Camera surgeon
C - Staff nurse

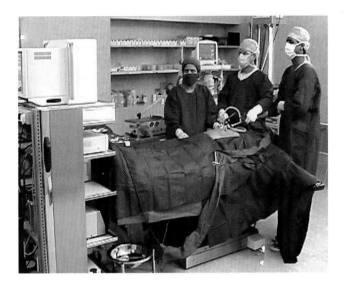

Figure 3 : Team Setup. Surgeon stands on right side of the head end of the patient, assisting surgeon on left side, staff nurse on right side of the surgeon and monitor in the foot end of the patient.

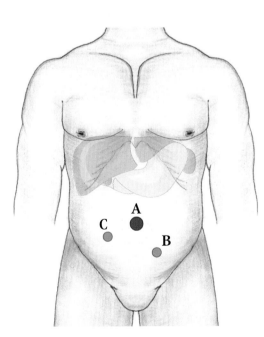

Figure 4 : Position of Ports for Right Inguinal Hernia

A - Subumbilical 10 mm optical port
B - 5 mm left hand working port just to the left of midline
C - Right pararectus 5 mm right hand working port

subcutaneous tissue is dissected carefully using Mayo's clamp to expose the anterior rectus sheath which is identified by its glistening appearance. The specially designed retractor helps to retract the subcutaneous tissue and fat. The small vessels in the subcutaneous tissue should not be torn during this dissection because bleeding in the area of incision will obscure the identification of rectus sheath. The anterior rectus sheath is incised transversely and it is separated with a curved hemostat to expose the rectus muscle. The entire rectus muscle is retracted to anterolateral side to enter the space between the muscle and posterior rectus sheath. The curved hemostat is inserted and the space is widened for introduction of the trocar. Many surgeons use finger dissection before introduction of the balloon in the preperitoneal space. The incidence of bleeding from tearing of the vessels is found to be high with the use of balloon dissector. We feel that use of balloon is not necessary and it also increases the cost of the surgery. The telescopic dissection with laparoscope is very effective in creation of extraperitoneal space.

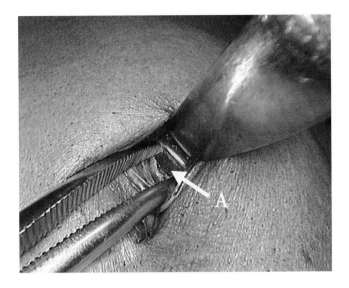

Figure 6 : Incision on the rectus saheath widened to expose rectus muscle

A - Rectus muscle

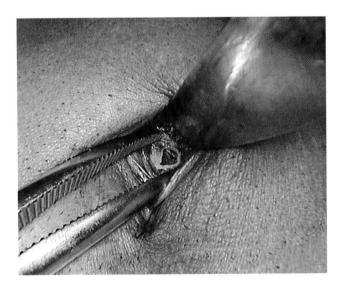

Figure 5 : Transverse incision in anterior rectus sheath

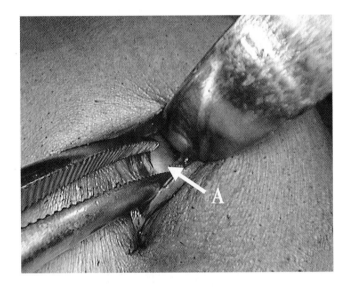

Figure 7 : Antero lateral retraction of Rectus muscle and exposure of extra peritoneal space

A - Posterior rectus sheath

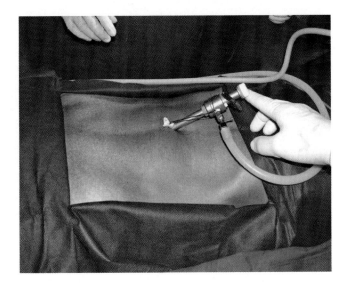

Figure 8 : Trocar in position. Wound is approximated with a silk suture with a wet gauze in between to prevent the gas leak. The same suture has been tied to the insufflation channel to prevent trocar slippage

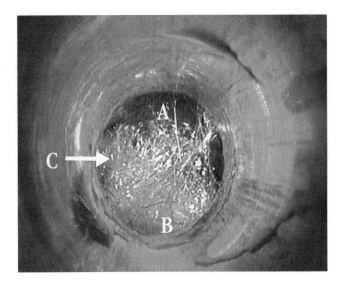

Figure 9 : Before creation of preperitoneal space

A - Inferior surface of rectus

B - Posterior rectus sheath

C - Cobweb appearance of areolar tissue

Placement of First Trocar

Keeping the rectus muscle retracted anteriorly and to the lateral side, the outer cannula of a 10 mm reusable trocar with its oblique end is carefully guided into the space between muscle and the rectus sheath. The wound is approximated with a thick suture material. A wet gauze is plugged between the suture and the wound to prevent leakage of gas. The same suture material is kept long and tied to the insufflation channel to prevent slippage of the trocar out of the incision.

Extra Peritoneal Dissection

A 10 mm telescope (0 degree) is introduced into the trocar. The scope is then moved downward on the sheath, allowing it to fall between the rectus muscle and the posterior rectus sheath. The telescope is moved forward and backward through the cobweb areolar tissue towards the pubic symphysis. These movements divides the transversalis fascia and the extraperitoneal space is entered. The dissected space is maintained by continuous CO_2 insufflation at 12-14 mm Hg. The space created is widened by moving the telescope at various directions.

Sweeping movement of the scope should be avoided below the arcuate, as injury to small vessels may cause bleeding in the preperitoneal space. This unnecessary bleeding causes further space creation difficult. The fascia transversalis can be identified by its attachment to the linea alba on the medial aspect. Once the space is created upto the pubis, the direction of the scope is turned laterally and the rectus muscle is displaced anteriorly by moving the scope on the posterior rectus sheath, upto to the attachment of rectus sheath on the lateral side. During this maneuver injury to the branch of the inferior epigastric vessel running over the sheath should be avoided. The dissection beyond midline is performed by dividing the ventral lamina of the transversalis fascia (fused with linea alba in midline). For unilateral hernias dissection upto 2-3 cms on the contralateral side of the midline is adequate.

In case of using balloons for extraperitoneal dissection, the following technique may be adopted. The balloon dissector is introduced posterior to the rectus muscle, upto the level of the pubis by

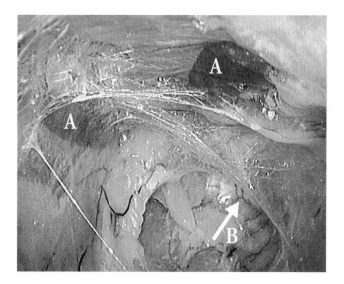

Figure 10 : Creation of preperitoneal space. Dissection in the midline using 0⁰ scope

A - Inferior surface of rectus
B - Right pubic ramus

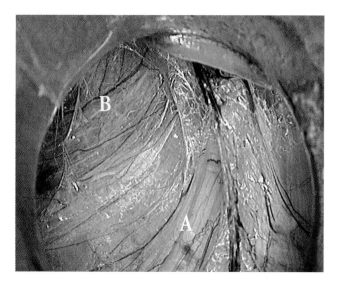

Figure 11 : Creation of preperitoneal space. Scope turned towards lateral direction

A - Posterior rectus sheath
B - Fascia transversalis

twisting motion. The tip is slightly elevated during this maneuver. The balloon should be directed towards midline to avoid injury to the epigastric vessels and inflated under vision. When the balloon is being inflated the Cooper's ligament, pubic bone, inferior epigastric vessels and the rectus muscle can be identified through the transparent balloon. Direct hernias can be completely reduced by balloon dissection alone. The transversalis fascia can be seen separating itself from the sac. The inferior epigastric vessels can be separated from the rectus muscle, particularly in older patients. This should be avoided by gentle introduction of the balloon trocar under vision. In cases of bilateral hernias, a bilateral (kidney shaped) balloon is used. This is introduced under the rectus muscle on the side with the larger hernia. We do not perform this technique mainly due to the costs involved. Moreover our technique of extraperitoneal space creation is easy to follow and the complete process can be completed within few minutes.

Creation of Working Ports

In case of right inguinal hernia the left hand working port is made just lateral to the midline about 5 cm below the level of the camera port. The extra peritoneal space is widened on the right lateral aspect and the right hand working port is placed on the right pararectus. In case of wide rectus muscle the lateral working port 5 mm is introduced in between the umbilicus and anterior superior iliac spine as laterally as possible (preferably just medial to the lateral rectus sheath fusion). The surgeon moves to the head end of the patient for the rest of the procedure.

The order of creation of port slightly differ in case of left sided hernias and bilateral hernias. For left inguinal hernia the right hand working port is created initially just to the right of the midline standing on the left side of the patient. The surgeon then moves to the head end for widening of the extraperitoneal space on the left side, creation of left hand working port and further dissection.

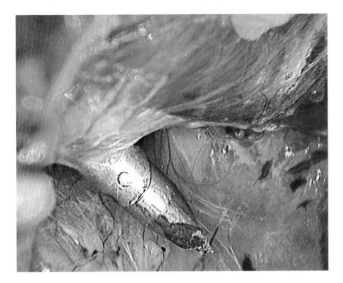

Figure 12 : Introduction of left hand working trocar (5 mm)

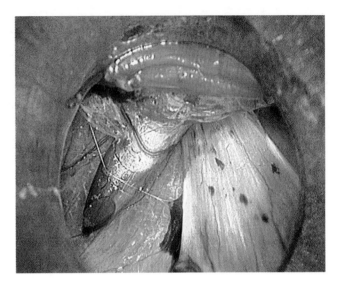

Figure 14 : Introduction of right hand working 5 mm trocar. (The surgeon moves to the head end of the patient after this stage)

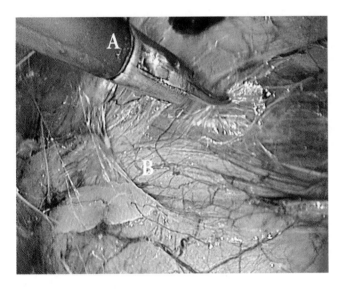

Figure 13 : Widening of extraperitoneal space on the lateral aspect for creation of right hand working port (Right inguinal hernia).

A - Instrument from the left hand working port

B - Peritoneum

In case of bilateral hernias the left hand working port is created at the level of rectus sheath attachment, after blunt dissection of the extraperitoneal space. Once the left hand port is created further port placement and dissection is carried out from the head end. The surgeon should carefully introduce the working trocars in the extraperitoneal space under vision to prevent laceration of small branches of inferior epigastric vessels and accidental entry into the peritoneal cavity.

Two Hand Technique

The position of the trocars in this technique is deserves special mention. Most of the techniques that have been described till now, have all the trocars in the midline. This arrangement of the trocars in the midline is associated with a relatively acute, unfavorable working angle resulting in crowding of the instruments. In our approach triangulation of instruments (70° angle between the working trocars) is maintained as in any other laparoscopic surgery.

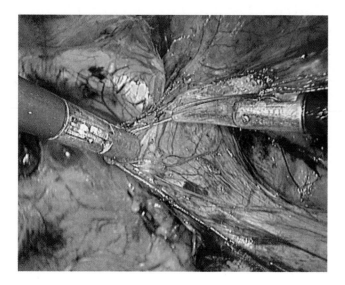

Figure 15 : Two handed dissection

This arrangement follows the basic ergonomic principles of laparoscopy. Dissection of preperitoneal space and placement of mesh is easier in this two hand technique. Even difficult hernias can be dealt with ease by this approach.[22,23]

The rectus muscle and posterior rectus sheath form a tunnel that opens into the dissected extraperitoneal space. When the tunnel is short, it does not interfere with the working trocars; if it is very long the available space will be limited and the exposure will be poor. In this case, the sheath should be incised with scissors. Usually there is minor bleeding from the small vessels during this maneuver. Mono or bipolar coagulation may be used before division of the sheath.

Medial Dissection

The exposure of Cooper's ligament begins with the dissection of the posterior aspect of the abdominal wall by gentle sweeping of the areolar tissue. By alternate blunt and sharp dissection with scissors on the right hand and counter traction with a blunt grasper on the left hand, the dissection is continued in the preperitoneal space. If a direct hernia is present, it is completely reduced at this point. This can be accomplished with gentle traction on the peritoneal attachments to the defect. The thinned out transversalis fascia also termed "Pseudo sac" is loosely attached to the peritoneum. The peritoneal layer is peeled off from the transversalis fascia, allowing it to balloon into the direct defect. When the sac is completely dissected, the pubic ramus and ilio pubic tract can be visualized on its entire extent. The direct sac should not be ligated as the bladder may form the medial wall of the sac.

After the dissection of the direct area, the femoral ring should be examined. The iliac vein is visible just lateral to Cooper's ligament. If it is not seen, either an incarcerated hernia or an enlarged lymph node is probably covering the view. If femoral hernia is present, it should be carefully reduced so that the small vessels in the femoral canal and corona mortis are not avulsed. If the contents are irreducible due to constriction at the neck of the sac, then an incision in the medial and superior edge of the femoral ring will release the constriction.

Lateral Dissection

The dissection into the lateral inguinal fossa (Space of Bogros) begins by dividing the transversalis fascial extension at the level of the inferior epigastric vessels. The fat and loose areolar tissue are dissected from the anterior abdominal wall just lateral to the vessel until the peritoneum is identified. The transversalis fascial sling is identified medial to the sac. The attachment between the sling and the cord structures is divided by sharp dissection. The left hand grasper gives traction on the sling and curved dissector is used to dissect between the sling and the sac. By this careful dissection injury to the inferior epigastric vessels is avoided. At this stage the iliopubic tract must be identified clearly.

In case of direct hernias, the peritoneal edge will be easily separated from the internal ring. In certain patients, direct hernias are associated with the presence of an indirect hernia. The laparoscopic approach clearly eliminates the possibility of missed hernias by thorough dissection of all possible hernial sites.

In indirect hernia, the sac should be separated from the cord structures which is usually seen on the posterior aspect. If the sac is large and wide it usually covers the cord structures. We use hand-over-hand technique, keeping dissection close to the sac, to dissect the cord structures. In case of bubonocele where the sac is small, the entire sac can be dissected

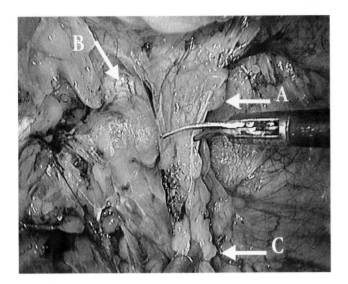

Figure 16 : Separation of pseudo sac from the peritoneum in direct hernia

A - Pseudo sac

B - Right side pubic ramus

C - Counter traction by left hand grasper

out of the internal ring. In cases of complete hernias, the sac is carefully separated from the cord structures. After the proximal sac is completely separated from the distal aspect and the cord structures, it is divided and ligated with an endoloop. But it may be difficult and more traumatic to completely dissect the cord structures from a large scrotal type of hernia. In these situations, particularly when the sac is adherent to cord structures, the sac should be transected and then mobilized circumferentially. The supero lateral edge is incised first as the cord structures may be the guide to the under surface of the sac. The vas deferens passes on the medial side and gonadal vessels on the lateral side. They must be identified and protected before incising the inferior wall of the sac.

Gentle dissection widens the lateral inguinal space (Bogros space) beyond the anterior superior iliac spine. The lateral femoral cutaneous nerve is usually seen beneath the thin transparent fascia on the lateral aspect. This fascia should be undisturbed to avoid injury to the nerve. The course of the nerve should be delineated completely before using any electrocoagulation in this area. The genito femoral nerve with its genital and femoral branches course along the medial margin of the psoas muscle and is not always visible. These nerves should be exposed only if there is need for coagulation in this area. Femoral nerve usually escapes injury as it is covered by the psoas muscle.

When dissecting the pubic bone and Cooper's ligament, the iliac vessels must be identified. The iliac vein is not usually visible due to its posterior location.

If the intraperitoneal CO_2 causes the peritoneum to balloon outward into the operative field, a Veress needle or mini trocar (3mm) is inserted into the right hypochondrium and the pneumoperitoneum is released. An endoloop can be applied to a button hole in any part of the peritoneum. Once the pneumoperitoneum, is released the surgeon can continue his dissection further without any hindrance. Indirect sac or any peritoneal rent is always closed in order to prevent internal herniation.

The entire posterior floor should be dissected in all cases of TEP. The edge of the peritoneum should be separated from the spermatic vessels and obturator vessels upto the level of obturator foramen and inferior vesical artery. Cord structures should be totally freed from the peritoneum at the end of the posterior dissection (Parietalisation). Inadequate parietalisation has been found to be a major cause for recurrence.

Placement of Mesh

A 15 x 12 cm sheet of polypropylene flat mesh is trimmed to fit the pelvic floor and introduced into the dissected space. As the dissected space is widest on the medial aspect when compared to the lateral aspect, the lateral half of the mesh.

Introduction of polypropylene mesh in the extraperitoneal space may be performed in two ways. The mesh is reverse loaded into the reducing sleeve and introduced through 10 mm port as described in TAPP approach. In the second method the scope is removed and the mesh is grasped on one end with a 5 mm grasper. The grasper is introduced through the 10 mm port along with the mesh. Once the mesh is inside the dissected space the grasper is removed. Either way we do not recommend rolling technique described by other authors. Once the mesh is fully in

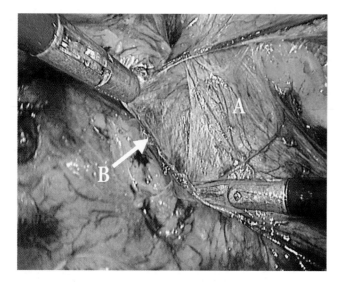

Figure 17 : Separation of sac from the transversalis fascial sling. Injury to inferior epigastric vessels can be avoided if the dissection is limited to the level of the sling

A - Sac
B - Transversalis fascial sling

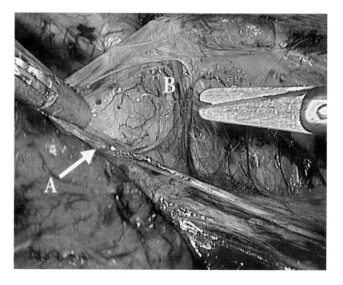

Figure 18 : Separation of sac from the cord structures

A - Sac
B - Cord structures

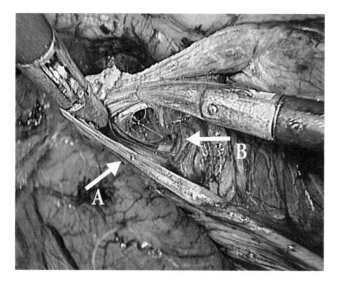

Figure 19 : Division of sac after separation. Care should be taken to avoid injury to the cord structures in this stage

A - Sac
B - Cord structures

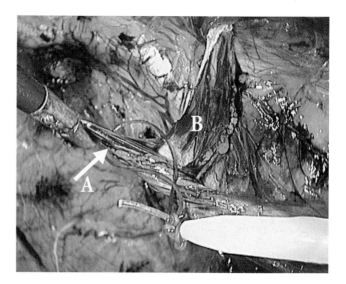

Figure 20 : Endoloop applied to the proximal sac after division

A - Sac
B - Cord structures

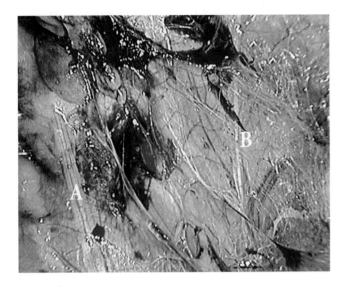

Figure 21 : Location of the nerves on the right side

A - Genito femoral nerve

B - Lateral femoral cutaneous nerve

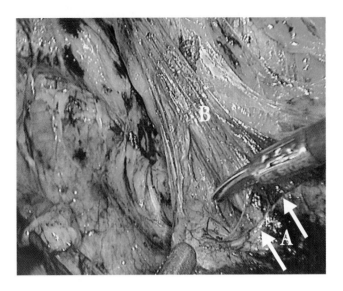

Figure 22 : Parietalisation. This prevents rolling of the mesh at the edges after release of CO_2

A - Peritoneal margin

B - Cord structures are separated from the peritoneum

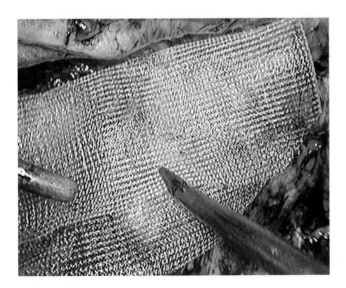

Figure 23 : Unfolding the mesh inside the peritoneal cavity

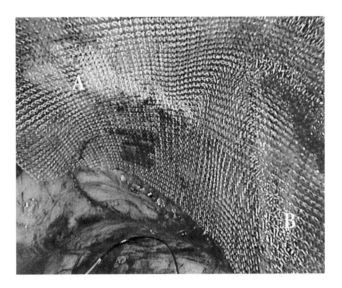

Figure 24 : Positioning of the mesh in the dissected space. The wider end of the mesh is placed medially and the narrower end on the lateral aspect

A - Symphysis pubis

B - Testicular vessels

the extraperitoneal compartment, it is repositioned using two graspers. Any folding or wrinkling of the mesh should be completely avoided.

The size of the mesh must be tailored to the size of patient's pelvis and should be large enough to cover all the potential hernia sites. The properly placed mesh should cover the entire dissected area extending beyond the midline on the medial aspect to anterior superior iliac spine on the lateral aspect. On the vertical axis it extends from just beyond the obturator foramen (inferior limit) to the level of the working trocars (superior limit).

Fixation of Mesh

Even though many prefer use of anchors or tackers for fixation of mesh, we prefer suturing the mesh to the Cooper's ligament and anterior abdominal wall with prolene sutures. Even though endo suturing is technically difficult, it is advantageous as it is cost effective and has lesser side effects when compared to anchors, tackers or 12 mm staplers. The practice of stapling is almost given up at many centres.

The mesh is initially sutured to the Coopers ligament. This helps in easy spreading of the mesh as one end is anchored. The mesh is spread over the entire area without any wrinkles or folds. The second area of fixation is on the superomedial aspect of the mesh. It is sutured to the under surface of the rectus muscle.

If there is a lipoma of the cord, it should be dissected from the canal and the cord structures, left in the retroperitoneum out of the operative field. Once the mesh is fixed, the lipoma of the cord can be positioned between the mesh and peritoneum.

Finally the CO_2 is released slowly by opening the side channel of a 5 mm port while the inferior aspect of the mesh is held against the psoas muscle. This ensures that the peritoneum covers the mesh without unrolling of the mesh. If CO_2 is trapped within the peritoneum, it is evacuated with the help of a Veress needle or 3 mm trocar.

The rectus sheath is approximated and the trocar wounds are closed with subcuticular sutures. In case of minimal bleeding we keep a small vacuum drain through the 5 mm port which is usually removed in a day or two depending on the drainage.

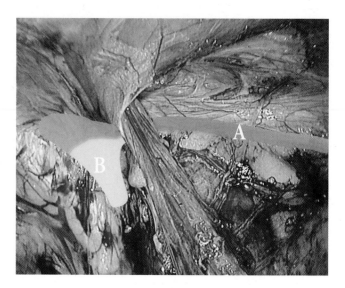

Figure 25 : Identification of Cooper's ligament

A   -   Iliopubic tract
B   -   Cooper's ligament

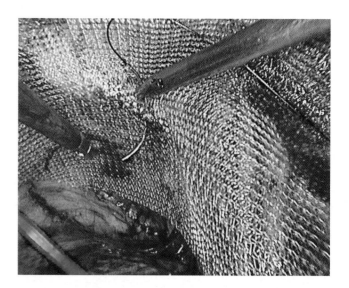

Figure 26 : Fixation of mesh to the Cooper's ligament by intracorporeal suturing using 1 0 prolene

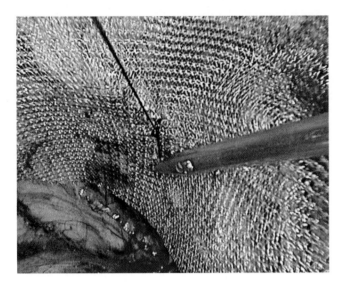

Figure 27 : Mesh fixed to the right Cooper's ligament

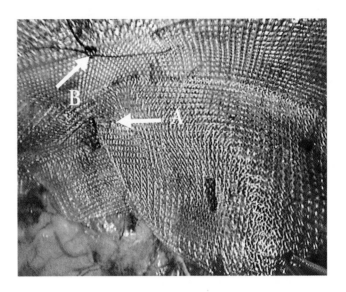

Figure 28 : Completion of fixation of mesh

A - Stitch to the right Cooper's ligament

B - Stitch to rectus muscle

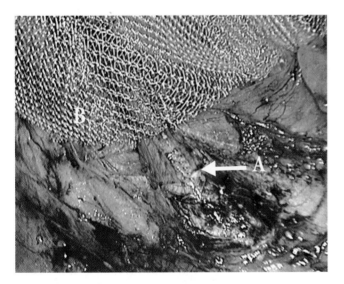

Figure 29 : Parietalisation

A - Peritoneal reflection on right side

B - Mesh

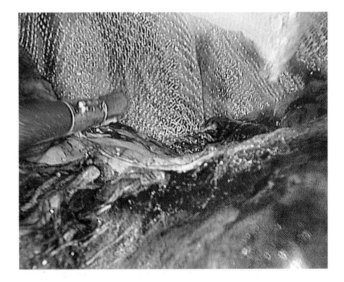

Figure 30 : Mesh being held at the lower border during the desufflation of CO_2 to prevent rolling of the mesh

POST OPERATIVE MANAGEMENT

We allow the patient to take liquids after the recovery from general anesthesia and encourage moving in the room by evening. The patients usually use the toilet by evening. Adequate analgesia is given through rectal (diclofenac) suppositories. We tend to keep the patients for a day in the hospital and discharge them on the 1st postoperative day. Patients are allowed to take normal diet on the 1 post op day and advised to carry on with their normal routine work as per their level of comfort.

OUR EXPERIENCE

We started performing laparoscopic hernia surgery since 1992. Till now we have operated on 4196 adult patients with 4692 hernias. In our early experience, TAPP formed the majority of cases and now we have gradually shifted towards TEP procedure for most of the repairs.

Demographic Data		
No. of Patients	:	4196
No. of Hernias	:	4692
Age	:	16-80 years
Men / Women	:	61 : 39
Unilateral / bilateral	:	3518 : 1174
Right / Left	:	2815 : 1877

We routinely perform TEP procedure for almost of my patients and restrict TAPP to selected patients (as mentioned in TAPP chapter).

	TAPP	TEP
1992-95	750	-
1996-1999	300	950
2000-2002	240	1650
2002-2003	22	780

Types of Hernias		
Direct Hernia	:	1646
Indirect Hernia	:	2848
Recurrent Hernia	:	190
Following Conventional	- 185	
Following lap repair	- 5	
Femoral Hernias	:	8
Total	:	4692

	TAPP	TEP
Duration of Surgery (mts)		
Unilateral	30* (23-50♦)	20 (15-40) mts
Bilateral	40 (34-100)	32 (25-56) mts
Hospital Stay	1.5 (1.1 – 7)	1.3 (1 - 8) days
Return to normalcy	3 (2- 6)	2.3 (2 - 5) days
Return to work	5.2 (4-12)	4.5 (3 - 10) days
Conversion	Nil	Nil
Size of mesh used		
Before 1995	8 x 10 cm	-
After 1995	15 x 12 cm	15 x 12 cm

* Mean; ♦ Range

COMPLICATIONS

We had urinary retention in 3% of patients who needed catherisation in the postoperative period. The incidence of seroma was less than 1.5% of which most of them resolved on conservative measures and needle aspirations as an out patient procedure once. Only in 5 patients multiple aspirations of 2-3 times were performed.

The incidence of hematoma was less than 0.5%. One patient had persistant drainage (more than 200 ml of blood stained fluid/day) in the postoperative period following TEP repair. On relaparoscopy through the same ports (on 2nd post op day) we could not find any specific bleeding vessel. This patient was on aspirin for his cardiovascular disease. Even though he had stopped anticoagulant two weeks earlier, the diffuse ooze was probably due to the clotting abnormality. He recovered completely on the 6 th post operative day.

We had 2 patients with bowel injuries. One patient had jejunal perforation following TEP repair for right inguinal hernia. A 3 mm trocar was inserted in the right hypochondrium to release the suspected pneumoperitoneum. The patient did not progress well and was subjected to relaparoscopy on the 2nd day. We found a jejunal perforation about 6 feet from the duodenojejunal flexure. The perforation was closed by intracorporeal suturing. The mesh was undisturbed and he completely recovered on the sixth postoperative day. Due to the extraperitoneal approach, the mesh escaped contamination by the peritoneal fluid without any infection. On retrospective analysis, we subsequently arrived at the probable sequence of events that lead to this perforation. The patient had CO_2 only within the layers of abdominal wall which was mistaken as pneumoperitoneum. The forceful introduction of the 3 mm trocar might have lead to this perforation.

One patient had an ileal injury due to electrocautery during TAPP repair. This was probably due to the result of activation of electro surgical instrument while it was touching the bowel. This injury was recognized immediately (partial thickness burn) and the serosa was plicated by intracorporeal suturing. The patient recovered completely.

Inferior epigastric vessel injury was seen in about 10 patients. This was managed by percutaneous suture using suture passer needle in three and electro cautery coagulation in the remaining.

Mesh Infection

We had four cases of mesh infection following laparoscopic hernia repair. Two patients subsided with drainage of the abscess cavity and antibiotics. The biopsy from abscess wall revealed tuberculosis in two patients. We removed the meshes. These patients recovered completely with anti tuberculous treatment. One of the patients developed recurrent hernia.

Recurrence Rates

We had 5 recurrences following laparoscopic hernia repair which occurred before 1995 (in the early period). Two patients had medial recurrence and three patients had lateral recurrence. Two patients were operated by conventional Lichtenstein repair.

After 2000, we adopt laparoscopic approach for patients with recurrence following laparoscopic repair in three patients.

CONCLUSION

Our technique of extraperitoneal repair (TEP) is more comfortable and highly effective in the laparoscopic management of inguinal hernias. Our port placement and 2 hand technique maintains the triangular orientation which is considered vital as per the ergonomics of laparoscopy. Nearly 98-99% of inguinal hernias can be treated by TEP approach. With adequate training and thorough knowledge of the working anatomy, surgeons can perform this procedure with ease and produce excellent results.

References

1. Vogt DM, Curet MJ, Pitcher DE, Martin DT, Zucker KA. Preliminary results of a prospective randomized trial of laparoscopic onlay versus conventional inguinal herniorrhaphy. Am J Surg 1995;169:84-9; discussion 89-90.

2. Fitzgibbons RJ, Jr., Camps J, Cornet DA, Nguyen NX, Litke BS, Annibali R, Salerno GM. Laparoscopic inguinal herniorrhaphy. Results of a multicenter trial. Ann Surg 1995;221:3-13.

3. McCloud JM, Evans DS. Day-case laparoscopic hernia repair in a single unit. Surg Endosc 2003;17:491-3.

4. Cheek CM, Black NA, Devlin HB, Kingsnorth AN, Taylor RS, Watkin DF. Groin hernia surgery: a systematic review. Ann R Coll Surg Engl 1998;80 Suppl 1:S1-80.

5. Juul P, Christensen K. Randomized clinical trial of laparoscopic versus open inguinal hernia repair. Br J Surg 1999;86:316-9.

6. Barrat C, Surlin V, Bordea A, Champault G. Management of recurrent inguinal hernias: a prospective study of 163 cases. Hernia 2003;7:125-9.

7. Knook MT, Weidema WF, Stassen LP, van Steensel CJ. Laparoscopic repair of recurrent inguinal hernias after endoscopic herniorrhaphy. Surg Endosc 1999;13:1145-7.

8. Frankum CE, Ramshaw BJ, White J, Duncan TD, Wilson RA, Mason EM, Lucas G, Promes J. Laparoscopic repair of bilateral and recurrent hernias. Am Surg 1999;65:839-42; discussion 842-3.

9. Memon MA, Feliu X, Sallent EF, Camps J, Fitzgibbons RJ, Jr. Laparoscopic repair of recurrent hernias. Surg Endosc 1999;13:807-10.

10. Sayad P, Ferzli G. Laparoscopic preperitoneal repair of recurrent inguinal hernias. J Laparoendosc Adv Surg Tech A 1999;9:127-30.

11. Knook MT, Weidema WF, Stassen LP, van Steensel CJ. Endoscopic total extraperitoneal repair of primary and recurrent inguinal hernias. Surg Endosc 1999;13:507-11.

12. DeTurris SV, Cacchione RN, Mungara A, Pecoraro A, Ferzli GS. Laparoscopic herniorrhaphy: beyond the learning curve. J Am Coll Surg 2002;194:65-73.

13. Edwards, C C, Bailey, W R. Laparoscopic Hernia Repair: The Learning Curve. Surgical Laparoscopy, Endoscopy & Percutaneous Techniques. 7(1):49-50, February 1997. 2000;10:149-153.

14. Liem MS, van Steensel CJ, Boelhouwer RU, Weidema WF, Clevers GJ, Meijer WS, Vente JP, de Vries LS, van Vroonhoven TJ. The learning curve for totally extraperitoneal laparoscopic inguinal hernia repair. Am J Surg 1996;171:281-5.

15. Arregui ME, Davis CJ, Yucel O, Nagan RF. Laparoscopic mesh repair of inguinal hernia using a preperitoneal approach: a preliminary report. Surg Laparosc Endosc 1992;2:53-8.

16a. Crawford D, Phillips E, Laparoscopic extraperitoneal hernia. In: Zucker K, ed Surgical Laparoscopy, Philadelphia: Lippinott WIlliam & WIlkins, 2000:571-584

17. McKernan JB, Laws HL. Laparoscopic repair of inguinal hernias using a totally extraperitoneal prosthetic approach. Surg Endosc 1993;7:26-8.

17. Dulucq J. Terres des hernias de laine par mise en place d'un patch prothique sous-peritoneal en retroperitoneoscpie. Cahiers Chir 1991;79:15-16.

18. Palanivelu C. Laparoscopic Space Access. In: Palanivelu C, ed. CIGES Atlas of Laparoscopic Surgery. Second ed. New Delhi: Jaypee Brothers Medical Publishers Pvt. Ltd, 2003:11-16.

19. Palanivelu C. Laparoscopic Space Access and Physiological Significance. In: Palanivelu C, ed. Text Book of Surgical Laparoscopy. Coimbatore: Gem Digestive Diseases Foundation, 2002:31-39.

20. Palanivelu C. Totally Extraperitoneal laparoscopic Hernia Repair. In: Palanivelu C, ed. Text Book of Surgical Laparoscopy. Coimbatore: Gem Digestive Diseases Foundation, 2002:237-242.

21. Heikkinen TJ, Haukipuro K, Koivukangas P, Hulkko A. A prospective randomized outcome and cost comparison of totally extraperitoneal endoscopic hernioplasty versus Lichtenstein hernia operation among employed patients. Surg Laparosc Endosc 1998;8:338-44.

22. Palanivelu C. Laparoscopic Totally extraperitoenal Hernioplasty (TEP). In: Palanivelu C, ed. CIGES Atlas of Laparoscopic Surgery. Second ed. New Delhi: Jaypee Brothers Medical Publishers Pvt. Ltd, 2003:97-101.

23. Palanivelu C, Rajan PS, Sendhilkumar K, Parthasarathi R. Results of Hand Sutured Laparoscopic Hernioplasty : Effective method of Repair. Surg Endosc 1998;12:596.

72

Laparoscopic Repair of Ventral Hernia

INTRODUCTION

Ventral hernias present a challenge even for the experienced surgeon, because of the high incidence of morbidity and recurrence. Wound infection, malnutrition, morbid obesity, chronic cough, prostatism and larger incisions are considered as risk factors for developing incisional hernia.[1] Even though many repairs have been described, search is still continuing for an ideal technique which is patient and surgeon friendly with lesser morbidity and recurrence.

Traditional repairs require laparotomy with suture approximation of the strong fascial tissues on either side. But the recurrence rate was very high (41-52%) on long term follow up.[2] The reason for the underlying problem was that in all sutured repairs, the repair is under tension and this increases the risk of ischemia, suture cut through and failure. From sutured repairs, the concept has slowly moved towards prosthesis with much reduced recurrence rate

of 12-24%. Unfortunately, positioning of the mesh makes it necessary to perform an extensive surgical dissection of soft tissues. This is associated with increased incidence of postoperative pain, seromas, hematomas and wound infection.[3-5]

Along with the worldwide acceptance of various laparoscopic surgeries, its use in ventral hernia was first reported by LeBlanc in 1993.[6] Following this various reports have been published on laparoscopic ventral hernia repair using various techniques and prosthetic materials.[6-14] Patients undergoing laparoscopic treatment of ventral hernias have shorter postoperative stay, fewer analgesic requirements and fewer wound complications.[15] With the introduction of inert prosthetic materials such as PTFE[8, 14, 16-18] and dual sided meshes the laparoscopic repair of ventral hernias have gained more momentum.

Although incisional hernias are usually asymptomatic except for protrusion of the abdominal wall, with time it enlarges and becomes symptomatic. These patients often have pain with movement, straining or cough and it interferes with their routine work. Vomiting, obstipation and severe pain indicates incarceration or strangulation of internal structures.

Ultrasound, CT scan and barium meal series may be used to diagnose the presence of incisional hernia in obese individuals. Laparoscopy may be used as diagnostic as well as therapeutic tool. Multiple defects and associated adhesions can be detected by laparoscopy.

INDICATIONS

Laparoscopic ventral hernia repair (LVHR) can be accomplished in almost all patients with excellent results. The size of the hernia is a determining factor in the selection of type of repair. Defects less than 3 cm are better done by conventional approach and laparoscopy is reserved for patients with larger defects. In obesity and recurrent incisional hernias laparoscopy is indicated even in smaller sized defects. The "Swiss cheese" type of hernias (multiple smaller defects) is ideally managed by laparoscopy as the defects are more clearly delineated when compared to open repair.

CONTRAINDICATIONS

The presence of infection and peritonitis are absolute contraindications for laparoscopic ventral hernia repairs. Cases of acute and subacute obstruction merits scrutiny on case to case basis. In case of acute obstruction, laparoscopy can be performed to relieve the obstruction and further placement of mesh depends on the viability of the bowel. In the absence of contamination, mesh reinforcement can be accomplished during the same surgery. If the viability is in doubt, the procedure should be limited to suture approximation of the defect. Placement of a prosthetic material can be done at later date. Previous use of prolene mesh induces extensive intra abdominal adhesions. Laparoscopic repair of these cases should be attempted only by experienced surgeons as it is not possible to predict the severity of adhesions. The threshold for conversion to open method should be very low in order to prevent major fatalities like unrecognized bowel injuries and delayed perforations due to adhesiolysis. Other conditions like ascites, portal hypertension are relative contraindications. A large pendulous abdomen with major abdominal defect will benefit more from conventional abdominoplasty rather than laparoscopy in terms of cosmesis. The routine contraindications to general anesthesia also apply to the laparoscopic ventral hernia repair.

CONVENTIONAL REPAIRS

Primary closure is a simple technique which involves closure of the fascial defect with continuous nonabsorbable suture after thorough delineation of the defect. Defects less than 3 cm with strong fascial edge can be treated by this method. The recurrence rates are high in this method.[19, 20]

In onlay repairs, a mesh (usually polypropylene) is sutured over the anterior rectus sheath after primary closure of the fascial defect. The mesh is separated from the abdominal contents by the muscles and fascia. Seroma formation, wound infection are the common complications following this type of repair.

Absolute Contraindications	Relative Contraindications
Infection	Morbid obesity
Strangulation	Extensive adhesions due to prior mesh
Koch's or any infective pathology	Very large ventral hernia
Peritonitis	Severe cardiomyopathy
	Pulmonary disease
	Portal hypertension

Types of Repair

Conventional Repairs	Laparoscopic Repairs
Primary closure	Primary Closure
Prosthetic mesh repairs	Prosthetic mesh repairs
Onlay Mesh Repairs	Intraperitoneal onlay mesh repair[16]
Inlay mesh repairs	Intraperitoneal onlay mesh with primary closure
	Retro rectus mesh repairs

Inlay mesh repair is a surgical technique in which the mesh is placed in the intra-abdominal aspect, after excision of the sac. Fixation of the mesh to the abdominal wall is done by partial or full thickness sutures on the abdominal wall at least 5 cm lateral to the hernia defect. ePTFE meshes are ideal for these types of repair, though there are reports of prolene mesh being used as inlay graft.[21]

Stoppa's repair of ventral hernia is a type of repair suited for lower abdominal defects associated with thin musculature. A space is created under rectus sheath which is extended into the retropubic space. The mesh is placed in the dissected space and anchored to Cooper's ligament on either sides.[22]

LAPAROSCOPIC REPAIRS

There are various methods of laparoscopic repair of ventral hernias. Simple closure of the defect and closure with reinforcement by prosthesis either in the intraperitoneal aspect or the extraperitoneal aspect are the main types of laparoscopic repairs.

LAPAROSCOPIC INTRAPERITONEAL ONLAY MESH WITH PRIMARY CLOSURE (IPOM)

Patient Position

The majority of the ventral hernias are located in the midline. In case of lower abdominal hernias, the surgeon stands near the right shoulder of the patient, the assistant surgeon near the left shoulder with the monitor at the foot end. The patient is in supine position with 10-15 degree Trendelenburg tilt to allow the bowel loops to fall away from the pelvis. In upper abdominal defects, the patient is placed in modified lithotomy position with 10-15 degrees headup tilt. The surgeon stands between the legs of the patient with the monitor near the head end, while the camera assistant stands on the right side of the patient. Operations on lateral defects of the abdominal wall, such as those in subcostal or flank areas will need semi or full decubitus position.

Instrumentation

For laparoscopic ventral hernia repair a good camera with an optimum light source is essential to prevent inadvertent enterotomies during adhesiolysis. We use the latest 3 CCD digital cameras with Xenon light source for all our laparoscopic surgeries. 10 mm, 30 degree scopes are routinely used as they provide excellent view of anterior abdominal wall compared to 0 degree scope. The camera port is usually 10 mm and the working ports are 5 mm The camera port is also utilized for introduction of the mesh and suture materials.

The instruments required for ventral hernia repair are very few. Atraumatic graspers for holding the bowel, sharp scissors and curved dissection forceps for adhesiolysis and Ethicon endo needle holder for intracorporeal suturing are the main instruments. I use a specially designed suture passer for fixing the mesh to the fascial layers. The fixation devices such as staplers, anchors and tackers can be used as per the comfort level of the surgeons. ePTFE or Composite mesh (Parietex) are ideal for intraperitoneal onlay mesh repairs. Prolene meshes can be used in subfascial extraperitoneal repairs. Monopolar or bipolar diathermy should be used with caution. Harmonic scalpel is ideal for release of adhesions between the omentum and the sac as this has minimal thermal spread.

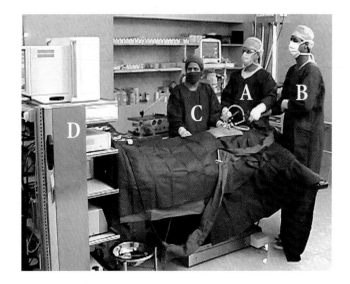

Figure 1 : Team setup for midline lower abdominal hernias

A - Surgeon
B - Camera surgeon
C - Staff nurse
D - Laparoscopic trolley

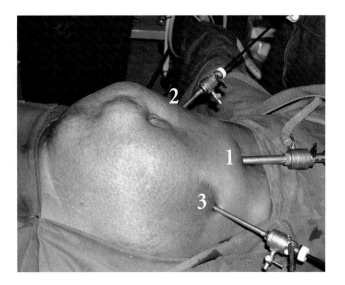

Figure 2 : Position of ports (midline lower abdominal hernias)

No.	Instruments	Place
1	Camera	Epigastrium 10mm
2	Right hand working port	Right Hypochondrium 5 mm
3	Left hand working port	Left hypochondrium 5mm

Technique

Port Placement

Pneumoperitoneum is created by Veress needle technique at an alternative site as the umbilicus is almost always included in the previous incision. The Veress needle is introduced in the left hypochondrium usually, but other sites like the right hypochondrium and areas remote to the previous incisions can also be used. We initially use a 3 mm trocar with 3 mm telescope to visualize the abdominal cavity for adhesions of the bowel loops. The 10 mm port is created under vision and the scope is changed to 10 mm. Subsequently all ports are created. Open laparoscopy is hardly needed for this purpose. The camera port is placed in the epigastrium and the left and right hand working ports in the left and right hypochondrium. The camera port is placed far enough from the defect so that there is no difficulty in visualizing the proximal area of the defect during fixation of mesh. The upper abdominal hernias which are usually rare are performed by placing similar ports in the lower abdomen. Trocars are placed on the lateral abdominal wall on the opposite side of the defect.

Adhesiolysis

The important and vital part of the surgery is the adhesiolysis. Usually structures like the bowel and omentum are adherent to the defect and the peritoneal sac. The release of the adhesions should be done carefully with sharp scissors, dissecting off the omentum and small bowel from the peritoneal wall. In case of extensive adhesions it might be a better option to leave some parts of the peritoneum and mesh on the bowel, rather risking injury during complete separation. The presence of the adhesions should not deter the surgeon from proceeding with the laparoscopic surgery, provided he has adequate experience. But the threshold for conversion should be low in these cases. If enterotomies are recognized during the surgery it can be closed either by intracorporeal suturing or after exteriorizing the bowel through a minilaparotomy (2-3 cm). The monopolar or bipolar cautery should be used as minimum as possible during adhesiolysis.

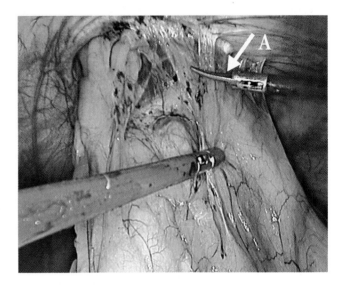

Figure 3 : Adhesiolysis. Adhesiolysis is performed by traction with left hand grasper while the inflated abdominal wall provides counter traction. The adhesions are divided with sharp scissors

A - Release of adhesions using scissors.

Assessment of Defect

Once adhesiolysis is complete and anterior abdominal wall is cleared off the fat, nature and extent of defect is assessed thoroughly. This assessment is more crucial than the preoperative assessment, as newer defects might be found during this stage. In cases of defects where reduction of the contents is not possible, minimal enlargement of the defect on the lateral side will help in easy reduction.

The defect is clearly delineated after releasing the pneumoperitoneum and the site of the defect and the area of proposed placement of the mesh is marked on the skin. The measurement of the defect is taken on the external surface of the abdominal wall rather than on the intraperitoneal side of the fascial defect. The entire circumference of the defect should be identified to ascertain its maximum dimensions. Then an adequate sized mesh that covers the entire defect and extending up to 3-5 cm from the edges of the defects is selected. The placement of the mesh over the entire area will prevent further development of hernias in the potentially weak areas.

To improve function of the muscle and quality of repair, we approximate the defective edges using intracorporeal continuous suturing with non absorbable sutures (1 ethilon loop). We have adopted this technique in over 160 patients. We introduce the needle through a 2 mm stab incision below the hernial defect. The length of the suture adequate enough to approximate the defect is pulled inside by holding with Ethicon Needle holder, while the tail end remains outside. The defect is closed by continuous suturing in 2 layers completing in the same area where it was started. The needle is cut from the thread and removed through the 5 mm port. The suture passer (thread grasper) is inserted through the previous stab incision, the suture material grasped and pulled out of the abdomen and tied extracorporeally. No attempt is made to dissect the sac.

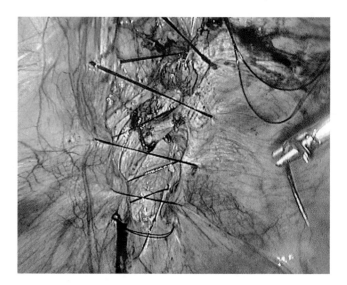

Figure 5 : Approximation of defect, started from lower margin of the defect. The sutures are continued till the upper margin of the defect in a continuous fashion.

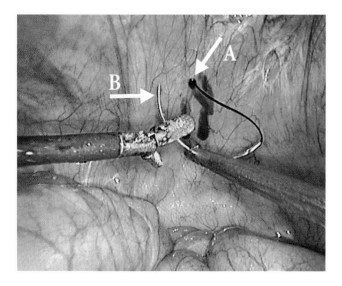

Figure 4 : Introduction of needle into the peritoneal cavity by percutaneous method

A - Site of needle entry

B - Large size needle (50 mm, half circle, heavy round body needle of 1 ethilon loop, Ethicon Needle Holder is heavy and sturdy for manipulation of even large needles)

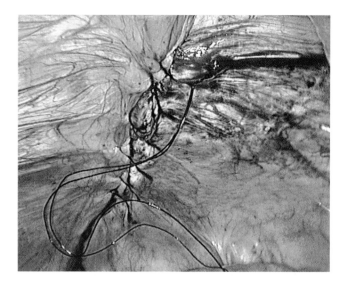

Figure 6 : Completion of closure of the defect (I layer). The sutures can be tightened at this stage by traction of the suture material present outside

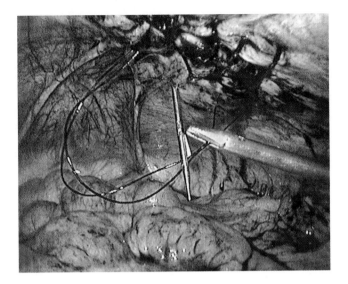

Figure 7 : Completion of closure of the defect (II layer). The needle has been removed and the tip of the suture being held by the thread grasper. Note the level of the entry and exit of the suture is very close to each other separated by few mms

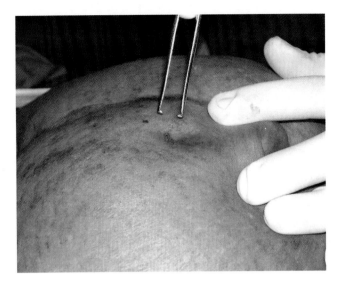

Figure 9 : External view after completion of knot (knot has been buried in the subcutaneous plane)

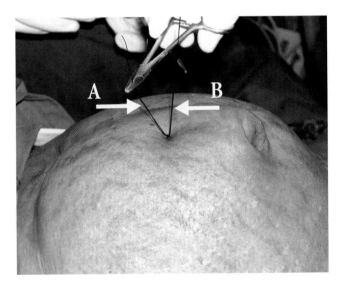

Figure 8 : Both the ends have been brought out through the same stab wound (2 mm) for extracorporeal knotting. When the knot is tightened it lies over the fascial sheath. Over tightening of the knot will result in necrosis of the intervening muscle and fascia

Choice of Mesh

Absorbable meshes have limited role in ventral hernia repair. It is mainly used in cases where mesh infection is a significant factor and primary closure is not possible. Polyester mesh has been associated with significantly higher enterocutaneous fistula formation and mesh infection and hernia formation, hence it should not to be used as intraperitoneal onlay graft. Polypropylene meshes prevents recurrence, unfortunately intestinal fistulization has been reported in many series. Expanded polytetrafluroethylene (EPT) has very few bowel complications. Even if adhesions develop, it can be separated because of smooth surface of the adhesions that are formed. Recently prostheses have been developed with both characteristics; tissue in growth on one side and nonadhesive surface on the other side. Composix, bilayer polypropylene (Parietex) and sepra mesh are examples of these types of meshes. In a study of the various complications following the use of polypropylene, polyester and PTFE mesh, the multifilamented polyester mesh had a significantly

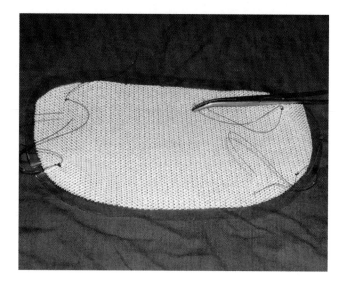

Figure 10 : Parietex composite mesh - Four corners tagged with prolene sutures

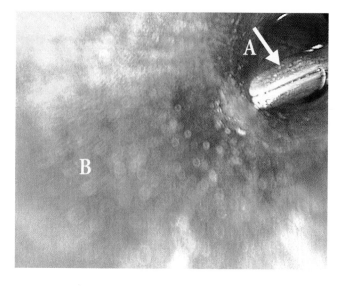

Figure 11 : Introduction of 5 mm grasper from the right hypochondrial port through the camera port under vision

    A - Tip of the grasper
    B - Lumen of camera port

higher mean number of complications per patient and higher incidence of fistula formation, infections, and the additional mean length of stay to treat complications.[5]

Introduction of Mesh

The selected mesh (Parietex) is taken and the four corners are tagged with 1-0 polypropylene sutures leaving 2 long threads in each side for fixation. The mesh is folded and reverse loaded on to a 10-5 mm reducer and then placed into the abdominal cavity through the 10 mm port after removing the camera. When reverse loading is not possible (when the mesh is larger in size) a second method is applied. Here the 5 mm needle holder from the right hypochondrium is railroaded into the camera port under vision while the telescope is slowly withdrawn. When the needle holder exists out of the port the top assembly (which holds the flap valve) is removed and mesh is grasped and pulled into the abdominal cavity. The scope is reintroduced and the remaining mesh is pushed into the abdominal cavity. With this method we are able to introduce all sizes of the mesh without the need to pull the mesh through the skin as recommended by some authors. This method is associated with potential risk of contamination of the mesh by microorganisms.

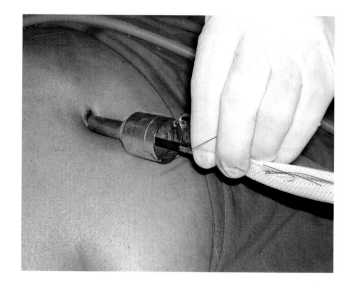

Figure 12 : Grasper exiting out through 10 mm camera port and introduction of folded mesh through the camera port

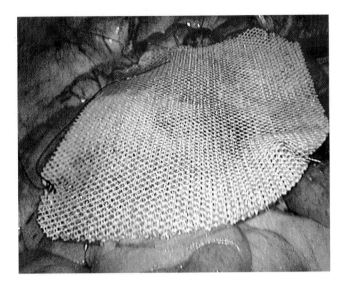

Figure 13 : Orientation of the mesh inside the peritoneal cavity (Hydrophilic coating facing the bowel and polyester surface facing the abdominal wall)

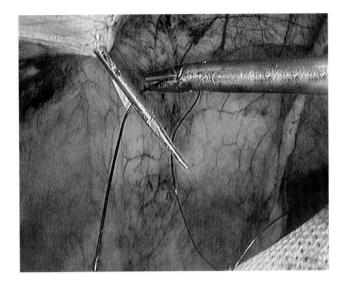

Figure 14 : Transfascial suturing. The suture passer (thread grasper) introduced through a 2 mm incision holding the prolene suture tagged to the mesh

Transfascial Suturing

Once the mesh is inside the abdominal cavity, we orient the mesh in proper direction and surface (hydrophilic coating should face the bowel and the polyester layer should face the peritoneum). Small skin incisions (2 mm) are made on the areas were transfixing sutures are planned. Subcutaneous fat is bluntly dissected with hemostats upto the fascia. The suture passer (thread grasper) is passed through incision obliquely; the suture material is grasped and broughtout. The thread grasper is again passed through the same incision few mms away from the previous track (in a different axis) and the other end of the suture material is brought out separately. The two threads are tied on the outer aspect. Since both the ends of the suture material are brought through the same wound, the knot lies on the fascia and is covered by the skin and subcutaneous fascia. The four corners of the mesh are sutured to the fascia in a similar manner. At this stage we deflate the pneumoperitoneum to check whether the placement of the mesh has been accomplished without any wrinkling or whether the mesh is too taut due to fixation beyond the edges of the mesh.

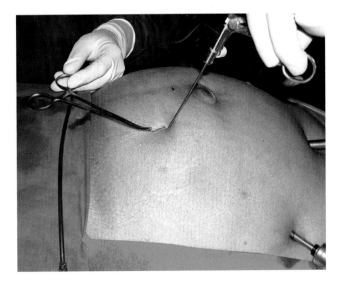

Figure 15 : Transfascial suturing. The prolene seen in the figure 14 has been pulled out and is held by the artery forceps. The thread grasper is again introduced through the same incision in a different track

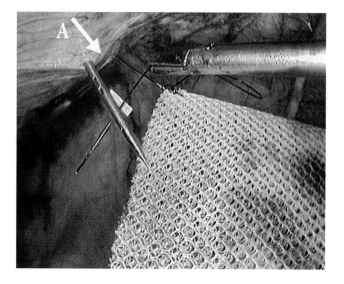

Figure 16 : Transfascial suturing. The entry of the thread grasper in a different point in the peritoneum.

A - Gap between the two entries

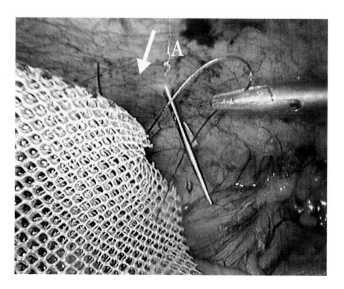

Figure 17 : Transfascial suturing

A - Gap between the two puncture sites

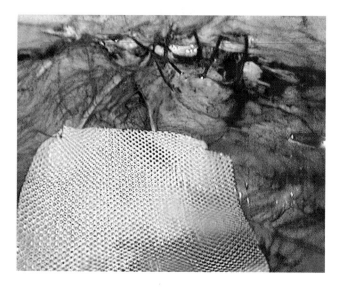

Figure 18 : Completion of transfascial suturing in lower border of mesh

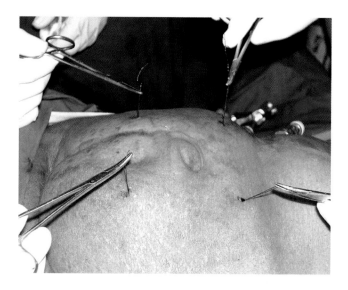

Figure 19 : Completion of transfascial suturing. Four prolene sutures are held separately

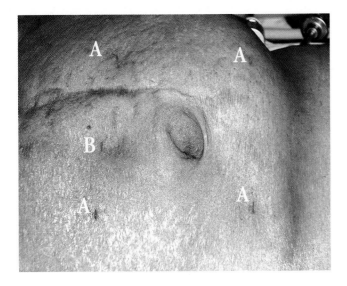

Figure 20 : External view after completion of transfascial suturing

A - Site of transfascial sutures

B - Site of needle entry for prolene suture used for closure of the defect

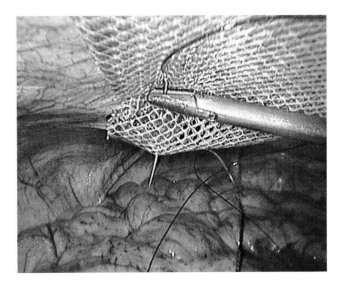

Figure 21 : Edges of mesh are fixed to the abdominal wall to prevent herniation of bowel between the mesh and the abdominal wall. (Endoanchors may also be used for this purpose).

Intracorporeal Suturing

We fix the edges of mesh to the abdominal wall by intracorporeal suturing using vicryl. We find the use of conventional sutures for this purpose are more cost effective when compared to devices such as staplers, anchors and tackers. However these devices are important as they fix the mesh effectively, especially for surgeons who are not well versed in endosuturing techniques. The sutures are placed 2-3 cm apart in all the four sides of the mesh. Once the suturing is completed, the pneumoperitoneum is deflated and the ports closed.

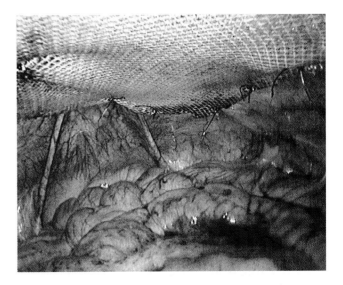

Figure 22 : Completed repair. Mesh seen over the abdominal wall covering the defect and extending beyond it in all directions

TRANSABDOMINAL EXTRAPERITONEAL REPAIR

In this method polypropylene mesh is placed in the preperitoneal space between the peritoneum and the muscular layer to prevent adhesions. This is mainly used in ventral hernial defects in the lower abdomen, where the preperitoneal fascia is loose. In this area placement of an onlay mesh is not ideal.

Principle of access to abdomen is the same as the previous technique. The peritoneum is incised along the edge of the defect and the peritoneal flap is raised as much as possible up to the lateral border of the rectus sheath. If possible, the sac is excised from the hernia by blunt dissection. The edges of the hernial defect are approximated with polypropylene interrupted mattress or continuous stitches. The subperitoneal dissection can be extended into the space of Retzius and a large size mesh can be placed. The polypropylene mesh of adequate size is placed over the defect extending for about 3 cm on all aspects. The mesh is anchored either by intracorporeal suturing or external mattress sutures with suture passer (thread grasper). Finally, the peritoneum is sutured over the mesh. The separation of the sac from the abdominal wall will be extremely difficult in some situations. If the peritoneum is lacerated to a large extent then it is advisable to convert the technique to intraperitoneal onlay mesh technique with ePTFE or Parietex meshes. We prefer this technique for small defects in the lower abdomen. This technique is not well suited for larger defects. In certain cases of ventral hernia a combination of intraperitoneal and extraperitoneal mesh repair may be ideal.

UMBILICAL HERNIA REPAIR

Umbilical hernia defects are common in adults and these are usually smaller defects which can be repaired either by open technique or by laparoscopic method. For defects more than 2 cm mesh repair is usually necessary. High incidence of recurrence and potentially increased risk of infection (if mesh is used) due to the incision in and around the umbilical crease are the problems involved in umbilical hernia repair. High bacterial flora counts in this area are thought to contribute to the increased incidence of wound infections when compared to other areas. Open

technique (Mayo) has shown high recurrence. In one third of patients, although the defect is small, the adjoining rectus sheath is defective or very thin. This cannot be assessed by open approach and might lead to recurrence. Several small series and case reports have demonstrated the feasibility of laparoscopic umbilical hernia repair as a potential means of avoiding these problems.

Laparoscopic approach enables to visualize the entire rectus sheath. If the defect is small and rectus sheath is well developed, excision of the sac and closure of the defect with prolene sutures is adequate. Even in smaller defects, if the surrounding rectus sheath is poorly developed, meshplasty is indicated.

Umbilical hernia repairs are performed in the same manner as ventral hernia repairs. The camera port is placed in the epigastric region and the two working ports on the lateral aspects in the pararectal area. The contents if any, are reduced with the help of external compression and simultaneous traction from inside. The defect is delineated and is closed with nonabsorbable sutures. If the defect is more than 2 cm, the defect is reinforced with a ePTFE or a Parietex mesh. The mesh is anchored to the abdominal wall either by intracorporeal suturing or by

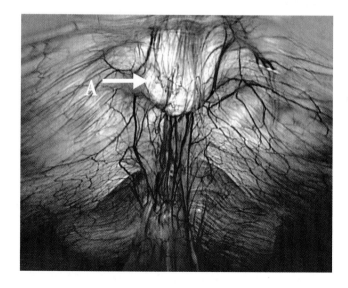

Figure 23 : Umbilical hernia

A - Defect is shown by external compression.
(Size of the defect - 3 cm)

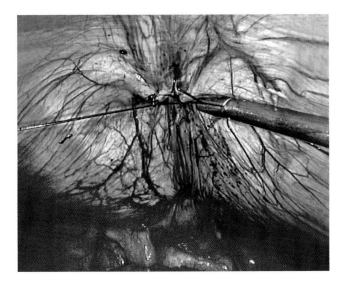

Figure 24 : Umbilical hernia. Approximation of the defect by intracorporeal suturing

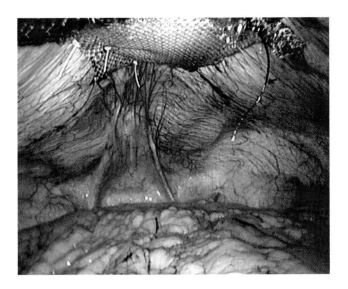

Figure 25 : Umbilical hernia. Reinforcement with parietex mesh

transfascial suturing as described in the ventral hernia repair. Laparoscopic umbilical hernia repair with mesh is a better alternative to conventional repair in terms of reduced recurrence and infections around the umbilical area.[23,24]

POSTOPERATIVE MANAGEMENT

We apply compression dressing in the area of the hernial defect to prevent seroma collection. The patient is advised to wear abdominal binder for 2 weeks. They are allowed to take fluids 4-6 hrs after the surgery. In cases of extensive adhesions the fluids are started after the movement of the bowel. The patient is encouraged to perform routine work without restrictions. Usually the patients are discharged on the second post operative day.

OUR RESULTS

Till now we have operated on 786 patients of ventral hernia in our institute. During the initial period we had performed ventral hernia repair by extraperitoneal approach with by keeping a prolene mesh in the preperitoneal area (65 patients). After 2000, we have shifted to 2 layered mesh (Parietex mesh) and we are using this mesh in all our patients now.

Out of 786 patients, 668 patients were females and 118 patients were male. The mean age group was 52 years (40-64 yrs). The indications for previous surgeries in these patients were mainly ceaserean section, hysterectomy and laparotomy for various other causes. Two patients had developed ventral hernia in the upper abdomen following sternotomy for coronary artery bypass grafting. 202 patients had undergone previous incisional hernia repair and of these 101 patients had undergone meshplasty. 25 patients had undergone surgery more than once for incisional hernia (2 - 7 surgeries). 455 (58.5%) of these patients were obese (BMI more than 35). Six hundred and thirty six patients had lower abdominal defects and the remaining 150 patients had defects in the upper abdomen. The lower abdominal defects were more commonly associated with multiple swiss cheese type defects when compared to upper abdominal defects.

The mean duration of surgery in these patients was 95 minutes (60-115mts). The average duration for passage of flatus was 1.5 days and the average hospital stay was 3 days (2-6 days). We had to convert to open surgery in 8 patients (1.01 %) due to the following reasons, extensive adhesions in 6 patients, inadverdant enterotomy in two. In three patients, there was difficulty in reduction of contents from the hernial sac due to dense adhesions to the mesh. We resorted to laparoscopic assisted approach in these patients. Through a minilaparotomy we reduced the contents and approximated the defect without any dissection. After creation of pneumopertioneum, the mesh was placed as routine.

Morbidity rate in our series was 8.76% (30 patients). There was trocar hematoma in 6 patients and respiratory infection in 8 patients. Sixty patients (7.71%) developed seroma in the immediate post operative period which was managed conservatively in most of the patients. Patients who had seroma for more then 8 weeks or symptomatic were aspirated by percutaneous needle aspiration (28 patients). 10 patients required repeated aspirations (2-5 times) for complete resolution of seromas. Out of these 2 patients who had recurrent seroma were drained by percutaenous trocar drainage. The drainage tube was removed after for 5 days and had an uneventful recovery.

Recurrence

We have had seven recurrences (0.89 %) in the mean follow up of 36 months. Three of these patients developed recurrence following intracorporeal suturing alone and 2 developed recurrence following laparoscopic intraperitoneal onlay mesh plasty with composite mesh. The recurrence was in these patients was found lateral to mesh. Small size of the mesh was probably the cause of recurrence in these two patients.

COMPLICATIONS OF LAPAROSCOPIC VENTRAL HERNIA REPAIR

The incidence of complications following laparoscopic repair are much less when compared to open repair.[15] Bowel injuries, seromas and mesh infection are the important complications.

Bowel injuries

Bowel injuries are the most important complications in laparoscopic ventral hernia repair with an overall reported incidence around 5%[25, 26] and occasionally around 15%.[27] This can occur either during the initial trocar entry or during adhesiolysis. The adhesiolysis is considered as the most crucial part of the laparoscopic ventral hernia repair. Avoidance of cautery, sharp dissection with scissors under good vision are some of the methods by which these can be prevented. In patients with previous history of peritonitis and previous mesh repair the incidence of dense adhesions is more and in these cases dissection should proceed with caution.

In case of bowel injury, it can be repaired either by laparotomy or laparoscopy. The mesh reinforcement should not be performed in these conditions and it should be deferred to a later date. The threshold for conversion in suspected bowel injuries and for deciding on relook laparotomy in patients who are not improving following dense adhesiolysis should be extremely low.

Seromas

The fluid accumulation in the retained hernial sac after laparoscopic approach is common and usually self limiting. Most of these fluid collections resolve with conservative management.[25,28] Aspiration of the seroma can be performed if it is continuously enlarging in size. This should be done under strict aseptic precautions, to avoid introduction of infection. Some patients have pain in the area of full thickness sutures. This usually subsides with conservative management like NSAIDs and injection of local anesthetics.

Mesh infection

The incidence of mesh infection is very low (about 1%[10]) when compared to 10-15%[29] incidence in conventional ventral hernia surgeries. All aseptic precautions should be taken to avoid this complication as managing this complication is very difficult. The infected meshes usually need removal for effective healing of the wound.

Table 1   Studies on laparoscopic ventral hernia repair

Reference	Patients (n)	Operating room time (min)	Hospital stay (days)	Seroma rate (%)	Infection rate (%)	Follow-up (months)	Recurrence rate (%)
Franklin et al[30]	176	-	-	0	2	30	1.1
Toy et al[31]	144	120	2.3	16	3	7	4.4
Carbajo et al[32]	100	62	1.2	10	0	30	2
Heniford et al[10]	415	97	1.8	5	2	23	3
LeBlanc et al[33]	100	-	1.2	7	2	51	6.3
Bageacu et al[33]	159	89	3.5	16	3	49	16
Ben Haim et al[28]	100	119	5	11	1	19	2
Heniford et al[1]	850	120	2.3		0.7	20	4.7
Palanivelu	786	95	3	7.71	-	36	0.89

DISCUSSION

The laparoscopic repairs have shown to be safe and effective in the management of ventral hernia. Most of the laparoscopic approaches have shown a decrease in complications like infection, seroma and wound dehiscence. (Table 1) The shorter hospital stay reported constantly in these studies is one of the important advantage of these repairs. This is mainly due to decreased pain, fewer complications, early mobility and faster return of bowel movements. The cost comparison between laparoscopic and open ventral hernia has been found to be less in one study, when the costs involved in treating the complications were taken into account.[8]

In one of the largest series of laparoscopic hernia repairs, Heniford et al has reported a low rate of conversion, shorter hospital stay and low risk for recurrence[10]. In an analysis of 850 patients who underwent laparoscopic ventral hernia repair over 9 years, the following results were published. Mean operating time was 120 min, mean estimated blood loss was 49 ml and hospital stay averaged 2.3 days. There were 128 complications in 112 patients (13.2%). The most common complications were ileus (3%) and prolonged seroma (2.6%). During a mean follow-up

time of 20.2 months, the hernia recurrence rate was 4.7%. Comparing patients who had a hernia recurrence with those who did not, the authors found significant associations between recurrence and larger hernias, longer operating times, previous hernia repairs and higher complication rates. Patients who were morbidly obese (BMI > 40) were also more likely to have recurrence as compared with those of more normal weight.

A series of comparative trials have shown persistent benefits in terms of shorter hospital stay, decreased infection and recurrence rates compared to open repairs. (Table 2)

In a review of comparison of lap and open ventral hernia studies, all seven studies reported higher complication rates and longer hospital stay in the open group. The conclusion from these studies was that laparoscopic incisional hernia is at least as effective and as safe as open mesh repair. Chari[27] and colleagues found no statistically significant difference between the two groups in terms of hospital stay or complication rate and concluded that there was no demonstrable advantage of laparoscopic over open repair (although no demonstrable disadvantage either), while the other authors suggested

Table 2   Randomized controlled trails of ventral hernia repair (Laparoscopy vs open)

Reference Team	Patients (n)		Operating time (min)		Length of stay (days)		Postop complication rate (%)		Infection rate (%)		Seroma rate (%)		Follow-up (months)		Recurrence rate %	
	Open	Lap	Open	Lap	Open	Lap	Open	Lap	Open	Lap	Open	Lap	Open	Lap	Open	Lap
Holzman et al [25]	16	20	98	128	5	1.6	31	23	6	5	0	5	19	10	13	10
Park et al [34]	49	56	78	95	6.5	3.4	37	18	2	0	2	4	54	24	35	11
Carbajo et al. [32]	30	30	112	87	9.1	2.2	50	20	18	0	67	13	27	27	7	0
Ramshaw et al [35]	174	79	82	58	2.8	1.7	26	15	3	0	-	-	21	21	21	3
DeMaria et al. [8]	18	21	-	-	4.4	0.8	72	57	33	10	50	19	24	24	0	6
Chari et al. [27]	14	14	78	124	5.5	5	14	14	0	7	-	-	-	-	-	-

Table 3: Issues in Transfascial Suturing

Concerns	Explanations
Prolonged duration of surgery	With adequate experience the duration is significantly reduced
Requires multiple incisions in the skin	Less than 2 mm in size, has excellent cosmesis when seen after 3-4 weeks
?? Increased rate of infection from the cutaneous flora due to the passage of needle	Not proven in any studies Contact with skin is avoided
Increased discomfort during early post	Probably due to over tightening the suture
Dragging sensation on long term	Probably due to nerve entrapment.

that laparoscopic repair was better in terms of complications and duration of hospital stay.

Carbajo et al in their only published prospective randomized study comparing Lap ventral hernia repair and open repair[32] provided evidence for the existence of many of the advantages mentioned in the reports on noncomparative investigations. This study assigned 60 patients to undergo either LVHR or open surgery. The 2 groups did not differ significantly in age, sex distribution, incisional hernia type, or size of defect. Both operating times and hospital stays were significantly shorter in the LVHR group. The author also found that the patients in the LVHR group had fewer complications and a significantly lower hernia recurrence rate during a

Causes of recurrence (Earlier studies)
Transfascial sutures not employed.
Use of smaller sized meshes.
Scar tissue reaction and encapsulation.
Ineffective anchoring of the mesh
Steep learning curve.

mean follow-up period of 27 months. These results again show that laparoscopic repair is more safe and reliable operation in terms of recurrence and complications.

Chioce of Mesh

The choice of mesh in these repairs has to be decided carefully in view of tendency to form adhesions. Polypropylene mesh is better avoided and use of inert materials is more favored. In the reports published so far about 80% have used ePTFE, rest have used other meshes like polypropylene and polyester. Franklin et al. who used prolene mesh in repair of ventral hernias, report approximately one third of patients with severe adhesions to the mesh when relaparoscopy was done.[30] Now recently more reports are published with double layered meshes like Parietex. In our experience of recurrent ventral hernias (operated with polypropylene mesh earlier), we found extensive adhesions that were difficult to release

Obesity

The laparoscopic ventral hernia repair in obesity is particularly useful as it avoids the wound related complications. Numerous reports have been published on the advantages of laparoscopy in patients with ventral hernia.[36]

Method of fixation

Several investigators have stressed the importance of mesh fixation to prevent hernia recurrence in laparoscopic repairs. This can be either by tackers or by sutures or with both. The tackers have been implicated as one of the causative factors in some reports. Heniford et al[10] reported results from consecutive patients from four surgeons, all at different centers, over a 6 year period. Of the 14 recurrences in this series, 6 occurred in patients in whom only tackers (no sutures) were used to fix the mesh. The total number of patients in whom only tackers were used was not reported, but the authors changed their practice early in the study as a result of these failures. In a similar study of 100 cases reported by LeBlanc et al., all of the recurrences resulted from mesh fixation with spiral tackers alone[6]. Although it appears that mesh fixation probably had some effect on their high recurrence rate, not all of the recurrences can be attributed to isolated tacker placement.

Recurrence

Size of the defect, obesity, diabetes mellitus, lower midline incision and wound infection are considered as the risk factors for recurrence. In a study by Hesselink et al hernias smaller than 4 centimeters, had a significantly lower recurrence rate (25 percent) than larger hernias (41 percent).[2] Careful dissection, minimal bowel handling, proper fixation with either sutures or anchors and selection of ideal cases will reduce the recurrence rates considerably.

CONCLUSION

Laparoscopic mesh repair produces low recurrence rates (0-9 percent) with acceptable morbidity. The evidence available at present suggests that laparoscopic repair is feasible, safe and at least as effective as open mesh repair, although experience with the new meshes is still limited. With the existing data, it will be prudent to recommend laparoscopic repair as the first line treatment for incisional hernia where the facilities and expertise are available;[37,38] where it is not, open mesh repair remains a suitable alternative. As laparoscopic skills improve, it is likely that laparoscopic repair will be more widely performed.

References

1. Heniford BT, Park A, Ramshaw BJ, Voeller G. Laparoscopic repair of ventral hernias: nine years' experience with 850 consecutive hernias. Ann Surg 2003;238:391-9; discussion 399-400.

2. Hesselink VJ, Luijendijk RW, de Wilt JH, Heide R, Jeekel J. An evaluation of risk factors in incisional hernia recurrence. Surg Gynecol Obstet 1993;176:228-34.

3. Luijendijk RW, Hop WC, van den Tol MP, de Lange DC, Braaksma MM, JN IJ, Boelhouwer RU, de Vries BC, Salu MK, Wereldsma JC, Bruijninckx CM, Jeekel J. A comparison of suture repair with mesh repair for incisional hernia. N Engl J Med 2000;343:392-8.

4. White TJ, Santos MC, Thompson JS. Factors affecting wound complications in repair of ventral hernias. Am Surg 1998;64:276-80.

5. Leber GE, Garb JL, Alexander AI, Reed WP. Long-term complications associated with prosthetic repair of incisional hernias. Arch Surg 1998;133:378-82.

6. LeBlanc KA, Booth WV. Laparoscopic repair of incisional abdominal hernias using expanded polytetrafluoroethylene: preliminary findings. Surg Laparosc Endosc 1993;3:39-41.

7. Lanzafame RJ. Laparoscopic cholecystectomy combined with ventral hernia repair. J Laparoendosc Surg 1994;4:287.

8. DeMaria EJ, Moss JM, Sugerman HJ. Laparoscopic intraperitoneal polytetrafluoroethylene (PTFE) prosthetic patch repair of ventral hernia. Prospective comparison to open prefascial polypropylene mesh repair. Surg Endosc 2000;14:326-9.

9. Farrakha M. Laparoscopic treatment of ventral hernia. A bilayer repair. Surg Endosc 2000;14:1156-8.

10. Heniford BT, Park A, Ramshaw BJ, Voeller G. Laparoscopic ventral and incisional hernia repair in 407 patients. J Am Coll Surg 2000;190:645-50.

11. Goodney PP, Birkmeyer CM, Birkmeyer JD. Short-term outcomes of laparoscopic and open ventral hernia repair: a meta-analysis. Arch Surg 2002;137:1161-5.

12. Liberman MA, Rosenthal RJ, Phillips EH. Laparoscopic ventral and incisional hernia repair: a simplified method of mesh placement. J Am Coll Surg 2002;194:93-5.

13. Thoman DS, Phillips EH. Current status of laparoscopic ventral hernia repair. Surg Endosc 2002;16:939-42.

14. Larson GM. Ventral hernia repair by the laparoscopic approach. Surg Clin North Am 2000;80:1329-40.

15. Robbins SB, Pofahl WE, Gonzalez RP. Laparoscopic ventral hernia repair reduces wound complications. Am Surg 2001;67:896-900.

16. Araki Y, Ishibashi N, Kanazawa M, Kishimoto Y, Matono K, Sasatomi T, Ogata Y, Shirouzu K. Laparoscopic intraperi-

toneal repair of postoperative ventral incisional hernia using Composix mesh. Kurume Med J 2002;49:167-70.

17. Eid GM, Prince JM, Mattar SG, Hamad G, Ikrammudin S, Schauer PR. Medium-term follow-up confirms the safety and durability of laparoscopic ventral hernia repair with PTFE. Surgery 2003;134:599-603; discussion 603-4.

18. Koehler RH, Begos D, Berger D, Carey S, LeBlanc K, Park A, Ramshaw B, Smoot R, Voeller G. Minimal adhesions to ePTFE mesh after laparoscopic ventral incisional hernia repair: reoperative findings in 65 cases. Zentralbl Chir 2003;128:625-30.

19. Paul A, Korenkov M, Peters S, Kohler L, Fischer S, Troidl H. Unacceptable results of the Mayo procedure for repair of abdominal incisional hernias. Eur J Surg 1998;164:361-7.

20. van der Linden FT, van Vroonhoven TJ. Long-term results after surgical correction of incisional hernia. Neth J Surg 1988;40:127-9.

21. Vrijland WW, Jeekel J, Steyerberg EW, Den Hoed PT, Bonjer HJ. Intraperitoneal polypropylene mesh repair of incisional hernia is not associated with enterocutaneous fistula. Br J Surg 2000;87:348-52.

22. Stoppa RE. The treatment of complicated groin and incisional hernias. World J Surg 1989;13:545-54.

23. Wright BE, Beckerman J, Cohen M, Cumming JK, Rodriguez JL. Is laparoscopic umbilical hernia repair with mesh a reasonable alternative to conventional repair? Am J Surg 2002;184:505-8; discussion 508-9.

24. Lau H, Patil NG. Umbilical hernia in adults. Surg Endosc 2003.

25. Holzman MD, Purut CM, Reintgen K, Eubanks S, Pappas TN. Laparoscopic ventral and incisional hernioplasty. Surg Endosc 1997;11:32-5.

26. Koehler RH, Voeller G. Recurrences in laparoscopic incisional hernia repairs: a personal series and review of the literature. Jsls 1999;3:293-304.

27. Chari R, Chari V, Eisenstat M, Chung R. A case controlled study of laparoscopic incisional hernia repair. Surg Endosc 2000;14:117-9.

28. Ben-Haim M, Kuriansky J, Tal R, Zmora O, Mintz Y, Rosin D, Ayalon A, Shabtai M. Pitfalls and complications with laparoscopic intraperitoneal expanded polytetrafluoroethylene patch repair of postoperative ventral hernia. Surg Endosc 2002;16:785-8.

29. Houck JP, Rypins EB, Sarfeh IJ, Juler GL, Shimoda KJ. Repair of incisional hernia. Surg Gynecol Obstet 1989;169:397-9.

30. Franklin ME, Dorman JP, Glass JL, Balli JE, Gonzalez JJ. Laparoscopic ventral and incisional hernia repair. Surg Laparosc Endosc 1998;8:294-9.

31. Toy FK, Bailey RW, Carey S, Chappuis CW, Gagner M, Josephs LG, Mangiante EC, Park AE, Pomp A, Smoot RT, Jr., Uddo JF, Jr., Voeller GR. Prospective, multicenter study of laparoscopic ventral hernioplasty. Preliminary results. Surg Endosc 1998;12:955-9.

32. Carbajo MA, Martin del Olmo JC, Blanco JI, de la Cuesta C, Toledano M, Martin F, Vaquero C, Inglada L. Laparoscopic treatment vs open surgery in the solution of major incisional and abdominal wall hernias with mesh. Surg Endosc 1999;13:250-2.

33. LeBlanc KA, Booth WV, Whitaker JM, Bellanger DE. Laparoscopic incisional and ventral herniorraphy: our initial 100 patients. Hernia 2001;5:41-5.

34. Park A, Birch DW, Lovrics P. Laparoscopic and open incisional hernia repair: a comparison study. Surgery 1998;124:816-21; discussion 821-2.

35. Ramshaw BJ, Esartia P, Schwab J, Mason EM, Wilson RA, Duncan TD, Miller J, Lucas GW, Promes J. Comparison of laparoscopic and open ventral herniorrhaphy. Am Surg 1999;65:827-31; discussion 831-2.

36. Hashizume M, Migo S, Tsugawa Y, Tanoue K, Ohta M, Kumashiro R, Sugimachi K. Laparoscopic repair of paraumbilical ventral hernia with increasing size in an obese patient. Surg Endosc 1996;10:933-5.

37. Palanivelu C. Laparoscopic Repair of Incisional Hernias. In: Palanivelu C, ed. Text Book of Surgical Laparoscopy. Coimbatore: Gem Digestive diseases Foundation, 2002:255-262.

38. Palanivelu C. Laparoscopic Repair of Ventral Hernia. In: Palanivelu C, ed. CIGES Atlas of Laparoscopic Surgery. Second ed. New Delhi: Jaypee Brothers Medical Publishers Pvt. Ltd, 2003:107-114.

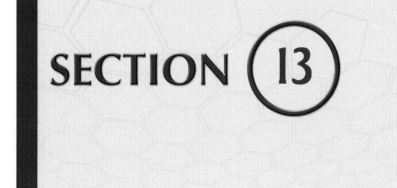

SECTION 13

Urology

73

Laparoscopic Adrenalectomy

INTRODUCTION

The adrenal glands are in most respects ideally suited to a laparoscopic approach, since most adrenal tumors are small in size and pathologically benign. Laparoscopic adrenalectomy was first described in 1992 by Petelin,[1] Gagner etal[2] and Higashihara etal.[3] It is a safe alternative to open adrenalectomy for carefully selected patients. Different laparoscopic approaches to the adrenal gland have been described, mirroring the approaches adopted in open surgery, viz., the transperitoneal anterior approach, the transperitoneal lateral approach and the retroperitoneal approach. The transperitoneal lateral approach was popularized by Gagner etal,[4] while the retroperitoneal approach was popularized by Mercan etal.[5] The laparoscopic approach has become the treatment of choice for benign adrenal tumors.[6, 7]

ANATOMY

Each adrenal gland weighs 4 to 6 grams and measures approximately 4 -5 cm. X 2-3 cm. X 0.5-1 cm. in size. The right gland is somewhat pyramidal in shape whereas the left gland assumes more of a flattened or crescent shape as it is closely applied to the kidney. The adrenal gland has a fibrous capsule & can be distinguished from the peri-renal fat by its golden orange color and the finely granular texture of the conical surface, friable consistency, ease of capsular disruption, fragmentation and bleeding. Both adrenals rest on the diaphragm, the right side one being related to the bare area of the liver and the hepato-renal ligament. A portion of the right gland (anteromedial) may lie posterior to the IVC. The left adrenal is related to the omental bursa, bordered medially by the stomach and superior pole of the spleen and inferiorly by the pancreas and the splenic vein.

The adrenal gland has rich blood supply from inferior phrenic artery, the aorta and the renal artery. All arteries enter into medial aspect of the gland. The adrenal vein is the most important to be considered. Each gland has got a single central vein. Right side adrenal vein is shorter (0.5 to 1 cm) and enters the IVC postero-medially. Occasionally there may be a second vein. The left adrenal vein is longer and drains into the left renal vein.

INDICATIONS

The indications and contraindications for laparoscopic adrenalectomy are enumerated in the following Table.[8]

Indications of laparoscopic adrenalectomy
1. Aldosteronoma.

2. Cushing's syndrome:
   i. Cortisol-producing adenoma.
   ii. Primary adrenal hyperplasia.
   iii. Failed treatment of ACTH-dependent cushing's.

3. Pheochromocytoma (sporadic or familial)
4. Nonfunctioning cortical adenoma (incidentaloma) - > 5 cm. or a typical radiographic appearance.
5. Adrenal metastasis.
6. Miscellaneous tumours (myelolipoma, adrenal cyst, ganglioneuroma

Contraindications to laparoscopic adrenalectomy
1. Adrenocortical carcinoma.
2. Malignant phaeochromocytoma.
3. Large adrenal mass >8-10 cm. in size.
4. Existing contraindication to laparoscopic surgery.

Hormone secreting adrenocortical tumors should be excised.[9, 10] Bilateral laparoscopic adrenalectomy has been reported in cases of Cushing's syndrome after failed trans-sphenoidal ablation for a pituitary adenoma,[11] Cushing's syndrome due to an ectopic ACTH-producing tumor,[12] macronodular adrenal hyperplasia,[13] congenital adrenal hyperplasia[14] and pheochromocytoma, either with or without MEN type 2.

In spite of successful laparoscopic resections of pheochromocytoma, the benefits of this procedure have been questioned. Intraoperative hypertensive crises are supposed to be more severe as a result of the increase in intra-abdominal pressure due to CO_2 gas insufflation.[15]

With advances in imaging techniques, the incidence of accidentally discovered adrenal tumors is increasing. These "incidentalomas" gradually increase in frequency with age and occur in 3-7% of aduts older than 50 years of age.[16] Per unit weight, adrenal is one of the most common sites for metastasis, especially from primaries in lungs and kidneys. Prolonged survival has been reported in a small percentage of cases after resection of unilateral adrenal metastasis.[17] Laparoscopic resection of adrenal metastases has been reported, but it is controversial.[18] Adrenocortical carcinomas are rare but exceedingly malignant. They account for 0.05% to 0.2% of all cases of cancer.[19] Tumors suspected of being malignant should be treated with conventional open surgery.[6] One should convert to open technique when a tumor whose removal is being attempted laparoscopically is suspected or confirmed to be malignant intra-operatively.[7]

PREOPERATIVE WORKUP

Ultrasound scan and CT Scan should be obtained preoperatively to know the exact size and location of the adrenal tumors and relationship to adjacent structures. Adrenal masses as small as 10 mm. can be reliably detected by CT although the relative lack of retroperitoneal fat in children might decrease the sensitivity of the test in them.[20, 21] If the operation is performed for a pheochromocytoma, the patient is pre-treated with alpha blockers like phenoxybenzamine and are hyperhydrated. In patients with Conn's Syndrome, the electrolyte imbalance has to be corrected and the blood pressure must be medically controlled. Patients with Cushing's Syndrome or Cushing's Disease due to cortisol-producing adrenal tumors should receive steroids preoperatively as the contralateral gland may be atrophied and suppressed.

OPERATIVE TECHNIQUE:[22, 23]

TYPE OF APPROACH

1. Transperitoneal
   i. Lateral flank approach.
   ii. Anterior approach.
B. Posterior retroperitoneal approach.

Regardless of the type of laparoscopic adrenalectomy, two basic principles for removal of the adrenal glands are observed:

1. Extra capsular dissection of the gland to avoid tearing and fragmentation, as this may result in implantation of adrenal tumor on the retroperitoneum.

2. A meticulous dissection technique and hemostasis with particular attention to safe and secure ligation of the adrenal vein first.

LAPAROSCOPIC LEFT ADRENALECTOMY

(Transperitoneal Lateral Flank Approach)

All operations are performed under general anesthesia. A 30 degree angled scope is important for visualization. The patient should be secured to the operating table with tape and safety straps to prevent movement and to allow tilting of the table to the reverse Trendelenburg position and to the left lateral position.

Position of Patient and Ports

Patient is placed in right lateral position with a sandbag underneath the iliac crest and ports are placed as in the Figure 2

Operative Technique

A pneumoperitoneum is created with closed Veress needle technique. The camera port is inserted in the umbilicus and the peritoneal cavity is explored.

First, the splenic flexure of the colon has to be mobilized by incising the splenocolic ligament. The

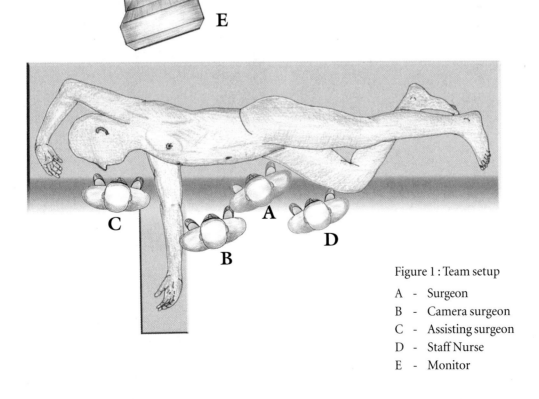

Figure 1 : Team setup

A - Surgeon
B - Camera surgeon
C - Assisting surgeon
D - Staff Nurse
E - Monitor

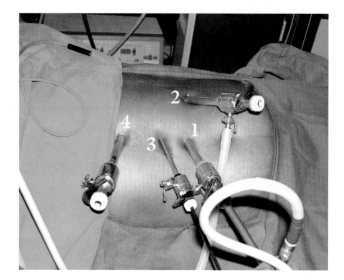

Figure 2 : Position of ports

1 - Camera port 10mm in Left midclavicular line
2 - Right hand working port 10 mm in Left anterior
       axillary line
3 - Left hand working port 5mm
4 - Retracting port 10mm

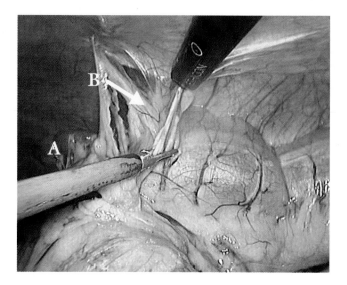

Figure 3 : Mobilization of splenic flexure of colon

A - Spleen
B - Splenic flexure

incision is extended along the anti-mesenteric border of transverse colon and extended down the left paracolic gutter along the line of Toldt using electrocautery scissors or Harmonic Scalpel®. Through the epigastric port, a fan shaped retractor is placed and the spleen and the tail of the pancreas are lifted cephalad and to the right. EndoBabcock's forceps introduced through the lateral port is used to retract the colon downwards and to the right. The dissection then proceeds superiorly between the spleen and kidney towards the diaphragm. The lieno-renal ligament is divided. If required, the attachments of the spleen to the diaphragm are divided to allow adequate retraction of the spleen.

Gerota's fascia is opened and the superior pole of the kidney is dissected free. It is very important to identify the upper pole of kidney which serves as the landmark for locating the adrenal gland. The adrenal gland itself is distinguishable from the surrounding peritoneal fat by its golden orange color and the granular texture of the cortical surface.

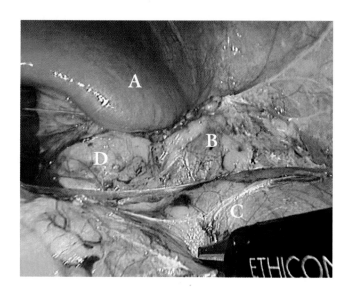

Figure 4 : Splenic flexure is mobilized completely and adrenal gland is exposed

A - Spleen
B - Left kidney
C - Colon
D - Left adrenal gland

The superior pole of the adrenal gland is mobilized first. Then the medial aspect of the gland where most of the arterial supply enters is carefully dissected using Harmonic Scalpel or Maryland's curved dissector with coagulating electro cautery. Vessels are controlled with clips and divided using scissors or Harmonic Scalpel. The inferior pole is then dissected carefully and the principle adrenal vein which drains into the left renal vein is clipped and divided. In pheochromocytoma, it is important to perform the manoeuver before the tumor itself is manipulated.

The adrenal vein is doubly ligated and divided. The lateral aspect of the adrenal is relatively avascular and may be mobilized after this. After the gland has been completely mobilized, it is placed in retrieval bag and removed. The operating field is re-inspected for hemostasis.

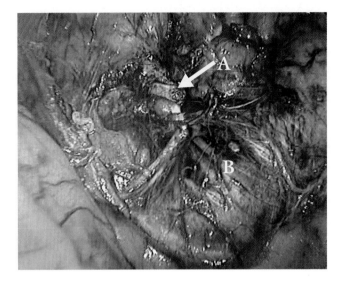

Figure 6 : Left adrenal vein is clipped close to the renal vein and divided

A - Divided end of left adrenal vein

B - Left renal vein

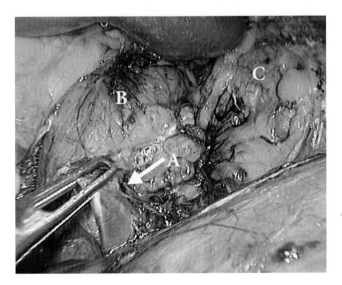

Figure 5 : Left adrenal vein is identified and dissected

A - Left adrenal vein

B - Adrenal gland

C - Left kidney

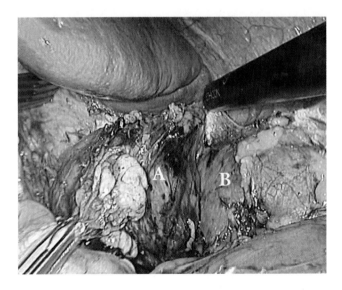

Figure 7 : Mobilization of adrenal gland from the upper pole of left kidney

A - Adrenal gland

B - Left kidney

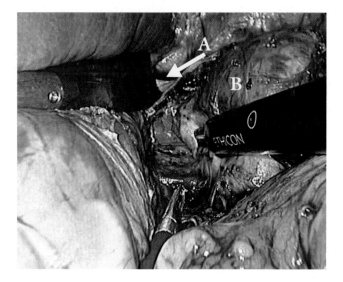

Figure 8 : Mobilization of the adrenal gland from the splenic attachment

A - Liver retractor is used to retract the spleen
B - Adrenal gland

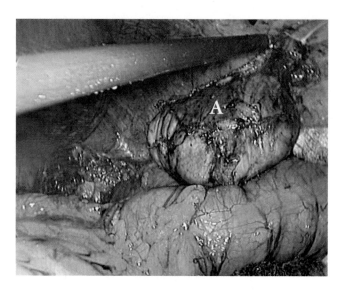

Figure 9 : Adrenal gland is excised completely

A - Excised left adrenal gland

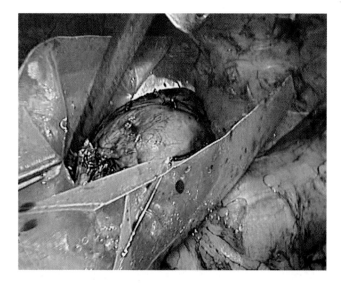

Figure 10 : Excised adrenal gland is placed in the endobag for extraction

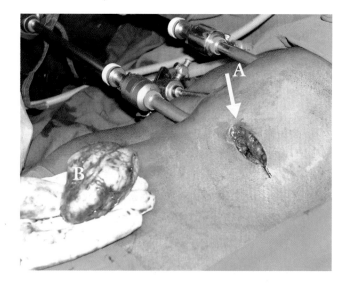

Figure 11 : By extending the right hand working port, excised adrenal gland is removed in toto

A - Exended right hand working port
B - Excised adrenal gland

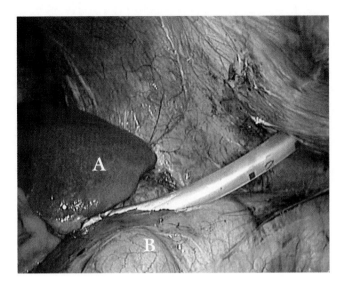

Figure 12 : Placement of drainage tube

A - Spleen
B - Splenic flexure of colon

LAPAROSCOPIC RIGHT ADRENALECTOMY

(Transabdominal Lateral Flank Approach)

The patient is placed on a rotatable table, on a bean bag in the left lateral position. The partial lateral position, allows the patient to be rotated to a supine position for initial trocar insertion, then rotated to a variable lateral position.

Operative Technique

Initial ports are placed in the umbilical or supra umbilical region, depending on the body habitus and the remaining ports are placed after initial exploration under visual guidance.

The hepatic flexure of the colon is mobilized from its parietal attachments using sharp and blunt dissection. The colon is retracted medially and inferiorly with the Endo Babcock and peritoneal attachment is divided with electrocautery scissor or Harmonic Scalpel. The right triangular ligament is divided sufficiently to allow retraction of the right lobe of the liver using a fan-blade retractor introduced through the epigastric port and visualisation of the IVC and adrenal gland.

After division of Gerota's fascia on the upper pole of the kidney, the adrenal gland should come into view. The principle central vein of the adrenal gland, if possible is divided first but in practice dividing the adrenal arteries facilitates exposure as the vein is approached. The adrenal arteries enter the medial surface of the adrenal gland and are carefully dissected and divided using the Harmonic Scalpel or Maryland's dissecting forceps with coagulating electrocautery. The adrenal vein should be dissected very carefully. Anatomically, it is difficult to control due to its short length and drainage into the postero-medial aspect of the IVC. It is also important to be aware of the anomalous drainage into the right hepatic or right renal vein. Clips are usually sufficient to control the vein, if necessary intracorporeal ligature may be applied. As an alternative technique, a clip can be placed on the gland side of the vein and endoloop can be preloaded over a grasper. The vein is divided and the endoloop is secured. Usually, another 3mm trocar has to be inserted to facilitate this manoeuver. After the adrenal vein is divided, the adrenal gland should be completely freed from the surrounding tissues using blunt dissection, electrocautery or Harmonic Scalpel. During this

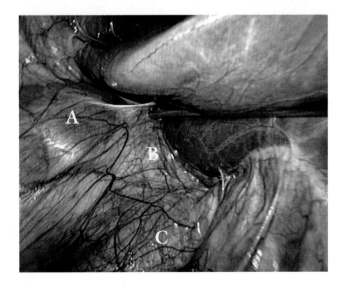

Figure 13 : Right lobe of liver is retracted up and right adrenal gland is exposed

A - Right kidney
B - Right adrenal gland
C - Inferior vena cava (IVC)

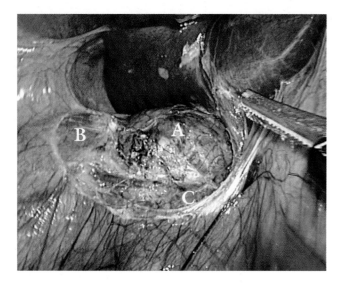

Figure 14 : Anterior peritoneal covering of the adrenal gland is dissected

A - Adrenal gland
B - Kidney
C - IVC

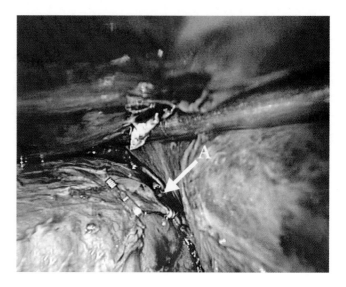

Figure 15 : Right adrenal vein is dissected and clipped

A - Clipped adrenal vein

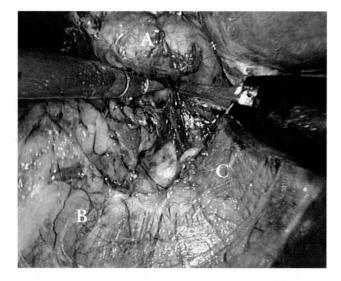

Figure 16 : Adrenal gland is lifted and mobilized posteriorly

A - Adrenal gland
B - Right renal vein
C - IVC

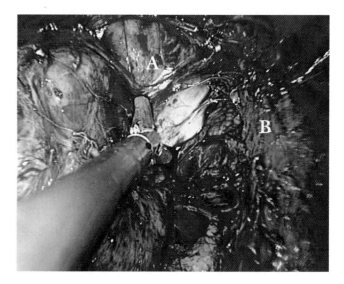

Figure 17 : Adrenal gland separated from the IVC

A - Adrenal gland
B - IVC

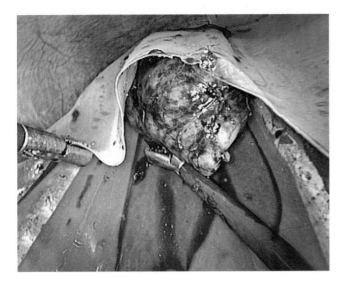

Figure 18 : Excised adrenal gland is placed in the endobag for extraction

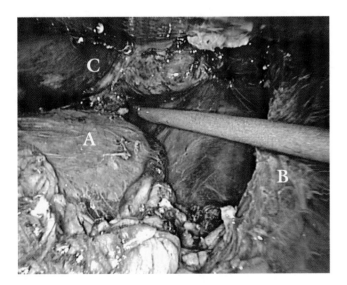

Figure 19 : Inspection of dissected area for hemostasis

A - Upper pole of left kidney
B - IVC
C - Inferior surface of thr right lobe of liver

process, any branches of the inferior phrenic vessels that are encountered can be divided. After the adrenal gland is completely freed, it should be placed into an impermeable bag to avoid contamination of the abdominal cavity during extraction. The adrenal bed is then copiously irrigated and haemostasis is secured.

ANTERIOR TRANS-PERITONEAL APPROACH

The advantage of this approach are that it provides a large working space and uses the traditional view with which the surgeons are familiar. The disadvantages of this approach is the difficulty in the retraction of the intestine. Right adrenalectomy is more difficult than the left adrenalectomy. For the right, mobilisation and retraction of the right lobe of the liver, hepatic flexure of the colon and second part of the duodenum may all be necessary and control of adrenal vein is more difficult due to inadequate exposure. The left adrenal can be approached through lesser sac, through mesocolon or laterally mobilizing the splenic flexure of the colon. The anterior transperitoneal approach is preferred for bilateral adrenalectomy.

POSTERIOR RETROPERITONEAL APPROACH

The retroperitoneal space is created initially by digital exploration, then by balloon dilatation. The retroperitoneal space is maintained by insufflating with CO_2 and the trocars are inserted into the retroperitoneum. The adrenal gland is endoscopically mobilized and removed.

Position of the patient and placement of ports

The patient is positioned prone with the ipsilateral flank raised slightly. The retroperitoneal space is identified under fluoroscopic guidance, insufflated with Verees needle and a trocar cannula is placed inferior to the lower pole of the kidney and just above the iliac crest. A 30 degree scope is inserted. Three additional ports are placed as follows. The location of the second port is at the lowest rib. Third port is placed at the mid portion of the kidney just lateral to the sacrospinalis. The fourth is inserted 2 cm lateral to the lateral border of the kidney. Then mobilisation and removal of adrenal is carried out as in the trans-peritoneal approach.

Alternatively, balloon can be introduced into the space created by digital dissection, inflated and retroperitoneal space can be created easily. Gaur has developed a new technique using a indigenous balloon for creating a retroperitoneal space.[24]

COMPARISON OF TECHNIQUES

Transperitoneal Lateral Flank Approach

Advantages

1. The lateral position allows gravity retraction of adjacent organs, thus facilitating exposure of the adrenals.

2. Placement of trocars subcostally provides cephalad and posterior access to abdominal cavity and retroperitoneum.

3. Allows large working space and examination of the rest of the structures.

4. Although the patient is in a lateral decubitus position, anatomic landmarks to help maintain orientation of the dissection are readily apparent.

5. Concomitant procedures such as cholecystectomy or liver biopsy can be easily performed.

Disadvantages

1. Control of right adrenal vein is difficult

2. Some retraction of the adjacent viscera is required and, on the left side, the colon has to be mobilized, which may cause post-operative ileus.

3. One is unable to approach the contralateral adrenal and so, for bilateral adrenalectomy, the patient has to be re-positioned.

Transperitoneal Anterior Approach

Advantage

1. Operating view port is same as for the opening.

2. Allows access to both the adrenal glands.

Disadvantages

1. More difficult and takes longer operating time.

2. Needs mobilization and retraction of the colon, liver and spleen, may also increase the risk of injury.

3. May require placement of additional trocars.

Posterior Retroperitoneal Approach

Advantages

1. Most direct access to Adrenal gland.

2. Avoids entry into the peritoneal cavity altogether and involves minimal retraction of adjacent organs.

3. Incidence of post-operative ileus is minimum.

Disadvantages

1. Limited working space, angle and working distance.

2. Posterior view may cause disorientation.

3. Injury to the pleura likely due to proximity.

4. Due to limited working space, larger tumors are difficult to manage. Moreover, if a peritoneal tear occurs during the operation, the working space may be further compromised.

DISCUSSION

This procedure requires advanced laparoscopic skills and a thorough understanding of adrenal anatomy and pathophysiology of adrenal disorders. The result depends upon the proper selection of individuals for the procedure.

An adrenal tumor of size of 8 cms. or more is considered the upper limit for laparoscopic adrenalectomy.[25, 26] Tumors larger than 6 cms should be approached cautiously for two reasons:

1. It is difficult to dissect the large masses. Control of the blood supply may be difficult particularly the right adrenal vein.

2. The risk of adrenal carcinoma increases as lesions increases in size beyond 6 cm in diameter. Suspicion of carcinoma is an indication for open surgery.

Although the size of an adrenal tumor has been shown to be an important indicator of the risk of it being malignant, many, if not most, large adrenal tumors are benign.[27-29] It has been estimated that for patients with adrenal tumors > 6 cms. in size, more than 60 adrenalectomies would have to be performed to remove 1 adrenocortical cancer.[30] At the same time, there are case reports of regional, peritoneal and distant recurrences after laparoscopic resection of unsuspected adrenocortical cancers in small sized tumors.[31-34] However, currently, tumor size > 6 cm. diameter and weight > 100 gms. are two of the best predictors of malignancy.[35] For patients with non-secretory tumors smaller than 5 cms. and no signs of malignancy, an observational approach should include follow-up with CT scan 3 months after diagnosis.[31]

Besides the traditional benefits of laparoscopic surgery, laparoscopic adrenalectomy may have other benefits:

1. The problem of widely fluctuating blood pressure is minimized in laparoscopic approach while operating on pheochromocytoma due to less manipulation.

2. More expeditious and definitive approach to the treatment of patients with intermediate sized adrenal lesions.

Of the three approaches used for laparoscopic adrenalectomy, the transperitoneal lateral flank approach is the most popular.[4] The retroperitoneal approach has yielded excellent results, although the exposure is sub-optimal and the learning curve is higher than that of transperitoneal approaches.[36, 37]

Laparoscopic adrenalectomy has been considered the gold standard for the treatment of benign adrenal tumors of small volume due to the better results obtained when compared to those of open surgery, in all aspects morbidity, hospitalization, convalescence, bleeding, pain, costs, etc.[6, 7, 38-41] Concerning the operative time, once the learning curve has been climbed, it is approximately the same as for open surgery.[42] The laparoscopic approach is superior to open surgery in cases of both unilateral and bilateral phaeochromocytoma,[43] bilateral tumors,[44] tumors in pregnancy,[45] and multiple tumors.[45] Actually, neither the laparoscopic or the open approach are risk factors themselves, if adequately employed, meaning avoiding the main risk factors of the procedure by

controlling the adrenal vein at the beginning, and doing minimal manipulation of the tumor.[46]

COMPLICATIONS

The complications associated with this procedure are enumerated in the following Table.[8]

Complications Of Laparoscopic Adrenalectomy

1. Hemorrhage.
2. Intraperitoneal Organ Injury
   i. Liver
   ii. Spleen
   iii. Pancreas
   iv. Kidney
   v. Colon
   vi. Diaphragm
3. Pancreatitis/ Pancreatic Fistula
4. Wound Problems
   i. Infection
   ii. Trocar Site Hernias
5. Neurological
   i. Nerve Compression
   ii. Compartment Syndrome
6. GI: Ileus
7. Urinary Tract: UTI
8. Pulmonary
   i. Pneumonia
   ii. Atelectasis
   iii. Pneumothorax
9. Thromboembolic: DVT/ Pulmonary Embolisation
10. Cardiovascular: Arrhythmias
11. Others
    i. Acute Adrenal Insufficiency
    ii. Lymphocele
    iii. Renovascular Hypertension
    iv. Tumor Recurrence

The most common complication of laparoscopic adrenalectomy has been hemorrhage, which, combined with poor exposure, was the most common reason for conversion to an open procedure.[8, 47] Deep vein thrombosis, hematoma (which required laparotomy or transfusion in several cases and pneumothorax are the most frequently reported complications after laparoscopic adrenalectomy.[6, 38]

CONCLUSION

Laparoscopic adrenalectomy is a safe and effective operation when performed by an experienced laparoscopic surgeon and can be carried out in a time comparable to that of open surgical technique. The transabdominal flank approach gives adequate exposure. Adrenal carcinoma is considered contraindication for laparoscopic approach.

Laparoscopic adrenalectomy is a challenging surgical procedure that requires advanced laparoscopic skills, an understanding of adrenal anatomy, proper patient selection and adherence to the principles of open adrenal surgery for proper and safe completion of the operation.

Finally, it should be remembered that open adrenalectomy is a safe, effective and proven technique. The morbidity associated with the open posterior approach is minimal and patient should not be subjected to the laparoscopic approach unless the well established principles of open adrenalectomy can be followed.

Referenes

1. Petelin J. Laparoscopic adrenalectomy. Proceedings, Third World Congress Endoscopic Surgery, Bordeaux, France, September 1992. Bordeaux, 1992.

2. Gagner M, Lacroix A, Bolte E. Laparoscopic adrenalectomy in Cushing's syndrome and pheochromocytoma. N Engl J Med 1992; 327(14):1033.

3. Higashihara E, Tanaka Y, Horie S, et al. [A case report of laparoscopic adrenalectomy]. Nippon Hinyokika Gakkai Zasshi 1992; 83(7):1130-3.

4. Gagner M, Lacroix A, Bolte E, Pomp A. Laparoscopic adrenalectomy. The importance of a flank approach in the lateral decubitus position. Surg Endosc 1994; 8(2):135-8.

5. Mercan S, Seven R, Ozarmagan S, Tezelman S. Endoscopic retroperitoneal adrenalectomy. Surgery 1995; 118(6):1071-5; discussion 1075-6.

6. Gagner M, Pomp A, Heniford BT, et al. Laparoscopic adrenalectomy: lessons learned from 100 consecutive procedures. Ann Surg 1997; 226(3):238-46; discussion 246-7.

7. Smith CD, Weber CJ, Amerson JR. Laparoscopic adrenalectomy: new gold standard. World J Surg 1999; 23(4):389-96.

8. Brunt L. Laparoscopic adrenalectomy. In B M, ed. pp. 213-237.

9. Flack M CG. Neoplasms of the adrenal cortex. In Holland JF BR, Morton DL etal., ed. Cancer Medicine. Baltimore: Williams & Wilkins, 1996. pp. 1563-70.

10. Schell SR, Talamini MA, Udelsman R. Laparoscopic adrenalectomy. Adv Surg 1997; 31:333-50.

11. Bax TW, Marcus DR, Galloway GQ, et al. Laparoscopic bilateral adrenalectomy following failed hypophysectomy. Surg Endosc 1996; 10(12):1150-3.

12. Ferrer FA, MacGillivray DC, Malchoff CD, et al. Bilateral laparoscopic adrenalectomy for adrenocorticotropic dependent Cushing's syndrome. J Urol 1997; 157(1):16-8.

13. Shinbo H, Suzuki K, Sato T, et al. Simultaneous bilateral laparoscopic adrenalectomy in ACTH-independent macronodular adrenal hyperplasia. Int J Urol 2001; 8(6):315-8.

14. Warinner SA, Zimmerman D, Thompson GB, Grant CS. Study of three patients with congenital adrenal hyperplasia treated by bilateral adrenalectomy. World J Surg 2000; 24(11):1347-52.

15. Joris JL, Noirot DP, Legrand MJ, et al. Hemodynamic changes during laparoscopic cholecystectomy. Anesth Analg 1993; 76(5):1067-71.

16. Kloos RT, Gross MD, Francis IR, et al. Incidentally discovered adrenal masses. Endocr Rev 1995; 16(4):460-84.

17. Lo CY, van Heerden JA, Soreide JA, et al. Adrenalectomy for metastatic disease to the adrenal glands. Br J Surg 1996; 83(4):528-31.

18. Heniford BT, Arca MJ, Walsh RM, Gill IS. Laparoscopic adrenalectomy for cancer. Semin Surg Oncol 1999; 16(4):293-306.

19. Lipsett MB, Hertz R, Ross GT. Clinical and Pathophysiologic Aspects of Adrenocortical Carcinoma. Am J Med 1963; 35:374-83.

20. Korobkin M. Overview of adrenal imaging/adrenal CT. Urol Radiol 1989; 11(4):221-6.

21. Dunnick NR. Hanson lecture. Adrenal imaging: current status. AJR Am J Roentgenol 1990; 154(5):927-36.

22. Palanivelu C. Laparoscopic adrenalectomy. In C P, ed. Textbook of Surgical Laparoscopy. Coimbatore: GEM Digestive Diseases Foundation, 2002. pp. 497-504.

23. Palanivelu C. Laparoscopic adrenalectomy. In C P, ed. CIGES Atlas of Surgical Laparoscopy: Jaypee Brothers Medical Publishers (P) Ltd., 2003.

24. Gaur DD. Laparoscopic operative retroperitoneoscopy: use of a new device. J Urol 1992; 148(4):1137-9.

25. Wells SA, Merke DP, Cutler GB, Jr., et al. Therapeutic controversy: The role of laparoscopic surgery in adrenal disease. J Clin Endocrinol Metab 1998; 83(9):3041-9.

26. Barnett CC, Jr., Varma DG, El-Naggar AK, et al. Limitations of size as a criterion in the evaluation of adrenal tumors. Surgery 2000; 128(6):973-82;discussion 982-3.

27. Khafagi FA, Gross MD, Shapiro B, et al. Clinical significance of the large adrenal mass. Br J Surg 1991; 78(7):828-33.

28. Terzolo M, Ali A, Osella G, Mazza E. Prevalence of adrenal carcinoma among incidentally discovered adrenal masses. A retrospective study from 1989 to 1994. Gruppo Piemontese Incidentalomi Surrenalici. Arch Surg 1997; 132(8):914-9.

29. Bernini GP, Miccoli P, Moretti A, et al. Sixty adrenal masses of large dimensions: hormonal and morphologic evaluation. Urology 1998; 51(6):920-5.

30. Copeland PM. The incidentally discovered adrenal mass. Ann Surg 1984; 199(1):116-22.

31. Suzuki K, Ushiyama T, Mugiya S, et al. Hazards of laparoscopic adrenalectomy in patients with adrenal malignancy. J Urol 1997; 158(6):2227.

32. Deckers S, Derdelinckx L, Col V, et al. Peritoneal carcinomatosis following laparoscopic resection of an adrenocortical tumor causing primary hyperaldosteronism. Horm Res 1999; 52(2):97-100.

33. Foxius A, Ramboux A, Lefebvre Y, et al. Hazards of laparoscopic adrenalectomy for Conn's adenoma. When enthusiasm turns to tragedy. Surg Endosc 1999; 13(7):715-7.

34. Bonjer HJ, Sorm V, Berends FJ, et al. Endoscopic retroperitoneal adrenalectomy: lessons learned from 111 consecutive cases. Ann Surg 2000; 232(6):796-803.

35. Page DL DR, Hough AJ. Tumors of the adrenal. Washington DC: AFIP, 1986.

36. Heintz A, Walgenbach S, Junginger T. Results of endoscopic retroperitoneal adrenalectomy. Surg Endosc 1996; 10(6):633-5.

37. Fahey TJ, 3rd, Reeve TS, Delbridge L. Adrenalectomy: expanded indications for the extraperitoneal approach. Aust N Z J Surg 1994; 64(7):494-7.

38. Henry JF, Defechereux T, Raffaelli M, et al. Complications of laparoscopic adrenalectomy: results of 169 consecutive procedures. World J Surg 2000; 24(11):1342-6.

39. Dudley NE, Harrison BJ. Comparison of open posterior versus transperitoneal laparoscopic adrenalectomy. Br J Surg 1999; 86(5):656-60.

40. Shen WT, Lim RC, Siperstein AE, et al. Laparoscopic vs open adrenalectomy for the treatment of primary hyperaldosteronism. Arch Surg 1999; 134(6):628-31; discussion 631-2.

41. Yoshimura K, Yoshioka T, Miyake O, et al. Comparison of clinical outcomes of laparoscopic and conventional open adrenalectomy. J Endourol 1998; 12(6):555-9.

42. Terachi T, Matsuda T, Terai A, et al. Transperitoneal laparoscopic adrenalectomy: experience in 100 patients. J Endourol 1997; 11(5):361-5.

43. Chigot JP, Movschin M, el Bardissi M, et al. [Comparative study between laparoscopic and conventional adrenalectomy for pheochromocytomas]. Ann Chir 1998; 52(4):346-9.

44. Manger T, Piatek S, Klose S, et al. [Bilateral laparoscopic transperitoneal adrenalectomy in pheochromocytoma]. Langenbecks Arch Chir 1997; 382(1):37-42.

45. Janetschek G, Finkenstedt G, Gasser R, et al. Laparoscopic surgery for pheochromocytoma: adrenalectomy, partial resection, excision of paragangliomas. J Urol 1998; 160(2):330-4.

46. Castilho LN, Medeiros PJ, Mitre AI, et al. Pheochromocytoma treated by laparoscopic surgery. Rev Hosp Clin Fac Med Sao Paulo 2000; 55(3):93-100.

47. Schlinkert RT, van Heerden JA, Grant CS, et al. Laparoscopic left adrenalectomy for aldosteronoma: early Mayo Clinic experience. Mayo Clin Proc 1995; 70(9):844-6.

74

Laparoscopic Nephrectomy

INTRODUCTION

Clayman et al first reported laparoscopic transperitoneal nephrectomy in 1991 for removal of an oncocytoma.[1] In 1992, Gaur reported the first successful retroperitoneal approach for renal surgery in India. He described a safe and easy technique for creation of retroperitoneal space by balloon.[2] This retroperitoneal approach can be used for several procedures like renal biopsy, nephrectomy, adrenalectomy, nephropexy, pyeloplasty, nephroureterectomy, renal cyst marsupialization, ureterolysis, retroperitoneal lymph node dissection, and ureterocutaneostomy.[3] Since the initial report by Clayman, several large series have reported the safety and efficacy of laparoscopic nephrectomy.[4-6] Laparoscopic nephrectomy has the advantages of shorter hospital stay, less postoperative pain and an earlier return to normal activities when compared to open surgery.[4-6] Long-term cancer control has also been reportedfollowing laparoscopic radical nephrectomy

and nephrourete- rectomy for renal malignancy.[7,8] Today laparoscopic nephrectomy has become a routine procedure in major urology centres for suitable patients having benign or malignant disease. Ratner et al first described laparoscopic living donor nephrectomy in 1995.[9] Since then laparoscopy is being increasingly utilized for live donor nephrectomies.

Laparoscopic simple nephrectomy is a safe alternative to open nephrectomy for the removal of nonfunctioning kidneys in benign diseases. Moreover, benign renal disease is the most common indication for laparoscopic nephrectomy. In a multicentre study by the German Urologic Association, Rassweiler et al showed that 92% of 482 laparoscopic nephrectomies were done for benign pathologies[5]. Laparoscopic nephrectomy produces a better cosmetic result with less morbidity and a shorter hospital stay. Complication rate depends upon the pathology affecting the kidney to be removed: post-inflammatory conditions have a higher complication

Types and Indications	
Simple Nephrectomy	Non-functioning kidney
	Renovascular end-stage disease
	Chronic pyelonephritis
	End-stage stone disease
	Renal dysplasia
	Xanthogranulomatous pyelonephritis
	Hydronephrosis
	Renal tuberculosis
Nephroureterectomy	Reflux nephropathy
	Primary obstructive mega-ureter
	Transitional cell cancer of Kidney/upper ureter
Radical nephrectomy	Renal cell cancer
Partial/hemi nephrectomy	Duplicated kidney with a Hydronephrotic or dysplasic part
	Small renal tumours
Live donor nephrectomy	

and conversion rate. Laparoscopic nephrectomy in chronic inflammatory renal disease may be technically more difficult due to perirenal adhesions and perihilar fibrosis.[10] Prior to renal transplantation, bilateral removal of the non-functioning kidneys can be suitably performed by laparoscopic approach. Fornara et al. compared the results of laparoscopic nephrectomy in dialysis and non-dialysis patients. Both groups had comparable results for operative times, analgesic consumption and post-operative times. However, only dialysis patients required transfusions indicating a higher complication rate for this group.[11]

PARTIAL NEPHRECTOMY

Partial nephrectomy with retroperitoneal laparoscopy is feasible, and has a reasonable operating time and blood loss. It is technically difficult but has the advantage of avoiding a large surgical incision for removal of a small piece of kidney. The use of biological glue may simplify haemostasis and closure of the collecting system but good quality drainage of the collecting system is still required to decrease the risk of urinoma.[12] This is an established procedure for benign disease. Recently, partial nephrectomy has become a generally accepted option for treating localised renal cell carcinoma of less than four cms in size. Direct vision and laparoscopic ultrasonography permit the surgeon to identify multifocal tumours and determine an adequate surgical margin.

Challenges associated with the laparoscopic approach, are particularly related to haemostasis and closure of the collecting system. Vascular occlusion and hypothermia are difficult to accomplish laparoscopically and the emphasis has been on techniques that allow simultaneous tumour resection and haemostasis. Electrocautery, the Cavitron ultrasonic surgical aspirator, the endovascular GIA stapler, the argon beam coagulator, topical agents, ultrasonic energy, and microwave thermotherapy have all been used to decrease bleeding during tissue removal.[13-15] Endoscopic retrieval pouches allow removal of the tumour specimen without tumour spillage. Only small series have been reported without long-term follow up.[16,17] It is not therefore recommended for use in clinical practice and should only be performed in controlled prospective trials.

RADICAL NEPHRECTOMY

The laparoscopic approach to renal cell carcinoma has evolved into a safe and effective minimally invasive alternative to open surgery. Laparoscopic radical nephrectomy is now almost the standard treatment for clinically localised renal cell carcinoma (T1 or T2). Studies have proven the oncological safety of this technique by the negative surgical margins in most patients and the low recurrence rate.[18,19] However, the follow up is still too short to confirm the validity of laparoscopic radical nephrectomy as an effective treatment for renal cancer. Laparoscopic radical nephrectomy has also been applied to patients with advanced stages of renal cell carcinoma.[20] Contraindications to laparoscopic radical nephrectomy include tumours with renal vein or vena cava thrombi.

The safety and efficacy of laparoscopic radical nephroureterectomy for the treatment of upper tract transitional cell carcinoma had been confirmed by a large multicentre study involving 116 patients.[21] Longer follow-up regarding oncological safety is still needed before laparoscopic radical nephroureterectomy can be considered as a standard treatment.

LIVE DONOR NEPHRECTOMY

Here the kidney and the renal vessels are completely dissected endoscopically and the entire specimen removed trough a small muscle-splitting incision 7 9 cms long. The donor has clear benefits in terms of pain reduction, cosmesis, shorter hospital stay and shorter recovery.[22] These benefits may increase the acceptance by potential kidney donors. The procedure is technically very demanding and should be performed by a very experienced surgeon well trained in laparoscopy. Preoperative multisection computed tomograghy could provide necessary anatomic information including the venous anatomy, helping the minimal access surgeon in safe performance of nephrectomy.[23]

LAPAROSCOPIC NEPHRECTOMY - APPROACHES

1. Transperitoneal
2. Retroperitoneal
3. Hand-assisted

Like in open surgery, the kidney can be approached through the peritoneum or retroperitoneally. In addition, hand-assisted surgery allows the use of one hand in the surgical field without losing pneumoperitoneum.

Transperitoneal Approach

Patient positioning

A bladder catheter and nasogastric tube is placed for decompression of the bladder and stomach and the patient positioned in a 45°, modified lateral decubitus position. The patient is taped in position with multiple strips of wide cloth tape/adhesive plaster so that the patient will remain securely in place while the table is tilted to one side or other to assist with retraction of the bowel. The axilla, knees, elbows, and ankles are padded. The entire flank and abdomen are included in the sterile skin preparation, in case conversion to an open procedure is required.

Trocar placement

Pneumoperitoneum is created using a Veress needle, which is inserted at the site where the first trocar will be placed and away from previous surgical sites. The

Advantages	Disadvantages
Transperitoneal Approach	
More familiar approach	Longer operative time (reported)
Anatomy easily recognizable	Risk of bowel injury during mobilization
Larger working space	
Retroperitoneal approach	
Quicker access to the renal hilum	Smaller working space
Avoids intraperitoneal irritation	Difficult to use endobags

initial 10-mm trocar is placed at the umbilicus. Remaining trocars are placed under direct vision. A 10-mm or 12-mm trocar is placed lateral to the ipsilateral rectus at the level of the umbilicus. The third trocar (5-mm) is inserted in the midline between the umbilicus and the xiphoid process. In obese patients, all ports are moved laterally for better purchase of instruments. Similarly, in very tall patients move all ports more superiorly. A three-trocar technique is usually utilized to complete the dissection. Additional trocars for retraction may be needed to complete the hilar dissection or assist with organ entrapment. For right nephrectomy, an additional 5-mm trocar is placed between the midline trocar and the xiphoid for liver retraction.

Mobilization of the colon

The white line of Toldt is identified and incised with scissors. The splenic ligaments should be incised to allow the spleen to fall medially along with the pancreas and the colon. For a right-sided nephrectomy, the peritoneal incision is continued cranially, above the hepatic flexure including the right triangular and right anterior coronary ligaments. Medial traction on the colon reveals colorenal attachments which are divided to complete the colon dissection. Remaining in the correct plane between colonic mesentery and Gerota's fascia is important. Once the colon is rolled medially, the duodenum is mobilised medially, exposing the inferior vena cava.

Identification and dissection of ureter and gonadal vessels

Once the colon is fully mobilized, the psoas muscle is seen. When this muscle is followed medially, the gonadal vessels are visualised. These vessels are swept medially, and the ureter is usually located just deep to them. Peristalsis of the ureter helps in differentiating it from the gonadal vessels. Once identified, the ureter is elevated and followed proximally to the lower pole and hilum of the kidney. Dissecting the gonadal vein and ureter superiorly helps in identifying the renal hilum. Following the left gonadal vein directly leads the surgeon to the left renal vein. The gonadal veins can be double clipped and divided. The ureter is not divided at this time because it can

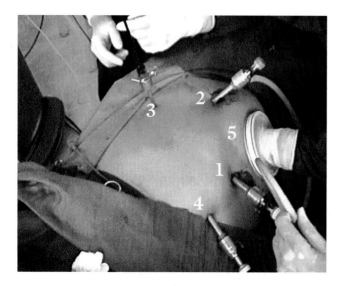

Figure 1 : Position of ports for laparoscopic left nephrectomy

1 - Supra umbilical camera port - 10mm
2 - Right hand working port - 10mm
3 - Left anterior axillary working port - 5mm
4 - Epigastric retracting port - 10mm
5 - Hand port (using Lap disc)

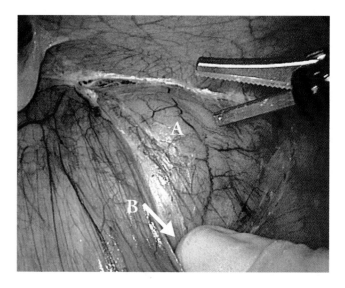

Figure 2 : Mobilization of descending colon by dividing the lateral peritoneal attachment

A - Lower pole of left kidney
B - Colon is retracted by hand

be used to elevate the kidney. Lower pole dissection can be easily performed at this point.

Dissection of the lower pole

For right nephrectomy, the left hand grasper is used to retract the kidney anterolaterally, and the suction aspirator is used in the right hand to detach any attachments between the lower pole and the psoas muscle. An additional trocar may be placed at the anterior axillary line subcostally to retract the liver superiorly as the dissection proceeds towards the renal hilum.

Dissection of renal hilum

With the ureter and lower pole of the kidney elevated, vessels entering the renal hilum can be identified and bluntly dissected using the tip of the irrigator-aspirator. Gonadal, lumbar, and accessory venous branches can be clipped and divided as necessary. Firm elevation of the lower pole of the kidney assists in identification and dissection of the renal hilar vessels. Gentle dissection with the tip of the suction-irrigator reveals the renal vein. By clearing off

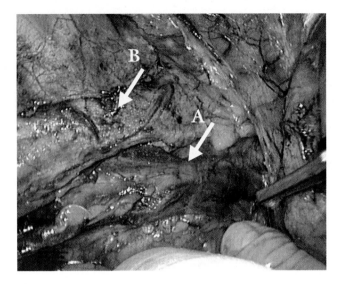

Figure 4 : Colon is mobilized medially and left ureter is exposed

A - Left ureter

B - Left gonadal vessel

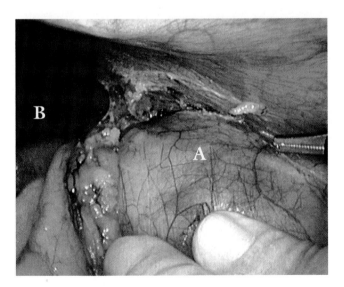

Figure 3 : Colon is mobilized medially upto the splenic flexure

A - Upper pole of kidney

B - Spleen

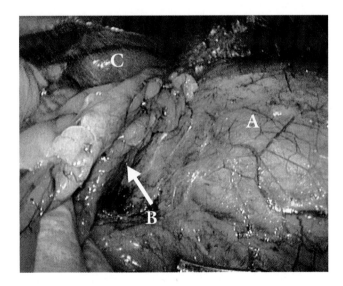

Figure 5 : Dissection carried out above, the upper pole of kidney is separated from the p\inferior border of pancreas

A - Left kidney

B - Pancreas

C - Spleen

inferior attachments and inferior lymphatics, one can identify the renal artery, which lies posterior to the vein. With an endovascular gastrointestinal anastomosis (GIA) stapler, the artery is divided first, followed by the vein.

Adrenalectomy

An adrenalectomy is also combined in patients undergoing radical nephrectomy for T2 or larger lesions or for upper-pole tumours of any size. Here the medial dissection is continued superiorly along the IVC until the adrenal vein is encountered. It is controlled with stapler, clips or by intra corporeal suturing. The dissection continues superiorly around the gland and adrenal artery branches are controlled with clips or cautery.

Dissection of the upper pole

The adrenal gland is preserved in cases of simple nephrectomy. For this the Gerota's fascia is incised anteriorly just above the hilum. Gerota's fat is then gently peeled off circumferentially above the upper pole of the kidney. At this point during the dissection, it may be necessary to clip and transect the ureter. This allows the kidney to be rotated anteriorly above the liver (right) or spleen (left) to facilitate incision of the uppermost attachments under direct vision. In cases of extreme fibrosis, a subcapsular nephrectomy can be performed once the artery and vein have been controlled.

Suction-aspirator or Endoshears are used to free the remaining renal attachments. Once the kidney is completely free, the ureter is divided last.

Specimen removal and closure

The kidney can be removed either intact or through morcellation. When morcellation is performed, the specimen should be placed into a sturdy entrapment sac. This minimizes the risk of rupture during mechanical morcellation of the tissue . Alternatively, the kidney can be removed intact through an incision after placement into a sac. The kidney can be delivered out of an extended trocar site or Pfannenstiel incision. The periumbilical incision is extended to approximately 5 cm, and the fascial incision to 7 cm. this usually allows easy removal of most kidneys.

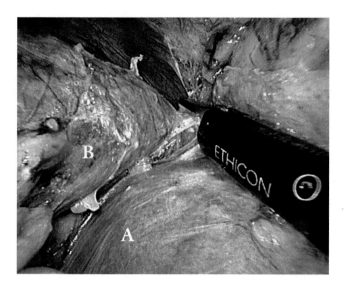

Figure 6 : Mobilization of upper pole of kidney from the spleen

A - Upper pole of left kidney
B - Spleen

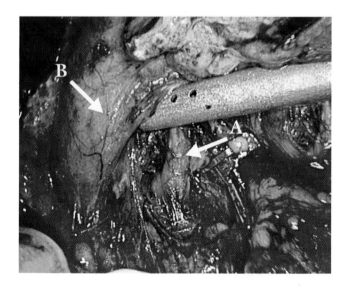

Figure 7 : Dissection in the renal hilum. Renal vein and artery is dissected

A - Left renal artery
B - Left renal vein

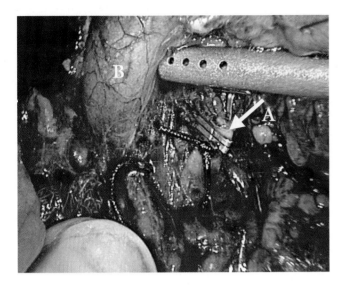

Figure 8 : Renal artery is ligated, clipped and divided

A - Divided end of left renal artery

B - Left renal vein

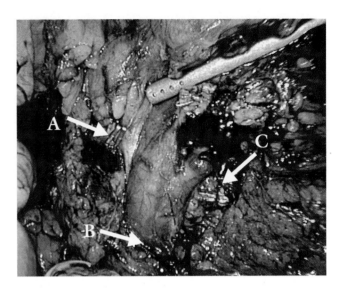

Figure 9 : Renal vein dissected and silk is passed around for ligation. Lumbar vein is clipped and divided

A - Clipped lumbar vein

B - Silk around the renal vein

C - Divided end of renal artery

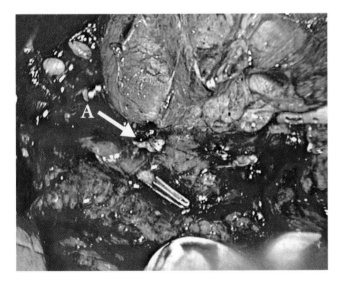

Figure 10 : Renal vein is ligated, clipped and divided

A - Divided end of renal vein

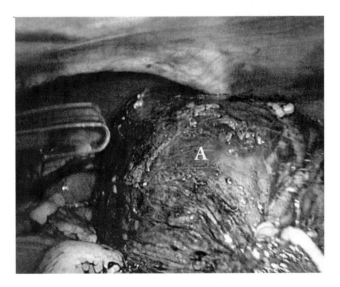

Figure 11 : Completely mobilized left kidney

A - Excised left kidney

For trocar sites greater than 5 mm, it is helpful to place the closure sutures before removing the kidney. Once the sutures are placed, trocars can be reinserted for kidney entrapment and removal. Once the specimen is removed, the umbilical fascia closed and pneumoperitoneum reachieved and hemostasis confirmed.

Postoperative care

The nasogastric tube is removed, immediately. On the first postoperative day, liquids are given and the urinary catheter removed. Adequate analgesics are given. The patients are discharged typically on the second or third postoperative day, once they are tolerating oral diet and their pain is under control.

Complications

The overall complication rate of laparoscopic nephrectomy is comparable to open nephrectomy.

Intraoperative

1. Bowel injury - Trocar injury

    Cautery injury

2. Liver laceration
3. Splenic laceration
4. Vascular injuries

RETROPERITONEAL APPROACH

Like in open surgery, the kidneys can also be approached extraperitoneally. Insufflation is initiated using a Veress needle or by an open technique. The Veress needle is directly inserted into the retroperitoneal space through a point two cms superior to the anterior-superior iliac spine. For open technique a small incision is made over the tip of the twelfth rib with the patient in the prone position and table flexed at the waist. The surgeon stands on the ipsilateral side and the subcutaneous layer and the muscle are incised. The retroperitoneal or Gerota's fascia is entered by digital dissection. A 10 mm laparoscope is inserted to assess proper positioning. After withdrawing the scope a balloon-dilating device is inserted into the space and the balloon inflated with 1 to 2 L of sterile normal saline. Further retroperitoneal dissection is performed under direct vision after placing the working trocars.

Another method of creating a retroperitoneal working space is by blunt dissection, using only the zero° laparoscopes.

Main advantage of the retroperitoneal approach is that the risk of injuring the intraabdominal organs is avoided. In addition, since the hilum is approached posteriorly, the renal artery can be controlled early.

HAND-ASSISTED LAPAROSCOPIC NEPHRECTOMY

In hand-assisted approach, a small laparotomy incision is created from the beginning to allow the non-dominant hand of the surgeon to be placed in side the abdomen for assistance. Pneumoperitoneum can be maintained using one of the hand- assist devices commercially available. The length of the incision is same as the surgeon's glove size in cms. For a right-handed surgeon performing right nephrectomy the incision can be placed in the right lower quadrant or in the periumbilical region. For a right-handed surgeon performing left nephrectomy the hand port incision is placed in the midline, periumbilically. The procedure is performed as in conventional transperitoneal laparoscopic nephrectomy.

The intra-abdominal hand provides the surgeon tactile sensation, aids in dissection, allows gentle traction-retraction, and increases the safety of the procedure. This decreases the operative time when compared to the totally laparoscopic technique. In addition, the intact specimen can be removed through the hand-port incision. This approach has got the postoperative benefits of laparoscopic surgery in addition to the above advantages.[24] The price paid is an incision 6-8 cms long, possibly more postoperative pain and a slower recovery when compared to a totally laparoscopic approach.

CONCLUSION

Laparoscopic nephrectomy is a viable alternative to open nephrectomy. The postoperative results of the laparoscopic nephrectomy are comparable to that of open surgery with much less pain and shorter convalescence. Hospital stays have decreased markedly. As with any new procedure, there is a learning curve and with experience and advances in techniques and equipment, the current operative times have decreased. Laparoscopic nephrectomy is a safe and efficacious approach for resection of benign non-functioning kidneys and localised renal tumours. However, the long-term cancer control needs to be confirmed.

References

1. Clayman RV, Kavoussi LR, Soper NJ, et al. Laparoscopic nephrectomy. N Engl J Med 1991; 324:1370-

2. Gaur DD. Laparoscopic operative retroperitoneoscopy : use of a new device. J Urol 1992;148:1137-9.

3. Rassweiler J, Manfred W. Laparoscopy and retroperitoneoscopy novel techniques of which clinical nephrologists should be aware. Nephrol Dial Transplant 1999;14:313-7.

4. Kerbl K, Clayman RV, McDougall EM, et al. Laparoscopic nephrectomy: the Washington University experience. Br J Urol 1994;73:231-6.

5. Rassweiler J, Fornara P, Weber M, et al. Laparoscopic nephrectomy: the experience of the laparoscopy working group of the German Urologic Association. J Urol 1998;160:18-21.

6. Hemal AK, Gupta NP, Wadhwa SN, et al. Retroperitoneoscopic nephrectomy and nephroureterectomy for benign non-functioning kidneys: a single-center experience. Urology 2001;57:644-9.

7. Portis AJ, Yan Y, Landman J, et al. Long term follow-up after laparoscopic radical nephrectomy. J Urol 2002; 167:1257-62.

8. Shalhav AL, Dunn MD, Portis AJ, et al. Laparoscopic nephroureterectomy for upper tract transitional cell cancer: the Washington University experience. J Urol 2000;163:1100-4.

9. Ratner LE, Ciseck LJ, Moore RG, et al. Laparoscopic live donor nephrectomy. Transplantation 1995;60:1047-9.

10. Machado MT, Lasmar MT, Batista LT, et al . Laparoscopic nephrectomy in inflammatory renal disease: proposal for a staged approach. International Braz J Urol 2005;31(1):22-28.

11. Fornara P, Doehn C, Miglietti G et al. Laparoscopic nephrectomy: comparison of dialysis and non-dialysis patients. Nephrol Dial Transplant 1998;13:1221-1225.

12. András H, Laurent S, , Patrick A, et al. Partial nephrectomy with retroperitoneal laparoscopy. The journal of urology: 1999; 162(11) 1922.

13. Yoshihiko T, Koike H, Takahashi K, et al: Use of the harmonic scalpel for nephron sparing surgery in renal cell carcinoma. J Urol 1998;159:2063.

14. Tanaka M, Kai N, Naito S: Retroperitoneal laparoscopic wedge resection for small renal tumor using microwave tissue coagulator. J Endourol 2000;14:569572.

15. Corwin TS, Cadeddu JA: Radiofrequency coagulation to facilitate laparoscopic partial nephrectomy. J Urol 2001;165:175176.

16. Tierney AC. Laparoscopic radical and partial nephrectomy. World J Urol 2000; 18: 249-256.

17. Hoznek A, Salomon L, Antipon P, Radier C, Hafiani M, Chopin DK, Abbou CC. Partial nephrectomy with retroperitoneal laparoscopy. J Urol 1999; 162: 1922-1926.

18. Gill IS, Meraney AM, Schweizer DK, et al. Laparoscopic radical nephrectomy in 100 patients: a single center experience from the United States. Cancer 2001;92:1843-55.

19. Rassweiler J, Tisvian A, Kumar AV, et al. Oncological safety of laparoscopic surgery for urological malignancy: experience with more than 1000 operations. J Urol 2003; 169:2072-5.

20. Walther MM, Lune JC, Libutti SK, Linehan WM: Laparoscopic cytoreductive nephrectomy as preparation for administration of systemic interleukin-2 in the treatment of metastatic renal cell carcinoma: A pilot study. Urology 1999;53:496.

21. El Fettouh HA, Rassweiler j, Schulze M, et al. Laparoscopic radical nephroureterectomy : results of an international multicenter study. Eur Urol 2002;42:447-52.

22. Ratner LE, Kavoussi L, Sroka M, et al. Laparoscopic assisted live donor nephrectomy: comparison with the open approach. Transplantation 1997; 63;229-233.

23. Rydberg F, Kopecky KK, Tann M, et al. Evaluation of prospective living renal donors for laparoscopic nephrectomy with multisection CT : The marriage of minimally invasive imaging with minimally invasive surgery. RSNA (RG) ,2001;21:S223-236.

24. Rudich SM, Marcovich R, Magee JC, et al. Hand-assisted laparoscopic donor nephrectomy: comparable donor/recipient outcomes, costs, decreased convalescence as compared to open donor nephrectomy. Transplant Proc 2001;33:1106-7.

SECTION ⑭

Gynecology

75

Laparoscopic Hysterectomy

INTRODUCTION

Hysterectomy is the commonest gynecological procedure encountered today. Palmer of France, who is called the father of the gynecological laparoscopy introduced laparoscopy to gyenocology in 1940. It was Kurt Semm of Germany who first performed laparoscopic assisted hysterectomy in 1974. Nearly two decades later, it is now possible to remove any size of uterus (even upto 32-34 weeks) by laparoscopy. Various other surgeries for chronic pelvic pain, infertility, pelvic malignancies, endometriosis, and adhesiolysis are routinely performed through laparoscopy.

ANATOMIC CONSIDERATIONS

We will discuss the main aspects of gynecological laparoscopic anatomy in this chapter. The uterus is situated between the bladder anteriorly and the rectosigmoid posteriorly in an anteflexed position.

The parietal peritoneum is applied directly over the uterus, fallopian tubes and ovaries, with little intervening adventitia. It reflects anteriorly over the bladder, forming the anterior cul-de-sac, and posteriorly over the upper vagina on to the rectosigmoid, forming the posterior cul-de-sac. The vesicovaginal and rectovaginal spaces are potential spaces that exist within loose areolar tissues along the endopelvic fascial planes.

Lateral reflections of the visceral peritoneum that are closely related to the adenexa and round ligaments form the broad ligaments on either side. The round ligaments are the condensations of perivascular fascia within the broad ligaments that pass anterolaterally from the anterior uterine cornu to exit the pelvis through the internal iliac rings. Samson's artery, is an anastomotic vessel that arises from the uterine vasculature that usually accompanies the round ligament. This must be controlled during division of the round ligament.

The anterior leaf of the broad ligament is a flat expanse of peritoneum covering the round ligament which also extends to the bladder. The medial aspect of the broad ligament is the triangular portion of peritoneum bounded by the round ligament anteriorly, the tube and infundibulopelvic ligament medially, and the pelvic sidewall laterally. When the anterior and middle leaves of the broad ligament are opened, the underlying loose areolar tissue can be easily dissected to expose the pelvic sidewall and retroperitoneal structures. The medial aspect of the broad ligament extends posteriorly to the fallopian tube, ovary and infundibulopelvic ligament. The ureter is loosely adherent to the medial leaf of the broad ligament throughout its course in the pelvis and can be readily visualized during laparoscopy through the normal peritoneum. The posterior boundary is formed by the uterosacral ligaments, which extends from the cervix to the rectum, inserting into the sacrum as the posterior rectal pillars.

The dominant uterine blood supply is from the uterine arteries which are the branches of internal iliac arteries. The uterine arteries courses anteromedially after its orgin, crossing anterior to the ureter approximately 2cm lateral to the cervix. Then they divide into ascending branches, that supply the uterine fundus and anastomose with vessels from the mesosalphinx, and descending cervicovaginal branches. The uterine veins coalesce and descend as a plexus and drain into the hypogastric vein. The vascular adventitia of the uterine vessels condenses to form the cardinal ligament, which transverses laterally. This provides a major lateral support to the uterine cervix. The ureter passes posterior to the uterine artery through the cardinal ligament within the ureteric tunnel.

The ovarian arteries from the aorta descend into the pelvis within the infundibulopelvic ligament. The ovarian artery continues medially, forming the arcade of the mesosalphinx and terminates by anastomosing with ascending branches of the uterine artery adjacent to the uterine cornu. The right ovarian vein drains into the inferior vena cava, whereas the left ovarian vein drains into the left renal vein.

The ureter must be isolated and visualized completely during pelvic laparoscopy. It enters the pelvis approximately at the level of the bifurcation of the common iliac artery, in proximity to the infundibulopelvic ligament. The pelvic ureter then courses anteriorly and medially in a shallow arc, close to the medial leaf of the broad ligament and enters the ureteric tunnel under the uterine artery. The most common sites of injury to the ureter are at the level of the uterine artery and uterosacral ligaments and at the level of infundibulopelvic ligament.

LAPAROSCOPIC HYSTERECTOMY

The word laparoscopic hysterectomy is used to denote various types with various proportions of the surgeries being performed by laparoscopic and vaginal approach. Apart from hysterectomy laparoscopy is also used in assessment of adnexal pathology, their staging and operability and biopsy of the suspected lesions. At present stage, even radical hysterectomy with pelvic lymphadenectomy can be performed effectively through laparoscopy. Laparoscopic hysterectomy is superior to conventional procedure as the imaging systems provide an excellent view of the anatomy by magnification. With the help of electrosurgical dissection devices like Harmonic scalpel and the procedures can be done in a bloodless manner. Endobags should be used to avoid any spillage of suspicious malignant tissues and dermoid. Recently combined hysteroscopy and laparoscopy is used for assessment of infertility.

TYPES OF LAPAROSCOPIC HYSTERECTOMY

There are various types of hysterectomies that are performed through laparoscopy. The following is the classification of these procedures.

Laparoscopic hysterectomy classification
1. Diagnostic Laparoscopy with vaginal hysterectomy.
2. Laparoscopic assisted vaginal hysterectomy (LAVH).
3. Total Laparoscopic Hysterectomy (TLH)
4. Laparoscopic supracervical hysterectomy (LSH) including CASH(Classical Abdominal Semm Hysterectomy)
5. Vaginal hysterectomy with laparoscopic vault suspension (LVS) or laparoscopic pelvic reconstruction (LPR)

6. Laparoscopic hysterectomy with lymphadenectomy
7. Laparoscopic hysterectomy with lymphadenectomy and omentectomy.
8. Laparoscopic radical hysterectomy with lymphadenectomy.

Laparoscopic hysterectomy denotes ligation of the uterine arteries either by electrosurgery desiccation, suture ligature, or staples. Maneuvers after uterine vessel ligation such as anterior and posterior colpotomy, division of cardinal and uterosacral ligaments, removal of uterus (either in toto or by morcellation) and vaginal closure can be done either by vaginal or laparoscopic approach. Laparoscopic ligation of the uterine vessels is the sine qua non for laparoscopic hysterectomy.

Laparoscopic assisted vaginal hysterectomy (LAVH)

Laparoscopic Assisted Vaginal Hysterectomy is a vaginal hysterectomy after laparoscopic adhesiolysis, endometriosis excision or oopherectomy. Unfortunately, this term is also used to refer to staple ligation of the upper uterine blood supply of a relatively normal uterus. In laparoscopic assisted vaginal hysterectomy the infundibulopelvic ligament and the broad ligaments are tackled through laparoscopy, while the uterine vessels and the vaginal incision, removal and suturing are done through the vagina. Some have recommended performing a laparoscopically assisted subtotal hysterectomy that leaves the cervix intact. In our opinion, the later procedure is rarely indicated, because most patients who are candidates for this procedure can be managed conservatively.

Indications for Laparoscopically Assisted Vaginal Hysterectomy

Refractory dysfunctional uterine bleeding.
Adenomyosis
Uterine Leiomyomas.
Chronic Pelvic inflammatory disease.
Endometriosis.
Refractory cervical dysplasia
Endometrial adenomatous hyperplasia
Benign adnexal masses and ovarian neoplasms.

We teach and use a modified LAVH technique. Laparoscopic dissection is used to lyse adhesions, control the round ligaments, open the pelvic side walls, control the infundibulopelvic ligament or utero-ovarian ligaments and tubes and partially develop the bladder flap. The procedure is then converted to a standard vaginal hysterectomy, with ligation of the uterosacral ligaments, cardinal ligaments, and uterine vessels and closure of the vaginal cuff performed vaginally. We believe that this is a safe technique to learn for surgeons who do not have advanced laparoscopic skills. It avoids the potential for ureteral injury.

Total Laparoscopic Hysterectomy (TLH)

The laparoscopic dissection continues until the uterus lies free of all attachments in the peritoneal cavity. The uterus is either removed through the vagina or through one of the ports (with morcellation if

Comparison of LAVH with Vaginal or Abdominal Hysterectomy

LAVH verses vaginal hysterectomy	LAVH versus abdominal hysterectomy
Superior visualization of abdominal contents	Abdominal incision avoided.
Reliable removal of adnexae	Reduced ileus
Can surgically approach adhesions, endometriosis, adnexal pathology	Reduced infectious morbidity
Higher cost	Concomitant repair of vaginal relaxation. Reduced hospital stay and convalescence.

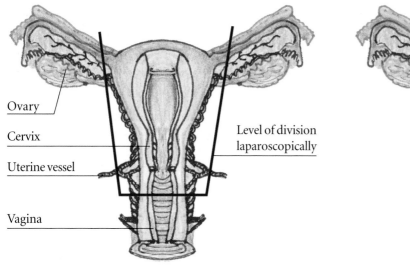

Ovary

Cervix

Uterine vessel

Vagina

Level of division
laparoscopically

Figure 1 : Total laparoscopic hystrectomy (TLH)

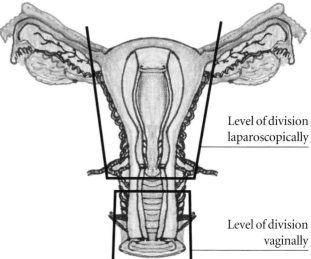

Level of division
laparoscopically

Level of division
vaginally

Figure 2: Laparoscopic Hystrectomy (LH)

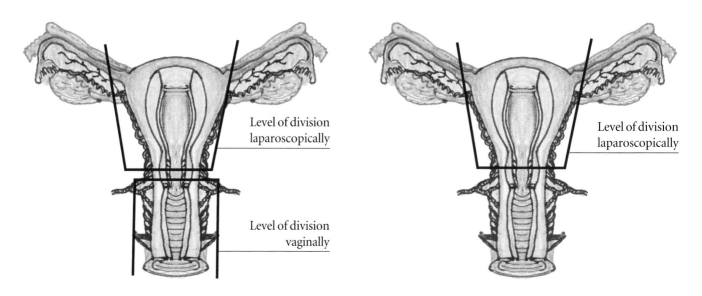

Level of division
laparoscopically

Level of division
vaginally

Figure 3 : Laparoscopic Assisted Vaginal
Hystrectomy(LAVH)

Level of division
laparoscopically

Figure 4 : Laparoscopic supracervical hystrectomy (LSH)

necessary) through laparoscopy. After removal, the vagina is closed by intracorporeal sutures laparoscopically.

Laparoscopic supracervical hysterectomy (LSH)

It has recently regained popularity after suggestions that total hysterectomy result in a decrease in libido. Kurt Semm's version of supracervical hysterectomy, called the CASH procedure (Classical abdominal Semm hysterectomy), leaves the cardinal ligaments intact while eliminating the columnar cells of the endocervical canal. After perforating the uterine fundus with a long sound-dilator, a calibrated uterine resection tool (CURT) that fits around this instrument is used to core out the endocervical canal. Thereafter, at laparoscopy, suture techniques are used to ligate the utero-ovarian ligaments. The uterus is divided at its junction with the cervix and removed by laparoscopic morcellation.

Laparoscopic pelvic reconstruction (LPR)

Laparoscopic pelvic reconstruction with vaginal hysterectomy is useful when vaginal hysterectomy alone cannot accomplish appropriate repair for prolapse. Ureteral dissection and suture placement before the vaginal hysterectomy aids in high plication of uterosacral ligament near the sacrum. Levator muscle plication from below or above is often necessary.

LAPAROSCOPIC HYSTERECTOMY

Preoperative Evaluation

Along with routine investigations, transvaginal ultrasound is also performed as it helps in mapping the fibroid, number of fibroids, defining the extent of the same, the presence of adnexal mass like endometrioma etc. In the case of mass in the pouch of Douglus eg : in severe endometriosis, recto vaginal adenomyosis, MRI or CT scan of abdomen will help in proper localization of the diseased tissue and its extent, involvement of the major vessels, ureter etc. In case of large uterus, broad ligament fibroids, ovarian tumours and in extended laparoscopic procedures preoperative ureteric stenting is advisable. Illuminated stents help in easy identification of the course of ureter and its entry into the bladder.

Preoperative Preparation

Preoperative preparation of the vagina with antiseptic vaginal pessaries for 3-5 days is ideal. Preoperatively broad spectrum antibiotics 2 hours prior to surgery are mandatory. In chronic cervicits and in high risk group preoperative biopsy of the cervix to rule out malignancy is essential. The bowel is prepared using polyethelene Glycol, so that it is empty during the procedure. This will help to maintain the bowels in a collapsed condition which in turn prevents bowel injury.

Anaesthesia

We usually prefer general anaesthesia as extreme positions such as, steep Trendelenburg position (20-25°) with pneumoperitoneum is difficult to achieve with regional anaesthesia.

Patient Position

The patient is placed in an extended semilithotomy position. We use the lithotomy rod designed by Dr.V.P. Pailey (India) with hip joint abducted, knee joint flexed and softly padded stirrup, which is used to hold the calf muscles. The gluteal region should be hanging a little outside the table as this will help in easy manipulation of the uterus especially during depression of the posterior vaginal wall. We use the specially designed single bladed SIM's speculum for this purpose.

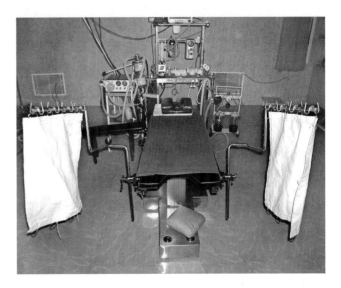

Figure 5 : Position of Lithotomy rod

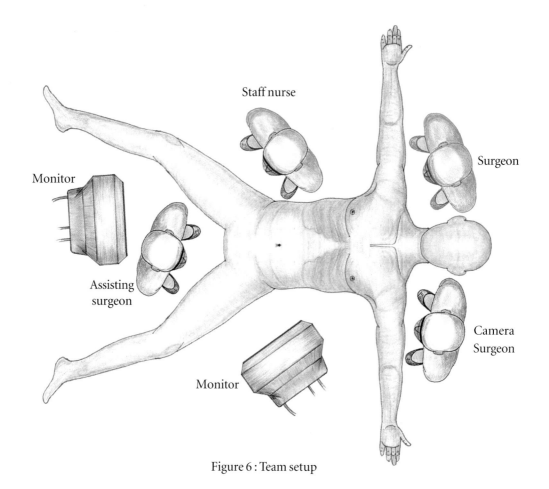

Figure 6 : Team setup

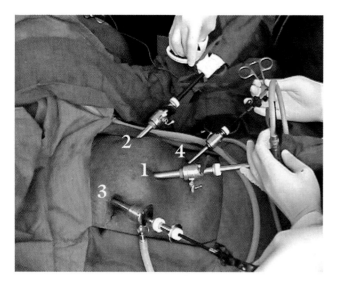

Figure 7 : Port position

No.	Instruments	Place
1	Camera	Umbilicus 10mm
2	Right hand working port	Right iliac fossa 10mm
3	Left hand working port	Left iliac fossa 5mm
4	Small bowel retraction port	Right lumbar 5mm

Instrumentation

Apart from routine laparoscopic instruments the following vaginal instruments are also essential for the surgery. Single bladed SIM's speculum, Bull dog Vulcellum, Uterine manipulator, Maingot's uterine clamp, Melsum Bawn scissors are some of the essential instruments. There are many types of uterine manipulators that are available now. We use Purandares Uterine manipulator in our surgeries. This consists of two blades in the upper end which fits into the uterine cavity. The knob at the external os level, prevents the instrument being pushed in invadvertantly into the uterus and thus prevents perforations. This instrument can be easily moved in all directions to antevert, retrovert and tilt the uterus laterally.

Position of Trocars

The bladder is catheterized after positioning the patient and draping. Pnueumoperitoeum is created by closed Veress needle technique and the initial 10 mm camera port is inserted in the umbilical area. Further ports are created under vision. Three trocars are placed including the umbilical camera port (10mm) 10mm right and 5mm left lower quadrants are the working ports. In presence of multiple scars, Veress needle is inserted in the epigastrium and using 3 or 5mm scope in the epigastric port, trocars are placed under guidance. In presence of adhesions right lumbar trocar is used for adhesiolysis. The working ports are placed lateral to the inferior epigastric vessels (2-3)cms and in a position that is medial to anterior superior iliac spines, to avoid over crowding of the instruments.

Initial assessment

As soon the camera trocar is inserted the abdominal cavity is assessed for intra abdominal adhesions, size and position of the uterus, tubes, ovaries, bladder, pouch of Douglas and hernial sac if any. Adhesion of the bladder over the anterior surface of the uterus should be expected in cases of previous ceserean sections.

Mobilisation of uterus

The dissection starts with the division of the infundibulo pelvic ligament and round ligament either with cautery or with one of the advanced electrosurgical devises like harmonic scalpel or ligasure. The dissection should be started over the ovarian and round ligament if the ovaries have to be retained back.

It is ideal to remove both tubes to prevent post hysterectomy chronic pelvic pain. Chronic pelvic pain is mostly due to hydrosalpinx and PID. The infundibulo pelvic ligament should be desiccated thoroughly, before division as it contains ovarian artery which is a direct branch of aorta. Otherwise, these vessels can retract inside and often form a hematoma. The position of the ureters should be identified properly before dissection, to avoid inadvertent injuries.

The two layers of the broad ligament are dissected apart to open up the plane between the two layers either with Harmonic scalpel or electrocatuery hook/scissor. The bladder is separated from the cervix after exposing the uterovesical fold of peritoneum. The bladder is lifted anteriorly and the cervix pushed down to separate the two structures. Retroversion of uterus by the vaginal surgeon with the help of the manipulator will help in proper exposure of the structures. After dissection n the anterior plane, the dissection proceeds to the lateral aspects of the

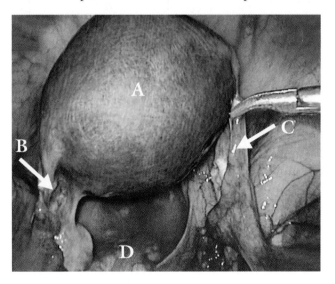

Figure 8 : Laparoscopic view of pelvis

A - Uterus

B - Right Adnexa

C - Left adnexa

D - Rectum

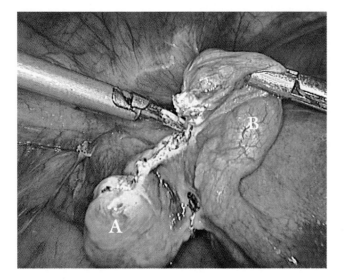

Figure 9 : Division of ovarian ligament and tube using harmonic ace on left side

A - Left ovary
B - Left uterine tube

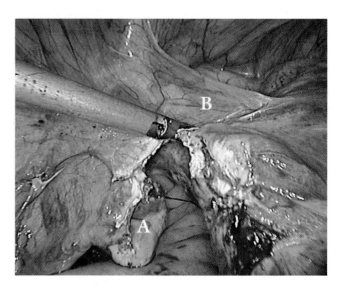

Figure 10 : Division of roung ligament

A - Left ovary
B - Broad ligament

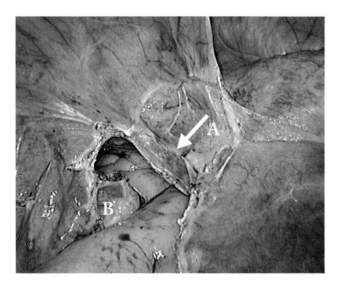

Figure 11 : Anterior leaf of broad ligament is divided and uterine vessels exposed

A - Left uterine artery
B - Left ovary

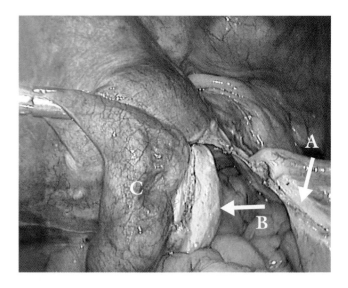

Figure 12 : Infundibulopelvic is divided on right side (in case of salphingo oopherectomy)

A - Infundibulo pelvic ligament
B - Right ovary
C - Right uterine tube

cervix in the same manner. Retraction of the vagina to opposite side of the dissection is very essential. The uterus is then anteverted to expose the posterior surface of brand ligament and uterosacral ligaments. The uterine artery is skeletonised after its identification. It can be easily identified by its tortuous course and branching into ascending, descending branches.

Control of uterine vascular pedicle

Control of uterine vascular pedicle can be performed in many ways. Ligature with conventional suture materials, bipolar cautery, Harmonic scalpel and ligature are some of the examples. The vessels can be ligated with Vicryl sutures, by intracorporeal suturing methods. At this stage No.1vicryl with curved needle is used to take a suture just lateral to the decending branch of the uterine artery. Extracoproreal surturing and knotting though described is not very effective and is more often time consuming and cumbersome. The pedicles should by doubly ligated to prevent accidental slipping and bleeding. Once both the vessels are ligated the color of the uterus becomes pale and the consistency becomes soft and flabby. The vessels can now be

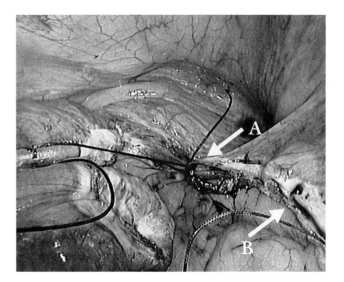

Figure 14 : Completion of ligation

A - Right uterine pedicle
B - Divided end of infundibulopelvic ligament

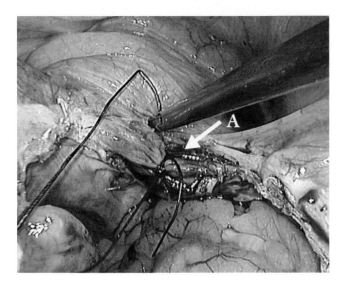

Figure 13 : Ligation of right uterine pedicle using 1 0 vicryl

A - Right uterine pedicle

divided using electro cautery hook. In case of tortuous vessels, bipolar coagulation may be used to dessicate the vessels before division. After perfect desiccation the uterine vessels are divided with scissors.

The pedicles are then dissected away from the uterus and cervix. Now high quality electrosurgical systems are available for the coagulation of the vessels. We have found that the harmonic scalpel is highly effective in laparoscopic gynaec surgery. The older shears (5mm/10mm) are highly effective for dissection in hysterectomy except uterine vessels. Harmonic ace, the new version of harmonic scalpel probe is highly effective in division of the vessels. Coagulation and cutting can be done without ligature in a faster manner. We have not used any ligature in the last few cases where the divisions of the vessels were done with Harmonic ACE probe. Ligasure is a specialized pulsed bipolar coagulation instruments with central knife. Simultaneous coagulation and division of the vessels can be performed using 10mm probes (Atlas). Unfortunately these are not cost effective due to disposable probes.

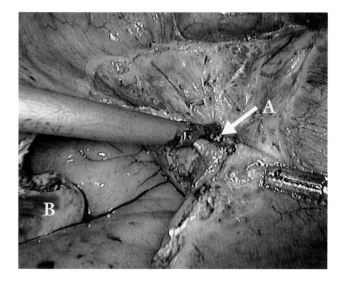

Figure 15 : Division of left uterine pedicle using harmonic ace

A - Left uterine pedicle
B - Left ovary

Circumferential Mobilization of Cervix

In this step we have to be cautious about ureter, which traverses just below uterine artery (Water under the Bridge). It is safer to confine the dissection close to the uterus to prevent any mishaps. At this sage the uterus remains attached only with Mackenrodt's ligament and this can be divided by bipolar cautery. Utero sacral ligaments are divided and pushed posteriorly.

The cervix can be readily identified in the anterior aspect by its coursing fibres. The bladder is carefully pushed down, especially in cases of previous caesarean sections. We have to be carefully and meticulously separate the bladder by sharp dissection. Harmonic scalpel is an ideal instrument in this maneuver. Similar difficulty is encountered in the posterior aspect in cases of endometriosis. The rectum and the ureter is pulled together and is densely adherent to the posterior surface of the uterus. All these dissections should be carried in a safe manner to avoid injury to these structures.

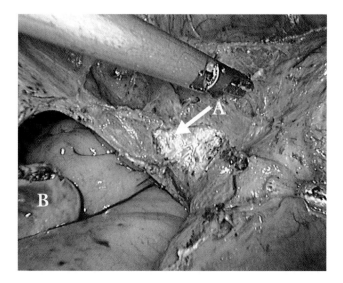

Figure 16 : Completion of division

A - Divided end of left uterine pedicle
B - Left ovary

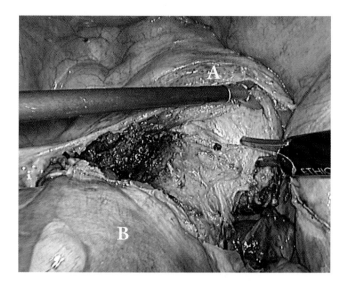

Figure 17 : Separation of bladder from the cervix

A - Urinary bladder
B - Uterus

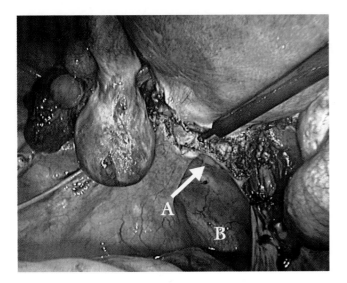

Figure 18 : Division of uterosacral ligament using monopolar electrocautery hook

A - Uterosacral ligament
B - Pouch of douglas

Vaginal dissection

The anterior lip of cervix is held with a vulcellum and a semicircle incision is made over the anterior lip of cervix close to the bladder. The bladder is pushed up by dissection with sharp scissors till the utero vesical fold of peritoneum is seen. The pouch of Douglas in opened by a transverse incision with the scissors after holding the posterior lip of cervix with vulcellum and the posterior fornix, with an Alies forceps. The lateral cervical or the cardinal ligament is and divided and ligated with No.1 vicryl. The pedicle is also anchored to the posterior vaginal wall at this stage. The same procedure is carried out in opposite side. The uterine vessels can be clamped at this stage if there is any bleeding. Uterus and adenexa retrieved through vagina. The Vault is inspected for active bleeding points. Meticulous heamostasis is obtained and the vault is closed with 1-0 vicryl continuous sutures. There is no need for suturing the peritoneum separately.

Re-evaluation

The pneumoperitoneum is recreated and a thorough lavage is done and hemostasis is again checked. The ports are removed under vision and closed. 10 mm and larger ports should be closed with a port closure needle.

Postoperative Management

No vaginal packing is necessary. Routine postoperative analgesic and anti-inflammatory and antibiotics are given. Indwelling catheter is removal after 8-10 hours. Most of the patients are comfortable after 24 hours. Liquids are started within few hours of surgery and solid diet is usually allowed in the 1st postoperative day and are discharged. Patients are allowed to resume routine work within 3- 5 days after surgery.

Removal of fallopian tubes

In conditions where both ovaries have to be retained back, it is better to remove fallopian tube along with the part of mesosalpinx. The ovary has got dual blood supply, from the uterine artery via mesosalpix and from the aorta directly via the infundibulo pelvic ligament. After hysterectomy the left out fallopian tubes usually lie in close contact with the vault. Any vaginal infection will ascend directly to the pelvis forming hydrosalpinx. Moreover because of the dual blood supply to the ovaries, removal of the tubes will not interfere with the ovarian blood supply. Another point of interest is if the meso salpinx is cut, the retained ovary with infundibulo pelvic ligament will recede back close to of the pelvic side wall. If the tubes are not cut the residual ovaries will directly lie over the over the vault. In this way residual pelvic pain can be reduced.

TOTAL LAPAROSCOPIC HYSTERECTOMY - TLH

The initial part of the surgery is similar to laparoscopic assisted hysterectomy in positioning of the patient and ports. An extra 5mm port is placed either on the right or left midclavicular line in the subcostal region for retraction of uterus. A 5mm myoma screw is placed through this port, which helps in retraction of the uterus. Apart from the instruments that are needed for laparoscopic assisted vaginal hysterectomy and additional CCL extractor is needed for total laparoscopic hysterectomy. This instrument helps in removal of uterus and suture of vagina without loss of pneumoperitoneum.

The initial dissection in the pelvis is very similar to that of laparoscopic assisted vaginal hysterectomy. After dissection of the broad ligament and isolation of uterine vessels, these are tackle either with intracorporeal ligation with vicryl sutures or with any one of the electro surgical devices such as bipolar coagulation or ligasure.

Circumferential Culdotomy

After division of the uterine vessels the 5mm myoma screw is introduced into the abdomen through the subcostal port and screwed into the uterus. Now with the myoma screw the uterus can be retracted to any position comfortably. The CCL extractor is introduced into the vagina after removal of the speculam, vulsulum and uterine manipulator. It is then pushed cranially so that the CCL extractor closely approximates the cervix and the fornices. The para cervical region along with the fornices are elevated well into the pelvic cavity, displacing the ureters laterally. At this stage the Mackenrodt's ligament is stretched on the lateral aspect. The uterus is retracted laterally and this ligament is divided either with harmonic scalpel or hook dissection.

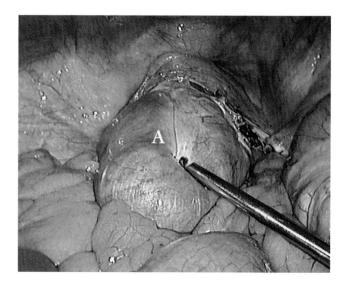

Figure 20 : 5 mm myoma screw is applied to the uterus for cranial traction

A - Uterus

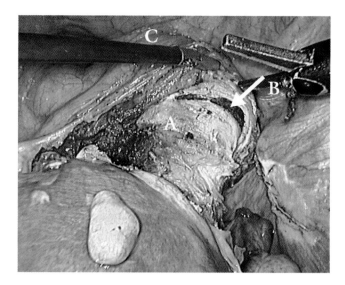

Figure 21 : Anterior vaginal wall is opened by harmonic scalpel, Methele blue soaked gauze piece is seen

A - Cervix
B - Methele blue soaked gauze piece
C - Urinary bladder

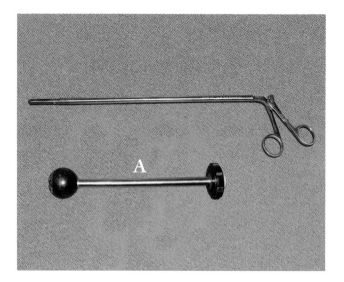

Figure 19 : CCL ectractor with 100mm claw forceps

A - CCL extractor

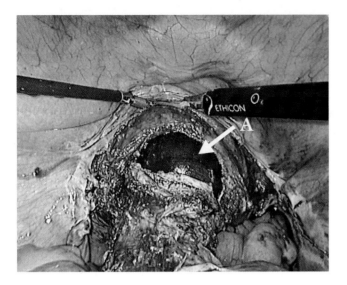

Figure 22 : Anterior vaginal wall is divided completely. Head of CCL extractor is seen

A - Head of CCL extractor

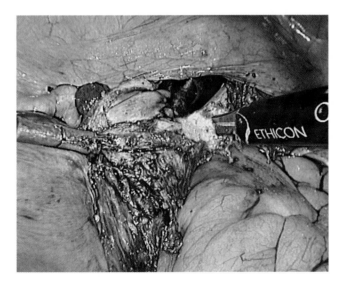

Figure 23 : Division of posterior vaginal wall

Maintaining the cranial traction on the uterus with the myoma screw, the bladder is mobilized well away from the anterior vaginal wall. After complete mobilization, the vaginal vault is incised over the CCL extractor. Entry into the vaginal space is confirmed by visualizing the black coloured CCL extractor. The incision is extended circumferentially over the entire vaginal vault.

At this stage pneumoperitoneum will start escaping through the incision. This can be controlled by keeping wet pads in vagina. At times minimal bleeding from the lateral fornix will be seen due to bleeding from decending cervical branch of uterine artery. This can be usually controlled by application of an endoloop. Once the uterus is entirely free from its attachments the myoma screw is removed from the uterus and taken out under vision.

Extraction of uterus through vagina

The CCL extractor is pushed cranially in to the opening in the vaginal vault and a 10mm claw forceps is introduced through its shaft. With the assistance from the laparoscopic surgeon, the vaginal surgeon holds the cervix firmly with the 10mm claw forceps. Maintaining firm pressure on the cervix the uterus is removed in toto through the vaigna. If the uterus is more than 10-12 weeks size, the conventional myoma screw is introduced into the uterine tissue through the vagina, taking care to protect the bladder and the rectum in the process. The uterine tissue is bisected around the myoma screw and debulked. At this stage it is easy to remove the uterus through the vagina.

Extraction of uterus with morcellator

In case of total laparoscopic hysterectomy, the uterus is debulked with a morcellator through the lateral working port. If morcellator is used, then port has to be enlarged to 15mm to accommodate the shaft of the morcellator. The uterus should be held by the myoma screw and morcellation should be started at one end of the uterus, proceeding carefully so as not to injure any of the abdominal organs. The morcellator is a very dangerous instrument and can cause disasterous complications like injury to hollow viscus and major vessels. The tip of the rotating morcellator tip should always be in the field of vision to prevent this complication.

Closure of vaginal vault

After extraction of the uterus, the entire vagina is again packed with wet abdominal pads to control the leakage of pneumoperitoneum. The pneumoperitoneum is recreated and vaginal suturing done. The vault is approximated by intracorporeal suturing with No.1 vicryl (continuous suturing). The suturing is started from one side and is completed on the other side. During suturing the tension on the suture line can be maintained by following the thread by the second assistant as shown in the figure. After completion of suturing a thorough peritoneal toileting is done and complete hemostasis is achieved. If at any stage bleeding from the pedicle is observed then it can be controlled by application of an endoloop.

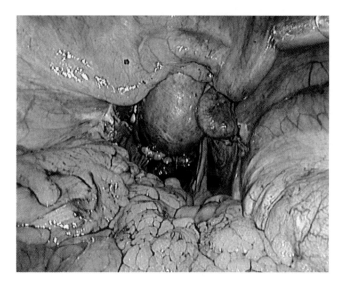

Figure 25 : Uterus is being pulled out through the vagina

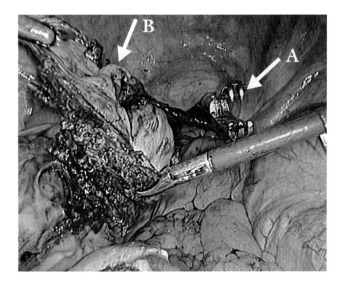

Figure 24 : 10 mm claw forceps is introduced through the CCL extractor and the excised uterus is being feeded.

A - Claw forceps
B - Excised uterus

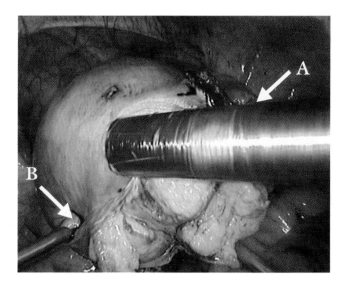

Figure 26 : Excised uterus is debulked by using morcellator (another method of extraction of large uterus)

A - Morcellator
B - Uterus is held by myoma screw

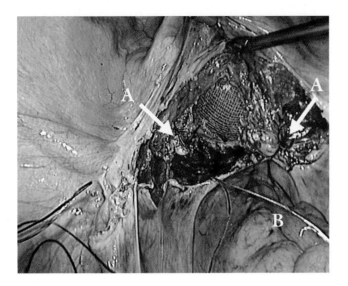

Figure 27 : Vagina is packed with pad and pneumoperitoneum is created, vault is inspected for hemostasis before suturing

A - Ligated uterine pedicle
B - Rectum

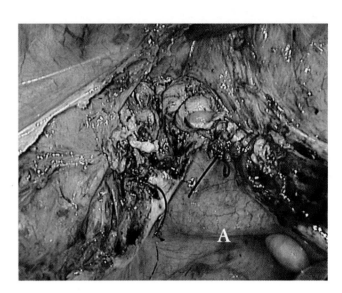

Figure 29 : Completion of vault closure

A - Rectum

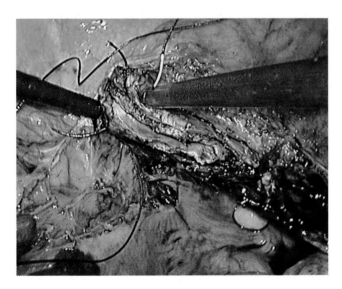

Figure 28 : Closure of the vault using 1 0 vicryl, continuous sutures

OUR EXPERIENCE

We have performed 635 laparoscopic hysterectomies in our institute since 1993. The mean age of the patients was 52 (40-68 yrs). The main indications were fibroid uterus, adenomyosis and dysfunctional uterine bleeding. Out of these 635 procedures, 410 procedures were done by laparoscopic assisted vaginal method and 225 procedures by total laparoscopic method. The mean duration of surgery in laparoscopic assisted vaginal hysterectomy was 120mts (range 86-160mts) and TLH was 100mts (65-140mts). There was no difference in the postoperative outcome between these patients. Urinary retention, wound infection, respiratory infection were the minor complications that were encounted in our series. We had two major complications, one bladder injury and one rectal injury.

The bladder injury occurred in a patient who had undergone two caesarean sections before. In this case the bladder was densely adherent over the anterior wall of the cervix. During mobilization, the bladder was injured and was confirmed by injection of methylene blue through the folley's catheter. The rent in the bladder was closed in two layers with 2-0 vicryl and the bladder was drained continuously for 8 days. The patient had an uneventful recovery.

We attempted total laparoscopic hysterectomy in a patient who had undergone myomectomy twice for infertility followed by unsuccessful abdominal hysterectomy due to dense adhesions. During the procedure we were able to release the adhesions completely all around. There was a small rent noticed in the anterior aspect of the rectum at the level of the uterine cervix at the end of the procedure. We sutured this in two layers by intracorporeal suturing. The patient recovered uneventfully and was discharged on the 5th post operative day. She is symptom free for the past one year.

We had also successfully operated a case of recto vaginal fistula following laparoscopic assisted vaginal hysterectomy done elsewhere. The fistula was demonstrated preoperatively by sigmoidoscopy. The fistulous area was dissected completely, the tract was excised. The rents were closed in two layers with 2-0 vicryl without any diversion colostomy. The patient recovered uneventfully.

CONCLUSION

Laparoscopic hysterectomy can be done in a safe and effective manner providing the maximum benefits of minimal access surgery to the patient. Though there are various versions of laparoscopic hysterectomies, the laparoscopic assisted vaginal hysterectomy and total laparoscopic hysterectomy are the commonest procedures that are performed in our institute. Based on our experience we feel that these two procedures can be offered to patients who need hysterectomy.

Selected references

1. Parker WH. Total laparoscopic hysterectomy and laparoscopic supracervical hysterectomy. Obstet Gynecol Clin North Am 2004; 31(3):523-37, viii.

2. Jenkins TR. Laparoscopic supracervical hysterectomy. Am J Obstet Gynecol 2004; 191(6):1875-84.

3. Wattiez A, Cohen SB, Selvaggi L. Laparoscopic hysterectomy. Curr Opin Obstet Gynecol 2002; 14(4):417-22.

4. Harkki P, Kurki T, Sjoberg J, Tiitinen A. Safety aspects of laparoscopic hysterectomy. Acta Obstet Gynecol Scand 2001; 80(5):383-91.

5. Summitt RL, Jr. Laparoscopic-assisted vaginal hysterectomy: a review of usefulness and outcomes. Clin Obstet Gynecol 2000; 43(3):584-93.

6. Parker WH. Total laparoscopic hysterectomy. Obstet Gynecol Clin North Am 2000; 27(2):431-40.

7. Lyons TL. Laparoscopic supracervical hysterectomy. Obstet Gynecol Clin North Am 2000; 27(2):441-50, ix.

8. Wakabayashi MT. Laparoscopic assisted vaginal hysterectomy/laparoscopic hysterectomy. Hawaii Med J 1999; 58(1):12-4.

9. Seidman DS, Goldenberg M, Nezhat C. 27 months follow-up study of 41 women who underwent laparoscopic supracervical hysterectomy. Jsls 1999; 3(4):335-6.

10. Moller C, Kehlet H, Ottesen BS. [Hospitalization and convalescence after hysterectomy. Open or laparoscopic surgery?]. Ugeskr Laeger 1999; 161(33):4620-4.

11. Hawe JA, Garry R. Laparoscopic hysterectomy. Semin Laparosc Surg 1999; 6(2):80-9.

12. Querleu D. [Laparoscopic and laparoscopically-assisted radical hysterectomy]. Contracept Fertil Sex 1998; 26(1):11-21.

13. Wood C, Maher PJ. Laparoscopic hysterectomy. Baillieres Clin Obstet Gynaecol 1997; 11(1):111-36.

14. Tsaltas J, Magnus A, Mamers PM, et al. Laparoscopic and abdominal hysterectomy: a cost comparison. Med J Aust 1997; 166(4):205-7.

15. Lipscomb GH. Laparoscopic-assisted hysterectomy: is it ever indicated? Clin Obstet Gynecol 1997; 40(4):895-902.

16. Chapron C, Dubuisson JB, Ansquer Y. Total laparoscopic hysterectomy. Indications, results, and complications. Ann N Y Acad Sci 1997; 828:341-51.

17. Masson FN, Pouly JL, Canis M, et al. [Laparoscopic hysterectomy. A series of 318 consecutive cases]. J Gynecol Obstet Biol Reprod (Paris) 1996; 25(4):340-52.

18. Martin J, Blanc JM, Pulton A, Allouard Y. [Vaginal hysterectomy. Role of laparoscopic preparation. Our experience]. Chirurgie 1996; 121(2):91-5.

19. Ben-Rafael Z, Orvieto R, Dicker D, Dekel A. [Laparoscopic hysterectomy--the future is here and now]. Harefuah 1996; 130(8):542-5.

20. Mage G, Masson FN, Canis M, et al. Laparoscopic hysterectomy. Curr Opin Obstet Gynecol 1995; 7(4):283-9.

21. Chapron C, Dubuisson JB, Aubert V, et al. [Total laparoscopic hysterectomy. Operative technique, results and indications]. J Gynecol Obstet Biol Reprod (Paris) 1995; 24(8):802-10.

22. Canis M, Mage G, Pouly JL, et al. Laparoscopic radical hysterectomy for cervical cancer. Baillieres Clin Obstet Gynaecol 1995; 9(4):675-89.

76

Laparoscopic Myomectomy

INTRODUCTION

Though the commonest treatment of symptomatic fibroids in a patient who had completed the family was hysterectomy earlier, increasing interests is now a days shown in organ preservation surgeries like myomectomy. Laparoscopic myomectomy is an advanced gynecological laparoscopic procedure that is gaining wider acceptance. These procedures need greater expertise and skill when compared to laparoscopic hysterectomy. With increased infertility problems in patients with uterine myoma, indications for laparoscopic myomectomies are gradually increasing. Laparoscopic myomectomies are proven to be safe and effective and offer all the advantages of minimal access surgery like shorter hospital stay, quicker recovery and faster return to normalcy.

Certain aspects make this procedure more technically demanding when compared to laparoscopic hysterectomy. Myomas, which are deeper in the myometrium are often difficult to locate and remove. Some of the patients who opt for myomectomy have usually taken a course of GnRH analogues which often make the myomas softer and pseudocapsules thicker, thus making the surgery difficult due to loss of tissue planes. Approximation of the uterine wound poses another problem as this needs adequate expertise. Closure of hysterotomy can be either performed by intracorporeal suturing or with the help of various suture assist devices like Endostitch.

INDICATIONS FOR MYOMECTOMY

The indications for laparoscopic myomectomy are similar to that of the conventional myomectomy. This is usually done in an infertile patient with multiple fibroids, when other causes for infertility have been ruled out. This can also be done in patients who have profuse periods associated with passage of clots or frequent periods lasting for more than 7 days with chronic anemia. The indication for laparoscopic myomectomy varies from author to author depending on the size and number of fibroids in the uterus. Few authors limit the size to less than 6cm and less than three in number, while others do not.

PREOPERATIVE EVALUATION

In patients with infertility, other factors for anovulation should be evaluated completely before taking a decision about laparoscopic myomectomy. Hysteroscopic evaluation should be done in all patients to assess for the presence of transmural and submucosal fibroids. These fibroids (upto 3-4cms) can be tackled by hysteroscopy alone. In case of broad ligament fibroids and larger sized fibroids, placement of a ureteric stent preoperatively will aid in easy identification of ureter. It is imperative that the patients hematological status is evaluated thoroughly before surgery as any bleeding diathesis can lead to disastrous hemorrhage during myomectomy.

The patient should be explained in detail about the possibility of recurrence following myomectomy, the possibility of inability to complete myomectomy and also the need for emergency hysterectomy in case of undue bleeding from the uterus which cannot be controlled by any other means. All these discussions should be documented properly and a written consent should be obtained before proceeding on with these surgeries.

TECHNIQUE

Position of patient and ports

The patient is placed in lithotomy position as in laparoscopic hysterectomy. The team setup and the position of ports are also similar to laparoscopic hysterectomy. The position of the ports might vary slightly, according to the size of the uterus and the fibroids. The ports should be placed more cranially depending on the size of the myoma or addition trocars are placed. In case of larger fibroids, the camera is placed in the supraumbilical position and the other two working ports are placed well above and lateral to the uterine myomas.

Initial Evaluation

Thorough evaluation of the peritoneal cavity is done after insertion of ports. After releasing the adhesions if any, the size, number and the exact location of the myomas in the uterus is ascertained. Although some authors describe about the use of Vasopressin in order to minimize bleeding, we do not routinely use this agent.

Hysterotomy and enucleation

The uterus is retracted well to the side opposite to that of the fibroid with the help of a uterine manipulator from the vaginal area. The uterus is fixed in this position and hysterotomy is made on the uterine surface overlying the myoma. We usually prefer transverse incisions as the blood vessels usually traverse horizontally in the uterus. The incision on the uterine wall can be done with monopolar hook or harmonic scalpel. The hysterotomy should be deep enough to incise the pseudo capsule of fibroid to aid in easy enucleation. Once the fibroid is visualized, the myoma screw is used to fix the fibroid and with traction from the myoma screw, the fibroid is slowly enucleated from the uterus by a combination of blunt and sharp dissection. Cranial traction often separates the fibroid from the uterus easily. Incase of larger fibroids the myoma screw should be placed at different positions on the fibroid before enucleation.

Monopolar cautery is usually not preferred in these cases. We routinely use ligasure or harmonic scalpel for this phase of dissection. Harmonic ACE the new probe, is a versatile instrument in dissection as well as control of uterine pedicle. Once fibroid is enucleated from its bed, hemostasis of the bed is achieved with bipolar cautery or Harmonic scalpel. Excess capsular tissue is trimmed off. Care should be taken not to disturb the tubal ostia in the fundus of the uterus.

Closure of Hysterotomy

The closure of the hysterotomy is usually performed by intracorporeal suturing with No.1 or 1-0 vicryl. Usually a single layer closure of the hysterotomy is sufficient. If the dead space following removal of the myoma is more, then multi layered suturing

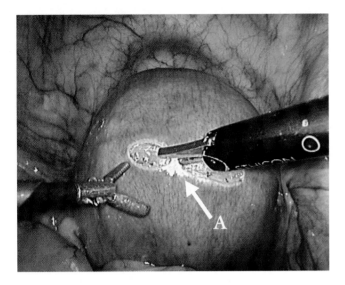

Figure 1 : Large fundal myoma. Uterus is opened transversely using harmonic scalpel.

A - Hysterotomy

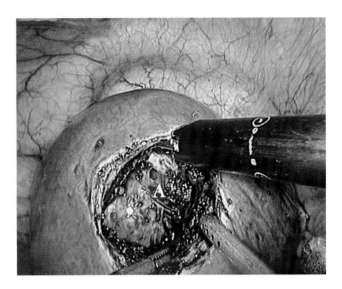

Figure 2 : Hysterotomy is widened and myoma is exposed

A - Myoma

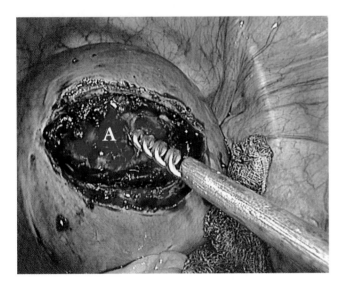

Figure 3 : 5 mm myoma screw is being applied to the myoma for cranial traction

A - Myoma

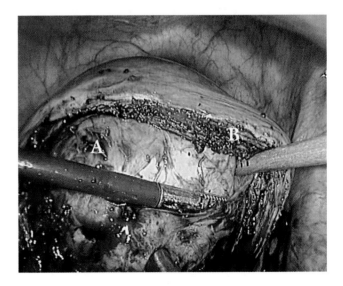

Figure 4 : Plane between the myoma and uterus is identified and the myoma is enucleated from the uterus

A - Myoma
B - Uterine wall

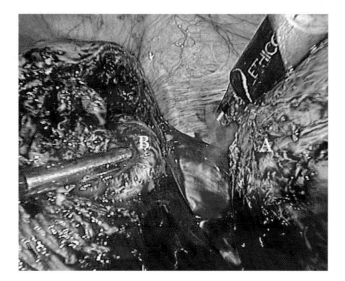

Figure 5 : Completion of myoma enucleation

A - Myoma
B - Endometrium

is advisable to prevent intramural hematoma. If endometrial cavity is inadvertently opened, it should be sutured separately with 2-0 vicryl to prevent fistulization.

Removal of fibroids

The enucleated fibroids can be removed from the peritoneal cavity either through posterior colpotomy or with the help of a morcellator.

Other myomas

Pedunculated myomas can be easily transected and the base cauterized with thermocoagulation. There is no need to suture the incision. Submucosal myomas can be tackled by hysteroscopy itself. Laparoscopic myomectomy in case of larger sized fibroids should not be attempted when proper visual field is not achieved.

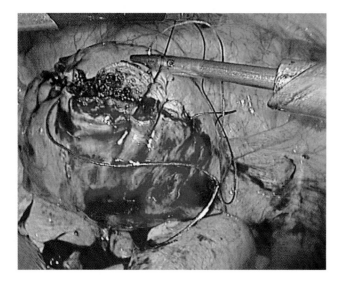

Figure 6 : Uterine wall is approximated using 1 0 vicryl stitches

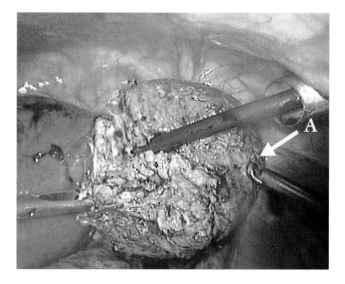

Figure 7 : Excised myoma is divided by using monopolar electrocautery hook for easy extraction

A - Myoma screw is holding the myoma

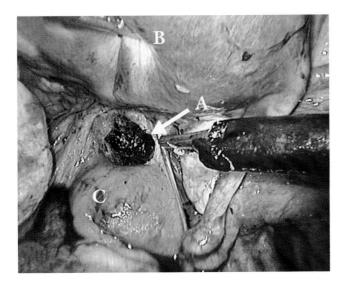

Figure 8 : Posterior colpotomy for extraction of myoma

A - Methylene blue soaked gauze piece is seen through the
       colpotomy wound
B - Posterior surface of the uterus
C - Rectum

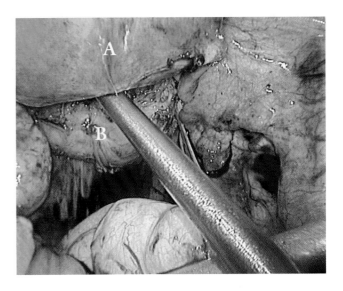

Figure 9 : Myoma is pulled out through posterior colpotomy

A - Uterus
B - Myoma

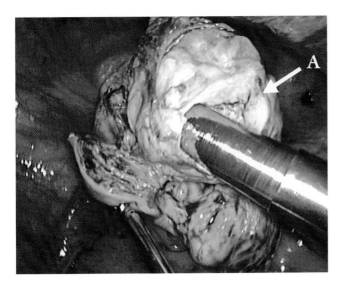

Figure 10 : In case of large myoma, morcellator is used for
extraction

A - Morcellation of myoma

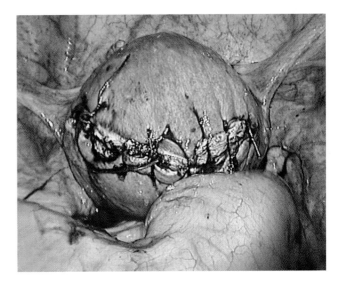

Figure 11 : View of the uterus after completion of laparoscopic myomectomy

POSTOPERATIVE MANAGEMENT

The postoperative management is similar to that of laparoscopic hysterectomy.

CONCLUSION

Laparoscopic myomectomy is safe, feasible and beneficial to the patients when compared to conventional myomectomy. This procedure needs adequate expertise in the field of advanced laparoscopic surgery and intracorporeal suturing.

Selected References

1. Benhaim Y, Ducarme G, Madelenat P, et al. [The limits of laparoscopic myomectomy]. Gynecol Obstet Fertil 2005; 33(1-2):44-9.

2. Hurst BS, Matthews ML, Marshburn PB. Laparoscopic myomectomy for symptomatic uterine myomas. Fertil Steril 2005; 83(1):1-23.

3. Koh C, Janik G. Laparoscopic myomectomy: the current status. Curr Opin Obstet Gynecol 2003; 15(4):295-301.

4. Dubuisso JB, Fauconnier A, Babaki-Fard K, Chapron C. Laparoscopic myomectomy: a current view. Hum Reprod Update 2000; 6(6):588-94.

5. Miller CE. Myomectomy. Comparison of open and laparoscopic techniques. Obstet Gynecol Clin North Am 2000; 27(2):407-20.

6. Miskry T, Magos A. Laparoscopic myomectomy. Semin Laparosc Surg 1999; 6(2):73-9.

7. Nezhat C. The "cons" of laparoscopic myomectomy in women who may reproduce in the future. Int J Fertil Menopausal Stud 1996; 41(3):280-3.

8. Reich H. Laparoscopic myomectomy. Obstet Gynecol Clin North Am 1995; 22(4):757-80.

9. Dubuisson JB, Chapron C. Laparoscopic myomectomy. Operative procedure and results. Ann N Y Acad Sci 1994; 734:450-4.

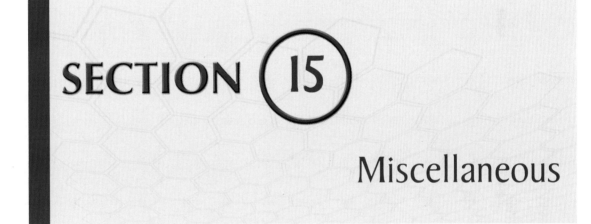

SECTION 15

Miscellaneous

77

Video Documentation

INTRODUCTION

Video documentation forms a integral part of the laparoscopic surgery. Properly recorded and edited videos can help the surgeon in many ways. It is a good learning tool for the surgeon in their initial laparoscopic surgical carrier. The surgeon can periodically review the surgeries performed by him, and modify his procedures till he attains perfection. Moreover it can also be used as an excellent teaching material in dissemination of the knowledge of laparoscopic surgery. At present time it is very essential that the laparoscopic surgeon has good knowledge about video documentation and editing. A properly edited high quality video that contains the entire procedure along with the external view is almost equivalent to witnessing live laparoscopic surgeries in a conference. Before seeing the technical details regarding video editing and recording we will see a few practical details about laparoscopic equip-

ments. Laparoscopic surgery is highly dependent on the image quality of the telescope, camera systems and light source. Laparoscopic surgeon should understand some of the basic functions of these equipments.

LAPAROSCOPIC EQUIPMENTS

Camera

The clarity of the recorded videos is directly proportional to the resolution of the cameras. Single chip cameras usually have a resolution of around 600 lines (the clarity of the video output is measured in terms of the number of horizontal lines). The three chip cameras have a higher resolution of 720 - 850, while the new generation digital cameras have a much higher resolution of around 1200 lines (Image 1, Pulsar). The output from the laparoscopic camera can either be in digital format or analog format. All the presently available cameras have analog output. Some of the new generation Laparoscopic digital cameras also have the option of digital output (Image 1, Striker HD, Olympus).

Laparoscope

The laparoscope can be rightly called as the eye of the laparoscopic surgeon as it is through which the surgeon sees the internal organs. The rod Hopkin's lens system offers the highest clarity when compared to the older generation laparoscopes and the currently available flexible tip laparoscopes. 0^0 laparoscopes give higher clarity than the thirty degree laparoscopes. 10mm laparoscopes are ideal for recording purposes. Even though 5mm and 3mm scopes offer a decent clarity during surgery, these are not ideal for recording purposes. Even if a surgeon starts the surgery with 5mm scope and later considers recording, it is better to change the telescope to 10mm rather than continuing with 5mm scope.

Light sources and Cable

Though various light sources are available, Xenon light sources are ideally suited for recording purposes as these provide a uniform distribution of light that is very similar to the sun light. Light cables also form an important part of video documentation. Even if the surgeon is using the highest possible laparoscopic camera, laparoscope and monitor the quality of the video will not be good if low quality light cables are used. The fluid filled cables are capable of transmitting the maximum amount of light without any loss. But these cables are rigid and difficult to manipulate during the surgery. This difficulty is more appreciated when 30° scopes are used. Though flexible cables transmit little lesser amount of light than the the fluid filled cables, these are ideal for routine use. These cables are more affordable and easier to handle. It is important to have a separate cable for purpose of recording apart from the routine cables. Adequacy of light can be checked by focusing the laparoscope towards the right hypochondrium. If the light is adequate, the surface of the liver and the diaphragm are seen with uniform illuminance otherwise the diaphragm will not be seen properly.

VIDEO SIGNAL FORMATS

There are various types of video signals that are used to transfer the video from one media to the other (for example from laparoscopic camera to monitor, camera to the recorder). Each of these formats have their own advantages and disadvantages. These signals can be broadly classified into analog video signal and digital video signals.

Analog Video Signals

The common analog video outputs that are used at present are the composite, S-video and RGB format.

Composite format

The composite format is the basic format of all the analog outputs. In this format the color response, synchronization and brightness are all encoded and sent through a single coaxial cable. The maximum resolution that can be obtain with this format is around 320 - 380 lines. This resolution is equivalent to the resolution of the ordinary television. So when a surgeon is using a television as the monitor, composite output is more than enough. This format can also be used for recording with video cassette recorders (VCR). Composite video cable has 2 types of connectors namely BNC and RCA. The usual connecting part in laparoscopic camera is BNC and RCA in televisions.

The main advantage of the composite output is the minimal loss of video quality even when long cables (upto 100mts) are used. This distance can be increased even upto few kms if proper amplifiers are used in between. Till recently this format was used in transmission of video signals in live laparoscopic surgical workshops.

S-Video (Y/C) format

This format offers better resolution than the previously described composite output, as the color and brightness of the signals are transmitted separately. The brightness is transmitted through the four single pins, while the color is transmitted through the other wire. A resolution of 450 lines can be achieved with this format. This format is usually used to record the surgeries in a digital video camcorder or in a computer through a video capture cord. All the presently available cameras have S-video output.

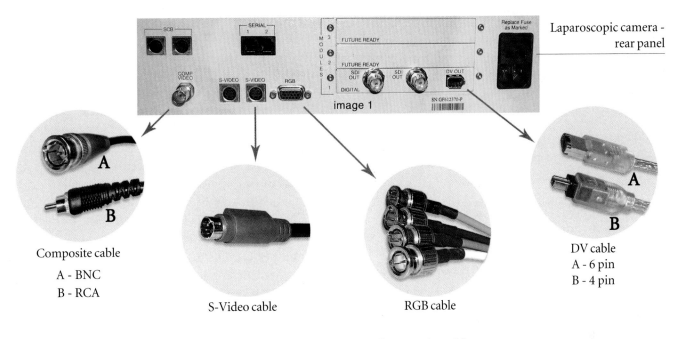

Figure 1: Types of video outputs and connecting cables

The main disadvantage of the S-video format is its restriction in the maximum length of cable that can be used. When S-video cables longer than 3 meters are used there is significant loss of visual clarity.

RGB format (Red, Green, Blue)

The RGB format offers the maximum resolution among all the analog formats. In this format the color signals are divided into the basic colors red, green and blue and these are sent through three different cables. An additional cable is used for synchronization. Altogether a set of 4 cables is needed for signal transmission in RGB format. To obtain the maximum resolution of this format it is essential to use a medical grade monitor along with three chip camera. The newer digital 3 chip cameras have digitized RGB video signals.

Though this format provides the maximum clarity of vision it cannot be used for recording purposes as most of the recording devices do not have RGB inputs. Higher end professional recorders with RGB input are available in the market, but the cost is prohibitive.

Digital Video Signals

Some of the recently available cameras have digital video inputs like digital video (DV) output, (also called as Firewire, 1394, iEEE), Digital video Interface (DVI) and Serial Digital Interface (SDI). Among all these formats the SDI offers the maximum clarity.

Digital Video (DV)

The video signals are transmitted in a digital form to the recording devices or the computers. This can be connected directly to devices like DV camcorder or computer through DV cable. It is an ideal format for recording in digital quality. We are using the standard DV format for all our recording for the past 3 years in our institution.

The signals are compressed (in a ratio of 5:1) and transferred through the DV cables. If this format is to be used for real time display in monitors then the signals have to be uncompressed. There will be a definite time delay of about $1/10^{th}$ of second in this process. So this format cannot be used for real time display in monitors.

Digital Video Interface (DVI)

This is an uncompressed high bandwidth digital video signal. This signal can be used for real time display during live surgery due to its uncompressed nature. DVI compatible flat monitors are now available in the market.

These signals offer the same clarity as that of the RGB in digitized format. It is also possible to record the DVI videos in the computers.

Serial Digital Interface (SDI)

This is also an uncompressed high quality digital format like DVI. This can also be used for real time display in monitors. Currently these signals are mainly used in television broadcasting.

VIDEO RECORDING AND EDITING

The captured video has to be edited in order to present in the conferences. This editing can be done either in analog format or digital format.

Basic recording and editing

This form of recording involves use of ordinary video tapes to capture the signals in analog format. This can be accomplished with a video cassette recorder (VCR). The composite video output from the camera can be connected to the video cassette recorder and the surgery can be recorded. The entire surgery is recorded in a VHS cassette and is named as master cassette. Subsequently editing can be done with the help of two video cassette recorders. The master cassette is played in one VCR and the necessary portions alone can be re-recorded in a cassette in the second VCR. The master cassette should not be disturbed during the editing process. The main disadvantage with this form of recording and editing is the loss of video clarity (about 10-15%) in the master cassette itself (when compared to clarity seen in the monitor) and subsequent loss during the second phase of recording in the process of editing. The end product has only about 1/3 of the visual clarity that is obtained in the laparoscopic camera. This loss can be prevented to a certain extent by using VHS PRO cassettes. This editing can be performed by the surgeon himself, though it might need some professional help from the audio visual personal.

High end professional recording devices are available like U Matic, Betacam, Digital betacam. These recording and editing units are very costly and used in TV stations.

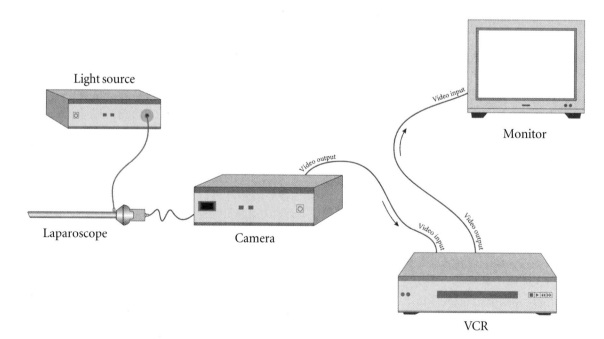

Figure 2 : Setup for VCR recording

Advanced Recording and Editing

Advanced recording usually involves capturing of the video in a computer hard drive. Digital editing requires dedicated video editing softwares like Pinnacle, Adobe Premier, Final cut pro etc. Digital video editing is more complex and time consuming. It needs a higher degree of patience and dedication to properly edit a surgery. It approximately takes more than 3 times the duration of the surgery for producing a high quality short video of an advanced procedure. For example producing a 10 minute video of a 2 hour long surgery like gastrectomy requires approximately 6 hours of dedicated editing in front of the computer. Even this is possible only if the operating surgeon himself edits the procedure. If the surgeon seeks professional help, then this duration will extend more as the audio video professionals are not well versed with the surgical procedures. Most of the time is spent in explaining the procedures to these professionals. Considerable amount of time can be saved if the surgeon learns the technique of editing.

Advantages

When compared to basic analog recording and editing, there is practically no loss of clarity in digital video recording and editing. The quality of the video remains the same irrespective of the number of editing a particular video passes through.

Addition of titles, graphics, photos, illustrations and 'Picture in Picture' is very easy with digital editing. Moreover text can be added as an overlay patch in the video without disturbing the quality of the video. Even though these are possible in analog VCR recording it needs a special devices like the title generator and video mixer. Use of intermediate devices like these will also result in decrease in the clarity.

In addition to these, the final edited version of the video can be produced in any of the available formats (CD, DVD, Digital video tape) with the digital editing software.

RECORDING DEVICES

The videos can be recorded either in the digital format or in analog format. The common recording device for analog signals is the video cassette recorders. Numerous devices are available for recording digital video signals.

Video Capturing Cards

Most of the presently available laparoscopic cameras have provision for analog video outputs (composite, S-video) only. For editing the videos in the computer these analog signals must be converted into digital video signal before storing in the hard drive. The video signals that are taken from the laparoscopic camera is fed into these capturing devices. The signals are converted into digital form and then stored in the computer.

Various devices are available in the market for this purpose (video capturing cards-Pinnacle, Canopus, Matrix, Pixel view, Aver capture etc). A reasonably good capturing card can be purchased within 10,000-15,000 Indian rupees.

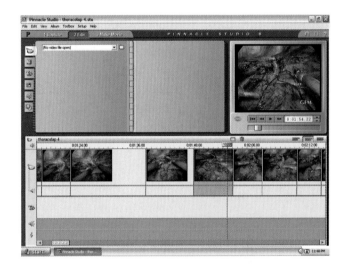

Figure 3 : Computer editing screen (using Pinnacle studio software)

Still Capture Cards

Capturing of stills during laparoscopic surgery with the help of still capturing cards through the computer is also possible. Many software companies have developed still capture devices with software. Stills can be capture during the surgery by activation of foot pedal.

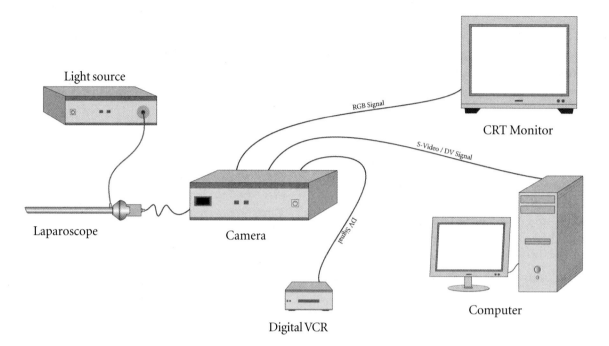

Figure 4 : Setup for digital recording

Figure 5 : Computer recording unit

A - Capturing device
B - External storage device

Usually there is a single computer with recording unit in the entire operating complex. Shifting this system is often tedious and cumbersome. With this trolley assembly we are able to conveniently shift the computer along with the recording equipment into the theatre for recording and subsequently to the editing room for further work.

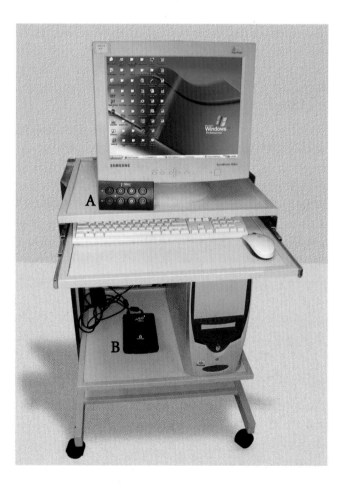

DV Camcorder

Recording of the videos in a digital camcorder is another simple way of capturing the video signals in digital format. The S-video output from the laparoscopic camera should be connected to the S-video input of the digital camcorder for this purpose. With this setup the surgery can be recorded in mini DV cassettes in digital video format. Even though this is a very simple procedure, direct editing is not possible. These digital signals should be transferred to the computer and then edited.

This transfer of data is time consuming. If a surgery is recorded directly in the computer, it will be immediately available for editing. This is not possible when digital tapes are used for recording. For example if a surgery of two hours duration is available in the tape, it takes another 2 hours for transferring the data from the digital tape to the computer. Hence recording in DV camcorder should be kept as an alternative way of capturing high quality of video only when the computer is not available inside the operating room during the time of surgery.

DV VCR

We found the portable digital video recorders like Sony DV VCR are very useful in recording the surgeries in digital video format. These devices have a decent sized LCD (4 inches) monitor which can be used for reviewing. Minor editing, addition of titles

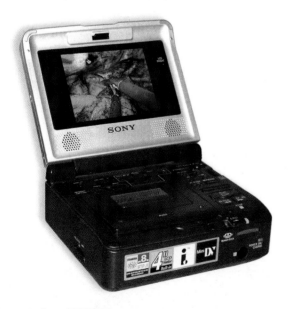

Figure 6 : Sony DV VCR

and transition effects can be done with these recorders. These have the complete range of output and input jackets like composite, S video and DV signals. Even memory cards can be used along with these digital recorders.

High definition video capture

Recently high definition video capture devices have been introduced in the market. There is no specific format like PAL, NTSC, SECOM in high definition videos. The main problem at present is the need for huge spaces in the hard drive for storing these videos when compared to the presently available digital video format (130 GB per hour of HDTV video versus 13 GB per hour of DV format video). The computers needed for capturing these high definition videos should have extreme configurations (Pentium 4 processor, minimum 1GB RAM).

To balance this problem a similar format called SD (Standard Definition) is available which requires lesser amount of space. These high definition capturing devices will become the standard method of recording of surgeries in the near future.

PRODUCTION OF VIDEOS AFTER EDITING

The final form of edited videos can be produced in any of the following formats for presentation and storage.

1	Full DV quality	Highest
2.	DVD quality (MPEG 2)	Intermediate
3.	CD quality (MPEG 1)	Lowest

Pitfalls in post editing production

Proper understanding of the video quality formats is essential in producing high quality videos. We have often observed some mistakes that routinely take place in digital editing. The surgery is initially captured in high quality digital video tapes, subsequently edited with the help of audio visual professionals and finally converted into CD format (MPEG 1) in compact disc. This usually results 3/4th loss of visual clarity as there is a compression of video 200 times in MPEG 1 format. Here eventhough the initial recording is in highest quality the end product is produced in the lowest quality which ultimately is of no use.

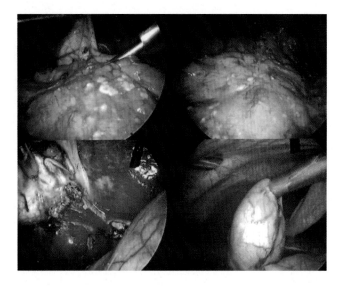

Figure 7 : Image captured with color video printer

Camera   -   3 chip camera
Light source -   Halogen 250 watts
Capture device -   Color printer

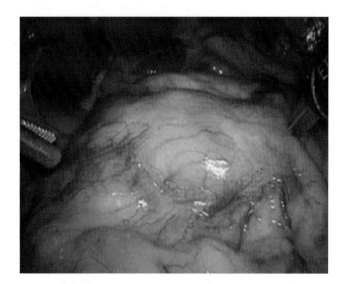

Figure 8 : CD quality image of 3 chip camera.

Camera   -   3 chip camera
Light source   -   Xenon 175
Capture device -   MPEG 1 capture card
Capture mode -   CD quality

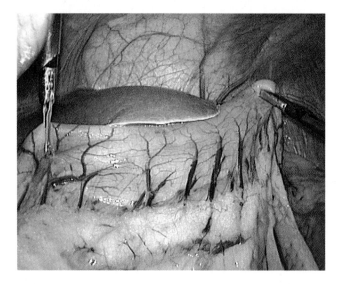

Figure 9 : DV quality image of 3 chip camera

Camera   -   3 chip camera
Light source   -   Xenon 300
Capture device -   DV capture card
Capture mode -   DV quality

TIPS TO PRODUCE HIGH QUALITY DIGITAL VIDEO

The signal from the laparoscope has to pass through various stages to ultimately reach the monitor and the recording device. All the components in these stages should work in perfect condition and coherence to obtain a clear video signal.

Lens Fogging

We often find that the laparoscope gets fogged as soon as it is introduced into the abdominal cavity. This is due to the sudden change in the temperature at the tip of the laparoscope (from cold atmosphere into the warm and moist abdominal cavity). This often results in reduction in the video clarity.

This happens more frequently if the CO_2 insufflation is connected to the camera port. The continuous insufflation of cold CO_2 by the side of the laparoscope further increases the fogging of the lens. Hence it is always better to connect the insufflation tubes to any of the ports other than that of the camera port.

Smudging of lens

It is a habit of all the camera surgeon to clean the tip of the lens by gently rubbing the scope over the organ such as the liver and the small bowel. Eventhough it is quick and effective at times, it is better avoided.

The thin film of tissue fluid sticks on to the surface of the lens. This fluid subsequently dries up resulting in image deterioration.

It is always a better practice to clean the tip of the lens with warm saline (kept in near body temperature). The saline can be maintained at body temperature by keeping it in a flask. The laparoscope should be carefully withdrawn from the port and the tip cleaned with a clean white gauze piece dipped in warm saline. Before introduction of cleaned scope into cannula, the port seal should be wiped of any blood stained fluid. If the inside of the trocar is stained with blood it should be cleaned with the help of a gauze piece before introducing of the laparoscope.

Problems with monopolar cautery

The field of vision usually is smoky when monopolar cautery is used during dissection. Intermittent letting out of the fumes during recording will help in evacuation of the smoke. It is a better practice to leave one of the 5 mm ports in a partially opened position during use of cautery.

Camera Head

At times the clarity of the picture remains the same even after cleaning the tip of the scope properly. This is usually due to the presence of dust particles in the camera head. The lens in the camera head should

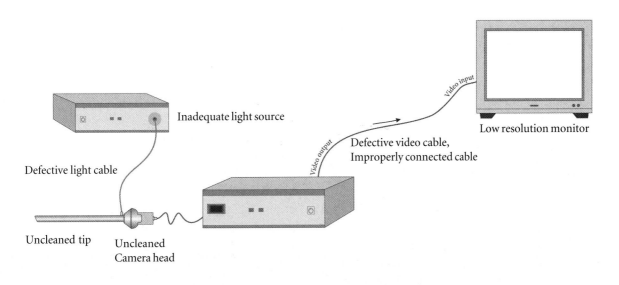

Figure 10 : Areas of potential degradation of video signal

the cleaned with a dry white gauze before it is connected to the laparoscope.

Role of Camera Surgeon

The camera surgeon plays a vital role in the production of a good quality video. An experienced camera assistant is a valuable asset especially when 30° scopes are used. It is better to use the services of an experienced camera surgeon or a staff nurse during the surgeries. It is always better to teach one particular theatre personal or assistant surgeon about the set up of camera, monitor and the recording system and continuously involve him in all the surgeries.

A panoramic view of the abdominal cavity should be shown in the initial phase and an intermediate view should be shown for dissection purposes. A close of view is ideal for inspection and division of tissues and endo suturing. The tip of the working instruments should always be in the center of the monitor irrespective of close up or panoramic view. A good camera surgeon can make difficult tasks easier and an average camera surgeon can make easier things more difficult.

OUR EXPERIENCE

We have gone through a process of complete evolution in video documentation and we feel that this might help the readers in better understanding of the procedures involved in recording and editing.

To begin with we started recording the surgeries in the video cassette recorders with VHS cassettes. We were using single chip cameras with halogen light sources and monopolar cautery for most of the surgeries. We were initially using analog video editing for presentation in the conferences. This was very cumbersome and there was significant loss of clarity. We then shifted over to 3 chip cameras and xenon light sources.

We captured still images and printed it with devices like Sony color printers and stored in the form of photographs.

We then shifted over to digital recording and editing in 1998. We were able to record, store and edit these videos in a more comfortable manner without any loss of video quality. We were using video capture cards like Dazzle for these purposes. Initially the format of recording was MPEG 1 quality. Even though provisions were available for recording in MPEG 2, the post capture editing was not easy due to the lack of proper editing software.

Later we moved on to DV format recording in 2002 with the help of DV capture cards like Pinnacle and Canopus. With this, we were able to convert the analog signals to DV form and store these either in DV tapes or in the the computer.

With the introduction of the 3 chip digital cameras (with DV output) in 2003, we started capturing the video signals from the camera directly into the computer or DV VCR.

We are planning to change the entire recording and editing system to the HDTV format in the near future. Even though this continuous acquiring of new technology has cost us more, this has definitely helped us to maintain the highest level of clarity. We can confidently say that quality of our videos in conferences and still images in our textbooks are rated as one among the best.

OUR RECOMMENDATIONS

We would like to share the lessons learnt from our experiences in video documentation with the readers. Our institute is often flooded with enquiries about practical tips for video recording and editing. Most of the surgeons want to start with basic recording system and then go for advanced recording.

In a set up where all the facilities are available, a 3 chip digital camera with digital output, xenon 300 watts light source, high resolution medical grade CRT monitor (1000 lines), high performance computer with advanced configuration (>1GB RAM, P4, 200 GB HDD), editing software, 3 CCD mini DV camera (for recording external video) and a 5 mega pixels digital camera will make a perfect recording and editing system at present. This system will help in producing the maximum clarity video for presentations.

A three-chip camera, Xenon 175 watts light source, medical monitors and a computer is an ideal set up for a basic recording purposes. We feel that recording with low-power light sources, cameras and recording system will not result in good quality videos. Most often, the surgeons feel that they will start with a basic system and then upgrade to more advanced systems. But we are of the opinion that utilizing ideal equipments from beginning will help the surgeon to progress fast in the field of laparoscopic surgery.

Selected Reading

1. Berci G, Schwaitzberg SD. The importance of understanding the basics of imaging in the era of high-tech endoscopy: part I. Logic, reality, and utopia. Surg Endosc 2002;4:377-380.

2. Berci G, Schwaitzberg SD. The importance of understanding the basics of imaging in the era of high-tech endoscopy: part II. Logic, reality, and utopia. Surg Endosc 2002;16:1518-1522.

3. Steven D. Schwaitzberg. Imaging systems in minimally invasive surgery. Mastery of endoscopic and laparoscopic surgery. Second edition. Chapter13., Lippincott Williams and Wilkins, USA, 2005;118-129.

4. SAGES Video protection guidelines. Society of American Gastrointestinal Endoscopic Surgeons (SAGES) Toolbox; 2004

78

Minimally Invasive Surgery - Is Future Perfect?

"Make the things simple, but not simpler."

Albert Einstien

The principle 'primum non nocere' is central to the practice of medicine. However, wounding is an inseparable component of the operation itself in surgery. It is a fact beyond doubt that in many surgeries, the trauma inflicted by the surgical access alone is greater than tissue damage caused by dissection of the organ to be operated on. The significant morbidity is mainly due to surgical access rather than surgery of the organ itself. The surgeon scientists all over the world have been working tirelessly to minimize this morbidity of the surgical procedure. Their efforts have made minimally invasive surgery (MIS) or minimal access surgery (MAS) as the "surgery of the 21st century". The tremendous leap of development on the technological front cannot be overemphasized to bring the MIS on the forefront of the art and science of surgery as compared to the surgery of yore.

The great skepticism of the past has now become welcome in almost all specialties of surgery. This brings great challenges and new complications, too. Now, due to peers' pressure and demand of educated patients coupled with a flood of information about the advantages of MIS, even reluctant surgeons of the past are turning into eager learners.

In the era of managed health care and evidence-based practice of medicine, safety of patients is obligatory and paramount. Therefore, to practice safe MIS, surgeon has to be properly trained in open surgery and qualified to perform MIS. The range of learning methods in the beginning, i.e., 1990s, was interesting. Some went abroad, some watched videos and started to perform MIS, some were taught by the instrument manufacturer's representatives and some went for weekend visits to some hospitals, saw one or two cases and got started. There were no guidelines and no credentialing. The mushrooming of so-called centers of laparoscopic surgery training has resulted in unprecedented incidence of complication. Learning and teaching at some of these centers are 'to see one operation, to perform one and to teach the next'. There seems to be reluctance to admit technical ignorance and to volunteer to get trained adequately.

In USA and Europe, where evidence-based practice of medicine is the norm rather than exception, credentialing and training issues have been adequately and promptly addressed. The Society of American Gastrointestinal and Endoscopic Surgeons (SAGES) has formulated the guidelines for privileges and credentialing in MIS. In India, though National Board has started MIS training as subspecialty of surgery at the post-doctoral level, no guidelines for privilege and credentialing in MIS for practicing surgeons exist; nor MIS has been included in the curricula of postgraduate surgical training.

HOW TO IMPROVE UPON

First, our attitude has to be changed. We have to enforce evidence-based medicine and structured training. Second, we have to understand and adapt the concept of continuing medical education (CME) and credit system. Third, we have to be responsive and adaptive to change in the practice of surgery. And last, age is no bar for learning; it is the mindset.

HOW TO ACHIEVE THESE OBJECTIVES

Discipline of Surgical Audit

Unfortunately, in many developing countries, there is no proper surgical audit, central registry or compulsory refresher-training program. Even in teaching hospitals, the teaching program is in the form of apprenticeship, 'do as I do' policy. This is no more tenable. Mere seniority in hierarchy does not ensure high quality of care and credential to train. It is the surgical audit that determines the actual outcome of surgeries from the hands of the consultant, resident and trainee. Here lies the core of evidence-based medicine and structured training program. Trainer has to be adequately trained and certified by peers or has credentials to do so.

Structured training program

Expensive training course in MIS is not the answer. It is at postgraduate level of surgical training, which will make the evolution of MIS a safe and sound practice of surgery. But training program must be structured and should be open for improvement. Mere apprenticeship is history now. Trainee must be adequately exposed to pathways of surgical training, i.e., observation, assistance, performance under supervision, and then independent performance of the procedure. This will ensure to produce competent minimally invasive surgeons. Animal training is a part of MIS training. Animal training alone is inadequate for independent practice of MIS. It does not have any credential credits.

CME and Refresher-Training Program

Medicine is an ever-changing science. Therefore, to keep pace with current practice of surgery, surgeons are needed to update themselves continuously and to adapt new and emerging technology to provide a better quality of care to their patients. CME and refresher-training programs are designed to meet these objectives. In the western world, especially in USA, this has becomes mandatory to acquire certain number of credit hours of CME each year to remain on legal roll of surgical practice.

Imbibing New Concepts

In this technological century, surgeons are needed to ensure that they understand and know well how to handle and operate newer high-tech instruments in open, and more so in laparoscopic surgery. Instruments like CUSA, Harmonic Scalpel, Argon Plasma Coagulator, etc., are turning surgeons into the technological surgeons. This knowledge of high-tech instruments has become 'the cry of the day'. The surgeon is also supposed to know adequately about information and digital technology for recording and presentation purposes. That is why computer literacy is a must for today's surgeon.

Training of Minimally Invasive Surgeon

SAGES has formulated guidelines for privileges and credentialing in Minimal Access Surgery. These guidelines can severe as a model for development of MIS training program at different levels, viz., resident level, post-doctoral level and practicing surgeon level.

GUIDELINES FOR PRIVILEGES IN LAPAROSCOPIC SURGERY

SAGES guidelines

1. Completion of residency or fellowship that incorporates structured experience in laparoscopic surgery. Competence should be documented by the laparoscopic training instructor.

2. Alternatively, demonstration of proficiency and clinical judgment equivalent to that obtained in a residency or fellowship program. Documentation and demonstration of competence with verification in writing from the experienced colleague is required.

3. For the surgeon who did not learn laparoscopic surgery during residency or fellowship, and who lacks prior documented experience in laparoscopic surgery, the basic minimum requirements for training are as follows.

    a. Completion of a residency in general surgery with privileging in the comparable open operation for which laparoscopic privileges are being sought.
    b. Privileges in diagnostic laparoscopy.
    c. Training in laparoscopic surgery by a surgeon experienced in these procedures or completion of a University sponsored or academic society recognized course which includes didactic instructions as well as animal experience.
    d. First assisting in laparoscopic operations performed by an experienced surgeon.
    e. Proctoring by a laparoscopic surgeon who is experienced in the same or similar procedure until proficiency is observed and documented in writing.

The basic promise underlying the SAGES guideline is that the surgeon must have training, ability and judgment to proceed immediately to a traditional abdominal procedure when circumstances so indicated.

Requirements for safe laparoscopic surgery

1. The individual must be fully trained and qualified general surgeon.

2. Must have practical experience in diagnostic laparoscopy.

3. Must acquire the basic skills of hand eye coordination. This is achieved much faster in Endotrainers.

4. Must practice the procedure in suitable animal model.

5. Must observe or preferably assist, at clinical laparoscopic procedures in centers where these operations are well established.

6. A system of quality assurance and peer review in the institute will ensure that the technical problems are identified early and corrected.

7. Continuing education in new techniques and the possibility of other will be of value.

Training of qualified surgeon

Only trained qualified surgeon should do laparoscopic surgery because as a trial inspection and dissection, if he considers it is technically not possible, he must be in a position to open and do it safely than looking and calling for another surgeon to come and do it.

Training in laparoscopic surgery

The general surgeon should be familiar with the basic steps of laparoscopy such as establishment of pneumoperitoneum, introduction of trocars and manipulation of instruments by performing diagnostic procedures.

This initiation into laparoscopy will give the surgeon an insight into the problems alluded to above, such as hand-eye co-ordination and depth perception. It also enables the surgeon to overcome the problems of overshooting targets, by introducing accessory trocars, blunt probe to move tissues, etc.

Endotrainers

These devices are ideal in assisting the surgeons to gain skill in manipulating long laparoscopic instruments. A number of training devices are available.

A number of tasks are available for the surgeon training on this device.

1. A chart with multiple drawing such as straight line, wavy line, dot, etc. can be marked and the surgeon himself can move the camera from one to another pre-fixure before attempting two hand manipulation. It is easy to learn to move the tip of the instrument right to left, up and down, focusing a point or having a panoramic view etc. Later, camera can be held by the assistant and surgeon manipulating the instruments accordingly.

2. Place different kinds of grain (half cooked) spread over a dish and to pick some specific grain and place at a pre-selected site.

3. Place some thin rubber tubes cut into small sizes, which can be picked up by one hand and given to the other alternatively. This gives two-hand manipulation.

4. Suspend a bunch of grapes within the cavity. Identify a given grape and cut it with scissors and remove it without damaging the grape.

5. Suspend a large size grape and grasp with the left hand, and peel the outer coat using the hand.

6. Suspend a piece of cooked chicken breast and carefully dissect the skin away from the flesh.

7. Fix a sheet of stomach wall of a sheep on cardboard and place it within a bench trainer. This can be cut in linear fashion on a premarked line. The left hand can assist while cutting.

8. Handling of needle and endosuturing can be learned easily within the trainer.

We have CD-ROMS on basic course based on the above techniques and endosuturing that serves as a master guide.

Animal experimentation

Most of the institutions do not have animal laboratory and it is too expensive for one or two training courses. This can be overcome by ex-vivo porcine liver gallbladder preparations. This may be used in the training box with an electrocautery earthing plate placed underneath this. The gallbladder may then be removed with standard fashion.

Suturing

Initially the co-ordination and orchestration of hand movements are so complex, suturing under video imaging is extremely frustrating. It is preferable first to perform the suturing in an endotrainer covered with perforated glass for instrument to go in with direct visualisation. Later, the surgeon may go to suturing under laparoscopic control. A good model is a sheet of stomach wall fixed on a wooden plate and later a piece of vascular graft with a slit may be sutured.

Depth perception

One of the most common problems in learning laparoscopic skill is orienting the instrument with the target. Keep the camera in panoramic view with the tip of the instrument within the field of vision and the target organ or object at the center of field of vision. Both the camera and the tip move towards the target. Repeating this maneuver and aiming at different targets, a surgeon may acquire the skill of depth perception. The movement of laparoscopic instrument is comparable to aeroplane take off and landing at different airport.

Training course

It is vital that a surgeon should attend a well-structured course; conducted by fully trained surgeons.

The knowledge of endosuturing and knotting is considered vital in performing complex laparoscopic procedures or in managing complications. This why we have included suturing and knotting lessons in the basic laparoscopic training course itself.

A suitable course should consist of:

1. Didactic session
2. Patient selection criteria
3. Instrumentation
4. Performance of the technique of laparoscopic procedure - live or videotapes
5. Indication and contraindication
6. Possible pitfalls and future development

Setting up a clinical program

Once a surgeon gained a background in diagnostic laparoscopy, worked on an endotrainer, attended a course, he is then ready to start work on a human. I personally feel, it is preferable to get adequate clinical exposure either as observer or as assistant a week or two in a center, where laparoscopic work is being carried out regularly to give more confidence to the surgeon.

Training in animals

Training in animal models is desirable because it provides the opportunity of executing the steps of the operation under laboratory condition, which closely resemble clinical practice. But this is not a must and not a substitute to the above-mentioned training program.

Minimal Invasive Surgical Trainer in Virtual Reality (MIST-VR)

Simulation has gradually become accepted as a vital part of surgical skills training. An increasing number of operative techniques and procedures can now be taught away from the operating room. A trainee can become familiar with a particular procedure and develop the pre requisite skills before operating on a real patient for the first time.

Advanced laparoscopic surgical training program

A surgeon knowing how to do a laparoscopic cholecystectomy is just a step into the field of laparoscopy. To perform laparoscopic cholecystectomy, it is not just sufficient to know the technique. One has to adopt various maneuvers and techniques to make laparoscopic surgeries safe. After adequate experience and confidence, one can start doing laparoscopic cholecystectomy in acute stage, difficult gall bladders and other procedures.

How safe is laparoscopic surgery ?

Many reports have shown that the incidence of complications are the same or less in comparison to those in open surgery. In fact we have seen since last few years some of the operations can be performed more perfectly and accurately, with less morbidity and mortality in laparoscopic surgery. Incidence of complications was alarming during the initial learning phase as per reports available. In our series, we do not have any bile duct injury and we have not converted any patients for managing complication. Even the few complications we had, these were managed by laparoscopy.

Does it take long time to perform?

Yes, only during the learning phase. After adequate experience common surgical procedures such as laparoscopic cholecystectomy, appendectomy, inguinal hernia repair and vagotomy, particularly straightforward cases are being performed at much shorter time than in conventional approach. Complex and advanced procedures take longer operative time by laparoscopy than open. Looking at the reduced postoperative morbidity and faster recovery, increased operative time becomes insignificant.

Prof. Rattner during his presidential address of 2005 annual meet of SAGES said "every surgeon should keep an open mind to look into the future development of surgery in the "disturbed technology". In late 1980's when laparoscopic surgery came into practice, many felt that we are deviating from the standard practice and adversely affecting the principles of surgery. Within few years, we realized that meaning of surgery has seen unprecedented change (i.e., from big incision for big surgery to small incision for big surgery), where high quality surgical care can be offered with least morbidity. This has brought great sense of satisfaction to the patients as well as to the surgeons. This is not only due to the minimally invasive approach but the introduction of high-tech equipments such as harmonic scalpel, pulsed bipolar coagulation, APC, CUSA, etc. too, made surgery bloodless. With accurate manifold magnification by digital imaging systems and newer endo-stapling devices used in reconstruction, MIS is state-of-the-art now.

Tremendous leap in technological and computer advancement in the medical field has led to introduction of robotic surgery, tele-presence surgery, Endo-assist surgery, Navigators, percutaneous interventional radiology, active isotope tracking system etc. This has resulted in the evolution of different treatment options for the same surgical disease. Hence, surgeon today faces tough times to find a unified and most rational system of treatment.

This so-called 'disturbed technology' will continue to grow further and will expand its influence on the process of clinical judgment. This increases the responsibility further on the shoulders of surgeon to keep updating himself and to adapt this disturbed technology rationally. It is of utmost importance to translate the benefits of this technology to highest quality of care with least morbidity and mortality.

The evidence-based practice of medicine changes as newer findings of class I evidence emerges. Therefore, newer technology and technique that are operator-dependent should be judged cautiously. In this regard, few points are noteworthy;

1. Early results of a study should be considered as a pilot study, and not conclusive evidence.

2. Randomized studies with currently available technology and techniques should be made as a reference point.

3. Dedicated and high-volume centers should be on the forefront to conduct large-scale prospective randomized study.

4. The practice of surgical audit should be made compulsory to ensure proper quality control.

The last 15 years of evolution of minimally invasive surgery has taught us some lessons:

1. Only class I evidence should be implemented in practice and protocols of treatment.

2. Class II evidence should be acceptable only when no class I evidence is available.

3. Surgical complications should make the basis for further research and nidus for improvement.

4. Technology and technique must be properly used to assess its full potentials and pitfalls.

It is surprising to note that in the era of evidence-based medicine, laparoscopic cholecystectomy had become gold standard for the treatment of gallstones diseases even before any randomized study was undertaken to assess its potentials and pitfalls. This is an exception rather than rule due to wide popularity and excellent results of laparoscopic cholecystectomy. But, this phenomenon is not continuing for other MIS.

The evolution of minimal access surgery can be understood in three phases:

1. Phase of development
2. Phase of improvement
3. Phase of standardization

During late 1980's and early 1990's, several new procedures were introduced in minimally invasive surgery. General laparoscopic surgical procedures were well accepted but complex procedures such as oncologic surgery were not accepted at this stage. This was due to some cumbersome technique and not-so-adequate achievement of oncological principles. The non-availability of advanced technology and techniques were major reasons.

With the emergence of newer and safer technology and advanced techniques across the globe, results of complex minimal access surgical procedures improved. A flood of information became available about improved outcomes and feasibility to perform more complex procedure successfully. This led to further improvement and refinement in technique, which paved the way to perform more complex procedure by MIS way that were previously thought to be 'not feasible'. The last 5 years has seen some unprecedented development in MIS. A number of techniques were available to perform a particular procedure. Comparative and randomized studies are being undertaken to determine the best technique. Now, almost all general surgical procedures in MIS have been standardized.

FUTURE

The blinding pace of development at technological front such as robotic surgery, human-computer interface, digitalization, virtual reality and artificial intelligence has far reaching and unimaginable implications on the development of art and science of surgery. Minimally invasive surgery has all the content to flourish in 21st century. The day is not far when MIS shall be performed by a machine with artificial intelligence which may even had the faculty of digitalized clinical judgments. Probably, surgeons' conscience and intuition can never be digitalized; that shall be only difference in human-surgeon and robot-surgeon.

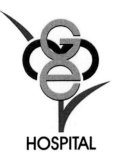

HOSPITAL

The Institution called GEM Hospital

(GastroEnterology Medical centre and Hospital)

Growth of an institution depends on the individuals working for the institution, inside and outside, and the infrastructure available with a considerable degree of freedom to improve. The story of this institution is parallel to the development of minimally invasive surgery itself. This institution, previously known as Coimbatore Institute of Gastro-endoscopic Surgery (CIGES), started laparoscopic surgery in 1991, soon after laparoscopic cholecystectomy became the sensation of surgical world. Initially, equipped with basic laparoscopic surgical instruments, this institution performed laparoscopic cholecystectomies, laparoscopic appendectomies and diagnostic laparoscopic procedures.

We adapted the philosophy of 'kaizen', i.e., to improve upon further and continuously. This single point focus on the art and science of laparoscopic surgery and work ethics with devotion and dedication have led the development and establishment of minimally invasive surgery in this institution as one of the most advanced institute worldwide with numerous firsts. With passage of time and dedicated following of philosophy of 'kaizen', several new dimensions were added in this institution. The faculty of 2 has now reached over 20 with equal number of trainees from length and breadth of India and other parts of the world. This is a substantial number considering single superspecialty services, viz., minimally invasive gastroenterological service. Now, this institution is equipped with state-of-the-art instruments and highly trained and reputed personnel providing endo-urology and endoscopic gynecologic surgical services in addition to medical and surgical gastroenterology incorporating minimal access oncologic surgery as well.

DEVELOPMENT OF MINIMALLY INVASIVE HEPATOBILIARY SURGERY

Laparoscopic modified subtotal cholecystectomy

One of the most significant achievement of this institution was the development of laparoscopic procedures for acute cholecystitis, gangrenous cholecystitis, cholecystectomy in cirrhotics, Mirrizzi's syndrome Type I and II and, cholecysto- and choledocho-enteric fistulae.

Type I: In acute cholecystitis, mucocele and empyema of the gallbladder where Calot's triangle anatomy is frozen, gallbladder content is aspirated first using subcostal midclavicular port and then neck of the gallbladder is transected. The cystic duct is dissected retrograde and suture closed. Cystic artery is coagulated. Mirrizzi's Type I and II are similarly dealt with.

Type II: In cirrhotics, after dissection of Calot's, if possible, gallbladder is transected at gallbladder-liver fusion plane and posterior wall mucosectomy is performed or mucosa is fulgurated. In gangrenous cholecystitis, similar technique is employed. These innovations have enabled us to achieve 0% conversion rate in the management of gallstone diseases without increasing the morbidity and mortality.

Laparoscopic choledochal cyst excision

With extensive experience in the complex laparoscopic procedures like CBD explorations and laparoscopic CBD injury management, we have been able to develop the technique of choledochal cyst excision and formation of the Roux-en-Y hepaticojejunostomy. The technique of this procedure is similar to open technique except the access route.

Laparoscopic hepatic hydatid cyst excision and the development of Palanivelu's cannula

High incidence of hepatic hydatid disease in this part of the country has prompted us to develop a new hepatic hydatid cannula-trocar system which is longer and wider in diameter with 2 suction port and hollow and fenestrated obturator. This cannula-trocar system, a closed extraction system, is unique and an excellent tool in the armamentarium of minimal access surgeons. This cannula-trocar system strictly follows the surgical principles of hydatid cyst evacuation and excision without permitting any peritoneal spillage, as suction pressure seals the contact area. This system also facilitates the evacuation of hydatid cysts from ruptured intrahepatic biliary radicals.

Laparoscopic hepatic resections

Availability of state-of-the-art laparoscopic instruments like CUSA probe and Harmonic Ace have led the development of anatomical and non-anatomical hepatic resection by minimal access route. With Argon Plasma Coagulator, control of bleeding form raw surface of the liver is a piece of cake.

Laparoscopic radio-frequency ablation of liver tumors

Laparoscopic ultrasonographic probes with real-time imaging and radio-frequency ablator has enabled us to treat unresectable, multicentric hepatocellular carcinoma as well as metastasis.

DEVELOPMENT OF MINIMALLY INVASIVE FOREGUT SURGERY

Thoracoscopic thymus and esophageal surgery

With increasing confidence and experience, we ventured into thoracoscopic surgery; now thymectomy and esophageal surgery for benign condition such as leiomyoma, removal of foreign bodies are routine procedures in our institution.

Laparoscopic foregut surgery

Laparoscopic management of achalasia cardia with Toupet fundoplication, Nissen's fundoplication, management of giant para-esophageal hernia, diaphragmatic hernia, and posterior mediastinal surgery such as esophageal diverticula have been standardized at our institution.

Minimally invasive esophagectomy

This institution has emerged as a world leader in the management of esophageal cancer in minimal access way. We have developed thoracolaparoscopic esophagectomy for middle third esophageal cancer in prone position with excellent ergonomics and comparable results to other techniques with largest series in this technique. The techniques of laparoscopic transhiatal esophagectomy and laparoscopic esophagogastrectomy with intrathoracic anastomosis, another first, have already been acknowledged worldwide.

Laparoscopic bariatic surgery

The laparoscopic bariatic surgery has been established as a standard of care in the field of weight reducing surgery at our institution, beneficiaries being around the world.

Laparoscopic Gastric and Duodenal Surgery

Apart from the management of several benign gastric and duodenal diseases such as gastric volvulus, superior mesenteric artery syndrome and other tumors of the stomach; laparoscopic D_2 gastrectomy is the standard therapy for resectable gastric cancers. We have developed a new technique of jejunal pouch formation after laparoscopic total radical gastrectomy.

DEVELOPMENT OF MINIMALLY INVASIVE PANCREATIC AND SPLENIC SURGERY

Laparoscopic distal pancreatectomy

The development of distal pancreatectomy has been a logical extension to laparoscopic management of pancreatic pseudocyst. We have also developed the technique of laparoscopic Roux-en-Y cystojejunostomy for difficult pseudocyst in infracolic as well as paracolic positions.

Laparoscopic Whipple's procedure

With increasing experience and confidence in gastric, biliary and pancreatic surgery; we graduated to laparoscopic Whipple's procedure and achieved the distinction of one of the foremost group in the world to perform this rare and very complex feat with excellent results.

Laparoscopic Mesh Splenopexy

For the laparoscopic management of wandering spleen, we have developed a technique of creating a pouch of prosthetic mesh and anchoring the spleen in its anatomical position.

DEVELOPMENT OF MINIMALLY INVASIVE COLORECTAL SURGERY

Laparoscopic appendicular abscess drainage

Since the beginning of laparoscopic appendectomy procedure, we were curious to develop a technique to deal with this complication of acute appendicitis. Now, we have successfully developed a technique to deal appendicular abscess laparoscopically; and we have never converted till date in the management of acute appendicitis and its complication.

Laparoscopic colorectal surgery

Laparoscopic colectomies, low anterior resections, abdomino-perineal resections, and colostomies have been routine surgeries at our institution. We have standardized the mesh rectopexy procedure for rectal prolapse as well.

Laparoscopic total proctocolectomy with ieal pouch-anal anastomosis

We have developed the technique to do total proctocolectomy and ileal pouch-anal anastomosis laparoscopically for familial polyposis and ulcerative colitis. This procedure has tremendously reduced the morbidity and hospital stay without compromising the quality of life.

DEVELOPMENT OF MINIMALLY INVASIVE HERNIA SURGERY

Laparoscopic inguinal hernia repairs

Totally extra-peritoneal approach is the standard of care for inguinal hernia at this institution; trans-abdominal preperitoneal approach being reserved for difficult cases.

Laparoscopic ventral hernia repair

Laparoscopic ventral hernia repair with Intra-peritoneal On-lay composite mesh is the treatment of choice for all operable ventral hernias. We always approximate the hernia defect with strong non-absorbable monofilament suture to achieve perfect anatomical alignment of abdominal muscles, thereby restoring their functional ability. This is considered as a landmark in laparoscopic ventral hernia surgery. We have successfully dealt with spegilean and obturator hernia laparoscopically.

DEVELOPMENT OF MINIMALLY INVASIVE PEDIATRIC SURGERY

The availability of mini-instruments, 2-3mm, has encouraged us to perform various pediatric procedures like herniotomy, appendectomy, cholecystectomy, splenectomy, midgut volvulus, intussusception, orchidopexy, etc., successfully. These procedures are in routine practice of the institution now.

Development of Endo-Urology

With working experience in general as well as urological surgery, we are now performing laparoscopic adrenalectomy and nephrectomy routinely. We also have experience of laparoscopic bilateral adrenalectomy.

Development of Endo-Gynecologic Surgery

With increasing experience in working in the female pelvis laparoscopically, we were attracted to totally laparoscopic hysterectomy and myomectomy, and now these laparoscopic procedures are in the routine OR list.

Increasing participation of our personnel at international meets demanded the acquisition of advanced knowledge and equipments for advanced tele-communication system, digital imaging and recording facility and maintenance of a digital library. Establishment of advanced digital telecommunication system at our institution has enabled us to beam live surgeries across the globe on a routine basis. Now, because of these high-tech and state-of-the-art facility, our presentation have fetched various top honors from international conferences and workshops.

Our institution, which was started on a leased OR, now has 3 fully equipped OR to perform advanced minimal access as well conventional procedure with facility of C-arm image intensifier, intra-operative laparoscopic Doppler and ultrasound and flexible endoscopy set-up. We also have fully equipped facility for therapeutic as well as diagnostic ERCP and endoscopic procedures such as luminal stenting of GIT. With over 150 beds and a fully equipped ICU, this institution is in the process of further expansion.

In addition, GEM Hospital has been accredited by National Board of Examinations, Ministry of Health, Government of India, for super-specialty training in surgical gastroenterolgy as well as post-doctoral fellowship training in minimal access surgery. Furthermore, the basic and advanced laparoscopic training courses of this institution have been endorsed by SAGES.

And finally, we pledge to keep on following the philosophy of 'kaizen'.

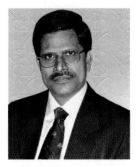

About the Author

Name	:	Dr. C. Palanivelu
Designation	:	Chair, Division of Surgical Gastroenterology and Minimal Access Surgery
		Director, Digestive Diseases Research and National Training Institute
		GEM Hospital, Coimbatore, India
Educational Qualifications	:	MS, DNB, MCh (GE), FRCS Ed., FACS

Dr. C. Palanivelu is a world-renowned surgical gastroenterologist and an advanced laparoscopic surgeon from Coimbatore. He has had his MS (Gen. Surgery) from Madurai, MCh (Surgical Gastroenterology) from Madras Medical College. He is among the first to popularize the field of laparoscopic surgery in India and other Asian countries. He is a fellow of various international colleges including the American College of Surgeons and the Royal College of Surgeons of Edinburgh. He was awarded the prestigious honor of the Royal College of Surgeons of Edinburgh, "Fellowship ad hominem" in May 2004. In College's transcript, this fellowship is awarded to the "doctors of distinction whose professional status is of a high order and who are deemed to have rendered special service to surgery in general or to the College, in particular". He is one among the very few people in India and youngest in the world to achieve this rare distinction. He is the Founder President of AMASI (Association of Minimal Access Surgeons of India), the association of laparoscopic surgeons of India. He is the Founder of GEM hospital, a dedicated center for Gastroenterology and Advanced Laparoscopic Surgery in Asia, which has Post Doctoral Fellowship in Minimal Access Surgery of 2 years duration and super specialty training in Surgical Gastroenterology of 3 years duration. This is accredited by National Board of Examination, Ministry of Health, Government of India. He is also the Director of Digestive Diseases Research and National Training Institute, a center of excellence that offers the most advanced and sought after laparoscopic training in India. This is the only center in Asia to be recognized by SAGES (Society of American Gastrointestinal Endo Surgeons) for training in basic and advanced minimal access surgery. Dr. C. Palanivelu has been recognized by SAGES for his outstanding videos and has been receiving the best video award from SAGES for the last 6 consecutive years. He has won the best Paper Award at the World Congress of Laparoscopic Surgery in Rome, 1998 the first and the only Indian surgeon to get this distinction till now. He has authored a number books in laparoscopic surgery of international standard, which include Art of Laparoscopic surgery, Ciges Atlas of Laparoscopic surgery, Text Book of Surgical Laparoscopy, Operative manual of Laparoscopic Hernia Surgery and Art of Laparoscopic Surgery: Text Book and Atlas. He has presented many research papers both in national and international fora and has developed many innovative techniques in the field of laparoscopic surgery. He has been the visiting faculty to various institutions in countries like USA, France, UK,

Sweden, Italy, Hongkong, Singapore, Argentina, China and South Korea.

OUTSTANDING CONTRIBUTIONS

- One of the leading surgeon to introduce the **"Key hole concept - Minimally Invasive (Laparoscopic) Surgery"** in India and other Asian nations.

- **Best Paper Award of World Congress of Laparoscopic Surgery,** Rome, 1998 for Laparoscopic Modified Subtotal Cholecystectomy.

- 9 innovative procedures had been selected and included in **SAGES video library** in last 6 consecutive years.

   - Received SAGES Best Video Awards for 3 consecutive years, i.e., 2003 through 2005.

   - Inclusion of 17 high quality video of the various laparoscopic procedures on knowledge and skill site of Royal College of Surgeons of Edinburgh's website

ORATIONS / AWARDS

1. Golden Jubilee Oration Award, Delhi State Chapter of Association of Surgeons of India, 2003

2. Prof. Hanumaiah Oration Award, Karnataka state Chapter of Association of Surgeons of India, 2003

3. Sivanandhan Oration Award, TN & P state Chapter of ASI, 2003

4. Fellowship ad hominem Award, 2003 by **Royal College of Surgeons of Edinburgh** the prestigious honor of the college in recognition of contributions to the field of laparoscopic surgery. This award was presented in February 2004 at Edinburgh, UK.

5. Prof. Ramaiah Oration Award, Andhra Pradesh Chapter of ASI, 1999

6. Rotarians Best Medico Award, 1998

7. International Man of the year Award by American Biographic Center, 1998

8. Man of the Millennium Award by International Biographic Center at Cambridge, 1999

9. Best Citizens of India Award, 2000

10. Vikas Rattan Award, 2000

11. Vocational excellence award of Rotary International, 2001

12. Gem of Coimbatore Citizen Award, 2002

13. Meritorious Service Award, Rotary Club of Coimbatore, 2004

MEMBERSHIP INTERNATIONAL SOCIETIES

1. Active member of Society of American Gastrointestinal Endoscopic Surgery (SAGES)

2. European Association of Endoscopic Surgery (EAES)

3. International Hepato-Biliary Pancreatic Association (IHBPA)

4. Member of International College of Digestive Surgery (ICDS)

5. Member of British Endo Paediatric Surgery (BAPS)

6. Member of Endoscopic and Laparoscopic Society of Asia (ELSA)

NATIONAL SOCIETIES

1. Founder President - Association of Minimal Access Surgeons of India (AMASI)

2. Fellow of Association of Surgeons of India (ASI)

3. Fellow of Indian Association of Colorectal Surgery (ACRSI)

4. Indian Association of Gastrointestinal Endoscopic Surgery (IAGES)

5. Indian Association of Surgical Gastroenterology (IASG)

6. Founder Member of Paediatric Endo Surgery-Indian Chapter

7. Founder Member of Hepato Pancreato Biliary Association-Indian chapter

Index

I

M

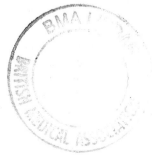